Thieme

The Chronic Ear

John L. Dornhoffer, MD, FACS
Professor and Vice Chair of Adult Services
Samuel D. McGill Chair in Otolaryngology Research
Director, Division of Otology and Neurotology
Director, Hearing and Balance Center
Department of Otolaryngology—Head and Neck Surgery
University of Arkansas for Medical Sciences
Arkansas Children's Hospital
Little Rock, Arkansas

Michael B. Gluth, MD, FACS
Associate Professor of Surgery
Medical Director, Comprehensive Ear and Hearing Center
Research Director, Bloom Otopathology Lab
Section of Otolaryngology—Head and Neck Surgery
University of Chicago Medicine and Biological Sciences
Chicago, Illinois

Thieme
New York • Stuttgart • Delhi • Rio de Janeiro

Library of Congress Cataloging-in-Publication Data

The chronic ear / [edited by] John L. Dornhoffer, Michael B. Gluth.
p. ; cm.
Includes bibliographical references and index.
ISBN 978-1-60406-864-1 (hardcover) – ISBN 978-1-60406-865-8 (eISBN)
I. Dornhoffer, John L., editor. II. Gluth, Michael B., editor.
[DNLM: 1. Ear Diseases–therapy. 2. Chronic Disease.
3. Ear Diseases–diagnosis. WV 200]
RF291.35
617.8–dc23 2015002879

Thieme Publishers New York
333 Seventh Avenue, New York, NY 10001 USA
+1 800 782 3488, customerservice@thieme.com

Thieme Publishers Stuttgart
Rüdigerstrasse 14, 70469 Stuttgart, Germany
+49 [0]711 8931 421, customerservice@thieme.de

Thieme Publishers Delhi
A-12, Second Floor, Sector-2, Noida-201301
Uttar Pradesh, India
+91 120 45 566 00, customerservice@thieme.in

Thieme Publishers Rio de Janeiro, Thieme Publicações Ltda.
Edifício Rodolpho de Paoli, 25º andar
Av. Nilo Peçanha, 50 – Sala 2508
Rio de Janeiro 20020-906 Brasil
+55 21 3172-2297 / +55 21 3172-1896

Cover design: Thieme Publishing Group
Typesetting by DiTech Process Solutions

Printed in China by Everbest Printing Co, Ltd 5 4 3 2 1

ISBN 978-1-60406-864-1

Also available as an e-book:
eISBN 978-1-60406-865-8

Important note: Medicine is an ever-changing science undergoing continual development. Research and clinical experience are continually expanding our knowledge, in particular our knowledge of proper treatment and drug therapy. Insofar as this book mentions any dosage or application, readers may rest assured that the authors, editors, and publishers have made every effort to ensure that such references are in accordance with **the state of knowledge at the time of production of the book.**

Nevertheless, this does not involve, imply, or express any guarantee or responsibility on the part of the publishers in respect to any dosage instructions and forms of applications stated in the book. **Every user is requested to examine carefully** the manufacturers' leaflets accompanying each drug and to check, if necessary in consultation with a physician or specialist, whether the dosage schedules mentioned therein or the contraindications stated by the manufacturers differ from the statements made in the present book. Such examination is particularly important with drugs that are either rarely used or have been newly released on the market. Every dosage schedule or every form of application used is entirely at the user's own risk and responsibility. The authors and publishers request every user to report to the publishers any discrepancies or inaccuracies noticed. If errors in this work are found after publication, errata will be posted at www.thieme.com on the product description page.

Some of the product names, patents, and registered designs referred to in this book are in fact registered trademarks or proprietary names even though specific reference to this fact is not always made in the text. Therefore, the appearance of a name without designation as proprietary is not to be construed as a representation by the publisher that it is in the public domain.

To my wife, Mary, for all her personal and professional support through all these years. To my patients, students, and friends in the field, all over the world, who have taught me, inspired me and made this career a fascinating journey of knowledge and friendship.

— *JLD*

To my parents, my wife April, and my sons Cameron, Christian, and Graeme for magnifying my life. To Marcus Atlas for teaching me the nuances of otologic surgery. To John Dornhoffer for his mentorship.

— *MBG*

Contents

Preface

The management of chronic ear disease is one of the most fascinating but difficult aspects in the field of otolaryngology. Not only is the surgical anatomy of the middle ear cleft and mastoid very challenging to grasp, even when not distorted by disease, but the underlying pathophysiologic mechanisms involved with chronic otitis media are poorly understood. The chronic ear may manifest itself in a variety of ways based on the degree of infection, extent of middle ear remodeling, severity of inflammation, and integrity of underlying Eustachian tube function. As such, the approach to the patient with chronic ear disease must be eclectic and complete. The purpose of this textbook is to focus specifically on this complicated area, and the audience would include any physician involved in the medical and surgical management of the ear. We feel that this book is unique, not only in its focus, but also in its broad scope covering all aspects of the chronic ear, its organization, and its unusually diverse panel of expert authors who have so kindly contributed content.

This book is organized into eight parts and begins with general fundamental principles of anatomy, physiology, and disease production. The chapters in this first part are comprehensive and didactic in nature. The second part deals with the diagnosis and office management of the chronic ear while the third part is an introduction to surgical management of chronic ear disease. Subsequent parts are presented in a roundtable format, with an overview and introduction by the editors at the beginning of each roundtable to concisely state the issues at hand. The subsequent chapters are generally short and practical, with authors depicting their respective techniques using a standardized format that includes patient selection, detailed description of technique, complications, and results. Finally, the last part deals with future considerations, such as Eustachian tuboplasty, endoscopic ear surgery, and tissue engineering.

There are a lot of different ways to approach chronic ear disease and in many respects no single "correct way." Our philosophy is that it is best for surgeons to understand multiple disease management strategies and to master as many surgical techniques as possible. Accordingly, this text endeavors to present a number of methodologies for engaging particular common chronic ear scenarios. For example, we have included chapters on traditional canal wall–up and canal wall–down mastoidectomy but have also included the new hybrid techniques of canal reconstruction and mastoid obliteration. There are descriptions of underlay fascia tympanoplasty as well as the use of cartilage and bioengineered materials. There is a chapter on grommet insertion for Eustachian tube dysfunction as well as one on balloon dilatation. We are pleased to have authors from 13 different countries and feel this textbook represents one of the most complete references for the treatment of the chronic ear.

Otology is an international field, with ongoing advances and innovations coming from all over the globe. The diverse nature of the contributing authors is truly unique and we believe a real highlight of this text. Both of the editors completed fundamental otolaryngology training in the United States as well as surgical fellowships in otology in Germany and Switzerland (JLD) and Australia (MBG). Some of the techniques we learned while abroad seemed clearly better than what we had previously done while some were worse and some just different. However, both of us feel strongly that our practices were heavily influenced by what our international mentors taught us and have since been strong advocates of open-mindedness and international collaboration in otology. We hope this spirit is passed along to the reader.

Acknowledgments

The editors wish to thank Mary Dornhoffer, ELS, for her editorial assistance during the preparation of this book. Her careful review of each chapter, thoughtful edits, and attention to detail made this a more readable and accurate text.

We would also like to thank artists Anthony M. Pazos and Sarah Faris for creating the illustrations in this book, and Eric Scherrer for the front cover artwork.

Contributors

Robert B.A. Adamson, PhD
Assistant Professor
School of Biomedical Engineering
Dalhousie University
Halifax, Nova Scotia, Canada

Shane R. Anderson, MBBS, M Phil, FRACS
Senior Lecturer
James Cook University
Consultant Adult and Paediatric Otologist
The Townsville Hospital
Townsville, Queensland, Australia

Samuel Atcherson, PhD
Associate Professor of Audiology
Interim Director of Audiology
Department of Audiology and Speech Pathology
University of Arkansas at Little Rock
University of Arkansas for Medical Sciences
Little Rock, Arkansas

Marcus D. Atlas, MBBS, FRACS
Winthrop Professor, Garnett Passe Rodney Williams Memorial Foundation
Chair of Otolaryngology
The University of Western Australia
Director, Ear Science Institute Australia
Subiaco, Western Australia, Australia

Patrick R. Axon, MD, FRCS (ORL-HNS)
Consultant Otologist and Skull Base Surgeon
Cambridge University Hospitals
Addenbrooke's NHS Foundation Trust
Cambridge, United Kingdom

Seilesh C. Babu, MD
Chief Financial Officer
Michigan Ear Institute
Farmington Hills, Michigan
Clinical Associate Professor
Wayne State University
Department of Otolaryngology
Detroit, Michigan

Manohar Bance, MBChB, MSc, FRCSC
Professor and Head
Department of Otolaryngology—Head and Neck Surgery
Dalhousie University
Halifax, Nova Scotia, Canada

Brent J. Benscoter, MD
Midwest Ear Institute
Indianapolis, Indiana

Alexander G. Bien, MD
Albany ENT & Allergy Services
Albany, New York

Bruce Black, MD, FRACS, FRCS, FRCSEd
Professor
Department of Surgery
University of Queensland Lady Cilentro Children's Hospital
Brisbane, Queensland, Australia

Robert J.S. Briggs, MBBS, FRACS, FACS
Clinical Associate Professor
Department of Otolaryngology
The University of Melbourne
Clinical Executive Director of Otolaryngology
The Royal Victorian Eye and Ear Hospital
Melbourne, Australia

Adva Buzi, MD
Assistant Professor
Division of Otolaryngology
The Children's Hospital of Philadelphia
Department of Otorhinolaryngology–Head and Neck Surgery
University of Pennsylvania Perelman School of Medicine
Philadelphia, Pennsylvania

Audrey P. Calzada, MD
California Head and Neck Specialists
La Jolla, California

Matthew L. Carlson, MD
Assistant Professor
Department of Otolaryngology—Head and Neck Surgery
Mayo Clinic
Rochester, Minnesota

Paula Casserly, MCh, FRCS (ORL)
Department of Otolaryngology, Head and Neck Surgery
St. James's Hospital and Royal Victoria Eye and Ear Hospital
Dublin, Ireland

Joseph M. Chen, MD, FRCS(C)
Head, Department of Otolaryngology—Head and Neck Surgery
Sunnybrook Health Sciences Center
Professor
University of Toronto
Provincial Coordinator
Ontario Cochlear Implantation Program
Toronto, Ontario, Canada

Richard A. Chole, MD, PhD
Lindburg Professor and Head
Department of Otolaryngology—Head and Neck Surgery
Washington University School of Medicine
St. Louis, Missouri

Sebahattin Cureoglu, MD
Associate Professor
Co-Director, Otopathology Laboratory
Department of Otolaryngology
University of Minnesota
Minneapolis, Minnesota

Stefan Dazert, MD
Professor and Chairman
Department of Otorhinolaryngology-Head and Neck Surgery
Ruhr-University of Bochum
Bochum, Germany

John L. Dornhoffer, MD, FACS
Professor and Vice Chair of Adult Services
Samuel D. McGill Chair in Otolaryngology Research
Director, Division of Otology and Neurotology
Director, Hearing and Balance Center
Department of Otolaryngology—Head and Neck Surgery
University of Arkansas for Medical Sciences
Arkansas Children's Hospital
Little Rock, Arkansas

Venkata S.P.B. Durvasula, MD, FRCS ENT
Instructor
Department of Otolaryngology-Head and Neck Surgery
University of Arkansas Medical Sciences
Little Rock, Arkansas

Howard W. Francis, MD, MBA
Professor and Vice Director
Department of Otolaryngology—Head and Neck Surgery
Johns Hopkins University School of Medicine
Baltimore, Maryland

Michael B. Gluth, MD
Associate Professor of Surgery
Medical Director, Comprehensive Ear and Hearing Center
Research Director, Bloom Otopathology Lab
Section of Otolaryngology—Head and Neck Surgery
University of Chicago Medicine and Biological Sciences
Chicago, Illinois

Jason C. Goodwin, MD
Staff Otolaryngologist
United States Air Force
Eglin Air Force Base, Florida

Richard K. Gurgel, MD
Assistant Professor
Division of Otolaryngology—Head and Neck Surgery
University of Utah School of Medicine
Salt Lake City, Utah

Marlan R. Hansen, MD, FACS
Marvin and Rose Lee Pomerantz Professor
Departments of Otolaryngology—Head and Neck Surgery and Neurosurgery
University of Iowa
Iowa City, Iowa

David S. Haynes, MD, FACS
Vice Chair and Chief Academic Officer
Professor of Otolaryngology, Neurosurgery, and Hearing and Speech Sciences
The Otology Group of Vanderbilt
Vanderbilt University Medical Center
Nashville, Tennessee

Florian Hoppe, MD
Professor and Chairman
Department of Otorhinolaryngology-Head and Neck Surgery
Klinikum Oldenburg
Medical Campus University of Oldenburg
Oldenburg, Germany

Karl-Bernd Hüttenbrink, MD
Professor and Head
Department of Otorhinolaryngology-Head and Neck Surgery
University of Cologne
Cologne, Germany

Brandon Isaacson, MD, FACS
Associate Professor
Co-Director of the Comprehensive Skull Base Surgery Program
Department of Otolaryngology—Head and Neck Surgery
University of Texas Southwestern Medical Center
Dallas, Texas

David H. Jung, MD, PhD
Instructor
Department of Otology and Laryngology
Harvard Medical School
Assistant in Otology
Massachusetts Eye and Ear Infirmary
Boston, Massachusetts

Shin-ichi Kanemaru, MD, PhD
Department of Otolaryngology–Head and Neck Surgery
Medical Research Institute, Kitano Hospital
Osaka, Japan
Department of Otolaryngology
Foundation for Biomedical Research and Innovation Hospital
Kobe, Japan

Jafri Kuthubutheen, MBBS (Hons), FRACS
Department of Otolaryngology–Head and Neck Surgery
Fiona Stanley Hospital
Princess Margaret Hospital for Children
Royal Perth Hospital
Perth, Western Australia, Australia

Bradley W. Kesser, MD
Professor and Director
Division of Otology/Neurotology
Department of Otolaryngology—Head and Neck Surgery
University of Virginia School of Medicine
Charlottesville, Virginia

Ilkka Kivekäs, MD, PhD
Research Fellow
Department of Otolaryngology
Harvard Medical School and Boston Children's Hospital
Boston, Massachusetts
Assistant Professor of Otorhinolaryngology
Department of Otorhinolaryngology
Tampere University Hospital and the University of Tampere
Tampere, Finland

J. Walter Kutz Jr., MD, FACS
Associate Professor
Department of Otolaryngology Head and Neck Surgery
University of Texas Southwestern Medical Center
Dallas, Texas

James Lin, MD
Assistant Professor
Department of Otolaryngology—Head and Neck Surgery
Kansas University Medical Center
Kansas City, Kansas

Thomas E. Linder, MD
Professor and Chairman
Department of Otorhinolaryngology—Head and Neck Surgery
Luzerner Kantonsspital
Luzern, Switzerland

Jan-Christoffer Lüers, MD
Associate Professor
Department of Otorhinolaryngology–Head and Neck Surgery
University of Cologne
Cologne, Germany

Michael J. McKenna, MD
Professor
Department of Otology and Laryngology
Harvard Medical School
Division Chief, Otology
Department of Otolaryngology
Massachusetts Eye and Ear Infirmary
Boston, Massachusetts

Cliff A. Megerian, MD, FACS
The Julius McCall Professor and Chairman
Department of Otolaryngology—Head and Neck Surgery
Case Western Reserve University School of Medicine
The Richard and Patricia Pogue Endowed Chair
President University Hospitals Physician Services
Chief Medical Officer Physician Practices
University Hospitals Health System
Cleveland, Ohio

Robert A. Mlynski, MD
Professor and Chairman
Dept. of Otorhinolaryngology–Head and Neck Surgery "Otto Körner"
Rostock University Medical Center
Rostock, Germany

Rick F. Nelson, MD, PhD
Assistant Professor
Department of Otolaryngology—Head and Neck Surgery
Indiana University School of Medicine
Indianapolis, Indiana

Michael M. Paparella, MD
Founder, International Hearing Foundation
Director, Otology/Neurotology Fellowship
Paparella Ear Head and Neck Institute
Director, Otopathology Laboratory
Clinical Professor and Chairman Emeritus
Department of Otolaryngology
University of Minnesota
Minneapolis, Minnesota

Dennis S. Poe, MD, FACS
Associate Professor
Department of Otology and Laryngology
Harvard Medical School
Department of Otolaryngology and Communications Enhancement
Boston Children's Hospital
Boston, Massachusetts

David D. Pothier, MSc, MBChB, FRCS(ORL-HNS)
Staff Neurotologist and Assistant Professor
Department of Otolaryngology, Head and Neck Surgery
University of Toronto
Toronto General Hospital
University Health Network
Toronto, Ontario, Canada

Alejandro Rivas, MD
Associate Professor of Otolaryngology–Head and Neck Surgery
Associate Professor of Neurological Surgery
Director of Endoscopic Ear Surgery
The Otology Group of Vanderbilt
Vanderbilt University Medical Center
Nashville, Tennessee

John J. Rosowski, PhD
The Eliasen Professor of Otology and Laryngology
Professor of Health Science and Technology
Harvard Medical School
Senior Scientist
Eaton Peabody Laboratory
Massachusetts Eye and Ear Infirmary
Boston, Massachusetts

Peter L. Santa Maria, MBBS, PhD
Instructor
Department for Otolaryngology, Head and Neck Surgery
Stanford University Hospital and Clinics
Stanford, California

Konrad Schwager, MD
Professor and Chairman
Department of Otorhinolaryngology–Head and Neck Surgery
Philipps University of Marburg, Campus Fulda
Fulda, Germany

Maroun T. Semaan, MD, FACS
Associate Professor of Otolaryngology—Head and Neck Surgery
Chief, Division of Otology and Neurotology
University Hospitals Case Medical Center
Cleveland, Ohio

Jeffrey D. Sharon, MD
Clinical Fellow in Otology, Neurotology, and Skull Base Surgery
Department of Otolaryngology–Head and Neck Surgery
Johns Hopkins School of Medicine
Baltimore, Maryland

Clough Shelton, MD, FACS
Professor and Chief of Otolaryngology
C. Charles Hetzel Jr., MD and Alice Barker Hetzel Presidential Endowed Chair in Otolaryngology
University of Utah School of Medicine
Salt Lake City, Utah

Juha Tapio Silvola, MD, PhD
Staff Surgeon and Senior Consultant in Otology, Otoneurology
ENT Department
Oslo University Hospital, Rikshospitalet
Oslo, Norway
Associate Professor of Otolaryngology
University of Tampere
Tampere, Finland

Henrik Smeds, MD
Senior Consultant in Otology and Neurotology
Department of Otolaryngology–Head and Neck Surgery
Karolinska University Hospital
Stockholm, Sweden

Hinrich Staecker, MD, PhD
Mary and David Zamierowski Professor of Skull Base Oncology
Department of Otolaryngology–Head and Neck Surgery
University of Kansas School of Medicine
Kansas City, Kansas

Holger H. Sudhoff, MD, PhD, FRCS, FRCPath
Professor and Chairman
Department of Otolaryngology—Head and Neck Surgery
Klinikum Bielefeld, Academic Teaching Hospital
Münster University
Bielefeld, Germany

Haruo Takahashi, MD
Professor and Chair
Department of Otolaryngology—Head and Neck Surgery
Nagasaki University Graduate School of Biomedical Sciences
Sakomoto, Nagasaki City
Nagasaki, Japan

Robert Vincent, MD, FRCSEd (Hon)
Causse Ear Clinic
Colombiers, France

Stefan Volkenstein, MD
Department of Otorhinolaryngology, Head and Neck Surgery
Ruhr-University of Bochum
St. Elisabeth-Hospital
Bochum, Germany

George B. Wanna, MD, FACS
Associate Professor of Otolaryngology—Head and Neck Surgery
Associate Professor of Neurological Surgery
Co-Director, Neurotology Fellowship Program
The Otology Group of Vanderbilt
Vanderbilt University Medical Center
Nashville, Tennessee

Cameron C. Wick, MD
Ear, Nose, and Throat Institute
University Hospitals Case Medical Center
Cleveland, Ohio

Richard H. Wiggins III, MD, CIIP, FSIIM
Director of Head and Neck Imaging
Professor
Departments of Radiology, Otolaryngology, Head and Neck Surgery, and BioMedical Informatics
University of Utah Health Sciences Center
Salt Lake City, Utah

Eric P. Wilkinson, MD
Surgeon/Partner
House Clinic
Research Scientist
Huntington Medical Research Institutes
Los Angeles, California

Heng-Wai Yuen, MBBS, MRCSE, MMed(ORL), DOHNS, FAMS
Director, Advanced Surgical Skills Training Centre
Senior Consultant and Director of Otology & Neurotology
Department of Otolaryngology–Head and Neck Surgery
Changi General Hospital
Clinical Senior Lecturer
Yong Loo Lin School of Medicine
National University of Singapore
Singapore

Matthew Yung, PhD, MS, MBA, FRCS, MBBS
Consultant Otolaryngologist
The Ipswich Hospital NHS Trust
Ipswich, Suffolk, United Kingdom

Yannick Zaugg, MD
Department of Otorhinolaryngology–Head and Neck Surgery
Centre Hospitalier Universitaire Vaudois
Lausanne, Switzerland

Master Glossary

5-FU: 5-fluorouracil
ABG: air-bone gap
ACE: angiotensin-converting enzyme
ADC: apparent diffusion coefficient
AMEI: active middle ear implant
ANCA: antibodies to neutrophil cytoplasmic antigens
c-ANCA: cytoplasmic-pattern ANCA
p-ANCA: perinuclear-pattern ANCA
AOM: acute otitis media
AOMT: acute otitis media with tympanostomy
BAHA: bone-anchored hearing aid
BC-FMT: bone conduction-floating mass transducer
BET: balloon Eustachian tuboplasty
bFGF: basic fibroblast growth factor
BMRM: Bondy modified radical mastoidectomy
CAA: congenital aural atresia
CBCT: cone-beam CT
CDC: Centers for Disease Control and Prevention
CF-HC: chloramphenicol/fungizone–hydrocortisone
CI: cochlear implant
COM: chronic otitis media
COME: chronic otitis media with effusion
CROS: contralateral routing of offside signaling
CSF: cerebrospinal fluid
CSF powder: chloramphenicol/sulfanilamide/fungizone powder
CSF-HC: chloramphenicol/sulfanilamide/fungizone–hydrocortisone
CSOE: chronic stenosing otitis externa
CSOM: chronic suppurative otitis media
CSS: Churg-Strauss syndrome
CT: computed tomography
CTV: CT venography
CWD: canal wall–down
CWR: canal wall reconstruction
CWU: canal wall–up
DACS: Direct Acoustic Cochlear Stimulator
DWI: diffusion-weighted imaging
DW MRI: diffusion-weighted magnetic resonance imaging
EAC: external auditory canal
ECoG: electrocochleography
EDTA: ethylenediaminetetraacetic acid
EES: endoscopic ear surgery
EGF: epidermal growth factor
EGFR: epithelial growth factor receptor
EOM: eosinophilic otitis media
EPI: echo planar imaging (also, non-EPI for non-echo planar imaging)
EPS: extracellular polymeric substance
ETD: Eustachian tube dysfunction
FGF: fibroblast growth factor
FLAIR: fluid-attenuated inversion recovery
FMT: floating mass transducer
FOM: footplate onto malleus
FOT: footplate onto TM
FTTP: Fisch Titanium Total Prosthesis
GPA: granulomatosis with polyangitis
GRE: gradient recalled echo
HA: hydroxyapatite
HB-EGF: heparin-binding EGF
HL: hearing level
HUA: hyaluronic acid
IAC: internal auditory canal
ICA: internal carotid artery
ICW: intact–canal wall
IGF: insulin-like growth factor
IL: interleukin
IMP: inferior musculoperiosteal
KGF: keratinocyte growth factor
LIMF: lateral incudomalleal fold
LPR: laryngopharyngeal reflux
LVP: levator veli palatini
MDGF: macrophage-derived growth factor
MERI: Middle Ear Risk Index
MIC: minimal inhibitory concentration
MMP: matrix metalloproteinase
MPO: myeloperoxidase
MRI: magnetic resonance imaging
MRM: modified radical mastoidectomy
MRP: malleus replacement prosthesis
MRSA: methicillin-resistant *Staphylococcus aureus*
MRV: magnetic resonance venography
MSSA: methicillin-sensitive *Staphylococcus aureus*
MTA: middle temporal artery
OME: otitis media with effusion
OOPS: Ossiculoplasty Outcomes Parameter Staging
PCR: polymerase chain reaction
PDGF: platelet-derived growth factor
PGOW: pressure gain at the oval window
PML: polymorphonuclear lymphocytes
PORP: partial ossicular replacement prosthesis
PTFE: polytetrafluorethylene
RANKL: Receptor Activator of NF-κB Ligand
RAST: Radioallergosorbant Test
RM: radical mastoidectomy
RoWPOWA: round window protection with oval window access
RS: receiver stimulator
SCC: semicircular canal
SDT: speech detection threshold

SHOM: stapes head onto malleus
SHOT: stapes head onto TM
SPGR: spoiled gradient recalled
SPL: sound pressure level
SRT: speech recognition threshold
SWI: susceptibility-weighted imaging
SWCR: soft wall canal reconstruction
TB: tuberculosis
TEES: transcanal endoscopic ear surgery
TGF: transforming growth factor
TIVA: total intravenous anesthesia
TM: tympanic membrane
TMJ: temporomandibular joint
TMM: tubomanometry
TNF: tumor necrosis factor
TOF: time of flight
TORP: total ossicular replacement prosthesis
TT: tympanostomy tube(s)
TVP: tensor veli palatine
VEMP: Vestibular Evoked Myogenic Potential
VORP: vibrating ossicular replacement prosthesis
VTE: venous thromboembolism
WHO: World Health Organization

Part 1

The Fundamentals of Chronic Ear Disease

1 Chronic Ear Disease in the Modern Era: Evolution of Treatment, Epidemiology, and Classification

Adva Buzi, Michael B. Gluth, and Bruce Black

Abbreviations used in this chapter:

AOM: acute otitis media
COM: chronic otitis media
CWD: canal wall-down
CWU: canal wall-up
ICW: intact–canal wall
PORP: partial ossicular replacement prosthesis
TORP: total ossicular replacement prosthesis

1.1 Historical Perspective

Prior to the modern era of antibiotics, otitis media was very often accompanied by deleterious outcomes, as evidenced by this quote from Hippocrates: "Acute pain of the ear with continued strong fever is to be dreaded for there is danger that the man may become delirious and die."[1] Surgery for chronic otitis media likely dates from antiquity, and drainage of abscesses by military surgeons and others was probably commonplace; however, little evidence of this remains. The history of chronic ear disease is well covered by the works of Milstein and Briggs.[2,3,4,5]

Recorded mastoid drainage dates from Rolianus (1671), followed by Petit (1774). The pain of the procedure probably dictated little more than a lancing or short incision. Drainage would have involved a proportion of cholesteatoma cases; these no doubt did worse than the non-cholesteatoma cases, but the earliest sources did not discern between cholesteatomatous or chronic infection conditions before the recognition of cholesteatoma in the 19th century. The modern era of mastoid surgery began with Wilde's (1853) postaural incision and drainage. Without anesthesia, these were very likely the rapid but agonizing procedures of the time. Before Lister and the advent of antiseptic technique, many would have suffered surgical sepsis and its consequences.

Advances in other fields (pathology, microbiology, anesthesia, and antiseptic technique) permitted the more complex cortical mastoidectomy techniques. In 1873, Schwartze and Eysell were the first to publish an article describing the procedure of mastoidectomy, including the utilization of a chisel and hammer to remove bone. They also postulated clear indications for performing a mastoidectomy, including active infection and hearing loss as well as tinnitus, the surgical treatment of which was controversial.[2] Despite this advance, cholesteatoma would have continued to cause problems until the underlying pathology became better appreciated; as such, mastoidectomy procedures of this era were primarily utilized to afford outward egress of pus.

Although likely first described by Duverney (in 1683), the term "cholesteatoma" was coined by Muller (1838), who noted the presence of cholesterol and fat in a tumor present in the ear. Much debate ensued in the 1800s as to the origin of this tumor in the ear canal. Several theories arose including dedifferentiation of bone cells (Virchow), direct extension of epidermal debris from the external auditory canal (Von Troeltsch), metaplasia of the middle ear mucosa (Gruber, Wendst, and Rokitansky), and others. At the end of the 19th century, Bezold and Habermann reached the conclusion, while examining pathologic specimens, that cholesteatoma could arise from skin migrating into the middle ear through a perforation and undergoing desquamation. Bezold also identified Eustachian tube dysfunction with resulting retraction pockets as a way for cholesteatoma to form.[6]

With a better understanding of cholesteatoma and chronic otitis media, the surgical aim of sac exteriorization arose and, with it, the development of "open" ear surgery as the radical mastoidectomy procedures of Kuester, von Bergmann and Zaufal, then Stacke (1888–90), in which the posterior canal wall was removed to permit drainage via the external canal. Subsequently, modified radical techniques, intending to preserve hearing by retention of some of the tympano-ossicular elements, emerged with the works of Bryant, Heath, and Bondy (1904–10). Variants of radical and modified radical mastoidectomy techniques remain in use today.[7,8] Despite the benefits of avoiding serious cholesteatoma-related morbidity and mortality, canal wall-down (CWD) procedures induced substantial alteration of normal anatomy. Resultant cavity symptomatology was often due to failure of another key function: epithelial migration. Split-skin (Thiersch)[9] and full-thickness (Wolfe) grafts failed to correct cavity problems; they did not self-clean, and they were prone to chronic dermatitic degeneration.[10] Canal wall-down surgery continued as the standard to the mid-twentieth century but progressively became more refined with the introduction of the operating microscope by Holmgren in 1923 and power drills.

Such refinement prompted the next phase of ear surgery that would endeavor to restore full ear function. This began with the introduction of "combined approach" canal wall-up (CWU) surgery by Jansen in 1958.[11] Also termed intact–canal wall (ICW) surgery, this was directed at maintaining both anatomy and function. Concurrently developed in several American centers by surgeons such as Sheehy and Jako,[12,13] CWU surgery was designed to avoid the above cavity problems of the CWD procedures, but it was quickly recognized that CWU surgery had its own inherent problems of residual and recurrent cholesteatoma.[14,15,16] In addition, continued Eustachian tube dysfunction often led to failure to achieve an aerated middle ear space.[15] These drawbacks made the procedure controversial at its inception. The principle of staging the surgical procedure alleviated some of these concerns and led to wider acceptance.[17] Despite improving outcomes, however, some surgeons remained skeptical and reverted to CWD procedures. The controversy between CWU and CWD procedures continues today.

With progressive focus on the function of the tympano-ossicular mechanism, the concept of tympanoplasty was introduced by Zollner and Wullstein in the 1950s, which not only addressed tympanic reconstruction by the application of skin grafts, but also further expounded on the "plastic technique" of shaping the external auditory meatus. This initial concept of tympanoplasty relied on principles of overlay grafting with skin grafts, a technique that was later refined by Sheehy in a form that is still utilized by some surgeons today as overlay or "lateral graft" tympanoplasty. Further development of tympanoplasty would explore the utility of other grafting materials. In 1958, Hans Heermann was the first to use temporalis fascia as a grafting material, which allowed placement of graft medial to the tympanic membrane in an underlay technique.

With the success of tympanoplasty came the advent of ossicular reconstruction to further rebuild the middle ear mechanism. Initially, various metallic and plastic implants were utilized. Results were promising, but poor long-term outcomes were achieved secondary to extrusion of implants. Autotransplantation of ossicles was the next step in the development of ossicular reconstruction. Removed ossicles were reshaped and reinserted to reestablish continuity. Incus transposition is a popular technique that is still used today,[18] although preparation of the graft for reimplantation is often cumbersome and time-consuming.

In search of a more simple technique and improved results, Janeke and Shea, in 1975, reintroduced the use of alloplastic materials in the form of biocompatible prostheses (partial ossicular replacement prosthesis [PORP] and total ossicular replacement prosthesis [TORP]).[19] Extrusion rates decreased when cartilage grafts were placed lateral to the prostheses.[20] Over the past several decades, the materials used for prostheses have undergone a variety of changes.

Still often driven by advances in technology and in other medical fields, otologic surgery continues its development in modern times. Hybrid tympanomastoid surgical techniques, which consist of the removal of part of the canal wall for cholesteatoma dissection followed by replacement or reconstruction to ultimately provide CWU anatomy, are evolving rapidly. Techniques to obliterate CWD mastoidectomy cavities have also advanced to minimize many of the negative factors associated with an open cavity. The use of rigid fiberoptic endoscopes is an example of an innovation that has begun to serve as an adjuvant to CWU and mastoidectomy-sparing techniques.[21] Advances in imaging, particularly MRI, have allowed the possibility of avoiding second-look surgery.[22] Tissue engineering poses the potential for reliable tympanic membrane reconstruction via a simple office procedure. Perhaps the most significant surgical aim pertaining to the chronic ear that remains elusive is correction of the dysfunctional Eustachian tube; nevertheless, efforts in this field are ongoing. The next century will likely see development of new strategies and continued innovations of existing techniques to improve the results of chronic ear surgery.

1.2 Epidemiology of Chronic Ear Disease

1.2.1 Risk Factors

Over time, a better understanding of the epidemiology of chronic ear disease is emerging. Risk factors for otitis media with effusion have been postulated to be associated with their underlying effects on Eustachian tube function and the middle ear environment. Chronic suppurative otitis media is much less common than acute otitis media. Studies linking risk factors to the incidence of chronic suppurative otitis media are lacking, and most of the data are inferred from the information evident about risk factors of acute otitis media. This is warranted, with the presumption that recurrent acute otitis media likely predisposes an individual to chronic suppurative otitis media.[23]

Age is a well-recognized risk factor for otitis media. Younger children are more prone to otitis media due to the short length, small caliber, and horizontal orientation of their Eustachian tube. In addition to this anatomical disparity, children are more likely to have an immature immune system, making them more susceptible to viral and bacterial pathogens.[24] Other risk factors include frequent upper respiratory tract infections, history of allergies, and family history of otitis media. Social and environmental influences are also important. These include exposure to smoking and day care attendance. Improvement of housing, hygiene, nutrition, and other social factors have shown to result in a significant decrease in prevalence of chronic suppurative otitis media in some societies.[25]

Several ethnic groups have been found to have a higher risk of developing otitis media and, consequently, going on to develop chronic suppurative otitis media. These include Southwestern American Indians, Australian Aborigines, Greenlanders, and Alaskan Eskimos.[25]

Eustachian tube dysfunction with resultant negative middle ear pressure has been established as a cause of acquired cholesteatoma. For this reason, risk factors of otitis media that lead to prolonged Eustachian tube dysfunction are thought to be coexistent in cases of cholesteatoma. These include craniofacial anomalies and cleft palate.

1.2.2 Prevalence

Otitis media has been examined heavily over the past several decades given that it is one of the most common diagnoses in primary care clinics worldwide. Its disease burden is pervasive; both developed and developing countries are affected. Studies examining the prevalence of the disease are usually population-based and, therefore, the overall prevalence is difficult to ascertain.

When reviewing the multiple population-based studies performed in the past several decades, it appears that several groups arise based on the prevalence rate of chronic suppurative otitis media. The populations with the highest prevalence (as mentioned previously) include Inuits (7% to 46%), Aborigines (12% to 33%), and Native Americans (4% to 8%), followed by populations in the South Pacific Islands (4% to 6%) and Africa (2% to 6%). A lower rate is found in the Asian and Middle Eastern countries (1% to 2%). The lowest prevalence rates occur in developed countries, including the United States, United Kingdom, Finland, Denmark, and Israel, all of which have prevalence rates of less than 1%.[26]

Fewer studies have examined the population prevalence of cholesteatoma. A study of patients in Iowa showed a prevalence of 0.01% and an incidence of 6 per 100,000.[27] Interestingly, the prevalence rates of cholesteatoma are often the reverse of those for chronic suppurative otitis media and are often found to be more common in developed countries. This may be secondary to the neutral middle ear pressure provided by a chronic perforation. As one example, a study performed in Sierra Leone, where the chronic suppurative otitis media rate among a population of 2,015 children was 6.4%, found only one child with cholesteatoma.[28]

1.3 Classification of Chronic Ear Disease

Several classifications of otitis media have been described. For several decades, an agreement on the consistency of definitions and terminology has been sought to standardize research efforts. The classification method most commonly used now relates to the timing of symptomology as well as the complications involved. Consequently, a great deal of overlap exists in the terminology used to refer to chronic ear conditions.

1.3.1 Acute versus Chronic Otitis Media

The spectrum of otitis media with an intact tympanic membrane is generally subdivided into three conditions: Eustachian tube dysfunction, otitis media with effusion (OME), and acute otitis media (AOM). Eustachian tube dysfunction refers to poor middle ear ventilation that may result in acute or chronic negative middle ear pressure, hearing loss, and otalgia.[29] Eustachian tube dysfunction may lead to OME, which describes a middle ear effusion without prominent signs of acute inflammation. This term has replaced designations such as serous otitis media or secretory otitis media. Within this category, a temporal classification also exists, with acute effusion lasting less than 3 weeks, subacute from 3 weeks to 3 months, and chronic for greater than 3 months. AOM refers to inflammation of the middle ear that has a rapid onset and resolution. It is often associated with one or more systemic symptoms including, but not limited to otalgia, fever, and irritability.

1.3.2 Tympanic Membrane Perforations

There is no universally accepted scheme to classify tympanic membrane perforations. Perforations of the pars tensa may be considered central or marginal depending on location relative to the annulus. At times, perforations are also described based on size (pinpoint, subtotal). Perforations of the tympanic membrane can also be considered acute or chronic in nature. An acute perforation is most commonly the result of a bout of AOM. The natural history of an acute perforation can follow several paths. The perforation can heal spontaneously, the inflammation of the middle ear can resolve with the perforation failing to close and become a chronic perforation, or the perforation can be associated with ongoing middle ear infection with otorrhea. When perforation and infection are present for at least 3 months, an ear may be classified as having chronic suppurative otitis media.[29]

1.3.3 Chronic Suppurative Otitis Media

Chronic suppurative otitis media has been informally subtyped according to several unofficial indicators. Infection, for example, may be regarded as active, intermittent, or quiescent depending on the frequency and duration of otorrhea.[30] A further division can also be made between a cholesteatomatous and non-cholesteatomatous chronic ear. Lastly, some surgeons have also classified COM as being predominantly tubotympanic (▸ Fig. 1.1), atticoantral (▸ Fig. 1.2), or mixed (▸ Fig. 1.3) in subtype. Tubotympanic chronic otitis media tends to be typified by disease of the pars tensa and mesotympanum, whereas atticoantral disease primarily involves the pars flaccida and epitympanum; however, this terminology is admittedly ambiguous and of uncertain utility.

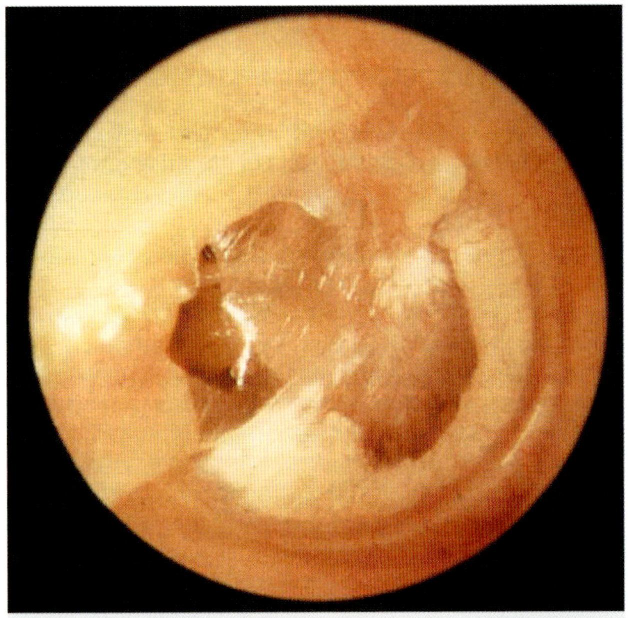

Fig. 1.1 Early tympanic membrane collapse invoving the pars tensa (Black Stage I). Limited posterior retraction into the mesotympanum and diffuse myringosclerosis are present. The pars flaccida is not involved. Pars tensa collapse such as this may progress to pars tensa cholesteatoma that originates within the posterior mesotympanum, having early involvement of the retrotympanum, most notably the sinus tympani. This collapse is commonly associated with ongoing Eustachian tube dysfunction.

Chronic suppurative otitis media has also been classified according to disease severity. Bellucci introduced a popular grading scale based on the frequency of otorrhea and whether or not the patient had a cleft palate.[30] Austin described a classification based on the underlying ossicular defect.[31] Eventually, Kartush modified Austin's classification and combined it with Bellucci's classification to create the popular Middle Ear Risk Index (▸ Table 1.1).[32] Other modern statistics-based rating scales have also been reported by Black[33] (Surgical Prosthetic Infection Tissue Eustachian) and Dornhoffer[34] (Ossiculoplasty Outcomes Parameter Staging Index) to better predict expected ossiculoplasty outcomes.

1.3.4 Drum Collapse (Atelectasis, Adhesive Otitis Media)

Although the diagnosis of chronic suppurative otitis media is often made based upon the presence of a chronically draining perforated tympanic membrane, chronic collapse of the tympanic membrane, often due to Eustachian tube dysfunction, may result in a sequence of symptoms that qualifies for inclusion. This condition has been referred to as adhesive otitis

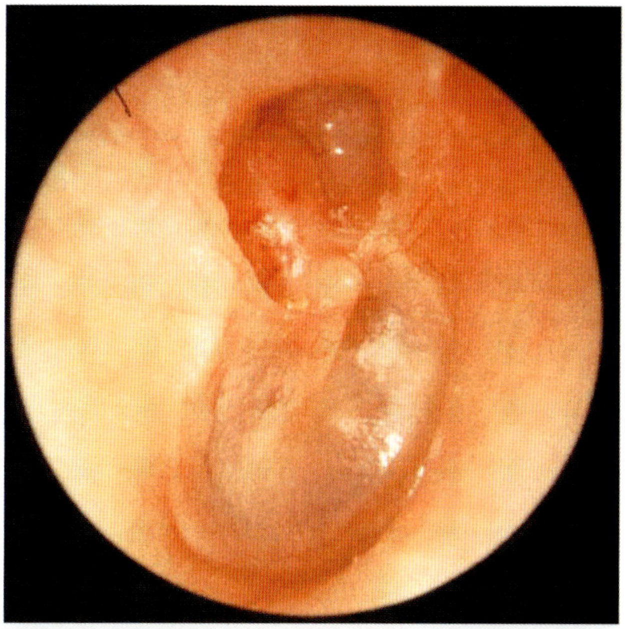

Fig. 1.2 Large attic retraction pocket. The pars flaccida has simultaneously collapsed into the posterior and anterior epitympanum. Aside from subtle anterior myringosclerosis that resulted from tympanostomy tube placement, the pars flaccida is reasonably normal and there is no underlying effusion of the mesotympanum. Attic retraction pockets may progress to form attic cholesteatoma and may be the result of selective epitympanic dysventilation (even in the setting of normalized Eustachian tube function) from blockage of the epitympanic diaphragm.

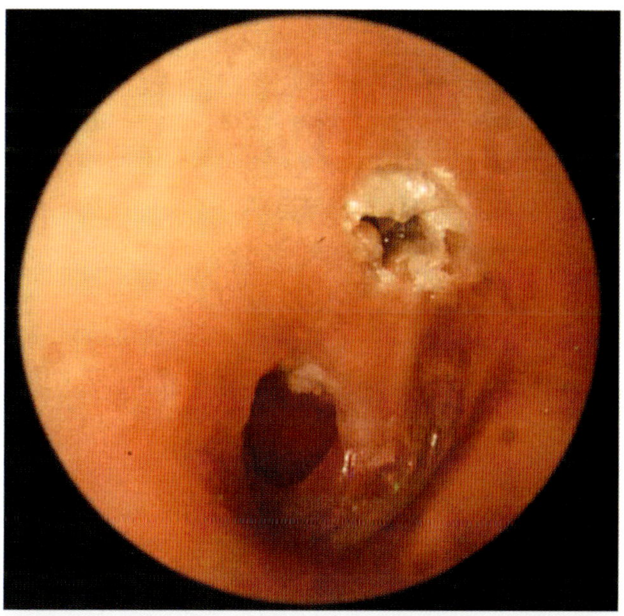

Fig. 1.3 Combined pars tensa-attic pattern. Simultaneous disease of the pars tensa and pars flaccida are noted in the form of attic cholesteatoma and pars tensa perforation respectively.

media when a combination of tympanic membrane atelectasis and adhesions between the tympanic membrane and underlying middle ear structures is present.

Table 1.1 Middle Ear Risk Index

	Risk Factor	Risk Value
Otorrhea (Belucci)	I. Dry	0
	II. Occasionally wet	1
	III. Persistently wet	2
	IV. Wet with cleft palate	3
Perforation	None	0
	Present	1
Cholesteatoma	None	0
	Present	1
Ossicular Status (Austin/Kartush)	0. M + I + S +	0
	A. M + S +	1
	B. M + S-	2
	C. M-S +	3
	D. M-S-	4
	E. Ossicular head fixation	2
	F. Stapes fixation	2
Middle Ear: Granulations or Effusion	No	0
	Yes	2
Previous Surgery	No	0
	Staged	1
	Revision	2
Smoker	No	0
	Yes	2

M, malleus; I, incus; S, stapes.

Several classification systems exist for tympanic membrane collapse depending on the site of tympanic membrane involvement; the most common among these[35,36,37] are outlined in Chapter 15. However, a practical and modern classification of the collapsed tympanic membrane, based on disease extent and its associated impact on disease management, has also been described by Black as a means of connecting classification to surgical decision-making.[38] For pars tensa collapse, classification is as follows (▶ Fig. 1.4): Stage I is collapse without hearing loss, treated by observation or tympanostomy tube placement; Stage II is collapse with hearing loss but no ossicular dysfunction, treated by tympanoplasty to reinforce the drumhead; Stage III is collapse with hearing loss and ossicular fixation/erosion, treated by tympanoplasty with ossicular reconstruction; Stage IV is acquired cholesteatoma, treated by one among a variety of tympanomastoidectomy or epitympanectomy techniques.

If an effusion is present, an asterisk is appended to warn of a possible poor hearing outcome (e.g., Stage III*).

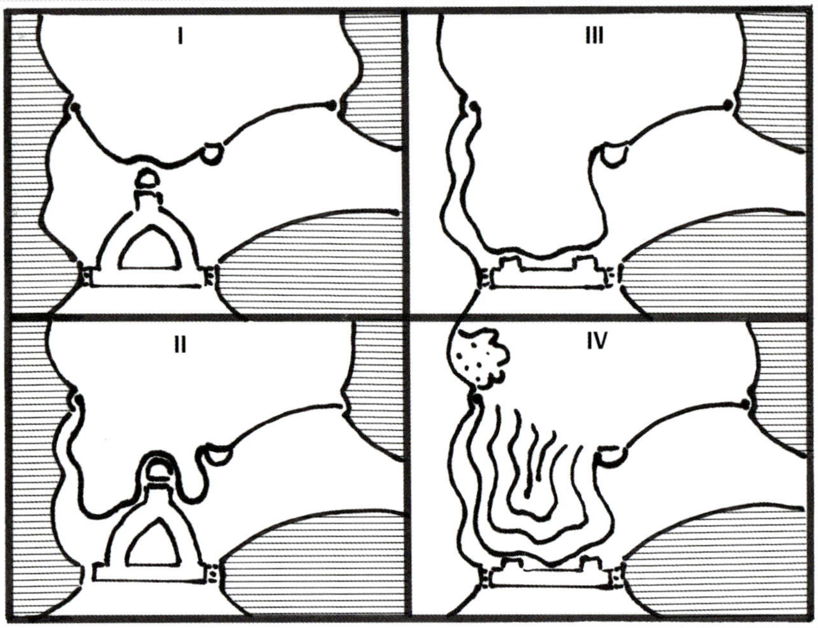

Fig. 1.4 Black classification of the collapsed pars tensa. Stage I is collapse without hearing loss, treated by observation or tympanostomy tube placement. Stage II is collapse with hearing loss but no ossicular dysfunction, treated by tympanoplasty to reinforce the eardrum. Stage III is collapse with hearing loss and ossicular fixation/erosion, treated by tympanoplasty with ossicular reconstruction. Stage IV is acquired cholesteatoma. If an effusion is present, denote with an asterisk (e.g., severe collapse with effusion: Stage II*). This indicates possible ongoing deafness.

1.3.5 Cholesteatoma

Cholesteatoma has been classified as being congenital or acquired, with further subdivision of the latter into primary and secondary acquired cholesteatoma. Nevertheless, Black and Gutteridge have proposed a modern system to replace these classic designations, with new practical groupings of attic, pars tensa, and combined type cholesteatomas.[39] This modern classification is essentially a further sub-classification of cases that fall into Stage 4 of the above-described tympanic membrane collapse classification. Each of these groups may then be further graded according to involvement of the mesotympanum, attic, aditus, and mastoid/antrum.

Acquired cholesteatoma typically originates from the pars flaccida (attic subtype) or posterior pars tensa (pars tensa subtype). In the former situation, a sac typically forms in the lateral epitympanic (Prussak's) space lateral to the malleus that expands and erodes some of the canal wall bone (scutum). With expansion, these most commonly exit the epitympanum by passing into the mesotympanum, via an inferior route, or into the mastoid, via a posterior route through the aditus ad antrum by taking an approach that passes lateral to the body of the incus. In contrast, pars tensa cholesteatoma usually arises from posterior retraction of the pars tensa into the mesotympanum, with early involvement of the oval window and posterior mesotympanic structures, such as the sinus tympani and facial recess. Extension of pars tensa cholesteatoma into the epitympanum typically takes a route medial to the incus that passes over the tympanic segment of the facial nerve. In contrast to most cases of acquired cholesteatoma, which are generally attributed to a tympanic membrane retraction pocket, some pars tensa cholesteatomas can be caused by direct epithelial ingrowth from the margin of a perforation (often retracted) into the middle ear cleft or undersurface of a perforation.

1.4 Conclusion

Chronic ear disease has plagued mankind for centuries, but dramatic advancements in surgical technology and our knowledge of pathophysiology have led to our modern understanding and management. Classification schemes endeavor to organize our descriptions and comprehension of what is a heterogeneous conglomeration of related entities that comprise what is commonly known by otologic surgeons as the chronic ear.

References

[1] Cawthorne T. The surgery of the temporal bone. Ann R Coll Surg Engl. 1953;12(6):403–423.

[2] Sunder S, Jackler RK, Blevins NH. Virtuosity with the Mallet and Gouge: the brilliant triumph of the "modern" mastoid operation. Otolaryngol Clin North Am. 2006;39(6):1191–1210.

[3] Milstein S. The history of mastoid surgery. Am J Otol. 1980;1(3):174–178.

[4] Mollison WM. A brief survey of the history of the mastoid operation. Proc R Soc Med. 1930;23(3):381–385.

[5] Briggs RJ, Luxford WM. Chronic ear surgery: A historical review. Am J Otol. 1994;15(4):558–567.

[6] Soldati D, Mudry A. Knowledge about cholesteatoma, from the first description to the modern histopathology. Otol Neurotol. 2001;22(6):723–730.

[7] Berrettini S, Ravecca F, de Vito A, Forli F, Valori S, Franceschini SS. Modified Bondy radical mastoidectomy: long-term personal experience. J Laryngol Otol. 2004;118(5):333–337.

[8] Sanna M, Facharzt AA, Russo A, Lauda L, Pasanisi E, Bacciu A. Modified Bondy's technique: refinements of the surgical technique and long-term results. Otol Neurotol. 2009;30(1):64–69.

[9] Morris MS, Mitchell CC, Snell SW, Sperling N. Contemporary skin grafting in otologic surgery. Ear Nose Throat J. 1992;71(12):652–654.

[10] Guilford FR, Wright WK, Draper WL. Controlled healing of mastoid and fenestration cavities. Trans Am Acad Ophthalmol Otolaryngol. 1958;62(3):455–466.

[11] Jansen C. The combined approach for tympanoplasty (report on 10 years' experience). J Laryngol Otol. 1968;82(9):779–793.

[12] Sheehy JL, Patterson ME. Intact canal wall tympanoplasty with mastoidectomy. A review of eight years' experience. Laryngoscope. 1967;77(8):1502–1542.

[13] Jako GJ. The posterior route to the middle ear: Posterior tympanotomy. Laryngoscope. 1967;77(3):306–316.

[14] Jansen C. Combined approach tympanoplasty in cholesteatoma surgery. In: Sade J. Cholesteatoma and Mastoid Surgery: Proceedings of the Second Interenational Conference. Amsterdam, Netherlands: Kugler Publications; 1982:455–459.
[15] Sadé J. Treatment of cholesteatoma. Am J Otol. 1987;8(6):524–533.
[16] Smyth GD. Surgical treatment of cholesteatoma: the role of staging in closed operations. Ann Otol Rhinol Laryngol. 1988;97(6 Pt 1):667–669.
[17] Tabb HG. The surgical management of chronic ear disease, with special reference to staged surgery. Laryngoscope. 1963;73:363–383.
[18] Hicks JN. Techniques in incus transposition and replacement. Laryngoscope. 1976;86(2):222–223.
[19] Janeke JB, Shea JJ. Self-stabilizing proplast total ossicular replacement prosthesis in tympanoplasty. Laryngoscope. 1975;85(9):1550–1556.
[20] Brackmann DE, Sheehy JL, Luxford WM. TORPs and PORPs in tympanoplasty: a review of 1042 operations. Otolaryngol Head Neck Surg. 1984;92(1):32–37.
[21] Marchioni D, Mattioli F, Alicandri-Ciufelli M, Presutti L. Transcanal endoscopic approach to the sinus tympani: A clinical report. Otol Neurotol. 2009;30(6):758–765.
[22] Jindal M, Riskalla A, Jiang D, Connor S, O'Connor AF. A systematic review of diffusion-weighted magnetic resonance imaging in the assessment of postoperative cholesteatoma. Otol Neurotol. 2011;32(8):1243–1249.
[23] Fliss DM, Dagan R, Houri Z, Leiberman A. Medical management of chronic suppurative otitis media without cholesteatoma in children. J Pediatr. 1990;116(6):991–996.
[24] Bluestone CD. Pathogenesis of otitis media: role of Eustachian tube. Pediatr Infect Dis J. 1996;15(4):281–291.
[25] Acuin J. Chronic Suppurative Otitis Media. Burden of Illness and Management Options. Geneva: World Health Organization, 2004.
[26] Bluestone CD. Epidemiology and pathogenesis of chronic suppurative otitis media: implications for prevention and treatment. Int J Pediatr Otorhinolaryngol. 1998;42(3):207–223.
[27] Harker LA. Cholesteatoma: an incidence study. In: McCabe B.F., Sade J., Abramson M. Cholesteatoma: First International Conference. Birmingham, AL: Aesculapius; 1977:264–267.
[28] Stewart IA, Byrne W. Letter: Discharing ears in Melanesian children.[Letter] N Z Med J. 1976;83(562):287.
[29] Bluestone CD. Definitions, terminology, and classification. In: Rosenfeld R.M., Bluestone C.D. Evidence-Based Otitis Media. 2nd ed. Hamilton, Ontario: BC Decker; 2003:120–135.
[30] Bellucci RJ. Selection of cases and classification of tympanoplasty. Otolaryngol Clin North Am. 1989;22(5):911–926.
[31] Austin DF. Reporting results in tympanoplasty. Am J Otol. 1985;6(1):85–88.
[32] Kartush JM. Ossicular chain reconstruction. Capitulum to malleus. Otolaryngol Clin North Am. 1994;27(4):689–715.
[33] Black B. Ossiculoplasty prognosis: the spite method of assessment. Am J Otol. 1992;13(6):544–551.
[34] Dornhoffer JL, Gardner E. Prognostic factors in ossiculoplasty: A statistical staging system. Otol Neurotol. 2001;22(3):299–304.
[35] Sadé J, Berco E. Atelectasis and secretory otitis media. Ann Otol Rhinol Laryngol. 1976;85(2) Suppl 25 Pt 2:66–72.
[36] Tos M, Poulsen G. Attic retractions following secretory otitis. Acta Otolaryngol. 1980;89(5–6):479–486.
[37] Borgstein J, Gerritsma T, Bruce I, Feenstra L. Atelectasis of the middle ear in pediatric patients: safety of surgical intervention. Int J Pediatr Otorhinolaryngol. 2009;73(2):257–261.
[38] Black B. The collapsed pars tensa: surgical classification and management. In: Magnan J, Chays A, eds. Proceedings of the Sixth International Conference on Cholesteatoma and Ear Surgery. Marseille: Label Production, 2001:267–278.
[39] Black B, Gutteridge I. Acquired cholesteatoma: Classification and outcomes. Otol Neurotol. 2011;32(6):992–995.

2 Eustachian Tube Dysfunction, Mucosal Gas Exchange, and Effusion

Holger H. Sudhoff

Abbreviations used in this chapter:

BET: balloon Eustachian tuboplasty
CT: computed tomography
ETD: Eustachian tube dysfunction
LPR: laryngopharyngeal reflux
MRI: magnetic resonance imaging
TMJ: temporomandibular joint
TMM: tubomanometry

2.1 Eustachian Tube Normal Physiology

The Eustachian tube is part of a structure comprising the nose, palate, nasopharynx, and middle ear spaces.[1] This includes the tympanic cavity, which contains the bony Eustachian tube and the mastoid cells system (▶ Fig. 2.1). The tympanic cavity and mastoid cells are connected via the Eustachian tube and permit gas and pressure exchanges. The Eustachian tube is a complex organ consisting of a dynamic canal with its mucosa, cartilage, surrounding soft tissue, peritubal muscles, superior bony support, and the sphenoid sulcus.

Clinical experience as well as numerous patient studies and animal models show that the Eustachian tube plays a significant role in various middle ear pathologies.[2,3,4] The understanding of its mechanical properties has improved significantly over the last years; however, there are still uncertainties due to its complex anatomy, various functions, and the impact of intrinsic and external factors (▶ Fig. 2.2).[5,6] Intermittent transitory tubal dilation is probably the major mechanism for equilibration of middle ear cleft pressure with the ambient atmospheric pressure.[7] Barometric and chemical receptors within the middle ear cleft are assumed to provide autonomic nervous system feedback that impact the frequency of involuntary tubal openings.[8,9]

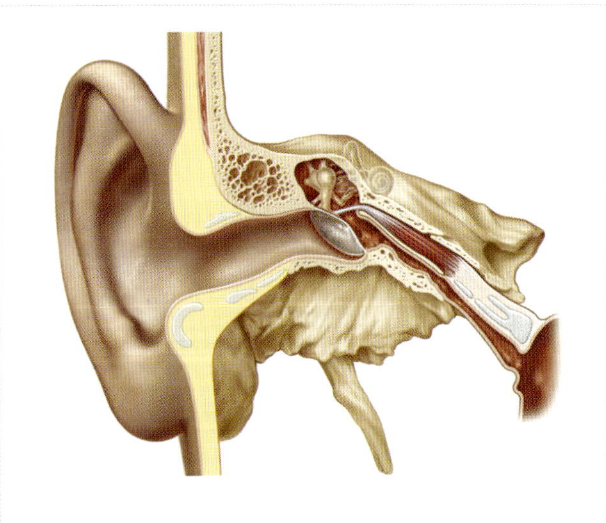

Fig. 2.1 Drawing of the cartilaginous and bony portions of the Eustachian tube and middle ear spaces.

Recently, McDonald and coworkers showed that the Eustachian tube may have a sequential peristaltic-like mechanism.[10] The proximal one-third of the tubal length is a bony funnel-shaped extension of the middle ear, which becomes narrowest at the isthmus region. The distal two-thirds of the tubal length is the pharyngeal portion, which is composed of cartilage. The cartilaginous portion is attached to peritubal muscles capable of a broad range of dynamic movements. Tubal dilation starts with the action of the levator veli palatine muscle to medially rotate the cartilaginous portion, primarily its mobile distal half of the medial cartilaginous lamina.[9] Tensor veli palatine muscle contraction follows, causing the resting convexity of the anterolateral wall to become concave as the concluding step to transiently opening the lumen.[10,11,12]

Currently, the surgical interventions available for chronic obstructive Eustachian tube dysfunction (ETD) have been expanded to include balloon Eustachian tuboplasty (BET), laser tuboplasty, and microdebrider tuboplasty, but long-term results still have to be established.[11,12,13,14,15,16,17]

2.2 Eustachian Tube Dysfunction

Eustachian tube dysfunction (ETD) can lead to clinical symptoms, such as aural fullness, impaired pressure equilibration, altered middle ear aeration, hearing loss, and autophony. Because the most common cause of obstructive dysfunction is mucosal inflammation within the cartilaginous Eustachian tube, patients should be questioned about inflammatory processes, such as allergic rhinitis, chronic rhinosinusitis, laryngopharyngeal reflux (LPR), and smoke exposure.[18,19] Pediatric ETD may be caused by adenoid tissue and mucosa swelling due to acute or chronic upper respiratory tract infections. Cleft palate, granulomatous disease, cystic fibrosis, Sampter's triad, or Kartagener's syndrome are facilitating factors. Eustachian tube dysfunction may be a contributing factor to vertigo.[1,20,21] It is important to distinguish ETD from other causes of aural fullness, such as a patulous Eustachian tube, temporomandibular joint (TMJ) disorders, superior semicircular canal dehiscence syndrome, Meniere's disease, and increased intracranial pressure.

Eustachian tube dysfunction is estimated to be present in about 1% of the general population.[22] Nearly 40% of all children up to the age of 10 years develop a temporary ETD.[23,24,25,26] Studies accessing pediatric and adult patient cohorts demonstrate that ETD is detectable in up to 70% of patients undergoing middle ear surgery.[25] Eustachian tube function is believed to be

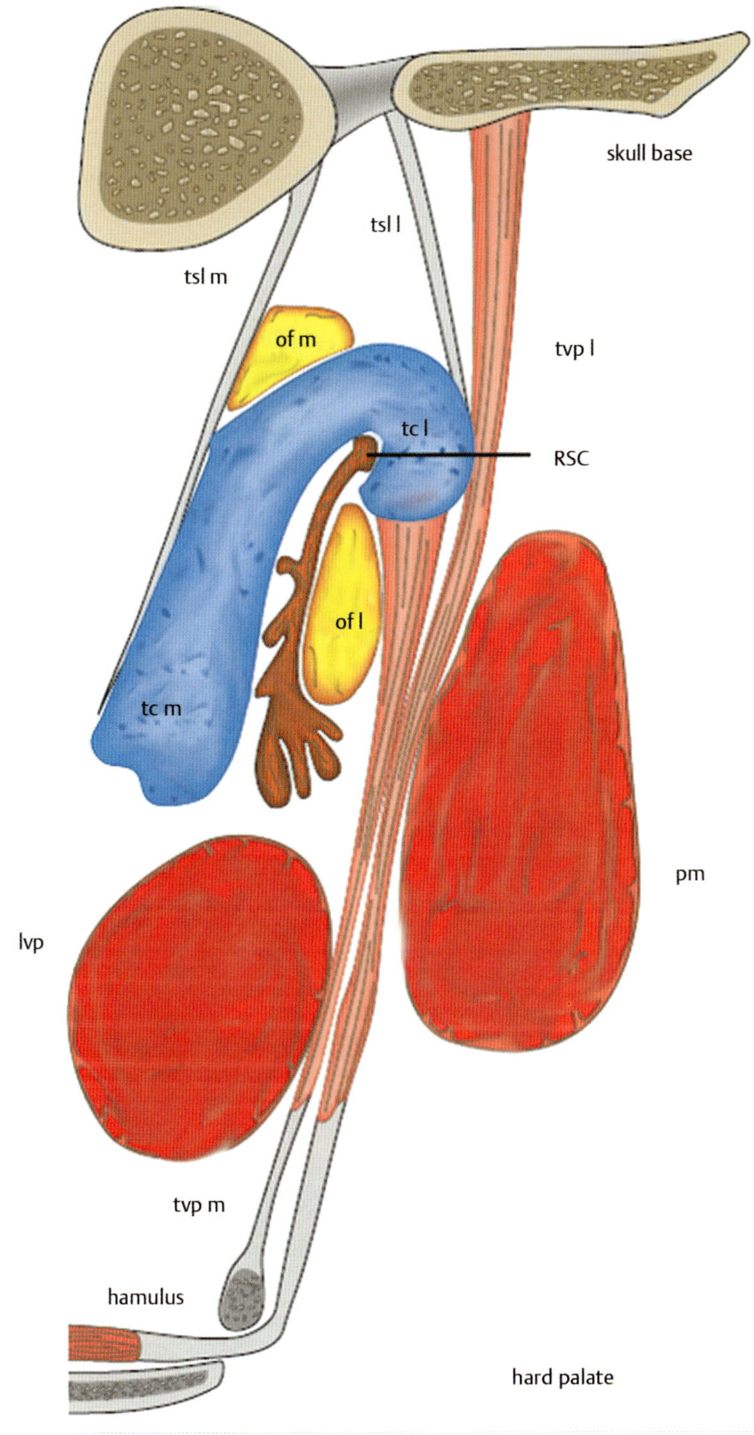

Fig. 2.2 Frontal view of the most important anatomic structures of the Eustachian tube.
tvp m, tensor velipalatini muscle, medial lamina
tvp l, tensor veli palatini muscle, lateral lamina
lvp, levator veli palatini muscle
pm, medial pterygoid muscle
tc l, tubal cartilage, lateral lamina
tc m, tubal cartilage, medial lamina
of l, lateral Ostmann's fat pad
of m, medial Ostmann's fat pad
RSC, Rüdinger's safety canal
tsl m, medial tubal suspensory ligament
tsl l, lateral tubal suspensory ligament

strongly related to the outcome of middle ear surgery.[25,26] Patients with a patulous Eustachian tube usually present with positional autophony, with autophony of both voice and breathing sounds, aural fullness, and, less commonly, otalgia.[27] The precise distinction between both forms of ETD (obstructive and patulous) is pivotal for an appropriate medical or surgical treatment. Patients with patulous Eustachian tubes may benefit from augmentation or reconstructive procedures.[27,28]

2.3 Eustachian Tube Assessment

A large number of methods have been employed to assess Eustachian tube function. More than 40 methods can be found in the literature.[29] None of these are proven to give detailed insights into all aspects of Eustachian tube physiology and pathology.[30] Clinical tests, such as otoscopy, nasal endosocopy, the Politzer test, the Valsalva maneuver, and the Toynbee maneuver, may give an initial assessment. Manometric tests, such as

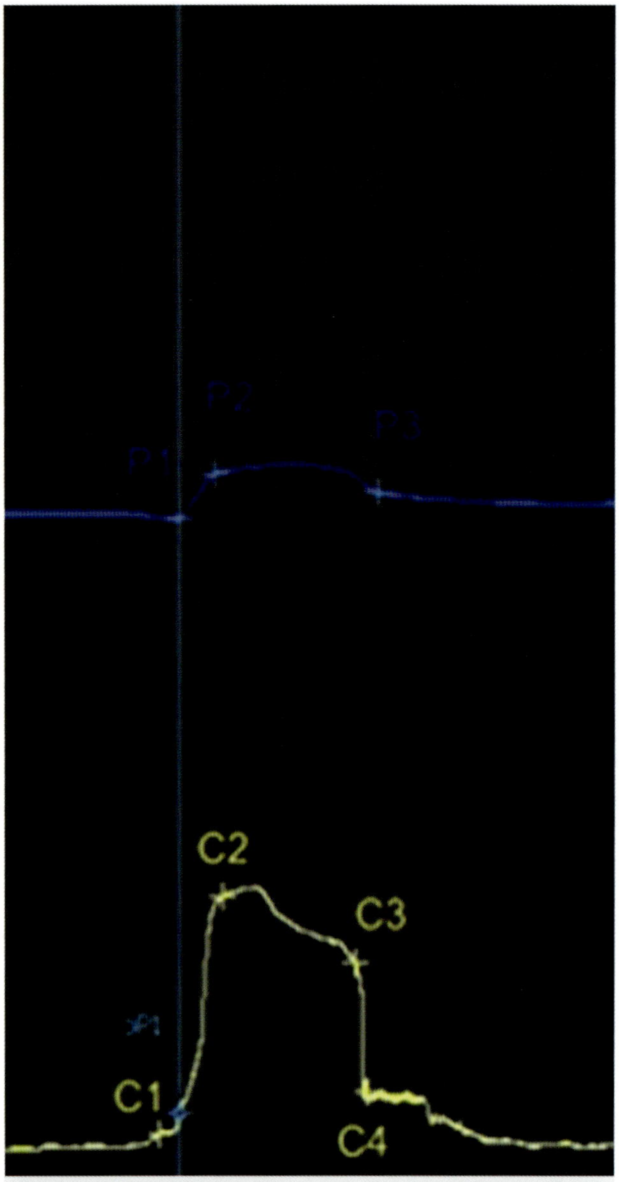

Fig. 2.3 Eustachian tube measurement by tubomanometry. The upper line represents the pressure in the nasopharynx, the lower line the pressure in the external ear canal.

tympanometry, reflex decay tympanometry, nine-step inflation-deflation test, modified inflation-deflation test, forced response test, and tubomanometry (TMM), are applicable diagnostic tests.[3,31,32]

TMM was described by Estève in 2001[33,34] and is a tool to measure the opening of the Eustachian tube and the transportation of gas into the middle ear by registering pressure changes (▶ Fig. 2.3). These are recorded by a pressure sensor in the occluded outer ear after applying the stimulus of a controlled gas bolus into the nasopharynx during swallowing. If tube opening is registered, the time of opening in relation to pressure applied can be measured (opening latency index or R). An R value of < 1 indicates early opening of the Eustachian tube, which is considered optimal.[32] The pressure chamber is an ideal device for simulating all possible situations regarding Eustachian tube function, regardless of an intact or defective ear drum.

Acoustic testing employing sonotubometry applies sound via a probe in the nose. At the same time, the changes of sound intensity during tube opening are recorded in the external ear canal. There are numerous other approaches to assess Eustachian tube function, such as phototubometry, scintigraphy, ultrasound, application of dye and taste-bearing substances, electromyography, flowmetry, and (opto)tensometry.[29,30] However, none of these methods has shown clinical significance.[30] Imaging using computed tomography (CT), cone beam tomography, and magnetic resonance imaging (MRI) have long been established to assess anatomic and functional deficiencies as well as to rule out pathology in the nasopharynx or superior canal dehiscence syndrome.[4,19,35,36]

2.4 Middle Ear and Mastoid Gas Exchange

The middle ear space and mastoid exchange gases with four different components: (1) the inner ear via the round window membrane; (2) the ambient atmospheric pressure via the tympanic membrane; (3) the resident blood via the middle ear mucosa; and (4) the nasopharynx via the Eustachian tube.[37,38] Gas exchange across pathways 1 to 3 is a passive, partial-pressure, gradient-driven, diffusion-based exchange process (▶ Fig. 2.4). The gas exchange via the Eustachian tube (pathway

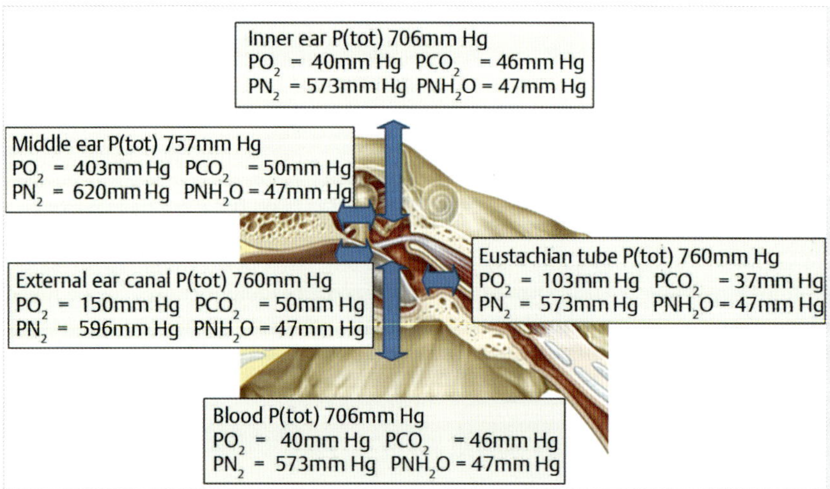

Fig. 2.4 Partial pressures (mm Hg) of the physiological gases for the middle ear spaces and surrounding structures.
Data are taken from Hergils L, Magnuson B. Regulation of negative middle ear pressure without tubal opening. Arch Otolaryngol Head Neck Surg 1988;114:1442–1444.

4) is an active, total-pressure, gradient-driven bolus exchange of mixed gases in the air phase.

The components that are present in the middle ear cleft are identical to those found in the blood and in the atmosphere: oxygen (O_2), carbon dioxide (CO_2), nitrogen (N_2), argon (Ar), and water (H_2O). Their relative quantities are expressed by their partial pressure P(x). Nitrogen is inert at the level of the middle ear cleft. The P(O_2) in the middle ear cleft is slightly lower and the P(CO_2) is slightly higher compared with venous blood. This hints at a modest consumption of O_2 and production of CO_2 within the middle ear cleft. Oxygen and nitrogen are removed by a passive, partial-pressure, gradient-driven, diffusive exchange via the mucosa into the blood compartment. Carbon dioxide and water vapor are diffused passively from the blood compartment, via the mucosa, into the middle ear cleft. The steady exchange of gas through the mucosa depends on the functional properties of the cells of the mucosal lining, the constant specific diffusion rate of the gas, and the underlying vascular system. The main purpose of the mucosa is to facilitate gas exchange between the middle ear cleft and the blood compartment.

Sound transmission via the ossicular chain requires a stable air compartment within the middle ear spaces. This means that the intra-middle ear cleft pressure must be equivalent to the atmospheric pressure (760 mm Hg). In ambient air, this equivalent value is obtained by calculating the sum of the partial pressures of the four main constitutive components in the air: O_2 (158 mm Hg), CO_2 (0.3 mm Hg), N_2 (596 mm Hg), and water vapor (5.7 mm Hg).[38] However, in the middle ear cleft, the composition of gas varies for two main reasons.[37] First, the middle ear cleft is a closed cavity that is connected with the nasal cavities by the Eustachian tube, and the gas in the nasopharynx consists of exhaled gas that contains less O_2 and more CO_2 compared with ambient air. The composition of gas in the middle ear cleft also varies because gas diffusion occurs between the middle ear spaces and the arterial and venous blood, via the mucosa. Arterial blood oxygen tension is approximately 93 mm Hg, whereas venous CO_2 tension is 44 mm Hg. The composition of gas tension in the middle ear cleft differs from that in the ambient air. The gradient from middle ear spaces to the capillaries is 57 mm Hg for O_2, and the gradient from the capillaries to the middle ear spaces is 39 mm Hg for CO_2.

Despite the differences in gas composition, the pressure in the middle ear spaces approximates the atmospheric pressure to enable optimal sound transmission. This is due to the sum of the partial pressures of O_2 and CO_2 being lower in the middle ear cleft (90 mm Hg) than in ambient air (150 mm Hg); N_2 exerts the higher partial pressure in the middle ear spaces (623 mm) because of its very slow diffusion to the capillaries. The composition of the exhaled gas that enters the middle ear spaces via the Eustachian tube contains less O_2 and more CO_2 compared with the ambient air. This reduces the passive diffusion of these gases through the mucosa. The blood flow through the middle ear mucosa is probably small. This limits the importance of gas diffusion and enables the P(O_2) and P(CO_2) to nearly equalize, due to their high diffusion rate. The same mechanism applies to water vapor.[39]

2.5 Middle Ear/Mastoid Volume Relative to Pressure Change

The behavior of the vascular system plays an important regulatory role in the physiologic balance of pressure variations in the middle ear spaces. Variations in the middle ear mucosa blood flow, associated with variations in the permeability of the vessels, allow ample adaptation to normal gas pressure fluctuations.[39,40,41,42] The normal extensive variations observed in middle ear cleft pressure over a 24-hour period, that appear regularly, are related to the vascular adaptations required by body position and sleep. The mastoid gas cell system constitutes the most important volume of the middle ear spaces and, therefore, represents the major part of the middle ear cleft mucosal area available for vascular gas exchange.[43]

The amount of gas present in the mastoid is important for regulating middle ear cleft pressure for two reasons. First, the physical, anatomical properties of mastoid volume affect compliance: the greater the volume, the more compliant the system. Second, the surface area affects mucosal gas exchanges. Both are important in the regulation of middle ear cleft pressure. The gas contained in the mastoid gas cells system acts as a physiological passive pressure buffer.[44]

The size of the mastoid gas cells system may vary between individuals to a great extent.[42] The genetic determination of growth, due to the time-dependent activation of morphogenetic genes and environmental factors, plays a pivotal role in the middle ear and mastoid volume. There is consent that a small mastoid gas cell system has an impact on future pathological predisposition. The smaller the system, the faster are the deviations from normal pressures. However, determining the volume of the mastoid to predict its pathological impact has no clinical significance. Under regular conditions, provided with healthy mucosa, a small adult mastoid is normal insofar as it constitutes the complete outcome of normal and standard development, that is, the individual simply possesses the morphological particularity of being "small."

A small mastoid in an adult is normal in that it is sufficient for the physiological balance of pressure variations in the middle ear spaces. The small mastoid is no more prone to develop middle ear pathology than is a mastoid of regular size. However, when the mucosa undergoes inflammatory processes, a small mastoid in an adult is much more likely to give rise to middle ear/mastoid pathology. Cinamon and Sadé studied how the aerated spaces of the middle ear and mastoid as well as the mobility of the tympanic membrane are capable of diminishing physiologic pressure changes that occur regularly in the middle ear spaces.[45] The mastoid air volume "dilutes" pressure changes relative to its size: the volume change required to alter a given pressure in an average (6-mL) mastoid is 6-fold that which is needed in a small (1-mL) mastoid. They found that it is the middle ear with a small mastoid that is most vulnerable to pressure changes and that may develop compensatory buffering mechanisms, such as additional tympanic membrane retraction or middle ear volume reduction by fluid accumulation.

Regarding the correlation between the gas exchange mechanism in the middle ear and the development of pathology in this area (otitis media with effusion and cholesteatoma),[44,46,47] Miura and coworkers described the influence of gas exchange function through the middle ear mucosa in the development of sniff-induced middle ear diseases.[48] Their findings suggested that impairment of gas exchange function through the middle ear mucosa, as well as ETD, might be closely related to the development of sniff-induced middle ear diseases.

2.6 Pathophysiology of Developing Negative Middle Ear Pressure and Effusion

An accentuated negative pressure created in the middle ear leads to the formation of an inflammatory exudate in the tympanic cavity and to impaired hearing. Moreover, the continued episodes of negative pressure are responsible for the formation of retraction pockets, atelectasis, and cholesteatoma formation.[38]

The next step in the sequence of events leading to otitis media is the development of middle ear effusion owing to the presence of lower pressures in the middle ear spaces; various mechanisms causing these pressures are discussed above. In 1878, Adam Politzer postulated that middle ear negative pressure can cause transudation of fluid from the middle ear mucosa into the cavity of the middle ear.[49] Since his time, subsequent observations and studies in humans and animals have provided evidence to support his hydrops *ex vacuo* theory.[1,3,44]

Traditionally, the formation of chronic negative middle ear pressure has been assumed to be due to a long-term imbalance between two main pressure regulators: the Eustachian tube function and the gas diffusion through the middle ear mucosa of the tympanic cavity. This was usually conceptualized by the relationship between baseline constant net gas absorption from the middle ear air into the mucosal blood, which then becomes pathologic if insufficiently counterbalanced by Eustachian tube–related pressure regulation. Nevertheless, more recent studies reveal that the perturbation of the mucosal gas exchange, not Eustachian tube function, may act as another cause for diminished middle ear pressure.[50]

At very low negative pressures, based on large hydrostatic pressure, a transudate can be forced to effuse from the blood vessels into the middle ear cavity. Basically, the impermeable basal membrane of the blood vessels allows fluid effusion. In addition, other complementary causes have been identified. Clinical practice has found that a diseased mastoid with sclerotic changes and decreased pneumatization has been correlated with cases of chronic otitis media and sequelae related to middle ear negative pressure. Another example of how middle ear negative pressure can cause transudation of an effusion was shown by Ingelstedt and co-workers in which they aspirated the middle ear and mastoid with a syringe in aviators and produced middle ear effusion.[51] This finding suggests an important role of the mastoid in the overall regulation of the middle ear pressure.[38,52]

2.7 The Nature of Various Subtypes of Effusion (Serous, Mucoid, Purulent)

Otitis media with effusion is one of the most prevalent childhood diseases. The consistency of the effusions can vary from watery to mucoid, the latter having a high viscosity. Many investigators have tried to determine how the secretion is generated.[53,54,55,56] The absorption of water and concentration of effusion are believed to be the cause of turning a serous fluid into a viscous fluid. Chemical analysis of middle ear effusions has shown a large quantity of mucin and higher levels of serous secretions, such as lysozyme and secretory immunoglobulin A, than in the serum. These results indicate that middle ear effusions are composed not only of transudate, but also of an exudate that is actively secreted from the middle ear mucosa.

Histological studies have also demonstrated the presence of hyperplastic secretory middle ear mucosa with a predominance of goblet cells in the setting of otitis media with effusion.[54] In addition, several inflammatory cytokines are present in the middle ear effusions; IL-6 and adhesion molecules, such as intercellular adhesion molecule-1, have been recently identified in the middle ear mucosa.[55] These findings support the belief that inflammation is closely involved in the development of chronic otitis media with effusion. All clinically distinguishable categories of otitis media with effusion (serous, mucoid, or purulent) probably represent different stages in a continuum of events,[56] with a degree of variability also based on the nature of any other underlying pathologic processes impacting the middle ear (allergy, infection, systemic inflammatory conditions).

2.8 Patterns of Middle Ear Ventilation, Selective Epitympanic Dysventilation

A selective epitympanic dysventilation syndrome was hypothesized by Marchioni and coworkers in 2010.[57] A normal Eustachian tube function appeared to be insufficient for complete ventilation of the middle ear, and an open tympanic isthmus or an incomplete tensor fold was necessary for epitympanic recess ventilation. The selective epitympanic dysventilation syndrome is supposed to consist of the contemporary presence of the following four conditions: attic retraction pocket or cholesteatoma, normal tubal function tests, complete epitympanic diaphragm, and isthmus blockage.[58]

2.9 Conclusion

Sound transmission necessitates a stable air compartment within the middle ear spaces maintained by a sufficient Eustachian tube function. In fact, functional impairment of the Eustachian tube plays a significant role in various middle ear pathologies. Despite a number of methods to assess Eustachian tube function, none provides detailed insights into all aspects of Eustachian tube physiology and pathology. Recent data reveals that not only Eustachian tube function, but also the perturbation of the mucosal gas exchange, may act as another cause for diminished middle ear pressure. At very low negative pressures, a transudate can be established in the middle ear cavity. The functional blockage of ventilation could be additionally selective within the epitympanic space. Eustachian tube physiology still exhibits uncertainties due to its complex anatomy, various functions, and the impact of intrinsic and external factors.

References

[1] Bluestone CD, Klein JO. Otitis media, atelectasis, and Eustachian tube dysfunction. In: Bluestone CD, Stool SE, Kenna MA, eds. Pediatric Otolaryngology, 3rd ed. Philadelphia: WB Saunders, 1996.

[2] Leuwer R, Koch U. [Anatomy and physiology of the auditory tube. Therapeutic possibilities in chronic disorders of tubal function] HNO. 1999;47(5):514–523.

[3] Bluestone CD. Introduction. In: Bluestone MB, editor. Eustachian tube: structure, function, role in otitis media. Hamilton, Ontario; Lewiston, New York: BC Decker; 2005. pp. 1–9.

[4] Sudhoff H. Eustachian Tube Dysfunction. Uni-Med Verlag Bremen, London, Boston: UNI-MED, 2013.

[5] Seibert JW, Danner CJ. Eustachian tube function and the middle ear. Otolaryngol Clin North Am. 2006;39(6):1221–1235.

[6] Pau HW. Eustachian tube and middle ear mechanics. Acta Otolaryngol. 2011;131:1279–1285.

[7] Sadé J, Luntz M, Levy D. Middle ear gas composition and middle ear aeration. Ann Otol Rhinol Laryngol. 1995;104(5):369–373.

[8] Eden AR, Gannon PJ. Neural control of middle ear aeration. Arch Otolaryngol Head Neck Surg. 1987;113(2):133–137.

[9] Rockley TJ, Hawke WM. The middle ear as a baroreceptor. Acta Otolaryngol. 1992;112(5):816–823.

[10] McDonald MH, Hoffman MR, Gentry LR, Jiang JJ. New insights into mechanism of Eustachian tube ventilation based on cine computed tomography images. Eur Arch Otorhinolaryngol. 2012;269(8):1901–1907.

[11] Ockermann T, Reineke U, Upile T, Ebmeyer J, Sudhoff HH. Balloon dilation eustachian tuboplasty: A feasibility study. Otol Neurotol. 2010;31(7):1100–1103.

[12] Ockermann T, Reineke U, Upile T, Ebmeyer J, Sudhoff H. Balloon dilatation eustachian tuboplasty: a clinical study. Laryngoscope. 2010;120(7):1411–1416.

[13] Caffier PP, Sedlmaier B, Haupt H, Göktas O, Scherer H, Mazurek B. Impact of laser Eustachian tuboplasty on middle ear ventilation, hearing, and tinnitus in chronic tube dysfunction. Ear Hear. 2011;32(1):132–139.

[14] Poe DS, Grimmer JF, Metson R. Laser Eustachian tuboplasty: Two-year results. Laryngoscope. 2007;117(2):231–237.

[15] Kujawski OB, Poe DS. Laser Eustachian tuboplasty. Otol Neurotol. 2004;25(1):1–8.

[16] Poe DS, Silvola J, Pyykkö I. Balloon dilation of the cartilaginous Eustachian tube. Otolaryngol Head Neck Surg. 2011;144(4):563–569.

[17] Metson R, Pletcher SD, Poe DS. Microdebrider Eustachian tuboplasty: A preliminary report. Otolaryngol Head Neck Surg. 2007;136(3):422–427.

[18] Takahashi H, Honjo I, Fujita A. Endoscopic findings at the pharyngeal orifice of the eustachian tube in otitis media with effusion. Eur Arch Otorhinolaryngol. 1996;253(1–2):42–44.

[19] Poe DS, Gopen Q. Eustachian tube dysfunction. In: Snow JB, Wackym PA, Ballenger JJ, editors. Ballenger's otorhinolaryngology: head and neck surgery. Lewiston, New York: BC Decker; 2009. pp. 201–208.

[20] Gudziol V, Mann WJ. [Chronic eustachian tube dysfunction and its sequelae in adult patients with cleft lip and palate] HNO. 2006;54(9):684–688.

[21] Goldman JL, Martinez SA, Ganzel TM. Eustachian tube dysfunction and its sequelae in patients with cleft palate. South Med J. 1993;86(11):1236–1237.

[22] Browning GG, Gatehouse S. The prevalence of middle ear disease in the adult British population. Clin Otolaryngol Allied Sci. 1992;17(4):317–321.

[23] Mewes T, Mann W. [Function of the eustachian tube in epitympanic retraction pockets] HNO. 1998;46(11):914–918.

[24] Choi SH, Han JH, Chung JW. Pre-operative evaluation of eustachian tube function using a modified pressure equilibration test is predictive of good postoperative hearing and middle ear aeration in type 1 tympanoplasty patients. Clin Exp Otorhinolaryngol. 2009;2(2):61–65.

[25] Podoshin L, Fradis M, Malatskey S, Ben-David J. Tympanoplasty in adults: A five-year survey. Ear Nose Throat J. 1996;75(3):149–152, 155–156.

[26] Dörrie A, Dommerich S, Pau HW. [Early postoperative middle-ear ventilation – risk for the transplant or guarantee for aeration of the tympanic cavity?] Laryngorhinootologie. 2003;82(2):102–104.

[27] Poe DS. Diagnosis and management of the patulous eustachian tube. Otol Neurotol. 2007;28(5):668–677.

[28] Schröder S, Lehmann M, Sudhoff H, Ebmeyer J. [The patulous eustachian tube-novel surgical approaches] HNO. 2013;61(12):1017–1025.

[29] Martino E, Di Thaden R, Krombach GA, Westhofen M. [Function tests for the Eustachian tube. Current knowledge] HNO. 2004;52(11):1029–1039, quiz 1040.

[30] Todd NW. There are no accurate tests for Eustachian tube function. Arch Otolaryngol Head Neck Surg. 2000;126(8):1041–1042.

[31] Sudhoff H, Ockermann T, Mikolajczyk R, et al. [Clinical and experimental considerations for evaluation of Eustachian tube physiology] HNO. 2009;57(5):428–435.

[32] Poe DS, Pyykkö I. Measurements of Eustachian tube dilation by video endoscopy. Otol Neurotol. 2011;32(5):794–798.

[33] Esteve D, Dubreuil C, Della Vedova C, Normand B, Martin C. Evaluation par tubomanometrie de la fonction douverture tubaire et de la réponse tympanique chez le sujet normal et chez le sujet porteur dune otide séro-muqueuse chronique. J Fr ORL. 2001;50:223–232.

[34] Ars B, Dirckx JJ. Tubomanometry. Den Haag: Kugler, 2003.

[35] Abdel-Aziz T, Schröder S, Lehmann M, Gehl HB, Ebmeyer J, Sudhoff H. Computed tomography before balloon Eustachian tuboplasty—a true necessity? Otol Neurotol. 2014;35(4):635–638.

[36] Tisch M, Störrle P, Danz B, Maier H. [Role of imaging before Eustachian tube dilation using the Bielefeld balloon catheter] HNO. 2013;61(6):488–491.

[37] Ars B, Ars-Piret N. Middle ear pressure balance under normal conditions. Specific role of the middle ear structure. Acta Otorhinolaryngol Belg. 1994;48(4):339–342.

[38] Sadé J, Ar A. Middle ear and auditory tube: Middle ear clearance, gas exchange, and pressure regulation. Otolaryngol Head Neck Surg. 1997;116(4):499–524.

[39] Yuksel S, Swarts JD, Banks J, Seroky JT, Doyle WJ. In vivo measurement of O(2) and CO(2) gas exchange across the human tympanic membrane. Acta Otolaryngol. 2009;129(7):716–725.

[40] Doyle WJ. The mastoid as a functional rate-limiter of middle ear pressure change. Int J Pediatr Otorhinolaryngol. 2007;71(3):393–402.

[41] Ranade A, Lambertsen CJ, Noordergraaf A. Inert gas exchange in the middle ear. Acta Otolaryngol Suppl. 1980;371:1–23.

[42] Raveh E, Sadé J, Mover-Lev H, Guney S. Mastoid buffering properties: I. Gas partial pressures. Ann Otol Rhinol Laryngol. 1999;108(8):750–755.

[43] Alper CM, Kitsko DJ, Swarts JD, et al. Role of the mastoid in middle ear pressure regulation. Laryngoscope. 2011;121(2):404–408.

[44] Hergils L, Magnuson B. Regulation of negative middle ear pressure without tubal opening. Arch Otolaryngol Head Neck Surg. 1988;114(12):1442–1444.

[45] Cinamon U, Sadé J. Mastoid and tympanic membrane as pressure buffers: a quantitative study in a middle ear cleft model. Otol Neurotol. 2003;24(6):839–842.

[46] Iwano T, Doi T, Hosoda Y, Ushiro K, Yamashita T. Transmucosal pressure regulation in the middle ear cavity. Pract Otol (Kyoto). 1993;86:1265–1272.

[47] Bhutta MF, Williamson IG, Sudhoff HH. Cholesteatoma. BMJ. 2011;342:d1088.

[48] Miura M, Takahashi H, Honjo I, Hasebe S, Tanabe M. Influence of the gas exchange function through the middle ear mucosa on the development of sniff-induced middle ear diseases. Laryngoscope. 1998;108(5):683–686.

[49] Politzer A. Lehrbuch der Ohrenheilkunde für Practische Ärzte und Studierende. Verlag von Ferdinand Enke, Stuttgart, 1878.

[50] Uchimizu H. Effects of inflammatory changes in the middle ear mucosa on middle ear total pressure. Acta Otolaryngol. 2007;127(10):1031–1037.

[51] Andréasson L, Ingelstedt S, Ivarsson A, Jonson B, Tjernström O. Pressure-dependent variation in volume of mucosal lining of the middle ear. Acta Otolaryngol. 1976;81(5–6):442–449.

[52] Tos M, Stangerup SE. Mastoid pneumatization in secretory otitis. Further support for the environmental theory. Acta Otolaryngol. 1984;98(1–2):110–118.

[53] Chung MH, Choi JY, Lee WS, Kim HN, Yoon JH. Compositional difference in middle ear effusion: Mucous versus serous. Laryngoscope. 2002;112(1):152–155.

[54] Bendek GA. Histopathology of transudatory-secretory otitis media. Preliminary report. Arch Otolaryngol. 1963;78:33–38.

[55] Yellon RF, Leonard G, Marucha PT, et al. Characterization of cytokines present in middle ear effusions. Laryngoscope. 1991;101(2):165–169.

[56] Paparella MM, Schachern PA, Yoon TH, Abdelhammid MM, Sahni R, da Costa SS. Otopathologic correlates of the continuum of otitis media. Ann Otol Rhinol Laryngol Suppl. 1990;148:17–22.

[57] Marchioni D, Alicandri-Ciufelli M, Molteni G, Artioli FL, Genovese E, Presutti L. Selective epitympanic dysventilation syndrome. Laryngoscope. 2010;120(5):1028–1033.

[58] Marchioni D, Mattioli F, Alicandri-Ciufelli M, Presutti L. Prevalence of ventilation blockages in patients affected by attic pathology: A case-control study. Laryngoscope. 2013;123(11):2845–2853.

3 Tympanic Membrane Wound Healing and Epithelial Migration

Peter L. Santa Maria

Abbreviations used in this chapter:

EGF: epidermal growth factor
EGFR: epithelial growth factor receptor
FGF: fibroblast growth factor
KGF: keratinocyte growth factor
HUA: hyaluronic acid
HB-EGF: heparin-binding EGF-like growth factor
IGF: insulin-like growth factor
IL: interleukin
MDGF: macrophage-derived growth factor
MMP: matrix metalloproteinase
PDGF: platelet-derived growth factor
TGF: transforming growth factor

3.1 The Normal Tympanic Membrane

3.1.1 Tympanic Membrane Structure

The tympanic membrane is composed of two parts, the pars flaccida and the pars tensa. The layers of the pars tensa (external to internal) are as follows[1]: epidermal layer of keratinizing squamous epithelium, connective tissue layer, and a single layer of mucosal cells.[2] The epidermis is three to five cell layers thick and lacks skin appendages.[3] The connective tissue layer is well developed and includes two main layers of fibers, an outer radial layer and an inner circular layer. There is a very thin layer of oblique fibers running in between these two layers of fiber.[4] The mucosal layer of the tympanic membrane, composed of ciliated columnar epithelial cells, is continuous with that of the middle ear cavity.[5] The pars flaccida, by comparison, contains a higher proportion of elastic fibers, lacks the organized separate connective tissue layers of the pars tensa, and lacks cilia on its mucous membrane.[3]

3.1.2 The Migratory Epithelium of the Tympanic Membrane and External Ear Canal

In humans, the epidermis migrates centripetally from the umbo and then outward to the external meatus (▶ Fig. 3.1),[6,7] facilitating a self-cleaning mechanism for the ear canal.[3] This process was first described by Burnett (1877) and later confirmed by Stinson (1936), Litton (1963),[7] Alberti (1964),[6] and Franz (1966).[8] The epithelia migrate at an average of 70–131 microns per day[6,9] with some diurnal variation.[10] The epithelial progenitor cells of the tympanic membrane responsible for this migration are likely to be located at the umbo and along the malleus.[11,12] Progenitor cells in the annulus are more likely to have a role in repair. Migration occurs via a plane of separation between more superficial cells sliding over ones below. The presence of intercellular spaces, cytoplasmic processes, and smaller numbers of desmosomes (points of intercellular adhesion) in the stratum basale and stratum spinosum suggest that

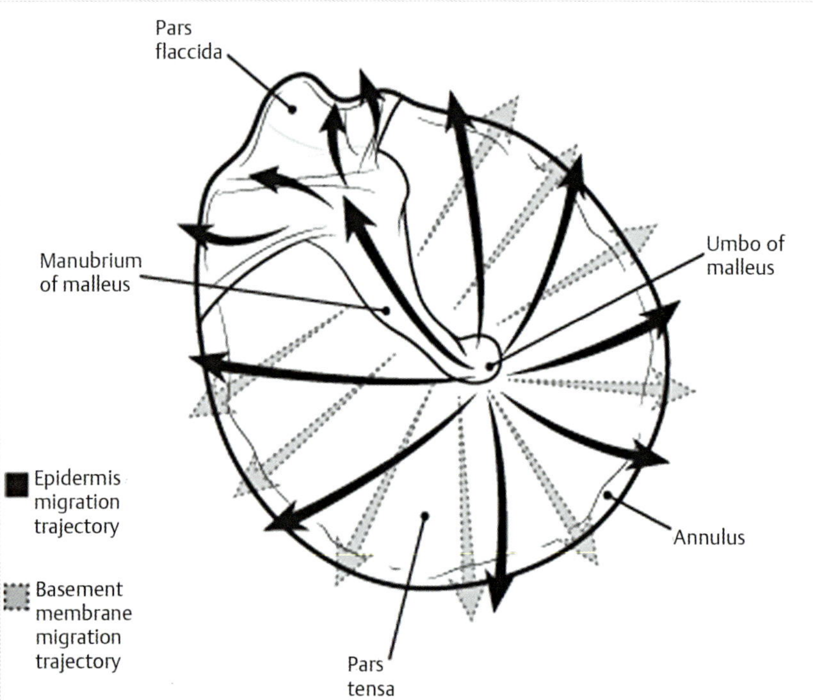

Fig. 3.1 The epithelial migration pattern of the tympanic membrane. The usual pattern of migration is marked in a solid line, with the alternate pathway seen in approximately 20% of subjects shown in broken lines. The migration pattern exactly at the umbo is directly up the handle of the malleus before fanning out radially.

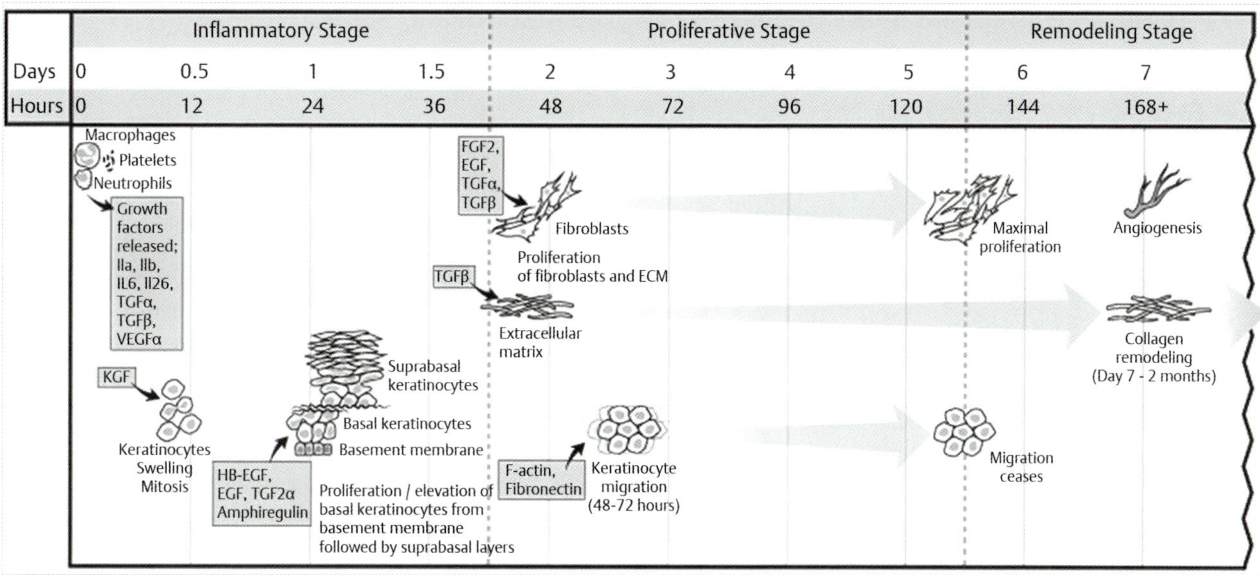

Fig. 3.2 Summary of the major events leading to perforation closure in the tympanic membrane. Wound healing in the tympanic membrane is divided into three stages, with keratinocyte migration beginning as early as 48 hours following perforation.

this is the plane in which migration occurs, along with movement on the basement membrane.[13,14] The speed of migration is relatively slower in the anterior and inferior quadrants.[15] Migration pathways spread outward from the tympanic membrane and out the external auditory canal to the bony cartilaginous junction, where desquamation occurs.[6]

Tympanic membrane migration can be affected by patient factors, including age, with children shown to have migration predominantly in a posterior-superior direction.[6] Animal studies show that older animals demonstrate slower migration.[16] In the presence of otitis media, the mitotic activity over the whole tympanic membrane increases.[17]

The migratory mechanisms are likely to involve a reduction in intercellular adhesion between layers of migratory cells.[18] The interaction between cell adhesion molecules is complex and includes selectins, desmocolin, F actin, fibronectin, integrin β-1, and cadherin-6.[19] Hemidesmosomes link keratin filaments of the basal layer to the underlying basement membrane and must be disassembled so that keratinocyte migration can occur.[20] The α3-β1 and α6-β4 integrins are important for maintaining the directional trajectory of cutaneous keratinocyte migration[21], and are likely to be important in tympanic membrane migration.

3.2 Tympanic Membrane Perforation

3.2.1 Etiology of Tympanic Membrane Perforation

Tympanic membrane perforations most commonly result from otitis media or trauma. Perforations associated with otitis media are typically small and usually heal spontaneously upon resolution of the infection. Ongoing infection may prevent a perforation from healing and is more common in developing countries, poor socioeconomic groups, and children.[22] During acute infection, the middle ear becomes full, with exudate putting pressure on the tympanic membrane, causing it to bulge outward. This pressure causes the central area to become ischemic and give way.[22] Traumatic causes include blunt injury, penetrating injury, barotrauma, and acoustic pressure (occurs between 195 dB and 199 dB at 30°C, with more sound pressure required at lower frequencies). Heat, corrosives, lightning, and water sports have the lowest incidence of spontaneous closure.[23]

3.2.2 Tympanic Membrane Wound Healing

The tympanic membrane is unique in that it is a structure suspended in air.[22] Repairing cells therefore have to bridge a gap. Unlike other wounds, there is no ready-made bed over which the cells can migrate[24] and no influx of reparative cells, nutrients, and fibroblasts as found in other epithelial healing.[25,26] Tympanic membrane perforations typically heal within 7–10 days.[27] The spontaneous healing rate of traumatic perforations is close to 80%.[23] Clinically, a perforation may be described as chronic when stable and present for 3 months. It can be divided into the following stages (▶ Fig. 3.2).[28]

The Inflammatory Stage (0–48 hours)

After acute injury, an acute inflammatory response occurs, with an exudate composed of interstitial fluid, lymph, and blood accumulating at the perforation margin. A crust layer forms, containing wound debris, providing a medium for the healing process. Within 12 hours the increased vascularity of the tympanic membrane can be observed along the handle of the malleus, the malleolar ligaments, and the annulus.[14] Mitotic activity can be demonstrated histologically 10–12 hours following perforation.[29,30]

The Proliferative Stage (48 hours to days 5–7)

Two days after perforation, the epithelium begins to migrate and the epithelia of the surrounding tympanic membrane becomes elevated from the connective tissue layer, with advancement of the wound edge beginning at 48–72 hours.[29,31,32,33] Perforation closure mainly occurs via proliferation of the epidermal layer from a distant origin, predominantly at the attachment of the tympanic membrane to the handle of malleus.[14,17] There is a small amount of local mitotic activity at the wound edge, but it occurs later in the process and is less intense.[22] Basal keratinocytes first spread and migrate, then proliferate, followed by migration of suprabasal keratinocytes.[25,34] Supporting granulation tissue beneath the proliferating squamous epithelium is a prerequisite for perforation closure. Without it, the epithelium shows only local hyperplasia and thickening without closure. The advancing keratinizing squamous epithelium occurs ahead of ingrowing connective tissue,[35] that is most pronounced on day 5, just prior to closure.[36] It is theorized that the rate of tympanic membrane closure is determined by the rate of advancement of the fibrous layer.[37]

Keratin was initially thought to act as a scaffold for the epithelium; however, it is not necessary for repair and is probably more a byproduct of the keratinocytes.[14] The mucosal cell layer could possibly provide a one cell-thick scaffold across the wound, with the other cells migrating over this.[38] The perforation is generally macroscopically closed by 5–7 days,[31] with pinpoint perforations often closing sooner than 4 days.[9,24] The final layer to migrate across the perforation, the connective tissue layer, may fail to migrate, leaving the perforation closed by two layers, not three (thin segment).[22]

The Remodeling Stage

After the perforation is closed macroscopically, the remodeling stage occurs, with the content of this area reducing over the next 7 days. The epithelium at this time is 3 or 4 times thicker than the uninjured tympanic membrane, taking approximately 2 months to return to a normal thickness.[30] The epithelium is of normal appearance, but the connective tissue layer is still thicker than normal, with a disorganized collagen framework and persistence of giant cells.[29,35] There is a macroscopically visible scar up to 6 months following perforation.

3.2.3 Pars Flaccida Healing

Perforations in the pars flaccida differ from the pars tensa in that they show greater exudation and bleeding. They show fibrous layer proliferation on the first day with no epithelial retraction. Epithelial proliferation is only seen around the perforation near the annulus, with none near the handle of the malleus.[39] Perforations in the pars tensa do not cause changes in the pars flaccida, whereas perforations in the pars flaccida cause epidermal hyperplasia in the pars tensa.[39]

3.2.4 Key Growth Factors in Tympanic Membrane Wound Healing

Immunohistochemical studies and microarray research have identified important growth factors in the healing of the tympanic membrane following perforation (▸ Table 3.1). Growth factors often require the presence of other growth factors, with little or no effect on their own.[19] Although the mechanisms are

Table 3.1 Expression of key growth factor RNA[a] as detected by microarray during tympanic membrane wound healing.

Growth factor	hours			day					
	12	24	36	2	3	4	5	6	7
KGF	↑↑	↓↓	↑	-	↑	↑	↑	↑↑	-
FGF2	↓	↓	↑	↑↑	-	-	-	-	-
HB-EGF	↑↑↑↑	↓	-	↑	-	-	↓	↑	-
EGF	↓	↓	↓	-	-	-	↑	↓	-
VEGFa	↑↑	-	-	-	-	-	-	-	-
TGFα	↑	↓	-	-	-	-	-	↓	↓
TGFβ	↑	↑	-	-	-	-	-	-	-
HA	↑	-	-	-	↑	↑	↑	↑	-
BMP6	↓↓	-	-	-	-	-	-	-	-
IL1a	↑↑	↓	↑	↑	↑	-	-	-	↑
IL1b	↑↑	-	-	↓	-	-	↑	↓	-
IL6	↑↑↑	↓	-	-	-	-	-	-	↓
IL24	↑↑↑↑	-	-	↓	-	-	-	-	↓

[a] Tympanic membrane wound healing relies on the expression of key growth factors with specific timing. Usually the gene expression precedes the detection by immunohistochemistry by 12–24 hours. Some growth factors, such as PDGF, do not significantly change their expression, but the receptor expression can change dramatically.

Data from Santa Maria PL, Redmond SL, McInnes RL, Atlas MD, Ghassemifar R. Tympanic membrane wound healing in rats assessed by transcriptome profiling. Laryngoscope. 2011;121(10):2199–2213. doi: 2110.1002/lary.22150. Epub 22011 Sep 22114.

multifactorial, the largest number of upregulated genes following injury are from the cystatin family, which are involved in epidermal development.[19]

During the inflammatory stage, growth factors, including platelet-derived growth factor (PDGF), epidermal growth factor (EGF), transforming growth factor (TGF)-β, and insulin-like growth factor (IGF)-1, are released from platelets; neutrophils then enter the wound, followed by macrophages.[40] These macrophages synthesize further growth factors, including TGF-β, TGF-α, macrophage-derived growth factor (MDGF), fibroblast growth factor (FGF)-2 (also known as basic FGF [bFGF]), and heparin-binding EGF-like growth factor (HB-EGF). These growth factors stimulate the migration of fibroblasts, epithelial cells, and vascular endothelium as the proliferative and repair phases begin. During these phases noninflammatory cells, such as keratinocytes (produce TGF-β, TGF-α, and keratinocyte-derived autocrine factor), fibroblasts (produce IGF-1, FGF-2, TGF-β, PDGF, and keratinocyte growth factor [KGF]), and endothelium (produce FGF-2 and PDGF), take over the synthesis of growth factors from the inflammatory cells. These growth factors are important for extracellular matrix formation and angiogenesis.[41,42]

A number of interleukins (ILs) are involved in the early stages of tympanic membrane wound healing, including IL-24, IL-19, IL-6, IL-1 β, IL-13r α, and IL-1 α. IL-6 in particular is important in initiating the healing process[19] via mitogenesis of wound-edge keratinocytes and is chemotactic for neutrophils.[32] Matrix metalloproteinases (MMPs) are enzymes that are able to break down elements of the extracellular matrix.[43] Both MMP-3 and MMP-12 are crucial for early tympanic membrane wound healing.[19]

Epidermal growth factor is mitogenic for epithelial and endothelial cells, fibroblasts, and keratinocytes. It is also chemotactic for epithelial cells and increases glycosaminoglycan production from fibroblasts.[44] Epidermal growth factor is detected in low levels in normal tympanic membranes, and, during healing, its detection corresponds to the times at which keratinocyte proliferation and migration occur.[33,45] TGF-α binds to EGF receptors and has essentially the same effects but may be more potent than EGF.[46,47] Its expression following perforation is similar to that of EGF.[48] Amphiregulin is also part of the EGF family and is one of the most upregulated growth factors in tympanic membrane wound healing.[19] Heparin-binding EGF-like growth factor is a relatively newly recognized factor in tympanic membrane wound healing.[45] It may be a key growth factor involved in keratinocyte migration as it has an emerging role in other areas of epidermal healing.[49]

Transforming growth factor-β exists in three isoforms (TGF-β 1, -β2, and -β3) and stimulates migration of inflammatory cells and fibroblasts, induces synthesis of extracellular matrix, inhibits proteases, can reversibly inhibit the division of keratinocytes, and has a role in coordinating vascularization and mesenchymal proliferation.[40,50] It induces proliferation of most cells but inhibits fibroblasts.[51]

The FGF family includes FGF-1 (acidic FGF), FGF-2 (basic FGF), FGF-10, and KGF (also called FGF-7), all of which are relevant to tympanic membrane healing.[52] Fibroblast growth factors stimulate the division and differentiation of cells, including keratinocytes, fibroblasts, vascular smooth muscle, vascular endothelium, and neurons. They also induce angiogenesis[40] and increase protease production, leading to matrix remodeling.[37] Although FGF-2 induces hyperplasia at epidermal proliferation centers, it does not increase proliferation at the perforation edge or affect epithelial cell migration.[22] Fibroblast growth factor-2 is not detectable in normal tympanic membranes.[33] Keratinocyte growth factor is mitogenic and chemotactic for epithelial cells (including keratinocytes), but not mesodermal cells (including fibroblasts). Keratinocyte growth factor promotes differentiation and organization of healing rather than rate of repair.[37]

Other factors thought to be important in tympanic membrane wound healing include hyaluronic acid (HA), fibronectin, and PDGF. Hyaluronic acid increases in quantity until the perforation heals.[53] Fibronectin is important for cell attachment and adhesion, facilitates cell migration, and is present at all stages of healing.[22] Platelet-derived growth factor increases the proliferation of fibroblasts, increasing the production of fibronectin and HA and initiating collagen production from fibroblasts.[54]

3.3 Factors Affecting Tympanic Membrane Wound Healing

3.3.1 Role of Perforation Size and Location

Most studies suggest neither the location of a perforation nor its size correlates to its chance of healing.[39] Greater perforation size probably leads to longer healing time, but research in this area generally does not show a significant difference in healing rates.[39] One study suggests the rate of healing correlates with the shape of the perforation, with large, kidney-shaped perforations being least likely to heal.[55]

3.3.2 Environmental Factors

Perforations heal differently depending on their environment. If accompanied by a sterile middle ear effusion (e.g., Eustachian tube obstruction), there is a higher likelihood of tympanosclerosis.[56] Perforations close more rapidly in the presence of infection, often before infection resolution and leading to long-lasting changes in the tympanic membrane. The state of the mastoid is also a factor, with a highly pneumatized mastoid promoting a higher likelihood of spontaneous healing of traumatic perforations.[23] Age, nutrition, and immunity influence cutaneous wound healing, and are likely to affect tympanic membrane wound healing as well[57,58].

3.4 Chronic Tympanic Membrane Perforations

Chronic tympanic membrane perforations[59] may be related to growth inhibition due to the epithelialization at the perforation edge,[22,35] insufficient blood supply in the central tympanic area,[60] connective tissue hyperproliferation,[28] or insufficient growth factors at the perforation border.[35,51] These exhibit marked epithelial hyperplasia, indicating continued efforts by the tissue to close the perforation, and the connective tissue layer will show excessive fibrosis and scarring. There is often associated chronic inflammation, either localized or diffusely spread throughout the connective tissue layer.[28] The normal migration of keratinocytes is disturbed, with remnants of keratinocytes seen in the keratin layer and the basal cells exhibiting cytoplasmic extensions into the papillary dermis.[35] Rete ridges and inclusion cysts can also be seen,[28] and growing epithelium will extend over the perforation edge to meet the mucosal layer.[35]

3.5 Current State of Regenerative Treatments For Tympanic Membrane Perforations

Office-based myringoplasty is yet to replace surgical tympanoplasty due to inferior results.[61] There are a number of growth factors currently under investigation.[62] Epidermal growth factor has been a focus of many studies, but it has complicated signaling, with many different receptors (EGFRs) that, in turn, allow multiple other growth factors (including HB-EGF, amphiregulin, and TGF-α) to act. A clinical trial of EGF in chronic tympanic membrane perforations had 0% success.[63] A number of other studies have failed to show a significant difference in healing time after EGF application.[40,64,65] This was likely because of the ability of EGFR to still be stimulated by a number of other routes.[66,67] EGF applied locally may lead to thinning and reperforation[68] and has the side effect of causing hypertrophy in the canal skin.[65] EGFR ligand shedding may be key in keratinocyte migration, and this can be enhanced with HB-EGF.[49,58] Factors such as HA and FGF-2 may play adjuvant roles.

Fibroblast growth factor-2 has received attention in the literature, with encouraging results in terms of closure rates,[69,70] but there are some concerns about epidermal hyperplasia and serous otorrhea. Compared with non-treated tympanic membranes, FGF-2-treated tympanic membranes exhibited fibroblast orientation that was more parallel to the tympanic membrane surface[71] and greater epidermal proliferation.[3] FGF-2 also induces vasodilation in the tympanic membrane, possibly explaining the acceleration of healing following application.[72]

Keratinocyte growth factor topical application does not enhance the closure rate of tympanic membrane perforation, but the repair process is reported to be more organized, showing greater hyperplasia and a thickened, healed area.[37] There was no statistical difference in healing between PDGF- and non-PDGF-treated ears.[73]

The effect of HA on healing time of tympanic membrane perforations is controversial.[74] Studies either show a reduction or no difference in healing time in perforations treated with HA.[74] It is postulated that HA acts by preventing dehydration of the perforation margins, by providing a supportive media for excess keratin and hyperplastic epithelium, and by regulating cell functions[75] or by influencing cell locomotion, which is likely needed to effect detachment so cells can move. Hyaluronic acid also has the side effect of causing canal skin hypertrophy.[65] Tissue-engineered tympanic membranes combining growth factors and scaffolds may soon be entering clinical trials.[76]

References

[1] Stenfors LE, Bloom GD, Hellström S. The tympanic membrane. Acta Otolaryngol. Suppl. 1984;414:28–30.
[2] Johnson FR, McMinn RM, Atfield GN. Ultrastructural and biochemical observations on the tympanic membrane. J Anat. 1968;103(Pt 2):297–310.
[3] Lim DJ. Structure and function of the tympanic membrane: a review. Acta Otorhinolaryngol Belg. 1995;49(2):101–115.
[4] Schmidt SH, Hellström S. Tympanic-membrane structure—new views. A comparative study. ORL J Otorhinolaryngol Relat Spec. 1991;53(1):32–36.
[5] Boedts D, Broekaert D. The keratinizing tympanic epithelium: an enigma. Acta Otorhinolaryngol Belg. 1991;45(1):21–26.
[6] Alberti PW. Epithelial Migration on the Tympanic Membrane. J Laryngol Otol. 1964;78:808–830.
[7] Litton WB. Epithelial migration over tympanic membrane and external canal. Arch Otolaryngol. 1963;77:254–257.
[8] Franz H. [Course, cause and action of epidermis migration of the tympanic membrane] Arch Klin Exp Ohren Nasen Kehlkopfheilkd. 1966;186(3):252–263.
[9] O'Donoghue GM. Epithelial migration on the guinea-pig tympanic membrane: the influence of perforation and ventilating tube insertion. Clin Otolaryngol Allied Sci. 1983;8(5):297–303.
[10] Reeve DR. Some observations on the diurnal variation of mitosis in the stratified squamous epithelium of wounded tympanic membrane. Cell Tissue Res. 1977;182(2):253–263.
[11] Knutsson J, von Unge M, Rask-Andersen H. Localization of progenitor/stem cells in the human tympanic membrane. Audiol Neurootol. 2011;16(4):263–269.
[12] Kakoi H, Anniko M, Kinnefors A, Rask-Andersen H. Auditory epidermal cell migration. VII. Antigen expression of proliferating cell nuclear antigens, PCNA and Ki-67 in human tympanic membrane and external auditory canal. Acta Otolaryngol. 1997;117(1):100–108.
[13] Johnson A, Hawke M. An ultrastructural study of the skin of the tympanic membrane and external ear canal of the guinea pig. J Otolaryngol. 1985;14(6):357–364.
[14] Santa Maria PL, Redmond SL, Atlas MD, Ghassemifar R. Histology of the healing tympanic membrane following perforation in rats. Laryngoscope. 2010;120(10):2061–2070.
[15] Revadi G, Prepageran N, Raman R, Sharizal TA. Epithelial migration on the external ear canal wall in normal and pathologic ears. Otol Neurotol. 2011;32(3):504–507.
[16] Yi ZX, Shi GS, Huang CC. Age-related epithelial migration on the tympanic membrane of the Mongolian gerbil. Otolaryngol Head Neck Surg. 1988;98(6):564–567.
[17] Boedts D. The tympanic epithelium in normal and pathological conditions. Acta Otorhinolaryngol Belg. 1978;32(4):295–419.
[18] Raja SK, Sivamani K, Garcia MS, Isseroff RR. Wound re-epithelialization: modulating keratinocyte migration in wound healing. Front Biosci. 2007;12:2849–2868.
[19] Santa Maria PL, Redmond SL, McInnes RL, Atlas MD, Ghassemifar R. Tympanic membrane wound healing in rats assessed by transcriptome profiling. Laryngoscope. 2011;121(10):2199–2213.
[20] Litjens SH, de Pereda JM, Sonnenberg A. Current insights into the formation and breakdown of hemidesmosomes. Trends Cell Biol. 2006;16(7):376–383.
[21] Russell AJ, Fincher EF, Millman L, et al. Alpha 6 beta 4 integrin regulates keratinocyte chemotaxis through differential GTPase activation and antagonism of alpha 3 beta 1 integrin. J Cell Sci. 2003;116(Pt 17):3543–3556.
[22] Gladstone HB, Jackler RK, Varav K. Tympanic membrane wound healing. An overview. Otolaryngol Clin North Am. 1995;28(5):913–932.
[23] Kristensen S. Spontaneous healing of traumatic tympanic membrane perforations in man: a century of experience. J Laryngol Otol. 1992;106(12):1037–1050.
[24] Taylor M, McMinn RM. Cytology of repair in experimental perforation of the tympanic membrane and its relationship to chronic perforations in man. Trans Am Acad Ophthalmol Otolaryngol. 1967;71(5):802–812.
[25] Johnson A, Hawke M. The function of migratory epidermis in the healing of tympanic membrane perforations in guinea-pig. A photographic study. Acta Otolaryngol. 1987;103(1-2):81–86.
[26] Johnson AP, Smallman LA, Kent SE. The mechanism of healing of tympanic membrane perforations. A two-dimensional histological study in guinea pigs. Acta Otolaryngol. 1990;109(5-6):406–415.

[27] Stenfors LE, Carlsoo B, Winblad B. Structure and healing capacity of the rat tympanic membrane after Eustachian tube occlusion. Acta Otolaryngol. 1981;91:75–84.
[28] Somers Th, Houben V, Goovaerts G, Govaerts PJ, Offeciers FE. Histology of the perforated tympanic membrane and its muco-epithelial junction. Clin Otolaryngol Allied Sci. 1997;22(2):162–166.
[29] McMinn RM, Taylor M. The cytology of repair in experimental perforations of the tympanic membrane. Br J Surg. 1966;53(3):222–232.
[30] Taylor M, McMinn RM. Healing of Experimental Perforations of the Tympanic Membrane. J Laryngol Otol. 1965;79:148–158.
[31] Clawson JP, Litton WB. The healing process of tympanic membrane perforations. Trans Am Acad Ophthalmol Otolaryngol. 1971;75(6):1302–1312.
[32] Werner S, Grose R. Regulation of wound healing by growth factors and cytokines. Physiol Rev. 2003;83(3):835–870.
[33] Mondain M, Ryan A. Epidermal growth factor and basic fibroblast growth factor are induced in guinea-pig tympanic membrane following traumatic perforation. Acta Otolaryngol. 1995;115(1):50–54.
[34] Boden P, Johnson A, Weinberger JM, Hawke M, Gotlieb AI. In situ localization of F-actin in the normal and injured guinea-pig tympanic membrane. Acta Otolaryngol. 1986;101(3–4):278–285.
[35] Spandow O, Hellström S, Dahlström M. Structural characterization of persistent tympanic membrane perforations in man. Laryngoscope. 1996;106(3 Pt 1):346–352.
[36] Govaerts PJ, Jacob WA, Marquet J. Histological study of the thin replacement membrane of human tympanic membrane perforations. Acta Otolaryngol. 1988;105(3–4):297–302.
[37] Clymer MA, Schwaber MK, Davidson JM. The effects of keratinocyte growth factor on healing of tympanic membrane perforations. Laryngoscope. 1996;106(3 Pt 1):280–285.
[38] Weinberger JM, Hawke M, Gotlieb AI. Repair of the wounded guinea pig tympanic membrane: organization of filamentous actin and spatial cellular reorganization. J Otolaryngol. 1988;17(7):352–358.
[39] Wang WQ, Wang ZM, Chi FL. Spontaneous healing of various tympanic membrane perforations in the rat. Acta Otolaryngol. 2004;124(10):1141–1144.
[40] Ma Y, Zhao H, Zhou X. Topical treatment with growth factors for tympanic membrane perforations: progress towards clinical application. Acta Otolaryngol. 2002;122(6):586–599.
[41] Bennett NT, Schultz GS. Growth factors and wound healing: Biochemical properties of growth factors and their receptors. Am J Surg. 1993;165(6):728–737.
[42] Bennett NT, Schultz GS. Growth factors and wound healing: Part II. Role in normal and chronic wound healing. Am J Surg. 1993;166(1):74–81.
[43] Krane SM. Clinical importance of metalloproteinases and their inhibitors. Ann N Y Acad Sci. 1994;732:1–10.
[44] McGrath MH. Peptide growth factors and wound healing. Clin Plast Surg. 1990;17(3):421–432.
[45] Santa Maria PL, Redmond SL, Atlas MD, Ghassemifar R. The role of epidermal growth factor in the healing tympanic membrane following perforation in rats. J Mol Histol. 2010;41(6):309–314.
[46] Koba R, Kawabata I. Immunohistochemical study of transforming growth factor-alpha expression in normal and perforated tympanic membrane. Ann Otol Rhinol Laryngol. 1995;104(10 Pt 1):793–797.
[47] Koba R. Epidermal cell migration and healing of the tympanic membrane: an immunohistochemical study of cell proliferation using bromodeoxyuridine labeling. Ann Otol Rhinol Laryngol. 1995;104(3):218–225.
[48] Ishibashi T, Shinogami M, Ishimoto SI, Yoshida K, Kaga K. Induction of KGF, basic FGF, and TGFalpha mRNA expression during healing of experimental TM perforations. Acta Otolaryngol. 1998;118(5):701–704.
[49] Tokumaru S, Higashiyama S, Endo T, et al. Ectodomain shedding of epidermal growth factor receptor ligands is required for keratinocyte migration in cutaneous wound healing. J Cell Biol. 2000;151(2):209–220.
[50] Hom DB. Growth factors in wound healing. Otolaryngol Clin North Am. 1995;28(5):933–953.
[51] Somers T, Goovaerts G, Schelfhout L, Peeters S, Govaerts PJ, Offeciers E. Growth factors in tympanic membrane perforations. Am J Otol. 1998;19(4):428–434.
[52] Santa Maria PLR, Redmond SL, Atlas MD, Ghassemifar R. Keratinocyte growth factor 1, fibroblast growth factor 2 and 10 in the healing tympanic membrane following perforation in rats. J Mol Histol. 2011;42(1):47–58.
[53] Laurent C, Hellström S. Extracellular matrix components reflect the dynamics of a healing tympanic membrane perforation—a histochemical study. Int J Biochem Cell Biol. 1997;29(1):221–229.
[54] Steed DL. The role of growth factors in wound healing. Surg Clin North Am. 1997;77(3):575–586.
[55] Kronenberg J, Ben-Shoshan J, Wolf M. Perforated tympanic membrane after blast injury. Am J Otol. 1993;14(1):92–94.
[56] Wielinga EW, Peters TA, Tonnaer EL, Kuijpers W, Curfs JH. Middle ear effusions and structure of the tympanic membrane. Laryngoscope. 2001;111(1):90–95.
[57] Griffin WL Jr. A retrospective study of traumatic tympanic membrane perforations in a clinical practice. Laryngoscope. 1979;89(2 Pt 1):261–282.
[58] Santa Maria PL, Varsak KY, Kim S, Yang YP. Heparin binding - epidermal growth factor-like growth factor for regeneration of chronic tympanic membrane perforations in mice. Tissue Eng Part A. 2015;21(9-10):1483–1494.
[59] Santa Maria PL, Atlas MD, Ghassemifar R. Chronic tympanic membrane perforation: a better animal model is needed. Wound Repair Regen. 2007;15(4):450–458.
[60] Masutani H, Nakai Y, Sugita M, Ohashi K, Moriguchi M, Matsunaga K. Microvasculature of the tympanic membrane. Acta Otolaryngol Suppl. 1991;486:99–104.
[61] Santa Maria PL, Oghalai JS. Is office based myringoplasty a suitable alternative to surgical tympanoplasty? Laryngoscope. 2013;124(5):1053–4.
[62] Hong P, Bance M, Gratzer PF. Repair of tympanic membrane perforation using novel adjuvant therapies: A contemporary review of experimental and tissue engineering studies. Int J Pediatr Otorhinolaryngol. 2013;77(1):3–12.
[63] Ramsay HA, Heikkonen EJ, Laurila PK. Effect of epidermal growth factor on tympanic membranes with chronic perforations: A clinical trial. Otolaryngol Head Neck Surg. 1995;113(4):375–379.
[64] O'Daniel TG, Petitjean M, Jones SC, et al. Epidermal growth factor binding and action on tympanic membranes. Ann Otol Rhinol Laryngol. 1990;99(1):80–84.
[65] Chauvin K, Bratton C, Parkins C. Healing large tympanic membrane perforations using hyaluronic acid, basic fibroblast growth factor, and epidermal growth factor. Otolaryngol Head Neck Surg. 1999;121(1):43–47.
[66] Kaftan H, Vogelgesang S, Lempas K, Hosemann W, Herzog M. Inhibition of epidermal growth factor receptor by erlotinib: wound healing of experimental tympanic membrane perforations. Otol Neurotol. 2007;28(2):245–249.
[67] Kaftan H, Reuther L, Miehe B, Hosemann W, Herzog M. The influence of inhibition of the epidermal growth factor receptor on tympanic membrane wound healing in rats. Growth Factors. 2010;28(4):286–292.
[68] Dvorak DW, Abbas G, Ali T, Stevenson S, Welling DB. Repair of chronic tympanic membrane perforations with long-term epidermal growth factor. Laryngoscope. 1995;105(12 Pt 1):1300–1304.
[69] Kanemaru S, Umeda H, Kitani Y, Nakamura T, Hirano S, Ito J. Regenerative treatment for tympanic membrane perforation. Otol Neurotol. 2011;32(8):1218–1223.
[70] Hakuba N, Iwanaga M, Tanaka S, et al. Basic fibroblast growth factor combined with atelocollagen for closing chronic tympanic membrane perforations in 87 patients. Otol Neurotol. 2010;31(1):118–121.
[71] Mondain M, Ryan A. Histological study of the healing of traumatic tympanic membrane perforation after basic fibroblast growth factor application. Laryngoscope. 1993;103(3):312–318.
[72] Mondain M, Ryan A. Effect of basic fibroblast growth factor on normal tympanic membrane. Am J Otolaryngol. 1994;15(5):344–350.
[73] Yeo SW, Kim SW, Suh BD, Cho SH. Effects of platelet-derived growth factor-AA on the healing process of tympanic membrane perforation. Am J Otolaryngol. 2000;21(3):153–160.
[74] Teh BM, Shen Y, Friedland PL, Atlas MD, Marano RJ. A review on the use of hyaluronic acid in tympanic membrane wound healing. Expert Opin Biol Ther. 2012;12(1):23–36.
[75] Güneri EA, Tekin S, Yilmaz O, et al. The effects of hyaluronic acid, epidermal growth factor, and mitomycin in an experimental model of acute traumatic tympanic membrane perforation. Otol Neurotol. 2003;24(3):371–376.
[76] Teh BM, Marano RJ, Shen Y, Friedland PL, Dilley RJ, Atlas MD. Tissue engineering of the tympanic membrane. Tissue Eng Part B Rev. 2013;19(2):116–132.

4 Pathophysiology of Cholesteatoma

Florian Hoppe and Michael B. Gluth

Abbreviations used in this chapter:

EGFR: epithelial growth factor receptor
IL: interleukin
MMP: matrix metalloproteinase
RANKL: Receptor Activator of NF-κB Ligand

4.1 Introduction

The word *cholesteatoma* is connected to Johannes Mueller, a German pathologist who introduced it in the year 1838 as a term for a "tumeur perleé," which had previously been described by the French pathologist Jean Cruveilhier in 1829.[1] Prior to this, in 1683, the French physician Joseph Guichard du Verney had observed and published a case of cholesteatoma and named it *steatome*. Also, Craigie in 1828 and Virchow in 1855 had each used the ancient Greek term *margaritoma*, which means "pearly tumor," to describe cholesteatoma.[2] Today the terms *epidermoid cyst* or *epidermoid*[3] are also widely used, especially by pathologists, to describe the microscopic findings of this pseudo-neoplasm. The term *epidermoid* is also commonly used in clinical medicine to describe these lesions when they are encountered outside of the tympanomastoid compartment, such as in the case of an epidermoid of the cerebellopontine angle.

4.2 Etiology

Two different types of cholesteatoma etiology can be distinguished: congenital and acquired. Congenital cholesteatoma is often located near the cochleariform process behind an intact tympanic membrane that has no past history of known perforation or otologic surgery. Congenital cholesteatoma is generally accepted to develop out of embryonic cell nests[4,5]; however, an alternate theory postulates that a reflux of amniotic cells into the middle ear space leads to congenital cholesteatoma. The prevalence of congenital cholesteatomas is 2% to 5%, and they are three times more likely to occur in males than in females.[6] An undiagnosed congenital cholesteatoma can eventually generate a perforation of the eardrum if allowed to grow into an advanced stage, which may then be difficult to differentiate from acquired disease.

In contrast to congenital cholesteatomas, acquired cholesteatomas develop from the epithelium of the tympanic membrane and clinically can be roughly divided into attic cholesteatomas, cholesteatomas of the pars tensa, and combined subtypes, according to Black.[7] Four main theories exist to account for the development of an acquired cholesteatoma. The first two of these, the retraction pocket theory and the proliferation theory, are the most widely accepted.

The retraction pocket theory posits that low pressure in the middle ear due to Eustachian tube dysfunction or epitympanic dysventilation leads to a retraction of the tympanic membrane, which eventually evolves into a trapped compartment that is unable to maintain a self-cleansing mechanism. The result is a medially advancing cholesteatoma sac.

With the proliferation theory, inflammation stimulates the basal cells of the stratum corneum of the pars flaccida of the tympanic membrane, resulting in papillary ingrowth into the attic space. Similar to the retraction pocket theory, the mechanism of this theory ends with a disrupted self-cleansing mechanism and medially advancing cholesteatoma sac.

The immigration theory proposes that, proceeding from a defect of the tympanic membrane, squamous epithelium grows into the middle ear space around the margins of a perforation. This theory of cholesteatoma development is consistent with what has been referred to as secondary acquired cholesteatoma due to the fact that the tympanic membrane perforation is the primary pathologic process that initiated the development of cholesteatoma secondarily. When encountered, this subtype of cholesteatoma usually consists of epithelium on the undersurface of the drumhead, the promontory of the cochlea, or the ossicular chain, as opposed to a cholesteatoma sac.

The metaplasia theory proposes that otitis media stimulates the middle ear mucosa into hyperplastic transformation and dedifferentiation that generates squamous epithelium, which starts to cornify and epidermalize. Evidence to support the metaplasia theory is weak.

Additionally, iatrogenic or implantation cholesteatomas are other possible etiologies for acquired cholesteatoma. These are cholesteatomas that develop secondary to displacement of unwanted epithelial tissue into the middle ear space during surgery or trauma.

4.3 Histology

Cholesteatomas comprise two layers: the matrix and the perimatrix (▸ Fig. 4.1). The structure of the matrix is similar to skin, with a stratum basale, stratum superficiale, and stratum corneum. This is often referred to as the epithelial layer. The perimatrix is characterized by connective tissue, with vessels and inflammatory infiltration of different extension. The extent of the matrix as well as the perimatrix varies tremendously from one part of a given cholesteatoma to another part and from one cholesteatoma to another. In cases of a so-called cholesteatoma pearl, the epithelial layer is thin and covered by a thin perimatrix on the outside, while inside there is only cell debris to account for the size of the cholesteatoma (▸ Fig. 4.2). In some cholesteatoma tissues, a papillary ingrowth of the matrix can be observed (▸ Fig. 4.3).

4.4 Proliferation

Monoclonal antibodies against various cell antigens within the cholesteatoma layers allow for the study of cholesteatoma cell subpopulations and differentiation status. Cholesteatoma is a proliferative disease with variable active periods. Using the monoclonal antibody Ki67 or Mib1 against a nuclear antigen in mitotic cells, expressed during the cell cycle in Phase S, late G1,

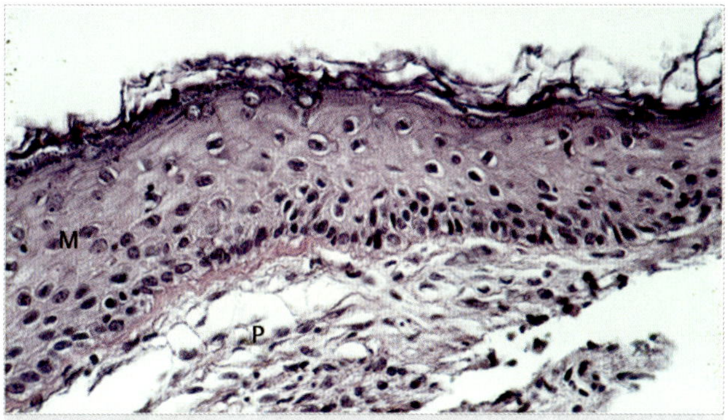

Fig. 4.1 Cholesteatoma matrix (M) and perimatrix (P).

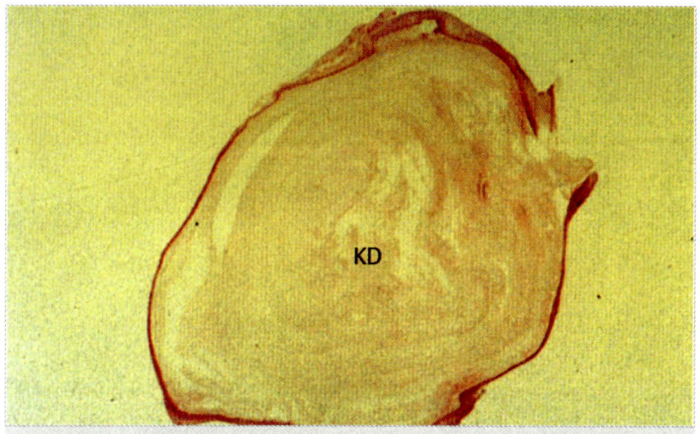

Fig. 4.2 Cholesteatoma pearl showing a thin matrix and perimatrix filled with keratin debris (KD).

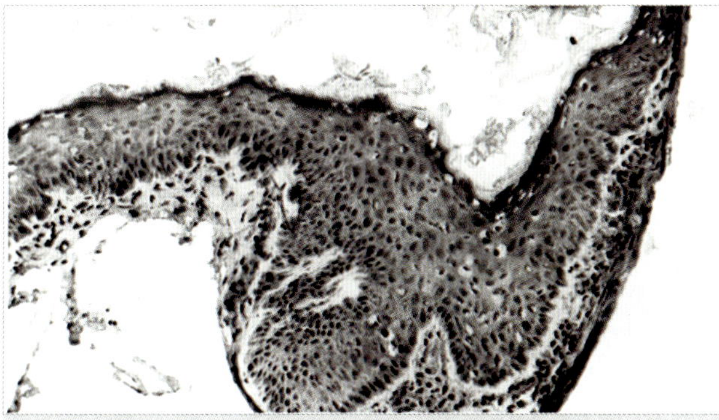

Fig. 4.3 Papillary ingrowth of the epithelium.

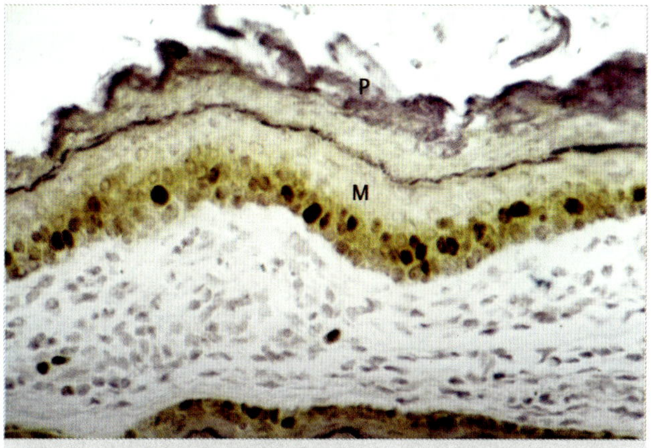

Fig. 4.4 Nuclear-stained (Ki67) proliferating cells in the basal and suprabasal layer of cholesteatoma matrix showing a high proliferation index. M, Matrix; P, Perimatrix.

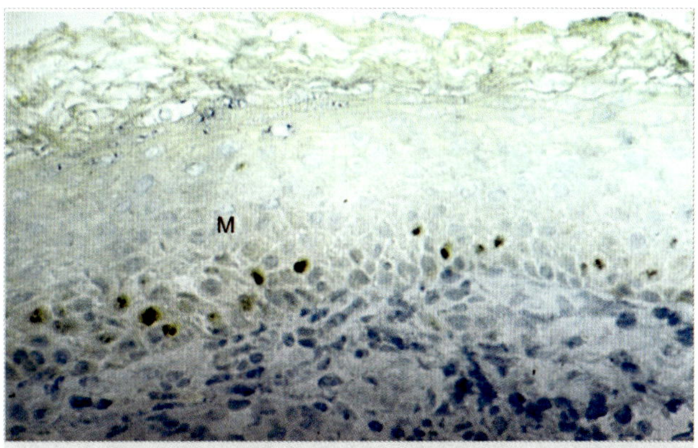

Fig. 4.5 Nuclear-stained (Ki67) proliferating cells in the basal and suprabasal layer of cholesteatoma matrix showing a low proliferation index. M, Matrix.

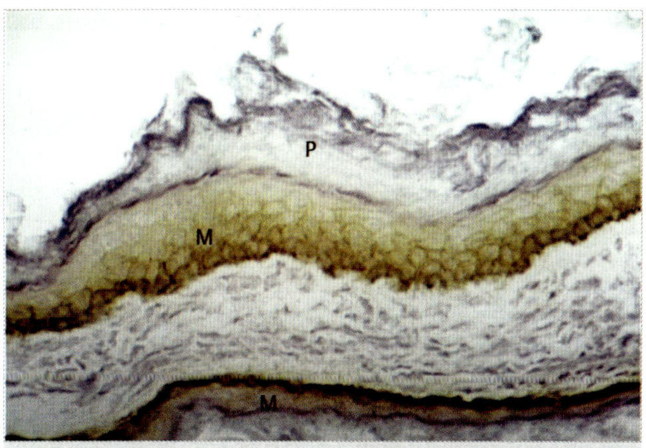

Fig. 4.6 EGFR staining in cholesteatoma tissue. M, Matrix; P, Perimatrix.

G2, and M, and an antibody against the epithelial growth factor receptor (EGFR), the proliferative activity of cholesteatoma can be analyzed.

In almost all cholesteatoma specimens, a nonhomogeneous staining is observed for Ki67 that depicts areas of high and low proliferative indices in the basal and suprabasal epithelial layer (▶ Fig. 4.4; ▶ Fig. 4.5). In contrast, EGFR staining shows a more homogeneous spread in all areas of the matrix and perimatrix independent of the thickness of the epithelium and degree of papillary ingrowth (▶ Fig. 4.6).[8] In addition, staining cholesteatoma for collagen IV and α-laminin, both components of a mature epithelial basal membrane, demonstrates gaps and interruptions of the collagen structure and basal membrane (▶ Fig. 4.7). Such interruptions suggest an immature basal membrane, as would be expected in a hyperproliferative disease state.[9]

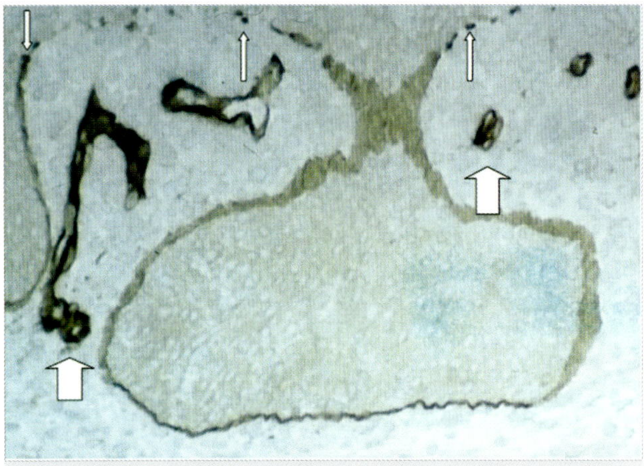

Fig. 4.7 Basal membrane stained with a laminin antibody showing a fragmented membrane (thin arrows) of the epithelial matrix and some vessels (thick arrows) in the perimatrix.

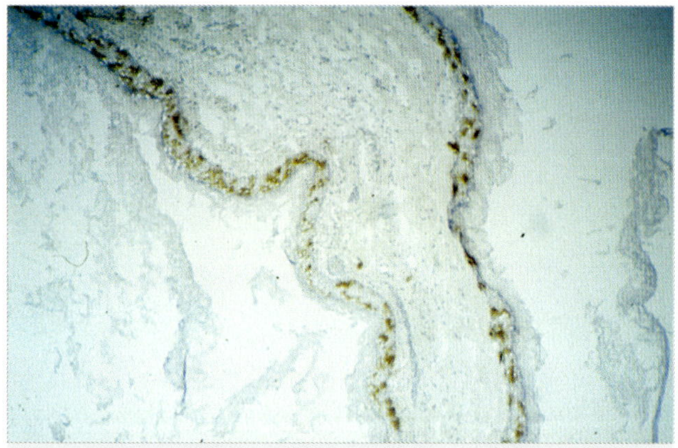

Fig. 4.8 CD1-positive Langerhans cells in the matrix of cholesteatoma.

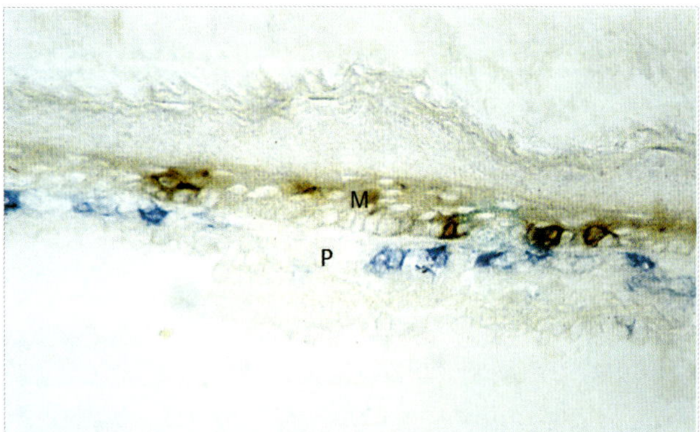

Fig. 4.9 Direct cell-cell contacts between CD1-positive Langerhans cells (brown) and CD4-positive T-helper cells (blue). M, matrix; P, perimatrix.

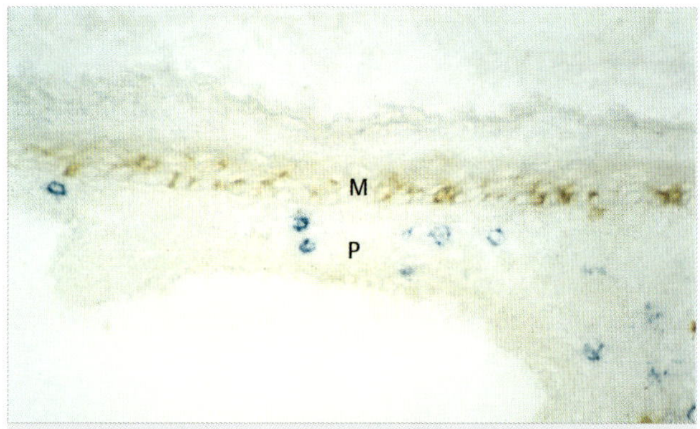

Fig. 4.10 CD 1-positive Langerhans cells (brown) show no contact to CD 8-positive suppressor cells (blue), parallel section to Fig. 4.9. M, matrix; P, perimatrix.

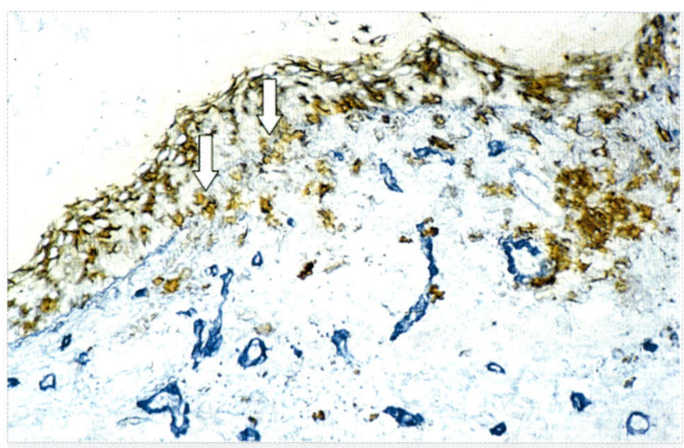

Fig. 4.11 Basal membrane-stained blue and CD1-positive Langerhans cells stained brown, showing cell migration through fragmented basal membrane parts (arrows).

4.5 Inflammation

Inflammation in cholesteatoma is characterized by the presence of CD1a-positive Langerhans cells, the most potent antigen-presenting cell in the matrix of cholesteatoma (▶ Fig. 4.8). Also present are a high number of T-helper cells (CD4), with a relatively lesser number of CD8-positive T-suppressor cells. Collectively, these findings compose a picture of an antigen/antibody-mediated host immune response to cholesteatoma. All components of the reaction are present, and cell-cell contacts between Langerhans cells and T-helper cells and between T-helper cells and macrophages in the perimatrix can be observed using double-staining techniques (▶ Fig. 4.9; ▶ Fig. 4.10). Gaps in the basal membrane allow the cellular migration of interdigitating cells as well as of T-cells (▶ Fig. 4.11).

B-cells and MHC class II-positive macrophages in higher numbers complete the findings of the immune response. Possible antigens, such as keratin,[10,11] bacterial antigens, viruses,[12,13,14] or foreign bodies, have also been considered to potentially play a role in the immune response. Via inflammation, various cytokines and mediators are produced that stimulate osteoclasts to resorb bone and fibroblasts to proliferate. Factors like interleukin (IL)-1, IL-2, IL-6, tumor necrosis factor, matrix metalloproteinase (MMP)-2, MMP-3, and MMP-9 have been detected in cholesteatoma tissues.[15,16,17,18,19,20,21,22] Recently, some publications have underlined the role of the fibroblasts in the perimatrix of cholesteatomas, noting their secretion of keratinocyte growth factor and MMP-2 and MMP-9.[23,24]

The higher occurrence of MMP and expression of CD31 as a marker for angiogenesis in children indicate a clear difference in the cholesteatomas of this age group and may explain a higher amount of recurrences and aggressive disease behavior in the younger patient.[25] However, the clinical findings of aggressive cholesteatoma do not clearly correlate with the immunohistochemical or molecular biological findings (author Hoppe's unpublished data).

4.6 Bone Destruction

Cholesteatoma can be observed to generate destruction of bone via a process of absorptive osteitis. Due to the inflammatory reaction spurred by exposure to various antigens, activated macrophages produce cytokines, such as IL-2, IL-6, and TNF-α, which in turn cause the expression of Receptor Activator of NF-κB Ligand (RANKL). This process leads to the activation of osteoclasts and the production of MMP-2, MMP-9, and endopeptidases, all of which can degrade the extracellular matrix of bone. These cytokines also interact with hexaminidase, an enyzme that induces the secretion of N-acetyl-d-hexosamine and influences bone resorption directly.[26,27] A stronger expression of MMP in the perimatrix correlates with a higher amount of bone destruction,[17,28] especially in sinus tympani cholesteatomas.

One question for surgeons is the possible use of autologous ossicles in patients undergoing surgery for cholesteatoma. In a group of 80 cases, 76% of specimens demonstrated ossicular bone destruction histologically. This was characterized by bone remodeling and a predominance of osteoclastic destruction. The epithelium never showed direct contact to the bony surface, but, instead, a layer of connective tissue was located between the bone surface and epithelium. Scanning microscope findings illustrate this clearly (▶ Fig. 4.12). Histology demonstrates the subepithelial inflammation typical of cholesteatomas and the osteitis in the haversian canals (▶ Fig. 4.13). In comparison to non-cholesteatomatous chronic otitis media, the findings of ossicular erosion in cholesteatoma are more severe (▶ Table 4.1).[29]

4.7 Spread of Cholesteatoma in the Temporal Bone

Due to the fact that cholesteatoma is a dynamic disease process, there is only a small amount of information about the direction

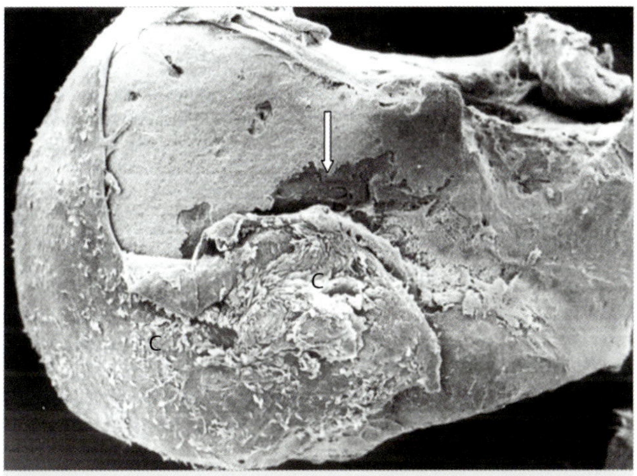

Fig. 4.12 Scanning microscopy showing head of the malleus with cholesteatoma tissue (C) and bone erosion (arrow).

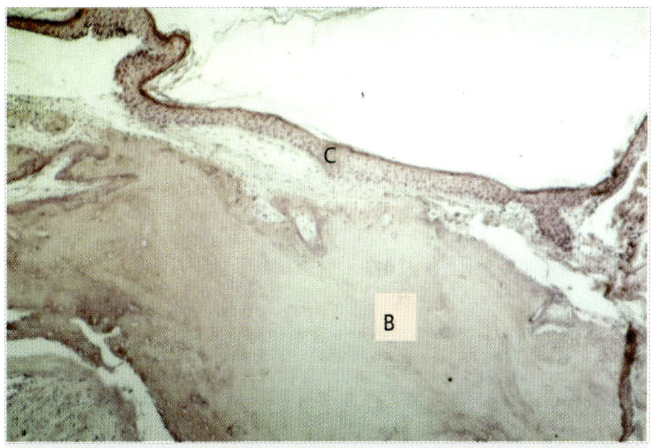

Fig. 4.13 Bone erosion with layer of cholesteatoma (C). B, bone.

Table 4.1 Histological findings in surgically removed ossicles

Histology	Otosclerosis	Cholesteatoma	Non-Cholesteatoma COM
	N=13	N=18	N=48
Thickened mucosa	1 (8%)	61 (76%)	36 (75%)
Squamous epithelium	0	19 (24%)	0
Subepithelial inflammation	2 (15%)	59 (74%)	27 (56%)
Osteitis	1 (8%)	42 (53%)	25 (52%)
Bone resorption	1 (8%)	61 (76%)	20 (42%)
Osteoclasts	0	20 (25%)	3 (9%)
Bone remodeling	0	22 (28%)	7 (15%)

COM, chronic otitis media
Used with permission from Peng JC, Hoppe F. Is reuse of autologous ear ossicles in cholesteatoma or chronic suppurative otitis media justified? Laryngo-rhino-otology. 1994;73(7):375-380.

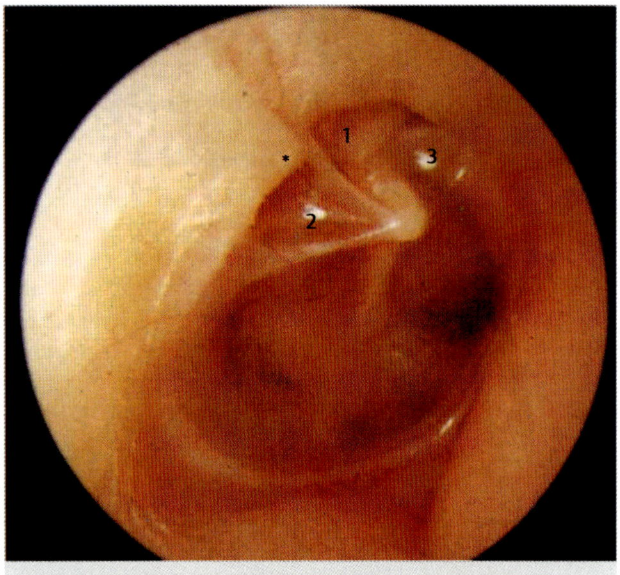

Fig. 4.14 Frequency of cholesteatoma site of origin. In order of frequency, acquired cholesteatoma forms from the (1) posterior epitympanum, (2) posterior mesotympanum, (3) anterior epitympanum. (*) posterior tympanic spine

of ingrowth into the mastoid and middle ear space. Clinical observations during surgery and radiological findings, as well as findings in post-mortem temporal bone examination, only reflect the final stage of the disease. Although there is no technique to confirm the stepwise pattern of cholesteatoma spread, Goycoolea and coworkers have highlighted the role of connective and granulation tissue present during otitis media with effusion as scaffolding for the ingrowth of cholesteatoma.[26] Furthermore, it has been surmised that acquired cholesteatoma has a tendency to spread according to planes of embryologic origin that are defined by the ligaments and mucosal folds of the middle ear, as highlighted by the work of Proctor.[30]

According to the retraction pocket theory, the most widely accepted sites of origin for primary acquired cholesteatoma are in the following order of frequency: posterior epitympanum, posterior mesotympanum, and anterior epitympanum[31] (▶ Fig. 4.14). However, it is quite possible for a single cholesteatoma to have elements of several of these subtypes simultaneously.[7]

4.7.1 Posterior Epitympanic (Attic) Cholesteatoma

Posterior epitympanic cholesteatoma may originate from retraction of the pars flaccida into the lateral epitympanic (Prussak's) space due to either diffuse negative middle ear pressure or selective epitympanic dysventilation (▶ Fig. 4.15). These cholesteatomas may spread posteriorly with penetration into the superior incudal space and then into the mastoid antrum, a route that extends lateral to the body of the incus. There is also the possibility of extension inferiorly into the mesotympanum and, subsequently, involvement of the sinus tympani and oval window niche by expansion through the posterior pouch of Von Troeltsch. Passage through this pathway generally involves erosion of the long process of the incus.

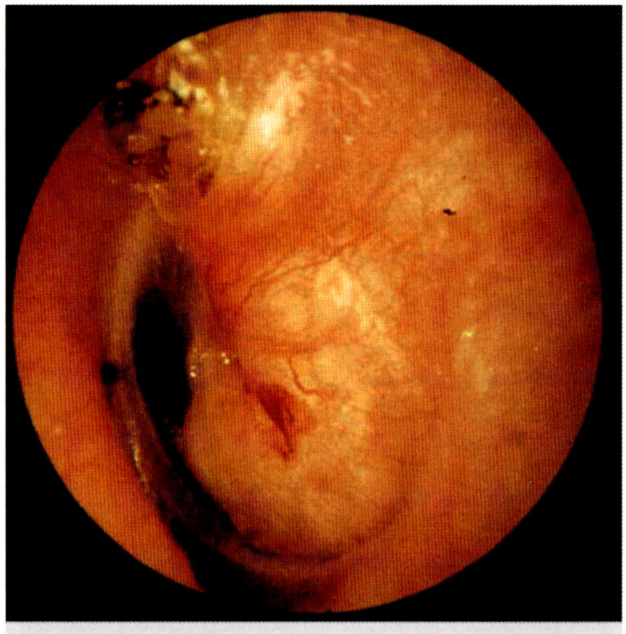

Fig. 4.15 Attic cholesteatoma. Attic cholesteatoma is most commonly derived from a posterior epitympanic retraction of the pars flaccida. These typically expand into the mesotympanum through the posterior pouch of Von Troeltsch, often behind an intact tympanic membrane such that a large white retrotympanic mass such as this is evident. Expansion into the mastoid antrum usually follows a posterior route through the superior incudal space that passes lateral to the incus body.

4.7.2 Mesotympanic (Pars Tensa) Cholesteatoma

Mesotympanic cholesteatoma is typically derived from the retraction of the posterior aspect of the pars tensa into the mesotympanum, which may be especially common in tubotympanic middle ear disease (▶ Fig. 4.16). These cholesteatomas may be associated with early erosion of the long process of the incus and possibly the stapes superstructure, with frequent deep penetration into the retrotympanum to involve the sinus tympani and facial recess at an early stage. If large, these cholesteatomas may also involve the round window niche and hypotympanum. Superior extension of posterior mesotympanic cholesteatoma into the epitympanum usually occurs through the posterior tympanic isthmus, with subsequent passage into the mastoid antrum medial to the body of the incus and growth over the tympanic segment of the facial nerve.

4.7.3 Anterior Epitympanic Cholesteatoma

Anterior epitympanic cholesteatoma, although less common, may expand to erode the head of the malleus and extend through the anterior epitympanic wall into the supratubal recess. Inferior extension into the mesotympanum may occur by expansion in the anterior pouch of Von Troeltsch, with subsequent passage anterior to the tensor tympani tendon into the protympanum. Anterior epitympanic cholesteatoma is also known to potentially extend into the medial epitympanic wall

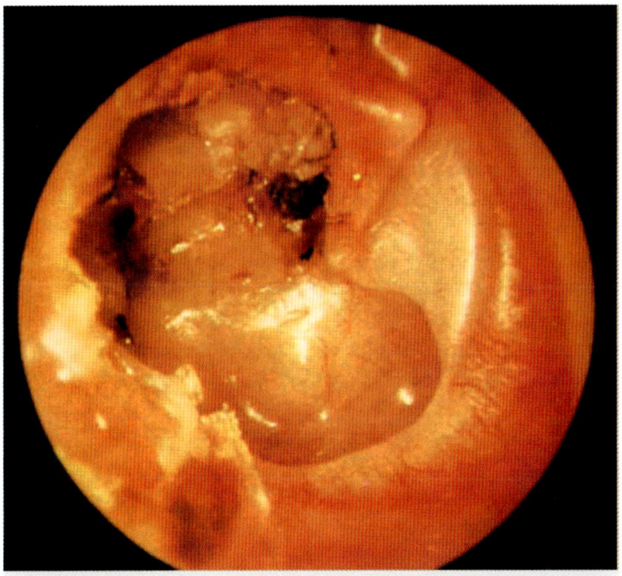

Fig. 4.16 Pars tensa cholesteatoma. Cholesteatoma derived from the pars tensa usually originates from a posterior retraction into the mesotympanum and retrotympanum. These cholesteatomas will involve the sinus tympani and oval window niche early. Expansion into the epitympanum and mastoid antrum usually follows a pathway over the tympanic segment of the facial nerve that is medial to the body of the incus.

through the anterior supralabyrinthine air cells,[32] with involvement of the perigeniculate aspect of the facial nerve, which may account for the proposed relative high rate of associated facial nerve morbidity in these cholesteatomas.[33]

References

[1] Sakuta M. [One hundred books which built up neurology (35)—Cruveilhier J "Anatomie Pathologique du Corps Humain" (1829–1842)] Brain Nerve. 2009;61(11):1354–1355.

[2] Virchow H. Über Perlgeschwülste. Virchows Arch. 1855;8:399.

[3] Schwartze H. Pathologische Anatomie des Ohres, in: Handbuch der pathologischen Anatomie, Hrsg. E. Klebs Berlin 1878: Bd.II S.16- 20.

[4] Michaels L. An epidermoid formation in the developing middle ear: possible source of cholesteatoma. J Otolaryngol. 1986;15(3):169–174.

[5] Persaud R, Hajioff D, Trinidade A, et al. Evidence-based review of aetiopathogenic theories of congenital and acquired cholesteatoma. J Laryngol Otol. 2007;121(11):1013–1019.

[6] Grundfast KM, Ahuja GS, Parisier SC, Culver SM. Delayed diagnosis and fate of congenital cholesteatoma (keratoma). Arch Otolaryngol Head Neck Surg. 1995;121(8):903–907.

[7] Black B, Gutteridge I. Acquired cholesteatoma: Classification and outcomes. Otol Neurotol. 2011;32(6):992–995.

[8] Hoppe F. Untersuchung zum Proliferationsverhalten von Cholesteatomen. HNO. 1995;43(12):710–715.

[9] Lang S, Nerlich A, Wiest I, Schreiner M. [Immunohistochemical basement membrane analysis of cholesteatoma epithelium] Laryngorhinootologie. 1994;73(7):371–374.

[10] Iino Y, Toriyama M, Ohmi S, Kanegasaki S. Activation of peritoneal macrophages with human cholesteatoma debris and alpha-keratin. Acta Otolaryngol. 1990;109(5–6):444–449.

[11] Iino Y, Toriyama M, Ogawa H, Kawakami M. Cholesteatoma debris as an activator of human monocytes. Potentiation of the production of tumor necrosis factor. Acta Otolaryngol. 1990;110(5–6):410–415.

[12] Stremlau A, Helms J. Müller- Hermelink H.K., Hoppe F., de Villiers E.M. Nachweis der DNS humaner Papillomviren (HPV) in einem "aggressiv" wachsenden Cholesteatom. HNO. 1995;43:3–5.

[13] Bergmann K, Hoppe F, He Y, et al. Human-papillomavirus DNA in cholesteatomas. Int J Cancer. 1994;59(4):463–466.

[14] Rydzewski B, Goździcka-Józefiak A, Sokalski J, Matusiak M, Durzyński L. [Identification of human papilloma viruses (HPV) in inflammatory states and ear neoplasms] Otolaryngol Pol. 2007;61(2):137–141.

[15] Vitale RF, Ribeiro FdeA. The role of tumor necrosis factor-alpha (TNF-alpha) in bone resorption present in middle ear cholesteatoma. Braz J Otorhinolaryngol. 2007;73(1):117–121.

[16] Suchozebrska-Jesionek D, Szymański M, Kurzepa J, Gołabek W, Stryjecka-Zimmer M. Gelatinolytic activity of matrix metalloproteinases 2 and 9 in middle ear cholesteatoma. J Otolaryngol Head Neck Surg. 2008;37(5):628–632.

[17] Wang J, Yu LS. [Expression of matrix metalloproteinase-2,9 in cholesteatoma from different positions] Zhonghua Er Bi Yan Hou Tou Jing Wai Ke Za Zhi. 2009;44(1):44–48.

[18] Juhász A, Sziklai I, Rákosy Z, Ecsedi S, Adány R, Balázs M. Elevated level of tenascin and matrix metalloproteinase 9 correlates with the bone destruction capacity of cholesteatomas. Otol Neurotol. 2009;30(4):559–565.

[19] Morales DS, Penido NdeO, da Silva ID, Stávale JN, Guilherme A, Fukuda Y. Matrix metalloproteinase 2: an important genetic marker for cholesteatomas. Braz J Otorhinolaryngol. 2007;73(1):51–57.

[20] Olszewska E, Borzym-Kluczyk M, Olszewski S, Zwierz K. Catabolism of glycoconjugates in chronic otitis media with cholesteatoma. J Investig Med. 2007;55(5):248–254.

[21] Breitkreutz D, Stark HJ, Mirancea N, Tomakidi P, Steinbauer H, Fusenig NE. Integrin and basement membrane normalization in mouse grafts of human keratinocytes—implications for epidermal homeostasis. Differentiation. 1997;61(3):195–209.

[22] Helgaland T, Engelen B, Olsnes C, Aarstad HJ, Vassbotn FS. In vitro cholesteatoma growth and secretion of cytokines. Acta Otolaryngol. 2010;130(7):815–819.

[23] Raffa S, Leone L, Scrofani C, Monini S, Torrisi MR, Barbara M. Cholesteatoma-associated fibroblasts modulate epithelial growth and differentiation through KGF/FGF7 secretion. Histochem Cell Biol. 2012;138(2):251–269.

[24] Barbara M, Raffa S, Leone L, et al. Characterization of primary cultures of cholesteatoma-associated fibroblasts. Otol Neurotol. 2012;33(6):988–995.

[25] Dornelles CdeC, da Costa SS, Meurer L, Rosito LP, da Silva AR, Alves SL. Comparison of acquired cholesteatoma between pediatric and adult patients. Eur Arch Otorhinolaryngol. 2009;266(10):1553–1561.

[26] Goycoolea MV, Hueb MM, Muchow D, Paparella MM. The theory of the trigger, the bridge and the transmigration in the pathogenesis of acquired cholesteatoma. Acta Otolaryngol. 1999;119(2):244–248.

[27] Olszewska E, Olszewski S, Borzym-Kluczyk M, Zwierz K. Role of N-acetyl-beta-d-hexosaminidase in cholesteatoma tissue. Acta Biochim Pol. 2007;54 (2):365–370.

[28] Rutkowska J, Olszewska E, Waniewska E, et al. [Hexosoaminidase gene expression in cholesteatoma in adults] Otolaryngol Pol. 2009;63(6):490–495.

[29] Peng JC, Hoppe F. [Is reuse of autologous ear ossicles in cholesteatoma or chronic suppurative otitis media justified?] Laryngorhinootologie. 1994;73 (7):375–380.

[30] Proctor B. The development of the middle ear spaces and their surgical significance. J Laryngol Otol. 1964;78:631–648.

[31] Jackler RK. The surgical anatomy of cholesteatoma. Otolaryngol Clin North Am. 1989;22(5):883–896.

[32] Gluth MB, Cohen MA, Friedland PL, Atlas MD. Surgical anatomy of the anterior supralabyrinthine air cell tract. J Laryngol Otol. 2011;125(10):1009–1013.

[33] Chu FW, Jackler RK. Anterior epitympanic cholesteatoma with facial paralysis: A characteristic growth pattern. Laryngoscope. 1988;98(3):274–279.

5 Microbiology of Chronic Ear Disease

Jeffrey D. Sharon and Richard A. Chole

Abbreviations used in this chapter:

AOM: acute otitis media
CDC: Centers for Disease Control and Prevention
CSOM: chronic suppurative otitis media
EDTA: ethylenediaminetetraacetic acid
EPS: extracellular polymeric substance
MRSA: methicillin-resistant *Staphylococcus aureus*
MSSA: methicillin-sensitive *Staphylococcus aureus*
OME: otitis media with effusion
PCR: polymerase chain reaction
TB: tuberculosis

5.1 Introduction

Chronic otitis media represents a fundamentally different process than acute otitis media, with different pathogenic organisms, immune responses, and complicating factors such as cholesteatoma and biofilms. Surgery is commonly required, in addition to antimicrobial therapy, for treatment of chronic drainage, pain, hearing loss, facial nerve paralysis, and intracranial complications.

5.2 Definitions

Otitis media is defined as inflammation of the middle ear and mastoid, and the duration of the process defines the subtype: acute (< 3 weeks), subacute (3–12 weeks), and chronic (> 12 weeks). *Acute otitis media* (AOM) (▶ Fig. 5.1) is the most common bacterial infection of children, affecting an estimated 72% of those age 3 years and younger.[1] Acute otitis media is considered to be recurrent if it happens 4 or more times in a year, or 3 or more times in a 6-month period. *Otitis media with effusion* (OME) is diagnosed when an effusion, which can be serous or mucoid, is present in the middle ear. This is commonly a sequela of AOM (▶ Fig. 5.2). *Chronic suppurative otitis media* (CSOM) refers to a draining ear due to chronic inflammation of the middle ear and mastoid, with tympanic membrane perforation or an ear tube present, with or without cholesteatoma (▶ Fig. 5.3). The duration of drainage necessary for diagnosis varies, but 3 months is a commonly accepted length of time to constitute a chronic condition. The prevalence of CSOM varies depending on the population being studied, with rates as high as 30% reported for high-risk populations like the Inuit, but estimated at < 1% for the United States.[2]

5.3 Microbiology

The pathogenic organisms responsible for AOM continue to evolve due to vaccination and antibiotic usage patterns. The 2013 vaccination schedule from the Centers for Disease Control and Prevention (CDC) recommends administration of the 13-valent pneumococcal vaccine at ages 2, 4, and 6 months, with a booster at age 12–15 months.[3] Recent data show that the most common bacteria responsible for acute otitis media, in order, are *Haemophilus influenza* (non-typeable), *Streptococcus pneumoniae*, and *Moraxella catarrhalis*.[4] Viruses are thought to contribute to infection by causing mucosal edema during upper respiratory tract infections but are not thought to be directly

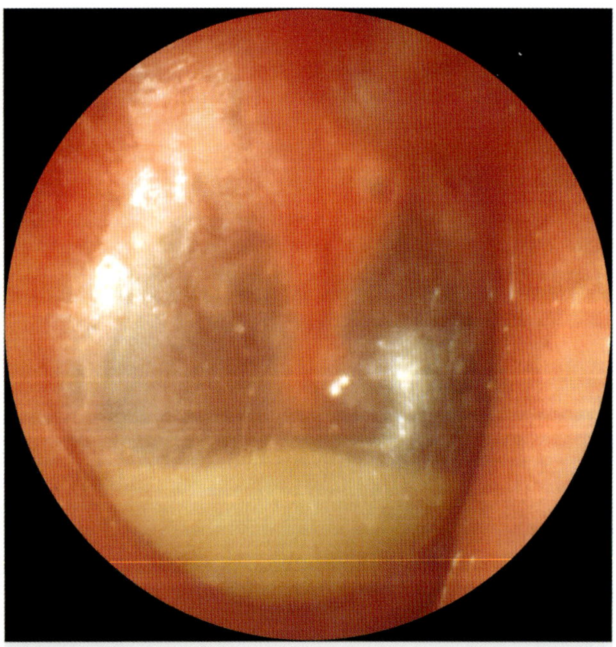

Fig. 5.1 Acute otitis media. A purulent exudate is visible behind an intact tympanic membrane.

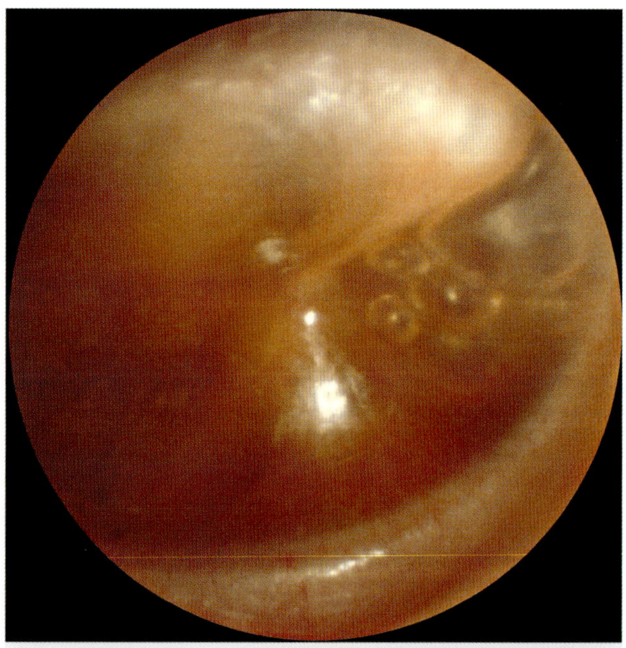

Fig. 5.2 Otitis media with effusion. Fluid appears behind an intact tympanic membrane. Gas bubbles can be seen anterior to the malleus.

causative. In fact, approximately 30% of viral upper respiratory tract infections in children are followed by AOM.[5] Chomaitree and colleagues found that 18.1% of middle ear fluid in patients with AOM had detectable virus, most commonly respiratory syncytial virus.[6] It is important to note that the bacteria responsible for AOM are upper respiratory tract organisms, and similar profiles of organisms are seen in other upper respiratory tract infections like sinusitis.

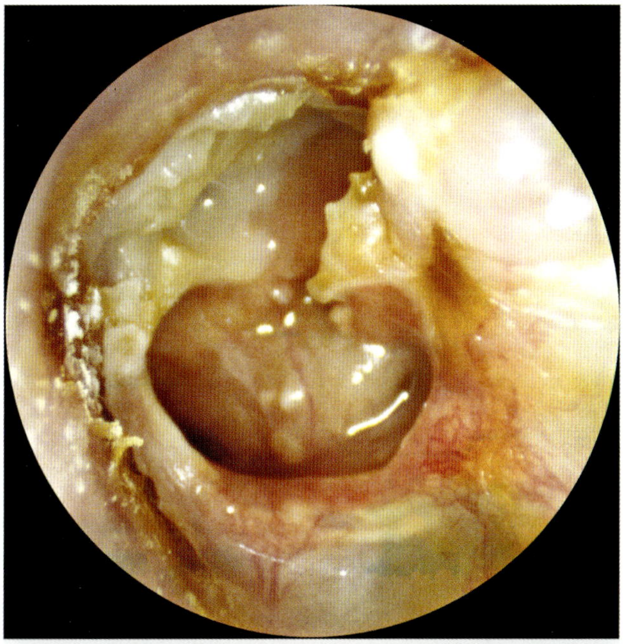

Fig. 5.3 Chronic suppurative otitis media. A near total tympanic membrane perforation is seen, with pus, mucosal edema, squamous debris, and lack of identifiable middle ear landmarks.

In contrast, the bacteria most commonly cultured from chronically draining ears due to CSOM are distinctly different aerobic and anaerobic organisms (▶ Table 5.1). The aerobic organisms identified most frequently are *Pseudomonas aeruginosa,* methicillin-resistant *Staphylococcus aureus* (MRSA), methicillin-sensitive *S. aureus* (MSSA), and coagulase-negative *Staphylococci.*[7] Different studies show variability in the frequency of those four species, but they are consistently reported as the most commonly cultured organisms from chronically draining ears, with *P. aeruginosa* and MRSA being the most common.[7,8,9,10,11,12,13] In addition, a host of other bacteria can be cultured, including *Enterobacter, Proteus, Acinetobacter, Klebsiella, Alcalineges, Serratia, Streptococcus,* and *Corynebacterium.* In one large study of 1102 patients in Korea, *P. aeruginosa* was cultured most frequently (31.8%), followed by MRSA (24.2%), MSSA (16.4%), and coagulase-negative *Staphylococci* (16.4).[10] Of interest, these percentages remained similar even when their cohort was divided into those with and without cholesteatoma.

In patients with cleft palate, the results were slightly different, with 35% *P. aeruginosa,* 15.5% *S. aureus,* 14% *Enterobacter faecalis,* and 12% *Proteus mirabilis.*[9] The higher percentage of gastrointestinal organisms suggests that nasopharyngeal reflux may play a role in the pathogenesis of infection in these patients.[14] Surgery may also change the microbial environment, with one study showing that, compared with preoperative cultures, postoperative cultures on ears that continued to drain

Table 5.1 Bacteriology of chronic suppurative otitis media (CSOM) with and without cholesteatoma

Bacteria	CSOM without Cholesteatoma		CSOM with Cholesteatoma	
	Yeo (N=692)	Prakash (N=204)	Yeo (N=234)	Ricciardiello (N=150)
Aerobes				
S. aureus	43.2%	48.69%	32.9%	19.1%
P. aeruginosa	31.7%	19.9%	32.1%	31.1%
CNS	9.5%	2.1%	18.4%	NR
K. pneumoniae	1%	9.4%	1.3%	1%
E. coli	0.6%	7.3%	1.1%	1.4%
Anaerobes				
Clostridium spp.	NR	26.1%	NR	3.8%
Peptococcus spp.	NR	23.2%	NR	12.1%
Peptostreptococcus spp.	NR	23.3%	NR	4.8%
Prevotella spp.	NR	15.9%	NR	NR
Bacteriodes spp.	NR	11.6%	NR	12.4

CNS, coagulase negative staphylococcus; NR, not reported
Data from
- Yeo SG, Park DC, Hong SM, Cha CI, Kim MG. Bacteriology of chronic suppurative otitis media–a multicenter study. Acta otolaryngol. 2007;127:1062–1067.
- Prakash R, Juyal D, Negi V, et al. Microbiology of chronic suppurative otitis media in a tertiary care setup of uttarakhand state, India. N Am J Med Sci. 2013;5:282–287.
- Ricciardiello F, Cavaliere M, Mesolella M, Iengo M. Notes on the microbiology of cholesteatoma: clinical findings and treatment. Acta Otorhinolaryngol Ital: organo ufficiale della Societa italiana di otorinolaringologia e chirurgia cervico-facciale 2009;29:197–202.

grew the same bacteria 22% of the time, different bacteria 51% of the time, and showed no growth 24% of the time.[8] There is some geographic variation in the microbiology, with a study showing that the three most commonly cultured bacteria in CSOM in Nigeria were *Klebsiella, Escherichia coli,* and *Streptococcus.*[15]

There is also evidence of changing microbiology over time, with one study showing an increase of community-acquired MRSA causing CSOM from 0.7% to 11.4% during the years 1998 to 2006.[16] Importantly, anaerobic bacteria have been cultured from 50% of chronically draining ears, including *Peptostreptococcus* spp., *Bacteriodes fragilis, Fusobacterium* spp., *Prevotella* spp., and *Porphyromonas* spp.[17] Of note, anaerobic bacteria have been shown to act synergistically with both *S. aureus* and *P. aeruginosa*, increasing their virulence.[18] Antibiotic coverage of anaerobic organisms has also been shown to improve time to resolution of ear drainage in CSOM.[19] It is interesting to note that the most commonly cultured aerobic bacteria, namely *S. aureus* and *P. aeruginosa*, are also the most commonly cultured organisms in otitis externa, suggesting that direct inoculation from the external auditory canal is responsible for some of the microbiological milieu in CSOM. Some have suggested that the nasopharynx may be a reservoir of pathogenic bacteria for ear disease, and one study comparing cultures from the middle ear and nasopharynx in patients undergoing operations for CSOM found that cultured bacteria were the same 26% of the time.[20]

Fungi are implicated in approximately 5% of cases of CSOM.[10] *Aspergillus* species, including *niger* and *fumigatus*, along with *Candida* species, including *albicans* and *parapsilosis*, are the most commonly cultured isolates.[12] These infections are commonly a result of prior antibiotic treatments for bacterial CSOM. Of interest, in one study 80% of fungal infections showed concurrent bacterial infections, and 62% of the time the classic otoscopic findings of fungal infection (e.g., visible spores) were absent (▶ Fig. 5.4).[21]

Tuberculous otitis is estimated to cause less than 1% of chronic ear infections.[22] It is difficult to diagnose because clinical signs and symptoms are variable. There is not always an association with pulmonary or systemic tuberculosis (TB), and TB is difficult to culture. However, diagnosis is important because treatment with anti-tuberculous medication can be successful. In a large study, including 53 cases of tuberculous otitis, the duration of symptoms varied between one and 10 years, with otorrhea reported most commonly, followed by hearing loss, otalgia, tinnitus, dizziness, and facial palsy.[23] Tympanic membrane perforations, which varied in configuration from total, subtotal, central, multiple, and marginal, were commonly observed. In addition, 70% of patients had erosion of the ossicular chain, most commonly the long process of the incus. In that series, histology obtained during surgery was the most reliable method of diagnosis, and it showed granulomas, Langerhans giant cells, and caseous necrosis. Stains for acid-fast bacilli and culture for *Mycobacterium tuberculosis* were frequently negative from both discharge fluid and operative specimens. Polymerase chain reaction (PCR) was positive in the 7 of 8 cases in which it was used. Of note, 11 patients who were diagnosed with TB did not undergo surgery and were treated medically with a combination of isoniazid, rifampin, ethambutol, and pyrazinamide. All of these patients were treated successfully after a mean of 6.5 months, arguing that anti-tuberculous medication alone is successful in treating uncomplicated tuberculous otitis.[23]

5.4 Cholesteatoma

Cholesteatoma is present in an estimated 40% of cases of CSOM.[24,25] Cholesteatomas (▶ Fig. 5.5) are keratinizing

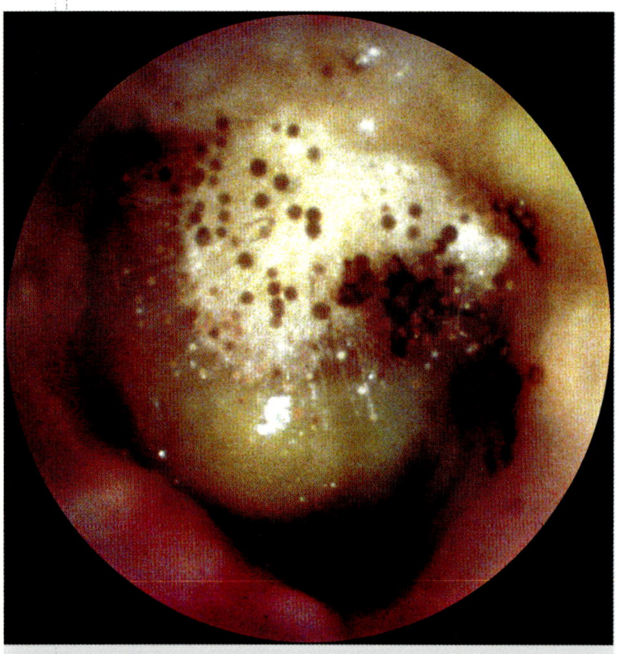

Fig. 5.4 Otomycosis. White and black fungal spores are visible in the external auditory canal, along with purulence.

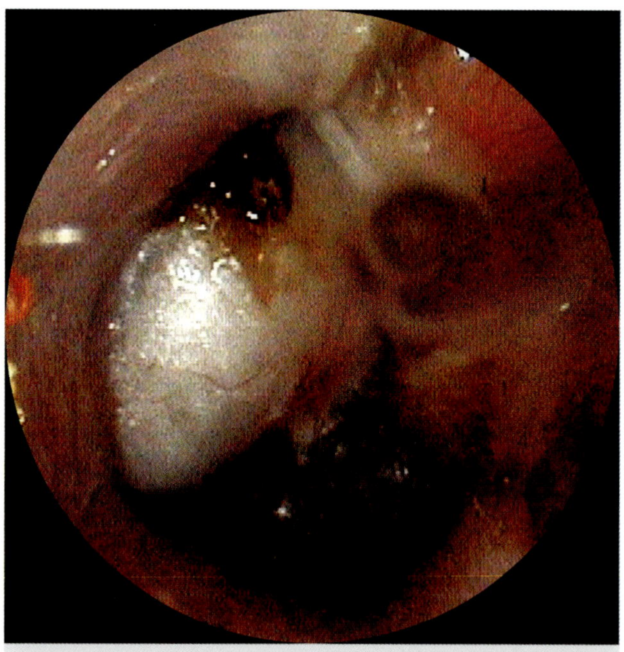

Fig. 5.5 Cholesteatoma. A white mass is seen in the posterior-superior quadrant, along with significant scutal erosion.

epidermal tissues within the middle ear or mastoid. Over time, they can grow, producing hearing loss and bone resorption, which can lead to facial nerve paralysis, labyrinthine fistulae, or intracranial complications.

Clinically, cholesteatomas can be infected or uninfected, and infected cholesteatomas seem to behave more aggressively. This observation is supported by data from experimental animals, in which induced cholesteatomas that were inoculated with *P. aeruginosa* were larger and demonstrated more bone resorption than uninfected cholesteatomas.[26] The bacterial profile of infected cholesteatoma is similar to CSOM, with several studies reporting similar culture results when comparing those patients with and without cholesteatoma.[10,13] In a recent study of 150 patients with cholesteatoma and CSOM, 58% of patients had polymicrobial infections, and of the remaining 42% with single-organism infections, 60.3% grew aerobes, 38.2% grew anaerobes, and 1.4% grew fungi.[27] The most common aerobic bacteria were *Pseudomonas* (31%), *Staphylococcus* (19%), and *Proteus* (8%), and the most common anaerobic bacteria were anaerobic gram-positive cocci (17.2%), *Bacteriodes* (12%), and *Clostridium* (4%). Inflammation in the vicinity of cholesteatomas may be due to multiple factors. Chronic infection, usually in the form of biofilms, may release lipopolysaccharide, which leads to the activation of osteoclastic bone resorption through a TLR-4-dependent pathway.[28,29]

5.5 Biofilms in Chronic Otitis

Chronic, recalcitrant infections in CSOM have been shown to be associated with bacterial biofilms. In contrast to the familiar single-cell bacterial phenotype, biofilm refers to a microcolony of bacteria growing within an extracellular matrix that has enhanced abilities to resist antibiotics and adhere to surfaces.[30] Bacteria in biofilms are able to resist antibiotics through a number of strategies, including having reservoirs of metabolically inactive cells deep within the biofilm that can repopulate if antibiotics kill off active cells at the periphery and by having extracellular polymeric substance (EPS) that physically protects the biofilm.[31]

Biofilms have been demonstrated in CSOM ears with and without cholesteatoma.[32,33] *P. aeruginosa, S. aureus, S. pneumoniae, H. influenzae,* and *M. catarrhalis* have all been shown to be capable of forming biofilms.[31,32] One study found evidence for biofilms in 6 of 10 patients undergoing surgery for CSOM, compared with 1 of 10 control subjects.[33] Another study examined middle ear and mastoid specimens for biofilms from patients with CSOM with and without cholesteatoma and found biofilms in 3 of 5 patients with cholesteatoma and in 1 of 7 patients without cholesteatoma.[34] Cultured *P. aeruginosa* from cholesteatoma was shown to be capable of several key features of biofilm bacteria, namely adherence to keratinocytes, quorum sensing, twitching motility, and production of extracellular matrix.[35] Because of their antibiotic resistance mechanisms, treatment of biofilm infections commonly requires physical removal in addition to antimicrobial therapy. However, there is evidence that some topical medications, like gentian violet, ethylenediaminetetraacetic acid (EDTA), and d-amino acids, inhibit biofilm growth *in vitro*.[36,37,38]

5.6 Antibiotic Resistance

P. aeruginosa is an aerobic gram-negative rod. It is resistant to many antibiotics through several mechanisms, including efflux pumps, inducible beta-lactamases, and mutations in the topoisomerase genes.[39,40,41] In a large study, *P. aeruginosa* isolates from the ear were sensitive to antibiotics as follows: ceftazidime (88.4%), amikacin (79.6%), piperacillin (79.3%), ciprofloxacin (39.5%), levofloxacin (37.8%), gentamicin (37.1%), and tobramycin (39.1%).[10] Another study showed high susceptibility to imipenem (79%), amikacin (78.9%), and ceftazidime (77.7%), and intermediate susceptibility to aztreonam (66.8%), ciprofloxacin (50.7%), and levofloxacin (43.8%).[39] These results certainly would question the common practice of using quinolone antibiotics as first-line therapy for pseudomonal otorrhea. Unfortunately, many of the other more effective antibiotics are not available in oral or topical formulations, instead requiring intravenous administration. Furthermore, topical quinolone antibiotics have been shown to be safe for administration in the middle ear whereas aminoglycosides are potentially ototoxic when in contact with the round window. Of note, there appears to be geographic variation in susceptibility, with studies from Iran, Spain, and Pakistan reporting high sensitivity to fluoroquinolones.[11,42,43]

Methicillin-resistant *S. aureus* is a gram-positive coccus that has increased dramatically in incidence since its first discovery in 1961.[44] It naturally resides on skin and along the upper aerodigestive tract. It is resistant to beta-lactam antibiotics through both the *blaZ* gene, which encodes a protein that hydrolyzes beta-lactams, and the *mecA* gene, which encodes a transpeptidase used for cell wall production that resists binding by beta-lactam antibiotics, rendering them ineffective.[45] In one large study, MRSA sensitivities for CSOM were as follows: vancomycin (100%), teicoplanin (85.3%), and sulfamethoxazole/trimethoprim (85.1%); there was very low sensitivity reported for oxacillin, clindamycin, and penicillin.[10] The differential resistance to antibiotics between MSSA and MRSA does not only include beta-lactams, with one study showing much higher susceptibilities for a variety of antibiotics for MSSA over MRSA, including ciprofloxacin (83% versus 7%), clindamycin (81% versus 11%), erythromycin (62% versus 4%), and tetracycline (71% versus 9%).[46] Interestingly, one study compared treatment of MRSA otorrhea with intravenous vancomycin, intravenous teicoplanin, and aural irrigations with dilute acetic acid, and similar cure rates were seen across all groups.[13]

5.7 Topical versus Systemic Antibiotics

Topical administration of antibiotics into the middle ear is generally preferred over systemic administration, not only for avoidance of systemic side effects, but also because drug concentrations in the middle ear are far higher.[47] A Cochrane review concluded that topical quinolone antibiotics were more effective in treating CSOM than systemic quinolone or non-quinolone antibiotics.[48] However, because drugs are being administered in high concentration into the middle ear space, ototoxicity is a very real concern. In experimental animals, aminoglycoside antibiotics have been shown to be ototoxic;

however, humans seem to be much less susceptible compared with experimental models.[49] The incidence of ototoxicity due to aminoglycoside-containing antibiotics is unknown, but has been estimated at 1 in 10,000 cases.[50] Controversy exists over the ototoxic potential of Cortisporin (Falcon Pharmaceuticals, LtD.), which contains neomycin, bacitracin, polymyxin B, and hydrocortisone.[51,52]

Potentially ototoxic topical preparations should be used sparingly when there is a possibility of contact with the round window membrane. The advantages of the use of these drugs must be weighed against the small potential of ototoxicity. Quinolone antibiotics, on the other hand, have been demonstrated in human and animal studies to be safe for administration.[53] Unfortunately, many of the antibiotics that are effective against quinolone-resistant *P. aeruginosa* and *S. aureus* are not available in topical formulations.

5.8 Conclusion

Studies of the microbiology of chronic otitis media with and without cholesteatoma have consistently shown a pattern of the presence of *P. aeruginosa* and *S. aureus* as the predominant organisms. There are local and regional variations in bacteria found in chronic otitis media, with gastrointestinal flora found in some locales. Antibiotic resistance of these organisms has changed over the last two decades with the appearance of quinolone-resistant *P. aeruginosa* and methicillin-resistant *S. aureus*. Furthermore, bacteria found in chronic otitis media are usually powerful biofilm formers; when bacteria assume the biofilm phenotype, they are up to 1000 times more resistant to antibiotics compared with the freely motile (planktonic) phenotype. New strategies for controlling these infections include more specific antimicrobials, such as those that disrupt biofilms.

References

[1] Hoffman HJ, Daly KA, Bainbridge KE, et al. Panel 1: Epidemiology, natural history, and risk factors. Otolaryngol Head Neck Surg. 2013;148(4) Suppl:E1–E25.
[2] Roland PS. Chronic suppurative otitis media: A clinical overview. Ear Nose Throat J. 2002;81(8) Suppl 1:8–10.
[3] Immunization Schedule 2015; accessed at http://www.cdc.gov/vaccines/schedules/hcp/imz/child-adolescent.html.
[4] Pichichero ME. Otitis media. Pediatr Clin North Am. 2013;60(2):391–407.
[5] Revai K, Dobbs LA, Nair S, Patel JA, Grady JJ, Chonmaitree T. Incidence of acute otitis media and sinusitis complicating upper respiratory tract infection: The effect of age. Pediatrics. 2007;119(6):e1408–e1412.
[6] Chonmaitree T. Viral and bacterial interaction in acute otitis media. Pediatr Infect Dis J. 2000;19(5) Suppl:S24–S30.
[7] Ahn JH, Kim MN, Suk YA, Moon BJ. Preoperative, intraoperative, and postoperative results of bacterial culture from patients with chronic suppurative otitis media. Otol Neurotol. 2012;33(1):54–59.
[8] Shim HJ, Park CH, Kim MG, Lee SK, Yeo SG. A pre- and postoperative bacteriological study of chronic suppurative otitis media. Infection. 2010;38(6):447–452.
[9] Weckwerth PH, de Magalhães Lopes CA, Duarte MA, et al. Chronic suppurative otitis media in cleft palate: microorganism etiology and susceptibilities. Cleft Palate Craniofac J. 2009;46(5):461–467.
[10] Yeo SG, Park DC, Hong SM, Cha CI, Kim MG. Bacteriology of chronic suppurative otitis media—a multicenter study. Acta Otolaryngol. 2007;127(10):1062–1067.
[11] Mozafari Nia K, Sepehri G, Khatmi H, Shakibaie MR. Isolation and antimicrobial susceptibility of bacteria from chronic suppurative otitis media patients in kerman, iran. Iran Red Crescent Med J. 2011;13(12):891–894.
[12] Prakash R, Juyal D, Negi V, et al. Microbiology of chronic suppurative otitis media in a tertiary care setup of uttarakhand state, India. N Am J Med Sci. 2013;5(4):282–287.
[13] Choi HG, Park KH, Park SN, Jun BC, Lee DH, Yeo SW. The appropriate medical management of methicillin-resistant Staphylococcus aureus in chronic suppurative otitis media. Acta Otolaryngol. 2010;130(1):42–46.
[14] Lieu JE, Muthappan PG, Uppaluri R. Association of reflux with otitis media in children. Otolaryngol Head Neck Surg. 2005;133(3):357–361.
[15] Adoga AA, Bakari A, Afolabi OA, Kodiya AM, Ahmad BM. Bacterial isolates in chronic suppurative otitis media: a changing pattern? Niger J Med. 2011;20(1):96–98.
[16] Park MK, Jung MH, Kang HJ, et al. The changes of MRSA infections in chronic suppurative otitis media. Otolaryngol Head Neck Surg. 2008;139(3):395–398.
[17] Brook I. The role of anaerobic bacteria in chronic suppurative otitis media in children: implications for medical therapy. Anaerobe. 2008;14(6):297–300.
[18] Brook I, Hunter V, Walker RI. Synergistic effect of bacteroides, Clostridium, Fusobacterium, anaerobic cocci, and aerobic bacteria on mortality and induction of subcutaneous abscesses in mice. J Infect Dis. 1984;149(6):924–928.
[19] Brook I. Management of chronic suppurative otitis media: superiority of therapy effective against anaerobic bacteria. Pediatr Infect Dis J. 1994;13(3):188–193.
[20] Chang J, Lee SH, Choi J, Im GJ, Jung HH. Nasopharynx as a microbiologic reservoir in chronic suppurative otitis media: preliminary study. Clin Exp Otorhinolaryngol. 2011;4(3):122–125.
[21] Saunders JE, Raju RP, Boone JL, Hales NW, Berryhill WE. Antibiotic resistance and otomycosis in the draining ear: culture results by diagnosis. Am J Otolaryngol. 2011;32(6):470–476.
[22] Vaamonde P, Castro C, García-Soto N, Labella T, Lozano A. Tuberculous otitis media: a significant diagnostic challenge. Otolaryngol Head Neck Surg. 2004;130(6):759–766.
[23] Cho YS, Lee HS, Kim SW, et al. Tuberculous otitis media: A clinical and radiologic analysis of 52 patients. Laryngoscope. 2006;116(6):921–927.
[24] Podoshin L, Fradis M, Ben-David Y, Margalit A, Tamir A, Epstein L. Cholesteatoma: an epidemiologic study among members of kibbutzim in northern Israel. Ann Otol Rhinol Laryngol. 1986;95(4 Pt 1):365–368.
[25] Benson J, Mwanri L. Chronic suppurative otitis media and cholesteatoma in Australia's refugee population. Aust Fam Physician. 2012;41(12):978–980.
[26] Jung JY, Lee DH, Wang EW, et al. P. aeruginosa infection increases morbidity in experimental cholesteatomas. Laryngoscope. 2011;121(11):2449–2454.
[27] Ricciardiello F, Cavaliere M, Mesolella M, Iengo M. Notes on the microbiology of cholesteatoma: clinical findings and treatment. Acta Otorhinolaryngol Ital. 2009;29(4):197–202.
[28] Nason R, Lee DH, Jung JY, Chole RA. Radiographic and micro-computed tomographic imaging of lipopolysaccharide-mediated bone resorption. Ann Otol Rhinol Laryngol. 2009;118(5):391–396.
[29] Zhuang L, Jung JY, Wang EW, et al. Pseudomonas aeruginosa lipopolysaccharide induces osteoclastogenesis through a toll-like receptor 4 mediated pathway in vitro and in vivo. Laryngoscope. 2007;117(5):841–847.
[30] Bjarnsholt T. The role of bacterial biofilms in chronic infections. APMIS Suppl. 2013;5(136):1–51.
[31] Post JC, Hiller NL, Nistico L, Stoodley P, Ehrlich GD. The role of biofilms in otolaryngologic infections: update 2007. Curr Opin Otolaryngol Head Neck Surg. 2007;15(5):347–351.
[32] Chole RA, Faddis BT. Evidence for microbial biofilms in cholesteatomas. Arch Otolaryngol Head Neck Surg. 2002;128(10):1129–1133.
[33] Lee MR, Pawlowski KS, Luong A, Furze AD, Roland PS. Biofilm presence in humans with chronic suppurative otitis media. Otolaryngol Head Neck Surg. 2009;141(5):567–571.
[34] Saunders J, Murray M, Alleman A. Biofilms in chronic suppurative otitis media and cholesteatoma: scanning electron microscopy findings. Am J Otolaryngol. 2011;32(1):32–37.
[35] Wang EW, Jung JY, Pashia ME, Nason R, Scholnick S, Chole RA. Otopathogenic Pseudomonas aeruginosa strains as competent biofilm formers. Arch Otolaryngol Head Neck Surg. 2005;131(11):983–989.
[36] Wang EW, Agostini G, Olomu O, Runco D, Jung JY, Chole RA. Gentian violet and ferric ammonium citrate disrupt Pseudomonas aeruginosa biofilms. Laryngoscope. 2008;118(11):2050–2056.
[37] Zenga J, Gagnon PM, Vogel J, Chole RA. Biofilm formation by otopathogenic strains of Pseudomonas aeruginosa is not consistently inhibited by ethylenediaminetetraacetic acid. Otol Neurotol. 2012;33(6):1007–1012.
[38] Kolodkin-Gal I, Romero D, Cao S, Clardy J, Kolter R, Losick R. D-amino acids trigger biofilm disassembly. Science. 2010;328(5978):627–629.

[39] Lee SK, Lee MS, Jung SY, Byun JY, Park MS, Yeo SG. Antimicrobial resistance of Pseudomonas aeruginosa from otorrhea of chronic suppurative otitis media patients. Otolaryngol Head Neck Surg. 2010;143(4):500–505.
[40] Poole K. Multidrug efflux pumps and antimicrobial resistance in Pseudomonas aeruginosa and related organisms. J Mol Microbiol Biotechnol. 2001;3 (2):255–264.
[41] Livermore DM. beta-Lactamases in laboratory and clinical resistance. Clin Microbiol Rev. 1995;8(4):557–584.
[42] de Miguel Martínez I, Del Rosario Quintana C, Bolaños Rivero M, Ramos Macías A. [Aetiology and therapeutic considerations in chronic otitis media. Analysis of a 5 year period] Acta Otorrinolaringol Esp. 2005;56(10):459–462.
[43] Aslam MA, Ahmed Z, Azim R. Microbiology and drug sensitivity patterns of chronic suppurative otitis media. J Coll Physicians Surg Pak. 2004;14(8):459–461.
[44] Lowy FD. Staphylococcus aureus infections. N Engl J Med. 1998;339(8):520–532.
[45] Lowy FD. Antimicrobial resistance: the example of Staphylococcus aureus. J Clin Invest. 2003;111(9):1265–1273.
[46] Park DC, Lee SK, Cha CI, Lee SO, Lee MS, Yeo SG. Antimicrobial resistance of Staphylococcus from otorrhea in chronic suppurative otitis media and comparison with results of all isolated Staphylococci. Eur J Clin Microbiol Infect Dis. 2008;27(7):571–577.
[47] Daniel SJ. Topical treatment of chronic suppurative otitis media. Curr Infect Dis Rep. 2012;14(2):121–127.
[48] Macfadyen CA, Acuin JM, Gamble C. Systemic antibiotics versus topical treatments for chronically discharging ears with underlying eardrum perforations. Cochrane Database Syst Rev. 2006(1):CD005608.
[49] Rizzi MD, Hirose K. Aminoglycoside ototoxicity. Curr Opin Otolaryngol Head Neck Surg. 2007;15(5):352–357.
[50] Haynes DS, Rutka J, Hawke M, Roland PS. Ototoxicity of ototopical drops—an update. Otolaryngol Clin North Am. 2007;40(3):669–683, xixi.
[51] Jinn TH, Kim PD, Russell PT, Church CA, John EO, Jung TT. Determination of ototoxicity of common otic drops using isolated cochlear outer hair cells. Laryngoscope. 2001;111(12):2105–2108.
[52] Berenholz LP, Rossi DL, Lippy WH, Burkey JM. Is there an ototoxicity risk from Cortisporin and comparable otic suspensions? Distortion-product otoacoustic emission findings. Ear Nose Throat J. 2012;91(3):106–135.
[53] Gates GA. Safety of ofloxacin otic and other ototopical treatments in animal models and in humans. Pediatr Infect Dis J. 2001;20(1):104–107, discussion 120–122.

6 Histopathology of Chronic Otitis Media

Sebahattin Cureoglu and Michael M. Paparella

Abbreviations used in this chapter:

AOM: acute otitis media
COM: chronic otitis media
PML: polymorphonuclear lymphocytes

6.1 Introduction

Otitis media is an inflammation of the middle ear cleft. It has been suggested that all types of otitis media represent different stages of a continuum of events, with the acute stage leading to a chronic stage.[1] In addition, one form of otitis media may resolve or lead to a more chronic stage of the disease. Although otitis media with effusion is characterized by the presence of a clear fluid in the middle ear cleft, there is no evidence of secretory cell proliferation at an earlier stage. Over time, the subepithelial space is widened by edema, vascular dilation, and the infiltration of host defense cells. With the reabsorption of watery components of the fluid, the increased density of goblet cells, and the formation of secretory glands, the middle ear effusion becomes mucoid and there are chronic inflammatory changes in the middle ear cleft.

Chronic otitis media (COM) has been clinically defined as a chronic discharge from the middle ear in the presence of a perforation of the tympanic membrane. Histopathologically, COM is defined when the inflammatory process has entered a chronic phase and permanent alteration of middle ear structures is seen (▶ Fig. 6.1; ▶ Fig. 6.2).[2] The pathologic changes in the tympanic membrane due to COM include perforation, retractions, myringosclerosis, pseudo-cystic spaces, and hemorrhage.[3]

The histopathological changes of the middle ear in COM are similar in the temporal bones with and without perforation of the tympanic membrane.[4] The most frequently encountered pathological tissues in the middle ear of patients with COM are granulation tissue; osteitis; fibrous thickening of the mucoperiosteum; fluid; cholesteatoma; and cholesterol granuloma;[2] with granulation tissue being the most common.[3]

Throughout the course of COM, osseous changes, including osteitis, necrosis, reabsorption, and osteoneogenesis, are occurring in the middle ear cleft (▶ Fig. 6.3).[2] The bony involvement parallels the severity of the inflammatory process. In the generalized form of active COM, although all three ossicles can show chronic changes, the incus is the most commonly involved, being followed in frequency by the stapes, and then the malleus.[2]

6.2 Chronic Silent Otitis Media

The clinical definition of COM that requires a tympanic membrane perforation and/or drainage from the middle ear excludes a large number of cases that show chronic pathologic changes in the middle ear cleft. Paparella, Schachern, and Cureogluintroduced the concept of chronic silent otitis media on the basis of histopathologic evidence of chronic infection in the middle ear

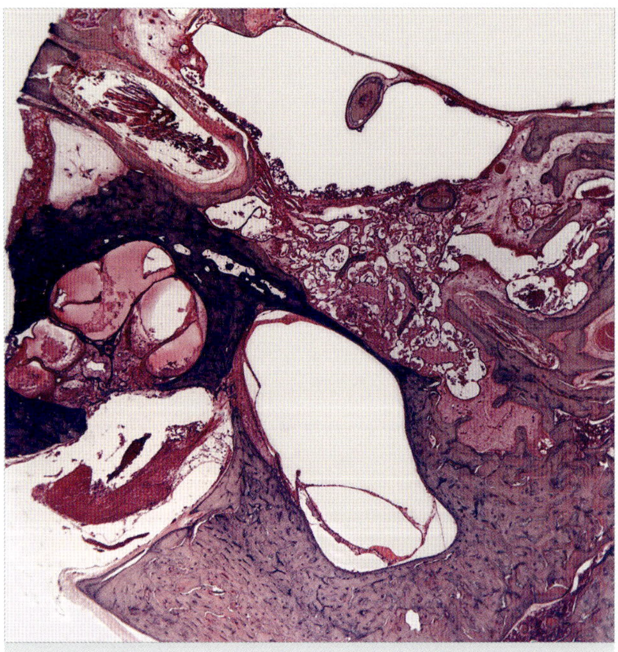

Fig. 6.1 This was an 18-month-old patient with chronic otitis media and seropurulent labyrinthitis. She had otogenic meningitis. Her right ear showed residual mesenchyme and chronic changes, including granulation tissue, fibrocystic changes, and cholesterol granuloma in the middle ear cleft. Note that the tympanic membrane was intact.

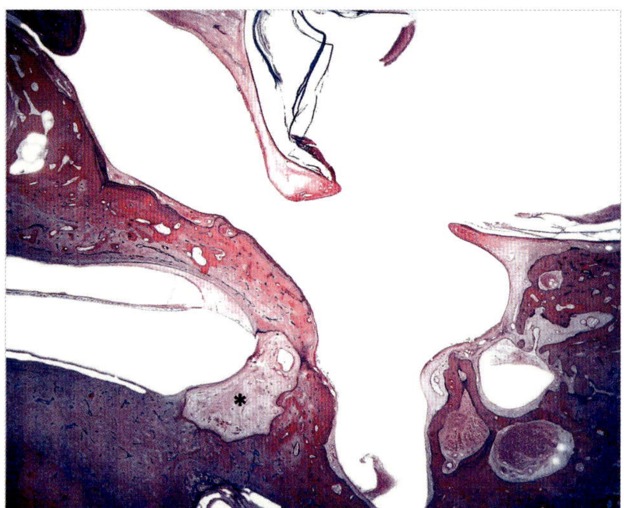

Fig. 6.2 This was an 82-year-old patient with a history of bilateral tympanic membrane perforation. Her right ear showed tympanosclerosis in the middle ear and tympanic membrane. The middle ear mucosa and subepithelial space were thickened. Granulation tissue was seen around the round window membrane (*).

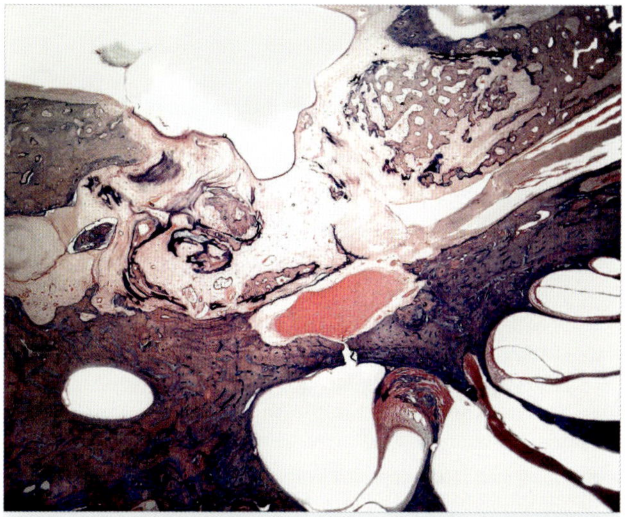

Fig. 6.3 This was a 75-year-old patient with a long history of chronic bilateral ear disease with frequent discharge since the age of 22 years. From age 72 years, he noticed episodic vertigo, which subsequently recurred. Histopathology evaluation showed chronic changes, such as ossicular erosion, new bone formation, and tympanosclerosis in the middle ear cavity.

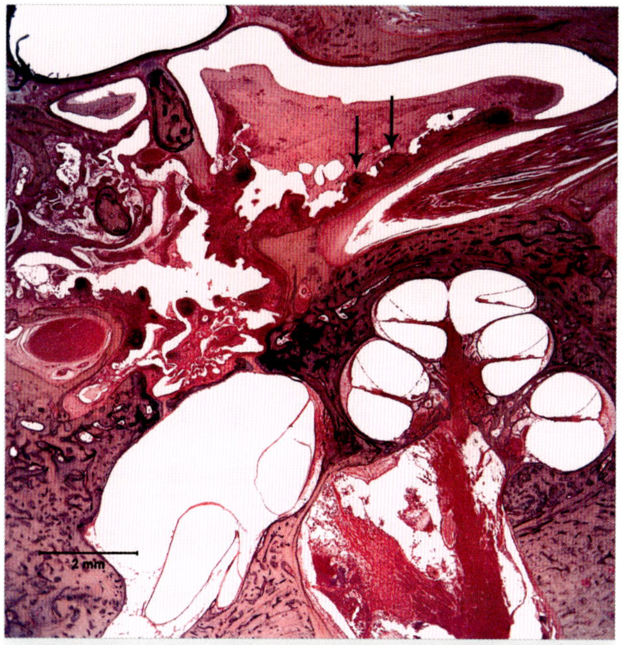

Fig. 6.4 This was a 10-month-old patient with otogenic meningitis. Histopathologic examination of his ears showed bilateral mucopurulent otitis media, polypoid middle ear mucosa (arrows), and purulent labyrinthitis. Fibrocystic changes can be seen in the facial recess and around the stapedial footplate. Note that the tympanic membrane is intact.

cleft in the absence of obvious ear-related symptoms and changes in the tympanic membrane (▶ Fig. 6.4).[5] In 1999, Jaisinghani, Paparella, Schachern, and Le studied 150 temporal bones from 97 patients with COM to correlate the presence of middle ear pathologies with the changes in the tympanic membrane.[3] Almost half of the temporal bones with middle ear pathology had no associated tympanic membrane pathology.

It has been stated that the incidence of COM associated with an intact tympanic membrane was four times more common than the incidence of COM with a perforated membrane.[5] In addition, the otopathological changes of the middle ear cleft in COM are similar in patients with and without perforation of the tympanic membrane.[5] In 1986, Paparella, Goycoolea, Bassiouni, and Koutroupas reported 10 temporal bones from 5 patients below the age of 2 years who died of *Hemophilus influenzae* meningitis.[6] None of the patients studied had documented clinical manifestations of any ear pathology before the onset of meningitis. Temporal bone findings included acute inflammatory disease as well as chronic pathologies such as granulation tissue, fibrosis, and mononuclear cell infiltration. These chronic irreversible pathologies in the middle ear and the presence of labyrinthitis in all cases indicated that the otitis media had been present for some time, suggesting meningitis of otogenic origin (▶ Fig. 6.5).

Because the chronic pathology is undetected, there is a lack of clinical treatment of otitis media, increasing the risk of complications due to the underlying problems (▶ Fig. 6.6).[5] As a result of the silent middle ear infection process, intratemporal problems, such as endolymphatic hydrops, labyrinthitis, facial palsy, and sensorineural hearing loss, and/or intracranial complications, such as meningitis or brain abscess, can be seen.[5,7] The clinician should, therefore, be aware that an intact tympanic membrane does not necessarily preclude the presence of pathologic changes in the middle ear cleft.

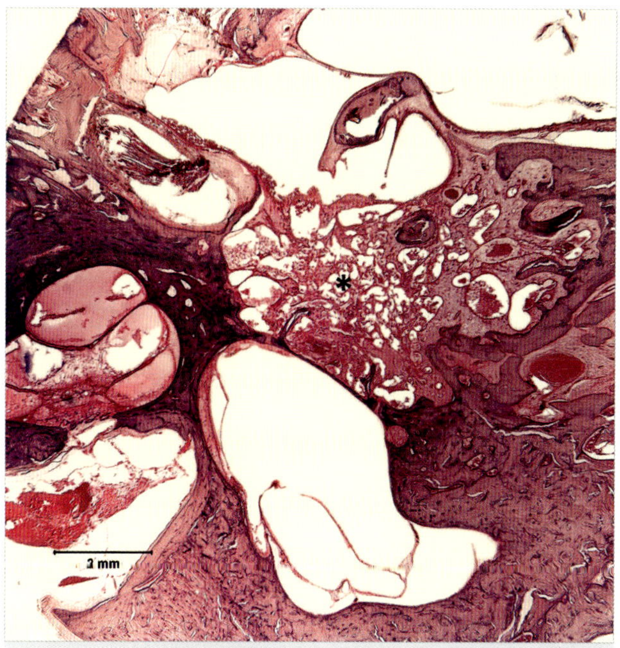

Fig. 6.5 This was an 18-month-old patient with otogenic meningitis. Histopathologic examination showed bilateral chronic otitis media with chronic changes, such as fibrocystic structures and granulation tissue as well as cholesterol granuloma in the middle ear cavity and seropurulent labyrinthitis (*).

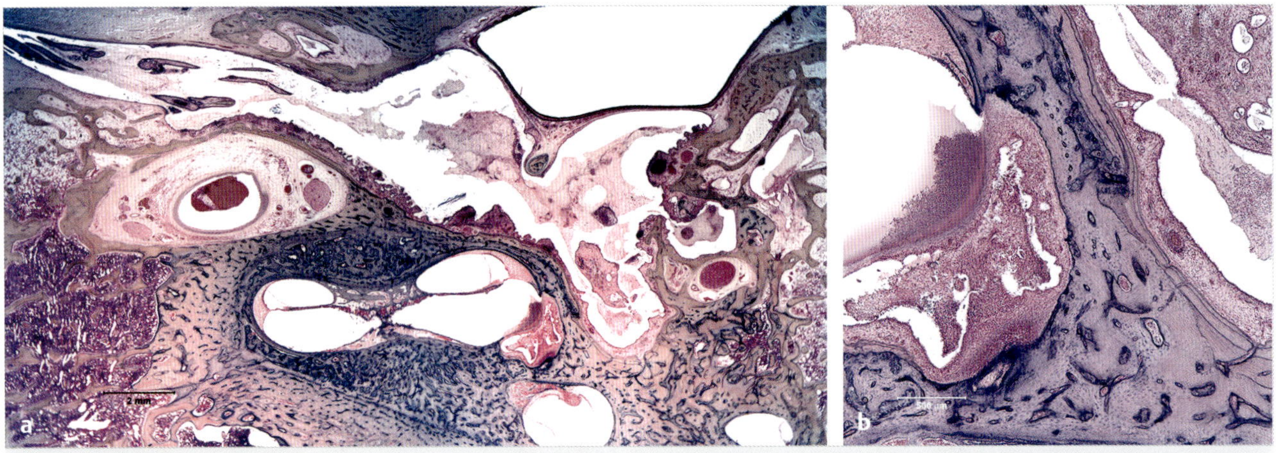

Fig. 6.6 (a) This was a 10-month-old patient with silent otitis media and otogenic meningitis. The tympanic membrane is intact. Histopathologic examination of his ears showed bilateral mucopurulent otitis media, polypoid middle ear mucosa, and purulent labyrinthitis. Note the presence of granulation tissue around the round window membrane. The mucopurulent secretions crossed the round window membrane into the scala tympani and the patient ended up with purulent labyrinthitis. (b) A higher magnification of the round window niche, which facilitates the accumulation of pus in the middle ear site (arrow).

6.3 Middle Ear/Inner Ear Interaction

The inner ear is intimately associated with the middle ear both functionally and anatomically. Functional changes of the middle ear mechanics affect the transmission of sound to the inner ear, whereas areas of anatomical connections allow for the passage of microorganisms, cytokines, toxins, or drugs from the middle to the inner ear, with potentially serious sequelae. The round window membrane, which is the only soft tissue barrier between the middle and inner ear and which lies within a niche and adjacent to the sinus tympani, facilitating the accumulation of pus, is vulnerable to toxic substances within the middle ear (▶ Fig. 6.6).

Inner ear sequelae that include labyrinthitis (▶ Fig. 6.1), endolymphatic hydrops (▶ Fig. 6.1),[8] outer hair cell losses, and as a result, sensorineural hearing loss and vestibular disturbances can occur in both acute otitis media (AOM) and COM.[9,10] In addition, a high-frequency sensorineural hearing loss can be clinically significant in cases of COM given that this denotes perilymphatic inflammation. The basal turn of the cochlea is the most common location of the pathologic changes in the inner ear during this middle ear interaction (▶ Fig. 6.7). This results in a temporary threshold shift, which may become permanent over time. Cureoglu et al showed loss of outer and inner hair cells, especially in the basal turn of the cochlea, and a decrease in the areas of the stria vascularis and spiral ligament in the basal turn of the cochlea of temporal bones with unilateral COM.[11]

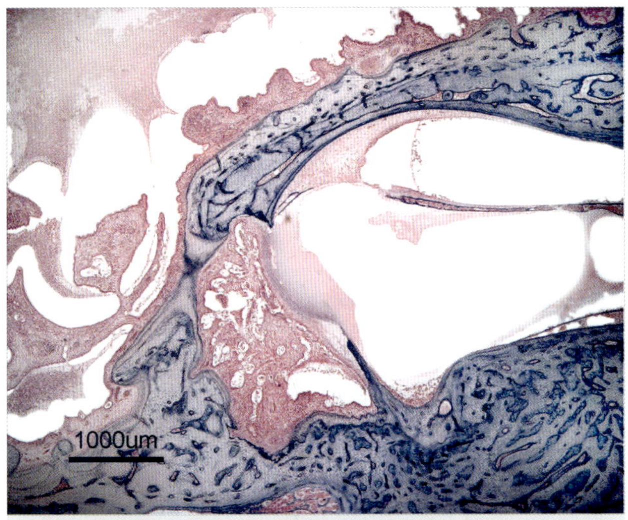

Fig. 6.7 This was another case involving a 10-month-old patient with otogenic meningitis. His left ear showed mucopurulent otitis media with polypoid middle ear mucosa as well as purulent labyrinthitis. Note that the basal turn of the cochlea is the most common location for pathologic changes in the inner ear during middle ear/inner ear interactions.

6.3.1 Serous (Toxic) Labyrinthitis

This is characterized by sensorineural hearing loss and vertigo that usually shows partial or complete recovery. It is usually a reaction to exotoxins rather than actual bacterial invasion (▶ Fig. 6.6).[12] The presence of vertigo in a patient with otitis media may indicate the presence of serous labyrinthitis. If it is diagnosed and treated before suppuration starts, the damage in the inner ear will be reversible. The histopathological markers of serous labyrinthitis can be described as endolymphatic hydrops, eosinophilic fluid staining due to increased proteinaceous content, and sero-fibrinous strands in the labyrinthine spaces without any associated host inflammatory cell invasion.[13]

6.3.2 Circumscribed (Localized) Labyrinthitis

The most common underlying problem of circumscribed labyrinthitis is cholesteatoma erosion. The erosion makes the membranous labyrinth sensitive to environmental changes such as temperature or pressure. The inflammation is localized to a bony surface of the labyrinth without the invasion of endosteum. If the patient starts to have sensorineural hearing loss in addition to a positional vertigo, treatment should be initiated for serous labyrinthitis to prevent suppurative labyrinthitis.

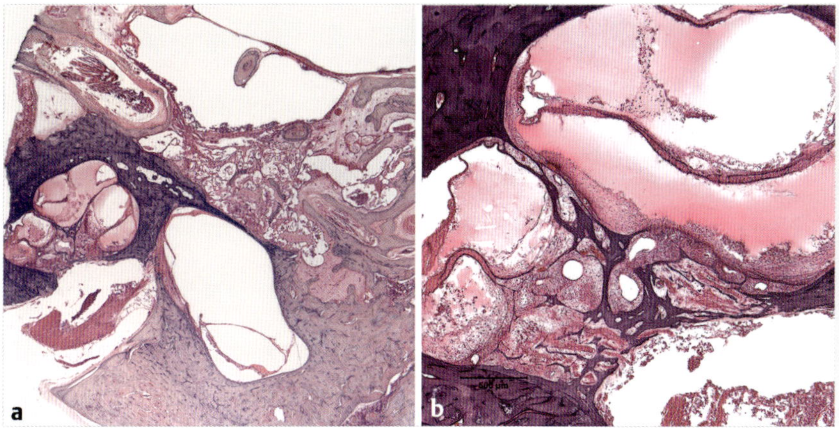

Fig. 6.8 (a) This was an 18-month-old patient with chronic otitis media. She had otogenic meningitis. Her right ear showed residual mesenchyme and chronic changes, including fibrocystic changes and cholesterol granuloma in the middle ear cleft. (b) A higher magnification of the inner ear showing seropurulent labyrinthitis and inner ear damage.

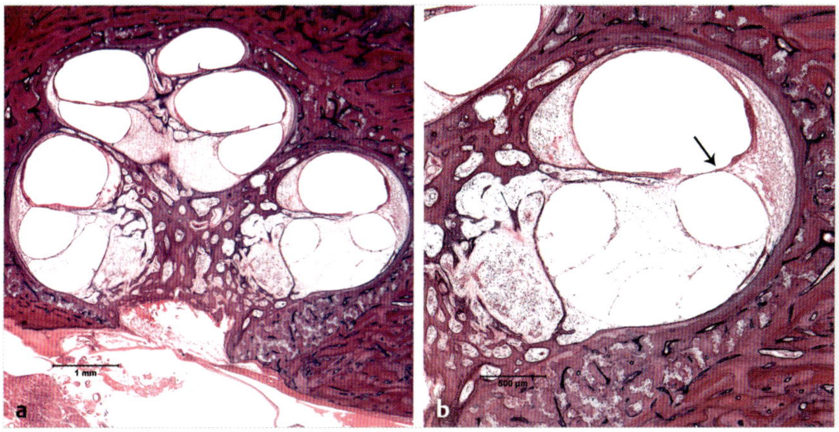

Fig. 6.9 (a) This was a 29-year-old patient with a diagnosis of acute leukemia. He had a history of dizziness and fluctuant hearing loss. Histopathologic exam showed bilateral fibrous labyrinthitis and profound endolymphatic hydrops. (b) A higher magnification of the basal turn of the cochlea showing severe organ of Corti damage, hair cell losses, reduced ganglion cells, and stria vascularis atrophy (arrow).

6.3.3 Suppurative Labyrinthitis

Hispathologically, suppurative labyrinthitis (▶ Fig. 6.8) has three stages; however, any intracranial complication may occur at any stage, and the patient may end up with a complete loss of labyrinthine functions.[14]

During the first stage, purulent effusion fills the perilymphatic spaces but spares the endolymph. The main symptoms are severe vertigo and hearing loss at this stage.

During the second stage, polymorphonuclear lymphocytes (PMLs) dominate in the area with fibrillar precipitates, especially in the perilymphatic space (▶ Fig. 6.9). Endolymphatic hydrops is also seen. This stage begins around 2 weeks after the onset of infection. Although vertigo subsides, sensorineural hearing loss progresses.

The third stage represents chronic labyrinthitis: fibroblasts predominate and small capillaries occur as a result of increased angiogenesis. Eventually osteogenesis may occur (in an animal model, around 2 months). After being stimulated by infection or inflammatory irritation following breakdown of cells, mesenchymal cells, which are located around capillaries, the undersurface of the basilar membrane, and endosteum that lines the perilymphatic space, rapidly differentiate into fibroblasts that produce collagen fibers, endothelial cells that form capillaries, and osteoblasts. The osteoblasts form trabeculae (lamellar or spongy bone) that join together and incorporate small blood vessels within them. Then, haversian canals form from the condensation of lamellar bone, which could be difficult to distinguish from the normal bone around it. Pathologic new bone formation within the otic capsule in response to inflammatory and/or destructive processes is called labyrinthine ossificans, which represents the terminal stage of repair of labyrinthitis. At early stages, only scala tympani of the basal turn of the cochlea is involved. Later, all parts of the inner ear are involved. In humans, it may take years to have a complete labyrinthitis ossificans (▶ Fig. 6.10; ▶ Fig. 6.11; ▶ Fig. 6.12).

6.4 Pathological Changes in the Middle Ear Cleft in COM

6.4.1 Granulation Tissue

Granulation tissue is the most common pathology encountered in chronic ears. It consists of vascularized connective tissue with a component of acute inflammatory exudation. The most common sites for granulation tissue are the epitympanum, mesotympanum, round window niche, and mastoid antrum (▶ Fig. 6.13).[2,3,5] During the formation of granulation tissue, the mucous membrane is thickened by edema, submucosal fibrosis, and infiltration with chronic inflammatory cells. Later, mucosal edema may progress to the formation of polyps.[1] With maturation, granulation tissue becomes more fibrous and less cellular, with increased collagen and reticular formation.[2] Granulation tissue may lead to adhesions or tympanosclerosis in the middle ear.[1] This activity, if unchecked, may lead to serious complications, including the destruction of the inner ear.

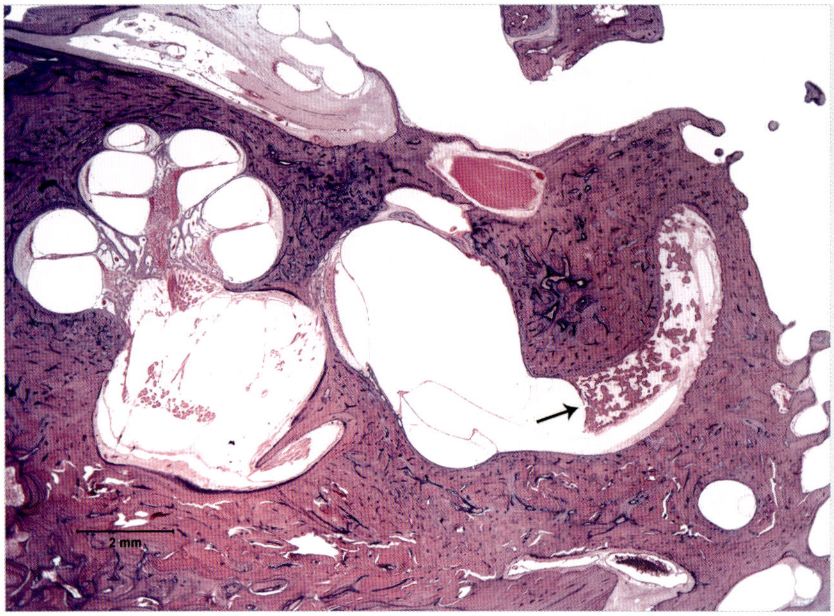

Fig. 6.10 This was a 49-year-old patient with acute leukemia. Histopathologic examination of her ears showed labyrinthitis ossificans in the lateral semicircular canal (arrow) and hydropic changes in the inner ear.

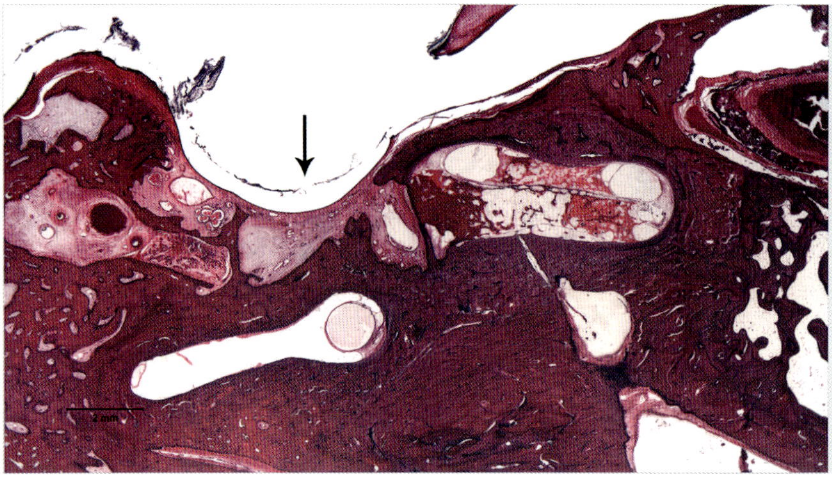

Fig. 6.11 This was a 74-year-old patient with a history of chronic otitis media dating back to childhood. At age 36 years, he experienced dizziness and total deafness in the right ear. He had a canal wall-down mastoidectomy (arrow) in both ears. At age 50 years, reactivation of chronic otitis media in his left ear occurred and caused vertiginous spells. In this section, labyrinthitis ossificans in the basal turn of the cochlea and granulation tissue at the round window niche can be clearly seen.

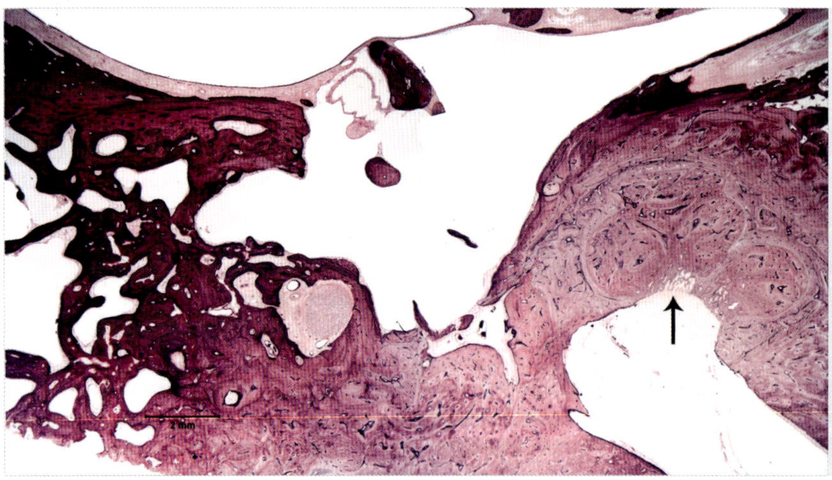

Fig. 6.12 This was a patient with recurrent episodes of chronic suppurative otitis media. Note the complete ossification of the cochlea (arrow).

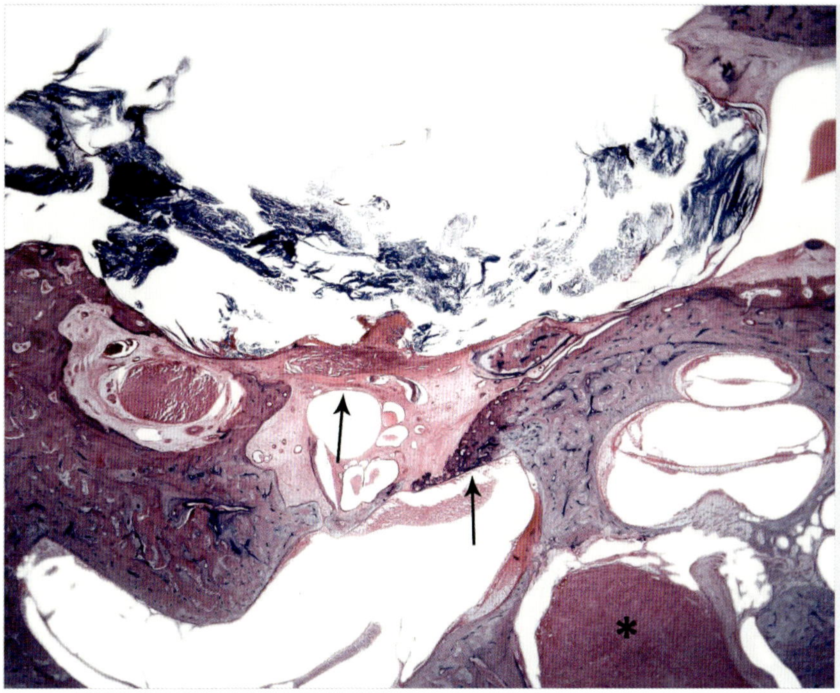

Fig. 6.13 This was an 86-year-old patient with a history of congenital deafness. Histopathologic examination showed bilateral chronic otitis media and cholesteatoma. The left ear showed granulation tissue, cholesterol granuloma, tympanosclerosis, otosclerosis (arrow), acoustic neuroma (*), and serous labyrinthitis.

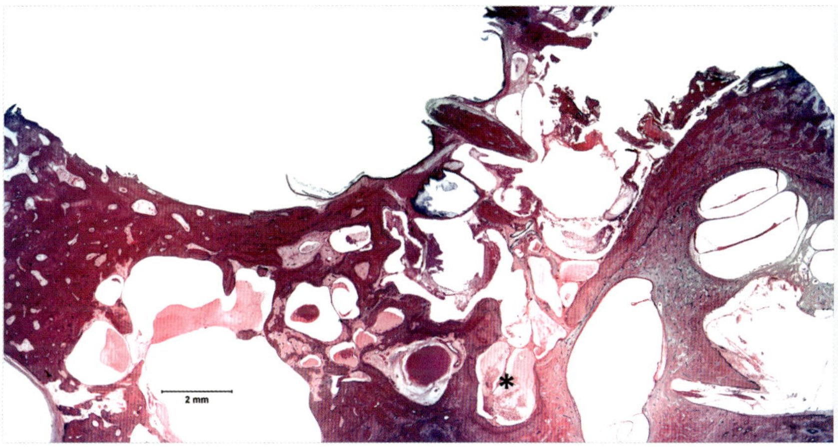

Fig. 6.14 This was an 83-year-old patient with carcinoma of the bladder. He had a history of bilateral decreased hearing beginning at the age of 60 years. Histopathologic examination showed bilateral chronic otitis media and cholesteatoma. His left ear showed chronic changes and cholesteatoma with seropurulent secretion in the mesotympanum and sinus tympani in the middle ear (*).

6.4.2 Cholesteatoma

Cholesteatoma can be described as a keratinized squamous epithelium in the middle ear cleft (▶ Fig. 6.14). It is classified as congenital or acquired based on its presumed etiology. The pathogenesis of cholesteatoma, outlined in Chapter 4, is multifactorial.

With acquired cholesteatoma, the pathogenesis is unclear and remains controversial. The most accepted theory is the invagination theory (also known as the retraction pocket theory) (▶ Fig. 6.15). Eustachian tube dysfunction creates negative pressure and causes loss of structural support for the tympanic membrane; eventually atelectasis results in retraction pockets (▶ Fig. 6.16). Keratin accumulates within these pockets and progresses to cholesteatoma (▶ Fig. 6.17).

Another commonly known theory is the epithelial invasion theory (also called the immigration theory) (▶ Fig. 6.18): there is an invasion of squamous epithelium into the middle ear cleft from the external auditory canal or tympanic membrane through a perforation, and subsequently that forms a cholesteatoma. In instances with lack of infection, the exfoliation rate is very slow; however, in the presence of infection, exfoliation grows rapidly and has a tendency to cause complications, potentially resulting in a smooth radical mastoidectomy cavity combining middle ear and mastoid cavities into one space (▶ Fig. 6.19).

Cholesteatoma may cause the erosion of the bone by two mechanisms: pressure exerted by the cholesteatoma mass or enzymatic activity. Even after a radical cleaning of cholesteatoma during surgery, residual cholesteatoma can occur in 7% to 50% of cases.[15,16] Residual cholesteatoma can be found in inaccessible areas, such as around the arch of the stapes, the sinus tympani, oval window area, retrolabyrinthine, and the perifacial regions.[17] Therefore, the removal of all accessible mastoid air cells and the pathologic tissue hidden in the inaccessible areas are necessary for reliable eradication of cholesteatoma. It has also been noted that many innocent-looking mucosal changes at a considerable distance from cholesteatoma can contain squamous epithelium (▶ Fig. 6.20).[18]

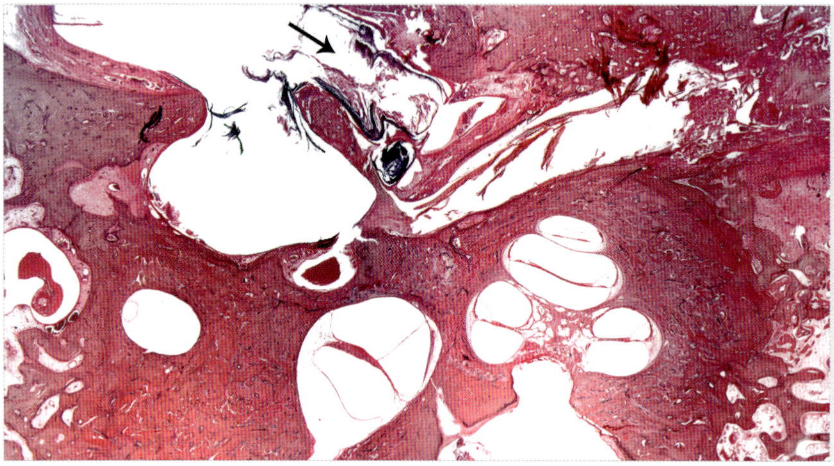

Fig. 6.15 This was a 50-year-old patient with metastatic carcinoma of the breast. Histopathologic examination of the ears showed bilateral chronic otitis media. The left ear showed chronic changes, including cholesteatoma, cholesterol granuloma, and a perforated tympanic membrane. Note the complete retraction of the tympanic membrane into the middle ear cavity and the accumulation of cholesteatoma in the anterior part of the retraction as well as a cholesteatoma mass in the anterior middle ear cavity (arrow).

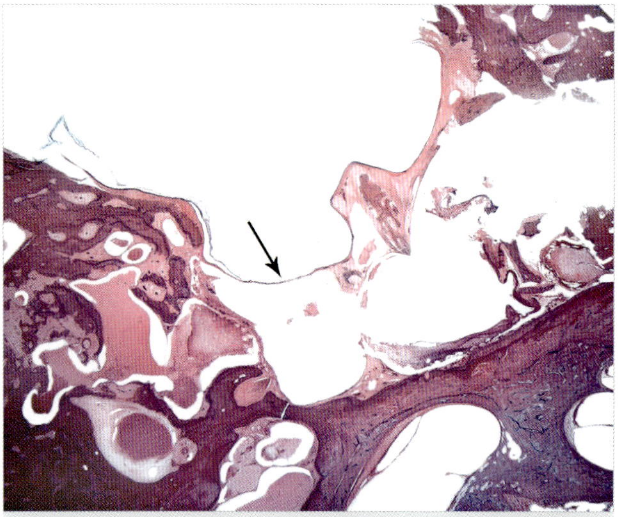

Fig. 6.16 This was an 83-year-old patient with carcinoma of the bladder. He had a history of bilateral decreased hearing that started at the age of 60 years. Histopathologic examination showed bilateral chronic otitis media and cholesteatoma. His left ear showed chronic changes, such as granulation tissue in the facial recess as well as seropurulent secretion in the middle ear. Note the posterior–superior quadrant of the tympanic membrane, which is also atrophied, is retracted into the middle ear cavity (arrow).

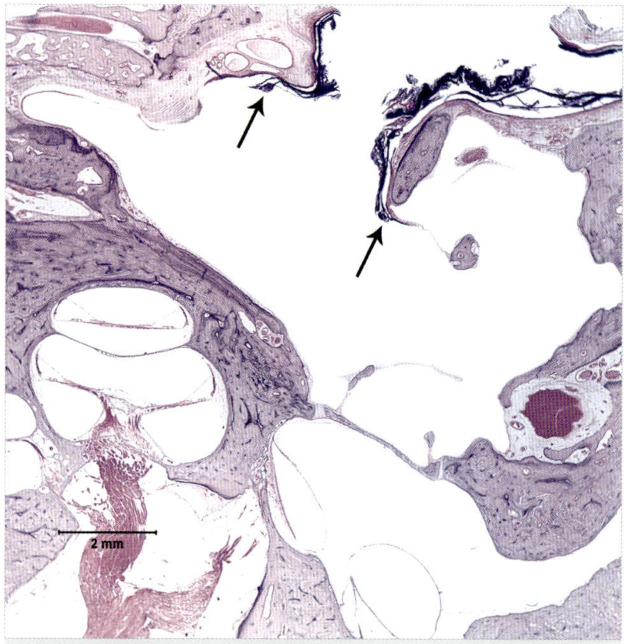

Fig. 6.18 This was an 88-year-old patient. The right ear showed attic cholesteatoma, tympanosclerosis in the middle ear, and an anterior perforation in the tympanic membrane. Note the invasion of squamous epithelium into the middle ear through the perforation (arrows).

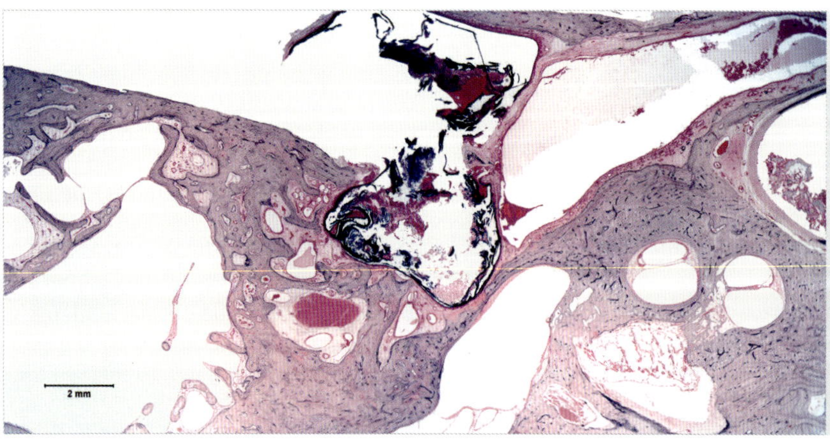

Fig. 6.17 This was a 64-year-old patient with acute bacterial meningitis. Histopathologic examination showed bilateral chronic otitis media. The left ear showed retraction of the posterior quadrants of the tympanic membrane and cholesteatoma. The middle ear showed chronic changes, including a glandular subepithelial space, tympanosclerosis, and granulation tissue around the facial recess and sinus tympani.

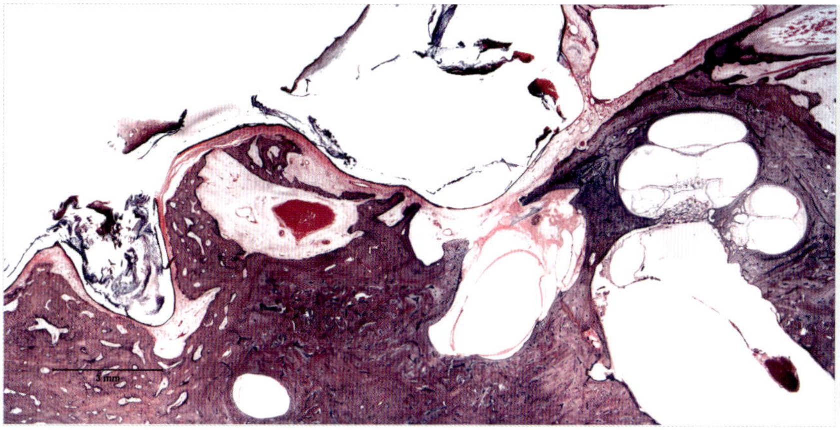

Fig. 6.19 This was a 74-year-old patient with a history of chronic otitis media dating back to childhood. Note that cholesteatoma caused a smooth radical cavity combining the middle ear and mastoid cavities into one. Note the significant damage in the inner ear, including fibrous changes, severe organ of Corti damage, and cochlear lateral wall atrophy.

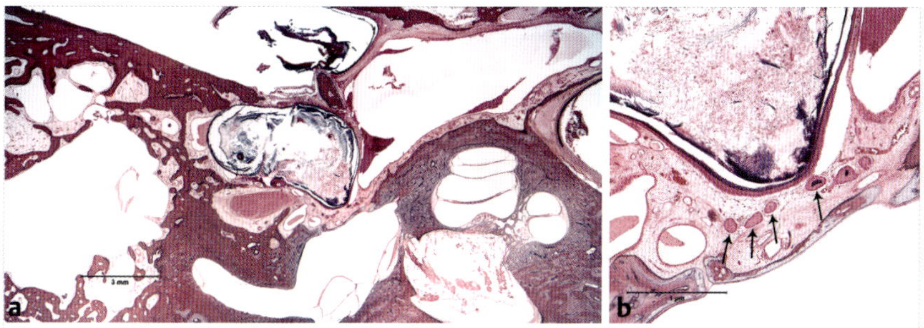

Fig. 6.20 (a) This was a 64-year-old patient with acute bacterial meningitis. Histopathologic examination showed bilateral chronic otitis media. The left ear showed chronic changes in the middle ear, including cholesteatoma located between the tympanic membrane and stapedial footplate. Note the glandular subepithelial space, tympanosclerosis, and granulation tissue around the round window niche. (b) A higher magnification of the footplate area shows small multiple cholesteatoma pearls located in the subepithelial space (arrows).

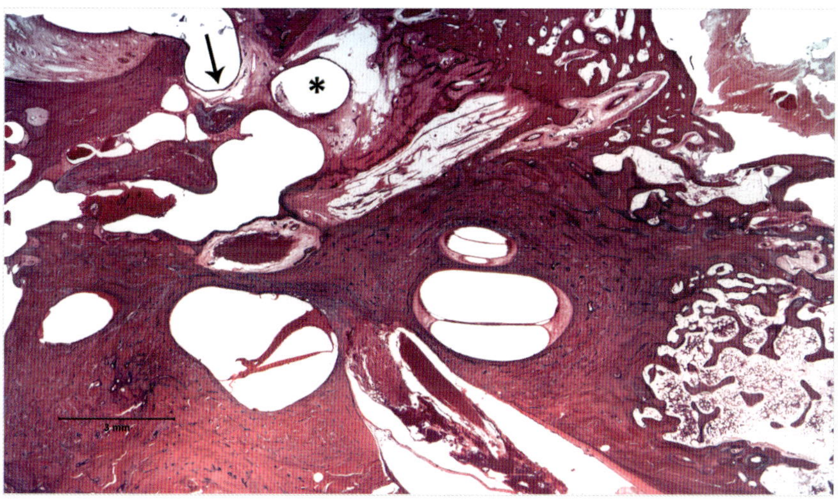

Fig. 6.21 This was a 54-year-old patient who died of hypnotic drug overdose. Histopathologic examination of the left ear showed the retraction of the pars flaccida (arrow), a pathology associated with fibrocystic changes, and granulation tissue in the attic and mesotympanum (*).

6.4.3 Atelectasis

Medial retraction of all or part of the tympanic membrane is known as atelectasis. It appears that a multifactorial imbalance in the middle ear pressure due to long-standing Eustachian tube dysfunction and/or dysregulation of middle ear gas diffusion may lead to the atelectatic state. This imbalance in the middle ear pressure may be caused by obstruction at different sites in the middle ear cleft.[19] Histopathologic evidence of obstruction in the tympanic isthmus was seen in most of the temporal bones with retraction pockets. The tympanic isthmus is the route by which air reaches the epitympanum. As a result, the tympanic membrane starts to be compressed at its weakest point, such as the pars flaccida or posterior-superior quadrant. The posterior aspect of the pars tensa is more prone to retraction than other parts of the pars tensa.[20] This may correspond with the difference between mucosa in the anterior and posterior aspects of the middle ear.[21] Anteriorly, the middle ear mucosa is dominated by pseudostratified ciliated cells, whereas the posterior middle ear is covered by flat cells.[22] The anterior mucosa is covered by a thick epithelial lining covered with mucus, whereas posteriorly the lack of cilia on the flat cells may lead to stagnation of inflammatory exudate.

Retractions of the pars flaccida tend to occur in conjunction with pars tensa pathology (▶ Fig. 6.21). Tos and Poulsen studied

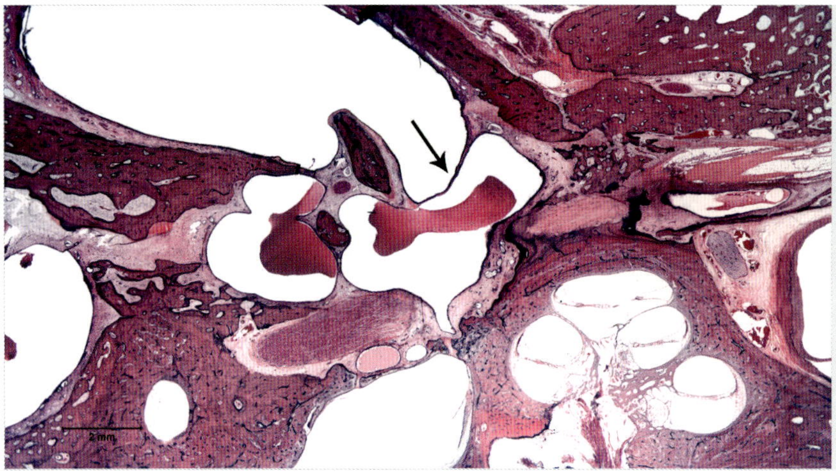

Fig. 6.22 This was an 84-year-old patient who died of pulmonary disease. Histopathologic examination of the left ear showed chronic changes, including tympanosclerosis, ossicular erosion, and mucopurulent secretion in the middle ear in addition to a retracted tympanic membrane (arrow).

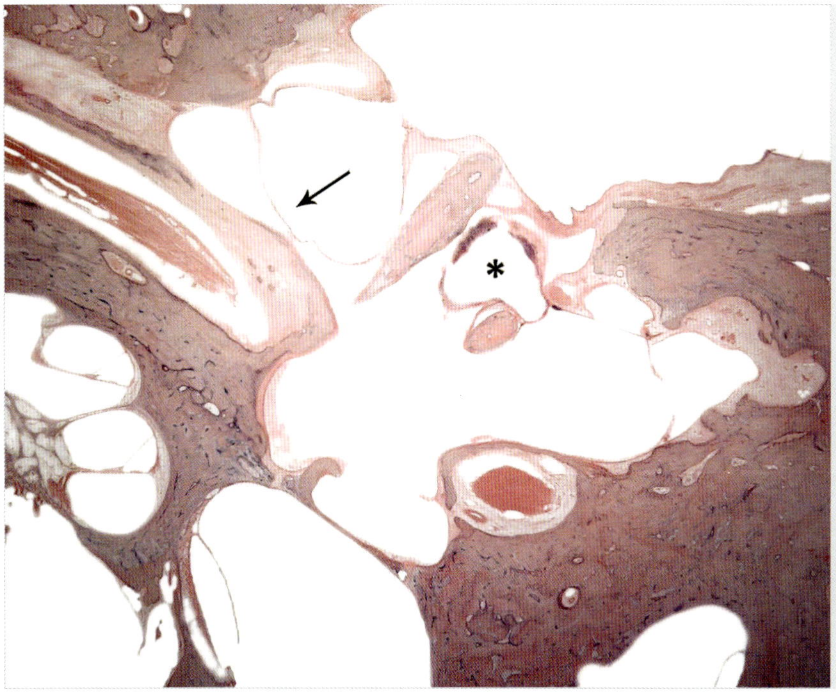

Fig. 6.23 This was a 50-year-old patient with metastatic carcinoma of the breast. Histopathologic examination of the ears showed bilateral chronic otitis media. The right ear showed retraction of the anterior tympanic membrane (arrow) as well as a cholesteatoma cyst (*) posteriorly located in the mesotympanum.

527 children under the age of 13 years who had undergone pressure equalizing tube insertion.[23] They found that in patients with a normal pars tensa, there were fewer retraction pockets in the pars flaccida. In 78% of ears with retractions of the pars flaccida, pathology of the pars tensa was present, which included atrophy, retraction, and tympanosclerosis. When mild retraction of the pars tensa was seen (Sade grade 1; ▸ Fig. 6.22), Shrapnell's membrane retraction was also seen in 74% of the ears. If Sade grade 2 retraction (▸ Fig. 6.23) was present (pars tensa adherent to the ossicles), 88% of the ears also showed pars flaccida retraction. There was a strong correlation between the degree of pars tensa disease and that of the pars flaccida.

The most common pathologies in temporal bones with retraction pockets include middle ear fluid, atrophy of the tympanic membrane, thickening of the mucoperiosteum, and cholesteatoma (▸ Fig. 6.24; ▸ Fig. 6.25). It has been shown that middle ear effusions have high concentrations of proteinases, especially collagenases.[24] The prolonged impact of these enzymes on that aspect of the tympanic membrane may cause the destruction in the collagenous layer of the tympanic membrane and resultant weakening.[21] Ruah, Schachern, Paparella, and Zelterman stated that the damage to the fibrous layer of the pars tensa was much greater in purulent otitis media than in the serous type.[25] This is most likely due to the increased neutrophilic infiltration and enzymatic content of the middle ear fluid in purulent otitis media compared with serous otitis media. The tympanic membrane becomes very thin, losing its lamina propria, the collagen-containing middle layer of the membrane (▸ Fig. 6.26).

6.4.4 Cholesterol Granuloma

Cholesterol granuloma is a foreign-body response to cholesterol crystals (▸ Fig. 6.27; ▸ Fig. 6.28). Microscopic evaluation shows cholesterol crystals surrounded by foreign body giant cells embedded in fibrous connective tissue,[26] with inflammatory cell infiltration and blood vessels. Erythrocytes and

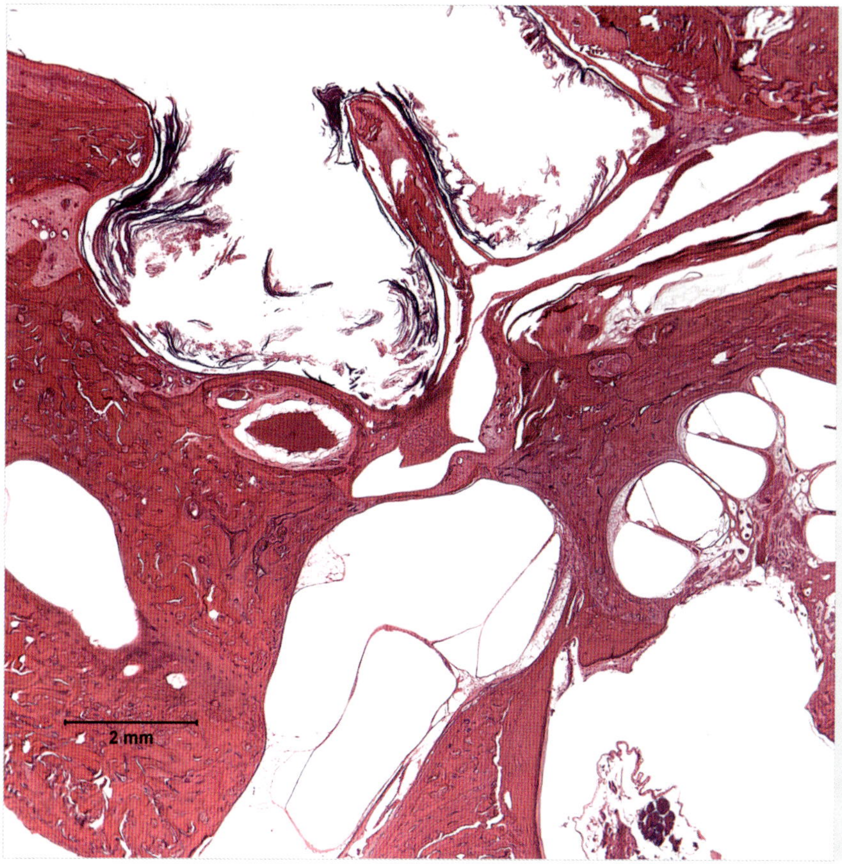

Fig. 6.24 This was a 50-year-old patient with bilateral chronic otitis media. The left ear showed severe retraction of the tympanic membrane. Note that the tympanic membrane is atrophied, the middle ear mucosa is thickened, and there is cholesteatoma formation in the retraction pockets.

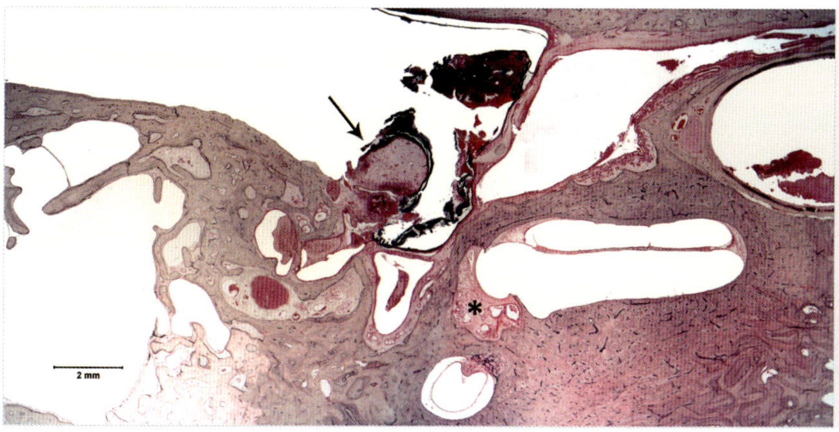

Fig. 6.25 This was a 64-year-old patient with bilateral chronic otitis media. The left ear showed a retracted tympanic membrane and chronic changes in the middle ear, including a glandular subepithelial space, middle ear polyp (arrow), tympanosclerosis, granulation tissue (*) around the round window niche, and cholesteatoma.

hemosiderin-laden macrophages are constant elements in the formation of cholesterol granuloma. Due to its pathogenesis, the most important factors of which are hemorrhage, impaired drainage, and ventilation blockage, cholesterol granuloma may also develop in cases of acute hemorrhagic otitis. Once ventilation to a bony space is blocked, negative pressure builds, with resultant transudation of blood. Regarding petrous apex cholesterol granuloma, it is possible that the sustained hemorrhage derived from exposed marrow elements is responsible for the progressive cyst expansion.

Cholesterol granuloma can be found in 12% to 20% of human temporal bones with COM. It can occur in any pneumatized bone in the body, in addition to the middle ear, petrous apex, and cerebellopontine angle, and can cause expansile changes in surrounding structures.[27,28] The locations where cholesterol granulomas develop have been confined to small, hollow, enclosed cavities, such as mastoid or petrous apex air cells, the facial recess, the oval window, and the round window niche.

Cholesterol granuloma may occur in isolation, without any previous history of infection.[29,30] This lesion is often called idiopathic hemotympanum in cases of middle ear cleft involvement and frequently coexists with cholesteatoma,[31] retraction, any type of COM, and COM with effusion.[32,33] The effusion in patients with cholesterol granuloma is mostly mucoid, suggesting a long-standing negative pressure in the middle ear cleft.

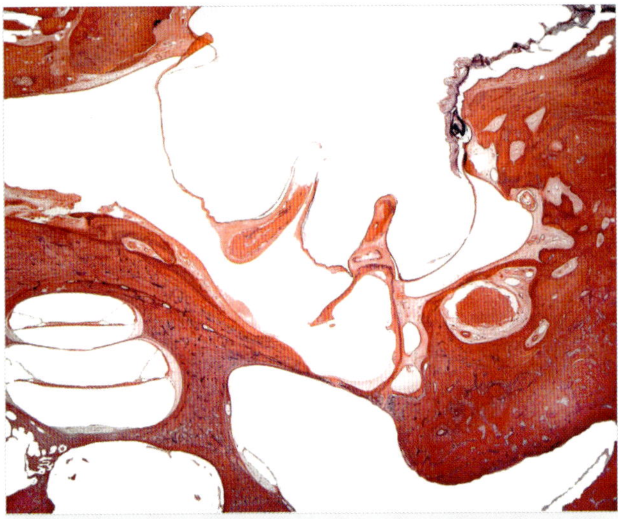

Fig. 6.26 This was a 50-year-old patient with metastatic carcinoma of the breast. Histopathologic examination of the ears showed bilateral chronic otitis media. The right ear showed chronic changes in the middle ear and a retracted tympanic membrane. Note that the tympanic membrane has lost its lamina propria and is very thin as a result.

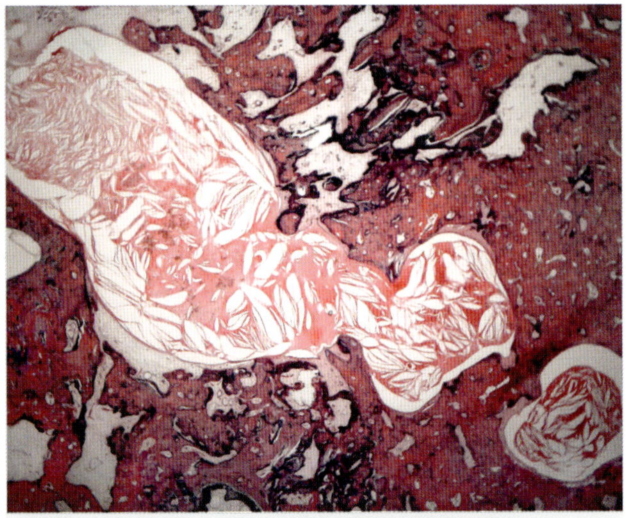

Fig. 6.27 This was a 73-year-old patient with chronic myeloid leukemia. Note the presence of a cholesterol granuloma in the mastoid region.

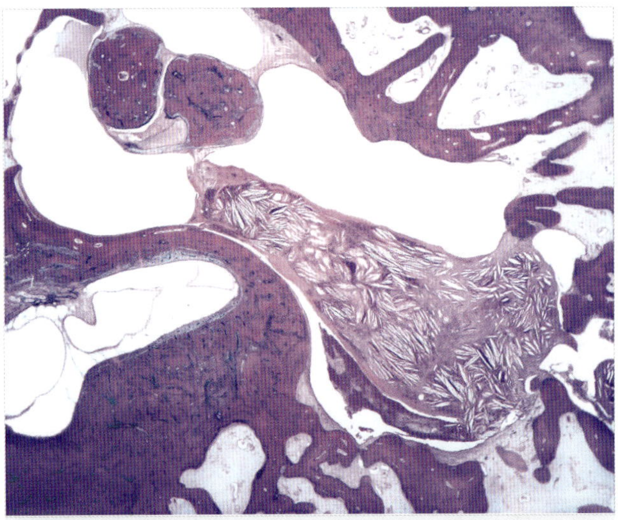

Fig. 6.28 Another asymptomatic cholesterol granuloma located at the aditus ad antrum is seen in the same patient as in ► Fig. 6.27.

Clinically, cholesterol granuloma is most often considered a harmless phenomenon found during surgery or pathologic studies. In rare cases, however, the slowly growing tumor becomes symptomatic. If it is associated with other middle ear diseases, such as cholesteatoma or otitis media with effusion, symptoms and signs become more obvious.

6.4.5 Biofilms

Biofilms are structured communities of microorganisms embedded in an extrapolysaccharide matrix.[34] Biofilms enhance the ability of microbes to evade host defenses and antibiotic medications.[35,36] Organisms causing otitis media, such as *Haemophilus influenzae, Streptococcus pneumoniae,* and *Pseudomonas aeruginosa,* have been shown to form biofilms.[37,38] Recent studies have shown that biofilms may be an important part of the pathology and pathophysiology of otitis media.[39,40] Increasing evidence indicates that bacterial biofilms play a role in chronic infections, and it has been proposed that biofilms are important in the establishment of COM that is resistant to medications and for which surgical intervention is often required (► Fig. 6.29).[41,42]

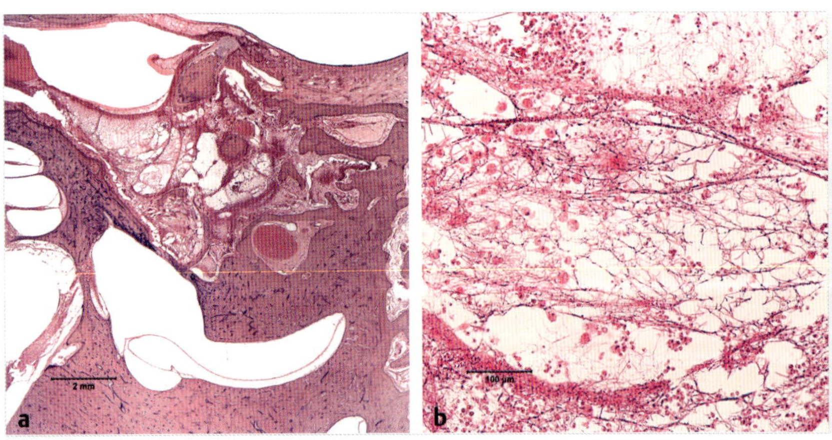

Fig. 6.29 (a) This was a 24-year-old patient who died of subdural hemorrhage and chronic myeloid leukemia. Histopathologic examination showed an intact tympanic membrane and chronic changes in the middle ear as well as bilateral otomycosis in the middle ear and tympanic membrane. (b) Higher magnification of the middle ear effusion shows bacterial communities within the extracellular matrix in the middle ear. The effusion is covered by round host cells and polymorphonuclear cells.

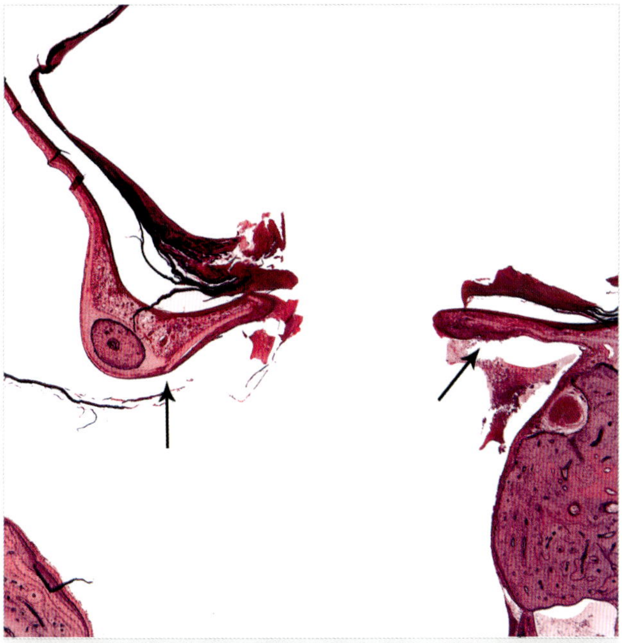

Fig. 6.30 This was a 64-year-old patient with a history of oropharyngeal carcinoma, bilateral pressure equalizing tube insertion, and radiation to the head and neck. Histopathologic examination showed bilateral central tympanic membrane perforations. Note the invasion of keratinized squamous epithelium into the middle ear through the perforation (arrows).

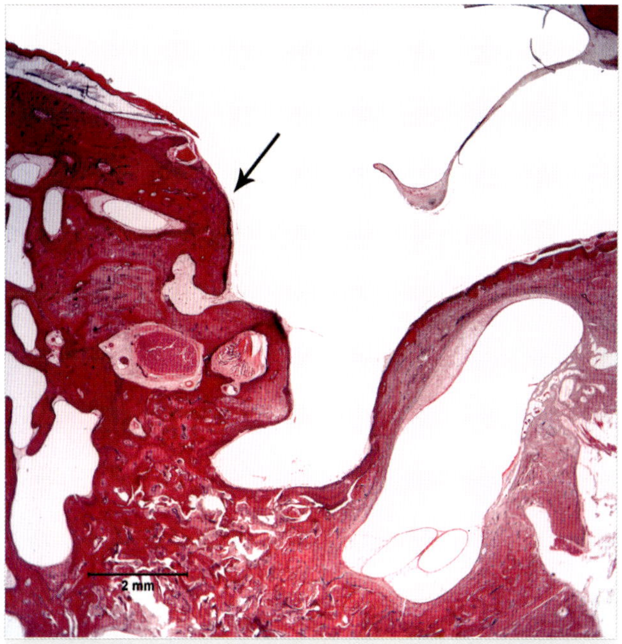

Fig. 6.31 This was a 66-year-old patient with a history of metastatic carcinoma of the ovaries, bilateral decreased hearing, and tinnitus. Histopathologic examination showed bilateral chronic otitis media. The left ear showed tympanosclerosis and marginal tympanic membrane perforation (arrow).

6.5 Tympanic Membrane Pathologies

6.5.1 Perforations

Conductive hearing loss due to tympanic membrane perforation involves mostly low frequencies; hearing loss increases with the size of the perforation but has no association with the location of the perforation (▶ Fig. 6.30).[43]

A central perforation, regardless of size, is a perforation in the pars tensa of the tympanic membrane. There is still a remnant of the tympanic membrane at all borders (▶ Fig. 6.30). A marginal perforation is a defect in the tympanic annulus (▶ Fig. 6.31). An attic perforation is located in the pars flaccida of the tympanic membrane.

6.5.2 Mucocutaneous Junction of the Perforation

The point of division between keratinized squamous epithelium and middle ear mucosa, in the presence of a perforation, is termed the mucocutaneous junction. In the presense of secondary acquired cholesteatoma, this junction is located within the middle ear cleft and may occur in marginal, attic, and even in central perforations (▶ Fig. 6.30). During surgery, the surgeon should look at the velvety appearance of the squamous epithelium to determine the location of the junction (▶ Fig. 6.18). Otherwise, iatrogenic cholesteatoma could occur.

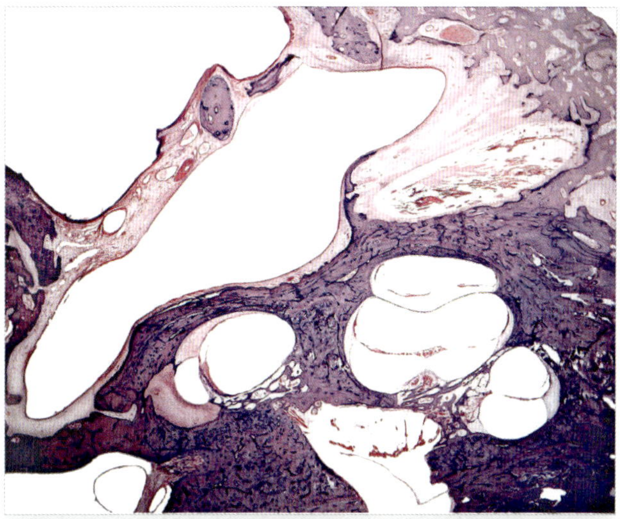

Fig. 6.32 This was a 51-year-old patient with metastatic carcinoma of the stomach. She had a history of a left canal wall-down mastoidectomy due to chronic mastoiditis at age 20 years. The tympanic membrane is intact and very thick, with hyalinization and fibrocystic changes. The middle ear mucosa is thickened. Granulation tissue is located around the round window niche. Note the Organ of Corti is damaged in all turns of the cochlea.

6.5.3 Dimeric Membrane

During the healing process of a tympanic membrane perforation, the thickness of the membrane will be determined by the fibrous tissue proliferation in the intermediate layer. If the proliferation of the fibrous tissue is abundant, a very thickened tympanic membrane will occur (▶ Fig. 6.32); otherwise, if the

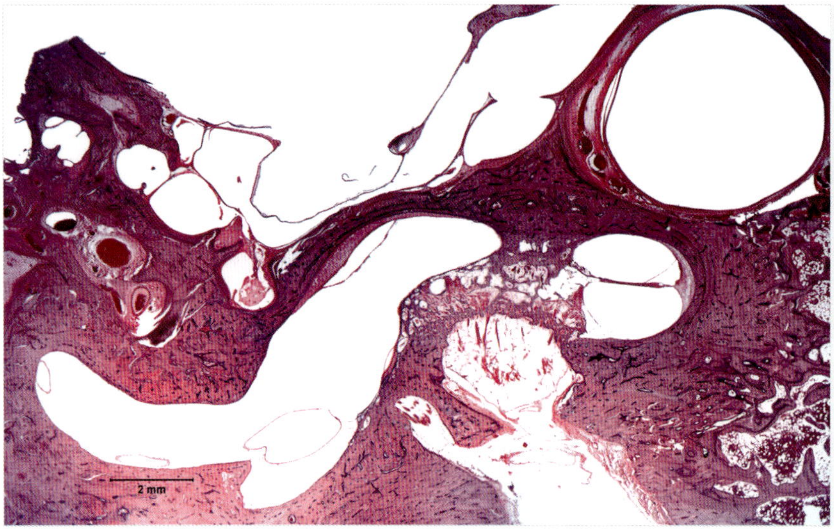

Fig. 6.33 This was a patient with chronic otitis media. The tympanic membrane is atrophied and retracted. Granulation tissue is seen in the middle ear and mastoid.

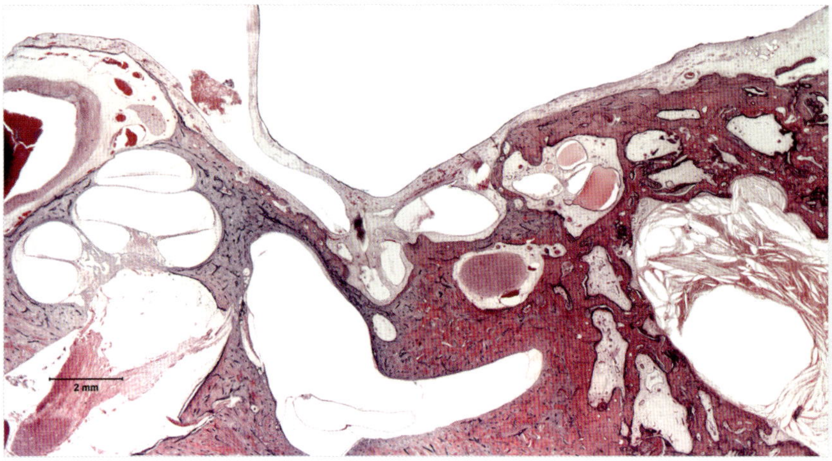

Fig. 6.34 This was a 73-year-old patient with chronic myeloid leukemia. He had a history of positional vertigo and acoustic trauma. Histopathologic examination showed bilateral chronic otitis media. The tympanic membrane is thickened and retracted. There are some fibrocystic structures and tympanosclerosis as well as granulation tissue in the middle ear and mastoid. The carotid artery was dehiscent and communicated with the cochlea in the right ear. There is a large cholesterol granuloma located in the mastoid antrum.

proliferation fails, there will be no fibrous layer in between the squamous and mucous membranes, which is called a dimeric membrane (▶ Fig. 6.33). It may also occur in the presence of chronic Eustachian tube dysfunction and negative pressure. As a result of a chronic negative vacuum into the middle ear, the whole tympanic membrane may become thin and retracted. These are the weak points of the tympanic membrane, so perforation may occur during irrigation of the external ear canal.

6.5.4 Epidermization

Epidermization occurs when middle ear mucosa is replaced with keratinized squamous epithelium that is usually in continuum with the external ear canal skin as a sequela of COM (▶ Fig. 6.33). There is usually retention of keratin debris or cholesteatoma formation. Otopathologic examination usually shows the resorption of scutum, the posterior-superior portion of the tympanic annulus, and the ossicles in the middle ear. In perforated membranes, the epidermis on the surface of the tympanic membrane or meatal skin may advance into the medial aspect of the tympanic membrane beyond the edge of the perforation; therefore, the perforation edges should be freshened with a small hook before elevating the tympanomeatal flap during tympanoplasty.

6.5.5 Tympanosclerosis

Fibrous proliferation and hyaline deposits in the submucosal layer or new bone formation (▶ Fig. 6.34; ▶ Fig. 6.35; ▶ Fig. 6.36) may occur during chronic inflammatory diseases of the middle ear and tympanic membrane, resulting in tympanosclerosis. The overlying mucosa may become very thin, with diminished vascularities, and eventually disappear.[44] Although purulent secretion is not common in an ear with tympanosclerosis, it often fixes the ossicles in the middle ear. Otoscopic examination shows white plaques in the tympanic membrane and a nodular appearance within the submucosa of the middle ear.

6.6 Complications of COM

6.6.1 Labyrinthine Fistula

The most common sites of erosion in the labyrinth are the lateral and posterior canals (▶ Fig. 6.37). The most common symptoms are vertigo, sensorineural hearing loss, and a positive fistula test. Surgeon should keep in mind that removal of the squamous epithelium that covers the fistula surface may cause sensorineural hearing loss.

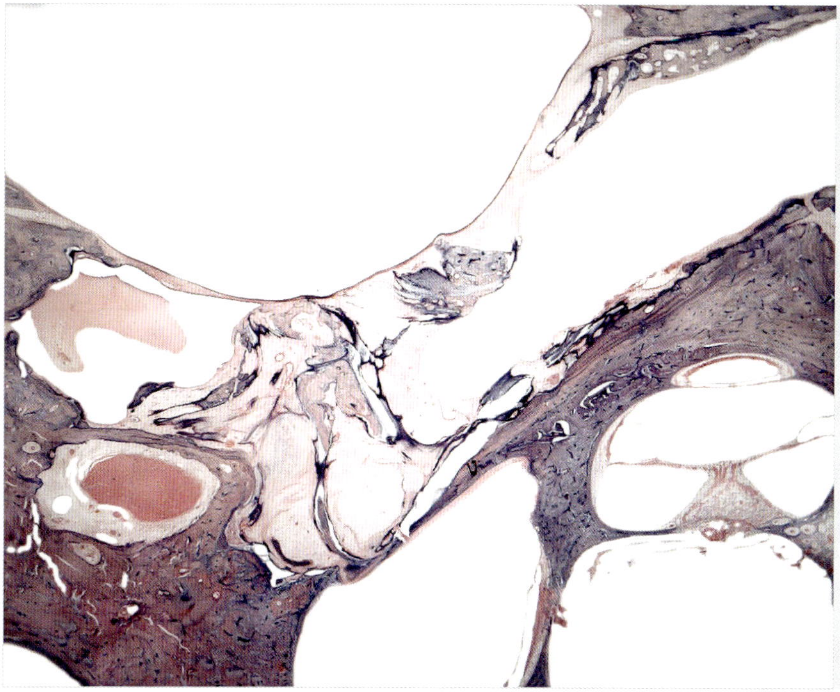

Fig. 6.35 This was a 75-year-old patient with bilateral chronic otitis media. Microscopic evaluation showed a retracted tympanic membrane, ossicular erosion, new bone formation, and tympanosclerosis in the middle ear as well as endolymphatic hydrops in the cochlea.

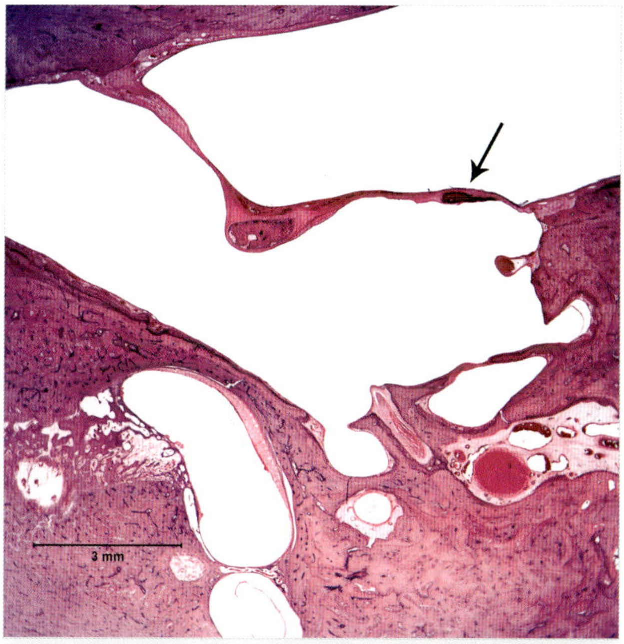

Fig. 6.36 This was a 63-year-old patient with a history of chronic otitis media. Histopathologic examination showed tympanosclerosis (arrow) of the intact tympanic membrane and granulation tissue in the mastoid as well as around the facial nerve.

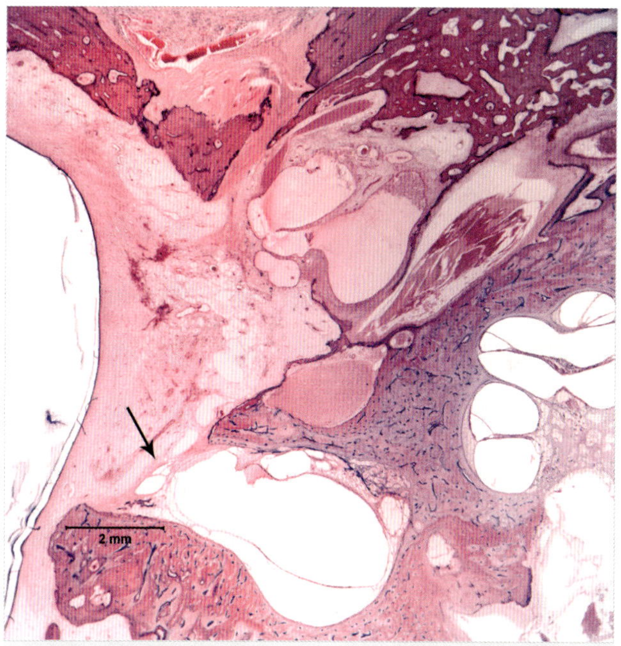

Fig. 6.37 This was a 68-year-old female patient with a history of bilateral chronic otitis media. Histopathologic examination showed large cholesteatoma, causing otomastoiditis, with granulation tissue just under it. There was a fistula of the bony wall of the lateral semicircular canal (arrow) in addition to mild endolymphatic hydrops in the cochlea.

A labyrinthine fistula may occur in about 10% of the operated cholesteatomas, and its presence should be assumed unless the contrary is proven given that it may not present any preoperative symptoms.

6.6.2 Facial Paresis or Paralysis

Facial paresis or paralysis may occur due to an insult anywhere along the course of the facial nerve; however, the tympanic portion of the nerve seems to be the most commonly involved site

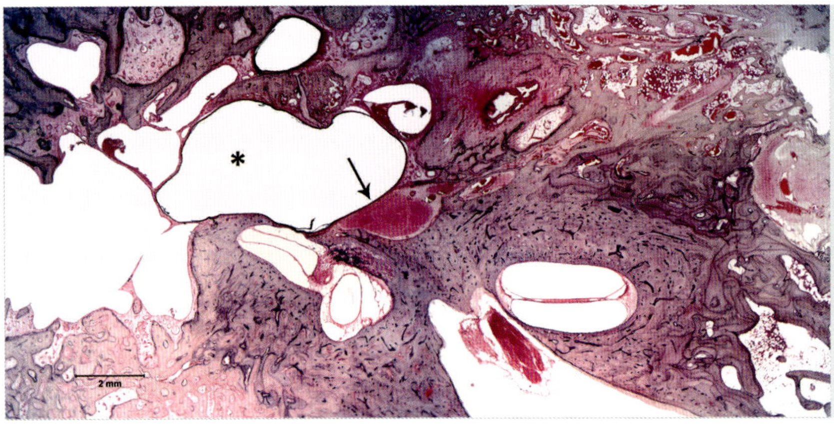

Fig. 6.38 This was a 64-year-old patient with acute bacterial meningitis. Histopathologic examination showed bilateral chronic otitis media. The left ear showed chronic changes in the middle ear, including a glandular subepithelial space, tympanosclerosis, granulation tissue around the mastoid cells, and cholesteatoma (*) that pushed the ossicular chain laterally and eroded the facial nerve bony canal (arrow).

(▶ Fig. 6.38).[45] Histopathologic observation shows the erosion of the bony canal of the nerve and osteitis.

References

[1] Paparella MM, Sipilä P, Juhn SK, Jung TTK. Subepithelial space in otitis media. Laryngoscope. 1985;95(4):414–420.

[2] Meyerhoff WL, Kim CS, Paparella MM. Pathology of chronic otitis media. Ann Otol Rhinol Laryngol. 1978;87(6 Pt 1):749–760.

[3] Jaisinghani VJ, Paparella MM, Schachern PA, Le CT. Tympanic membrane/middle ear pathologic correlates in chronic otitis media. Laryngoscope. 1999;109 (5):712–716.

[4] da Costa SS, Paparella MM, Schachern PA, Yoon TH, Kimberley BP. Temporal bone histopathology in chronically infected ears with intact and perforated tympanic membranes. Laryngoscope. 1992;102(11):1229–1236.

[5] Paparella MM, Schachern PA, Cureoglu S. Chronic silent otitis media. ORL J Otorhinolaryngol Relat Spec. 2002;64(2):65–72.

[6] Paparella MM, Goycoolea M, Bassiouni M, Koutroupas S. Silent otitis media: clinical applications. Laryngoscope. 1986;96(9 Pt 1):978–985.

[7] Tovi F, Leiberman A. Silent mastoiditis and bilateral simultaneous facial palsy. Int J Pediatr Otorhinolaryngol. 1983;5(3):303–307.

[8] Paparella MM, Goycoolea MV, Meyerhoff WL, Shea D. Endolymphatic hydrops and otitis media. Laryngoscope. 1979;89(1):43–58.

[9] Schaaf RC. The frequency of vestibular disorders in developmentally delayed preschoolers with otitis media. Am J Occup Ther. 1985;39(4):247–252.

[10] Golz A, Netzer A, Angel-Yeger B, Westerman ST, Gilbert LM, Joachims HZ. Effects of middle ear effusion on the vestibular system in children. Otolaryngol Head Neck Surg. 1998;119(6):695–699.

[11] Cureoglu S, Schachern PA, Paparella MM, Lindgren BR. Cochlear changes in chronic otitis media. Laryngoscope. 2004;114(4):622–626.

[12] Goycoolea MV, Paparella MM, Juhn SK, Carpenter AM. Oval and round window changes in otitis media. Potential pathways between middle and inner ear. Laryngoscope. 1980;90(8 Pt 1):1387–1391.

[13] Spratley JE, Schachern PA, Paparella MM, Yoon T, Le CT. Histopathologic study of serous labyrinthitis in human temporal bones. Folia Otorhinolaryngologica. 2000;6:39–46.

[14] Paparella MM, Sugiura S. The pathology of suppurative labyrinthitis. Ann Otol Rhinol Laryngol. 1967;76(3):554–586.

[15] Edelstein DR, Parisier SC. Surgical techniques and recidivism in cholesteatoma. Otolaryngol Clin North Am. 1989;22(5):1029–1040.

[16] Veldman JE, Braunius WW. Revision surgery for chronic otitis media: a learning experience. Report on 389 cases with a long-term follow-up. Ann Otol Rhinol Laryngol. 1998;107(6):486–491.

[17] Parisier SC. Management of cholesteatoma. Otolaryngol Clin North Am. 1989;22(5):927–940.

[18] Palva T, Mäkinen J. Why does middle ear cholesteatoma recur? Arch Otolaryngol. 1983;109(8):513–518.

[19] Paparella MM, Jung TT. Experience with tympanoplasty for atelectatic ears. Laryngoscope. 1981;91(9 Pt 1):1472–1477.

[20] Sadé J, Avraham S, Brown M. Atelectasis, retraction pockets and cholesteatoma. Acta Otolaryngol. 1981;92(5–6):501–512.

[21] Sadé J, Luntz M. Gaseous pathways in atelectatic ears. Ann Otol Rhinol Laryngol. 1989;98(5 Pt 1):355–358.

[22] Sade J. Middle ear mucosa. Arch Otolaryngol. 1966;84(2):137–143.

[23] Tos M, Poulsen G. Attic retractions following secretory otitis. Acta Otolaryngol. 1980;89(5–6):479–486.

[24] Granström G, Holmquist J, Jarlstedt J, Renvall U. Collagenase activity in middle ear effusions. Acta Otolaryngol. 1985;100(5–6):405–413.

[25] Ruah CB, Schachern PA, Paparella MM, Zelterman D. Mechanisms of retraction pocket formation in the pediatric tympanic membrane. Arch Otolaryngol Head Neck Surg. 1992;118(12):1298–1305.

[26] Manasse P. Über Granulationsgeschwülste mit Fremdkörperriesenzellen. Virchows Arch. 1894;136:245.

[27] House JL, Brackmann DE. Cholesterol granuloma of the cerebellopontine angle. Arch Otolaryngol. 1982;108(8):504–506.

[28] Matt BH, Myer CM III Bellet PS. Cholesterol granuloma presenting in the ear canal. Ann Otol Rhinol Laryngol. 1990;99(8):672–673.

[29] Miglets AW, Booth JB. Cholesterol granuloma presenting as an isolated middle ear tumor. Laryngoscope. 1981;91(3):410–415.

[30] Leonetti JP, Shownkeen H, Marzo SJ. Incidental petrous apex findings on magnetic resonance imaging. Ear Nose Throat J. 2001;80(4):200–202, 205–206.

[31] Plester D, Steinbach E. Cholesterol granuloma. Otolaryngol Clin North Am. 1982;15(3):665–672.

[32] Paparella MM, Lim DJ. Pathogenesis and pathology of the "idiopathic" blue ear drum. Arch Otolaryngol. 1967;85(3):249–258.

[33] Sadé J, Halevy A, Klajman A, Mualem T. Cholesterol granuloma. Acta Otolaryngol. 1980;89(3–4):233–239.

[34] Hall-Stoodley L, Stoodley P. Evolving concepts in biofilm infections. Cell Microbiol. 2009;11(7):1034–1043.

[35] Gilbert P, Das J, Foley I. Biofilm susceptibility to antimicrobials. Adv Dent Res. 1997;11(1):160–167.

[36] Mah TF, O'Toole GA. Mechanisms of biofilm resistance to antimicrobial agents. Trends Microbiol. 2001;9(1):34–39.

[37] Moscoso M, García E, López R. Biofilm formation by Streptococcus pneumoniae: role of choline, extracellular DNA, and capsular polysaccharide in microbial accretion. J Bacteriol. 2006;188(22):7785–7795.

[38] Jensen PØ, Givskov M, Bjarnsholt T, Moser C. The immune system vs. Pseudomonas aeruginosa biofilms. FEMS Immunol Med Microbiol. 2010;59(3):292–305.

[39] Bakaletz LO. Bacterial biofilms in otitis media: Evidence and relevance. Pediatr Infect Dis J. 2007;26(10) Suppl:S17–S19.

[40] Chole RA, Faddis BT. Evidence for microbial biofilms in cholesteatomas. Arch Otolaryngol Head Neck Surg. 2002;128(10):1129–1133.

[41] Lee MR, Pawlowski KS, Luong A, Furze AD, Roland PS. Biofilm presence in humans with chronic suppurative otitis media. Otolaryngol Head Neck Surg. 2009;141(5):567–571.

[42] Burmølle M, Thomsen TR, Fazli M, et al. Biofilms in chronic infections – a matter of opportunity – monospecies biofilms in multispecies infections. FEMS Immunol Med Microbiol. 2010;59(3):324–336.

[43] Mehta RP, Rosowski JJ, Voss SE, O'Neil E, Merchant SN. Determinants of hearing loss in perforations of the tympanic membrane. Otol Neurotol. 2006;27 (2):136–143.

[44] Nadol J Jr. Infections. In Schuknecht's pathology of the ear. 3rd edition. People's Medical Publishing House. Editors: Merchant SN, Nadol JB. 2010, USA, p 304.

[45] Yetiser S, Tosun F, Kazkayasi M. Facial nerve paralysis due to chronic otitis media. Otol Neurotol. 2002;23(4):580–588.

7 Surgical Anatomy Relevant to the Chronic Ear

Howard W. Francis and Alejandro Rivas

Abbreviations used in this chapter:

COM: chronic otitis media
CT: computed tomography
EAC: external auditory canal
IAC: internal auditory canal
LIMF: lateral incudomalleal fold
SCC: semicircular canal
TM: tympanic membrane

7.1 Introduction

Safe and effective surgery for chronic ear disease demands an understanding of temporal bone anatomy and its relevance to function and pathophysiology. Whereas knowledge of surgical anatomy informs the technical processes needed to navigate middle ear and mastoid structures without additional morbidity, an understanding of the mechanisms of chronic otitis media (COM) should guide decisions that reduce recrudescent disease.

Ventilation of the middle ear and mastoid air cells supports the transduction of sound to the cochlea. Whereas the Eustachian tube serves as the primary conduit of airflow into and out of this closed system of air spaces, continuity from one chamber to the other is required to preserve a healthy and functional ear. Acute otitis media usually follows the interruption of middle ear ventilation at the level of the Eustachian tube and consists of a metabolic cascade in the lining of the middle ear and other spaces within the temporal bone that leaves it susceptible to bacterial invasion and empyema. This series of acute and reversible events is comparable with post-obstructive changes in a lung segment after aspiration of a foreign body, for example.

Chronic hypoventilation of the middle ear and mastoid, however, can lead to COM characterized by persistent mucosal changes that support bacterial colonization and recurrent superinfection. Akin to the consequences of chronic obstructive lung disease, such as bronchitis, COM can be associated with an overproduction of secretions and the generation of purulent discharge. Degradation of the ossicular chain, particularly the long process of the incus, and the tympanic membrane (TM) occur during acute exacerbations of COM. A single nutrient vessel of the long process of the incus is susceptible to thrombosis and bone necrosis in the setting of otitis media.[1,2] When persistent hypoventilation occurs at the level of the Eustachian tube, changes in the mesotympanic area may include retraction of the pars tensa with effusion, TM perforation with mucosal hypertrophy, and polypoid changes of the middle ear with otorrhea. Similar mucosal changes occurring in the attic, antrum, and other temporal bone air cells result from hypoventilation in these areas but are not as readily appreciated on physical examination.

These hidden changes can occur even in the setting of normal Eustachian tube function if ventilation pathways between the mesotympanum and remaining air-filled spaces throughout the temporal bone are narrowed or obstructed. Restricted airflow through the attic to the antrum may, for example, result from space restrictions imposed by contracted bony walls of the attic and aditus ad antrum or by a relatively large incus body and malleus head. Restricted ventilation through the attic is more likely, however, the result of soft tissue stenosis imposed by inflammatory effects on the system of ligaments and mucosal folds associated with the ossicular chain. Whether congenitally narrowed or restricted by inflammatory changes and scarring following recurrent infections, obstruction of airflow in the attic region produces chronic mucosal changes in the mastoid. The resulting negative pressure in the attic region creates favorable conditions for attic retraction of the TM and migration of keratinized epithelium, leading to cholesteatoma formation. In addition to eliminating cholesteatoma and its health risks, the goal of otologic surgery should be to establish a healthy well-ventilated ear.

7.2 Temporal Bone Osteology

As the epicenter of chronic ear disease, the attic and the antrum are the primary targets of surgical intervention (▸ Fig. 7.1). From the beginning of the mastoidectomy procedure, the goal of establishing a well-ventilated ear should at all times be guided by landmarks and surgical principles that preserve the cortical lining of the middle fossa and, depending on the approach, the external auditory canal (EAC).[3] Starting with the soft tissue dissection, the cortical surface of the mastoid process should be exposed as far anteriorly as the root of zygoma, thereby giving access to the region immediately superior to the bony EAC, deep to which the attic will be found. Review of coronal computed tomography (CT) scans through this area will provide information about the space available between the middle fossa and EAC cortex to access the attic. If too narrow, limited access through the mastoid can still be accomplished. Appropriate placement of the anterior-posterior periosteal incision adjacent and tangential with the EAC, followed by the elevation and retraction of the temporalis muscle, provides access to important cortical landmarks needed to perform a safe mastoidectomy.

Following placement of a superior-inferior incision and elevation of the mastoid periosteum to the bony EAC, landmarks for the underlying mastoid antrum become visible. The spine of Henle is a cortical extension of the bony EAC that presents as a ridge at the superior posterior edge of the canal rim (▸ Fig. 7.2a).[3,4,5,6] Posterior to the spine of Henle is a depression in the cortical bone known as Macewen's triangle, also known as the cribrose area for the multiple bony perforations that accommodate small emissary veins from the antral mucosa found deep to this area. The linear ridge oriented in an anterior to posterior direction superior to the EAC is known as the temporal line and serves as an estimate for the lowest level at which the middle fossa floor can be found within the mastoid. The so-called mastoid tegmen corresponds to the cortical lining of the middle fossa and starts laterally above the temporal line

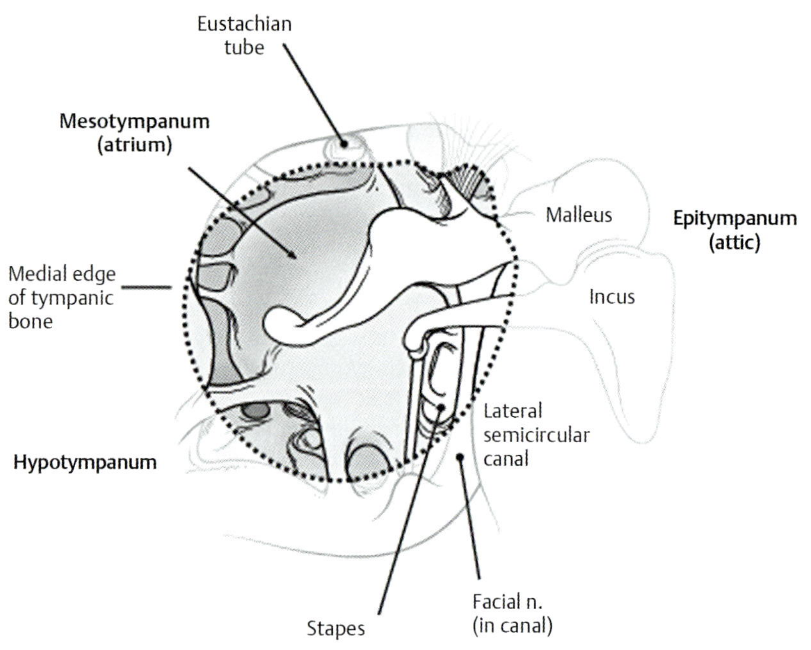

Fig. 7.1 The aperture normally occupied by the tympanic membrane encompasses the mesotympanum. The epitympanum is the superior space occupied by the head of malleus and body of the incus, and which communicates posteriorly with the mastoid antrum.

before it curves inferiorly to form the roof of the mastoid and attic spaces. With this in mind, the tegmen should first be identified superficially above the temporal line and followed inferiorly and medially into the mastoid cavity, where it often bows before ascending to take a more superior position within the antrum (▶ Fig. 7.2b).[3]

Other lateral landmarks of importance include suture lines within the EAC where the tympanic ring connects with the mastoid bone inferiorly (tympanomastoid suture line) and the squamous bone superiorly (tympanosquamous suture line). The canal skin is often caught within these suture lines. Efforts should be made to broadly elevate the canal skin and disengage it from these suture lines laterally so as not to create tears with deeper dissection. The canal skin terminates at the annular ligament of the TM, except superiorly where it transitions to the pars tensa at the edge of the scutum or notch of Rivinus.

The temporal bone has a pyramidal shape with the squamous, mastoid, and tympanic portions forming the base and the petrous bone forming the apex medially (▶ Fig. 7.3a). Medial to the labyrinth, the petrous apex is marrow-filled in children and becomes ventilated to varying degrees with maturation (▶ Fig. 7.3b).[5] Meckel's cave is located within a depression on the superior (middle fossa) surface of the petrous apex. The internal auditory canal (IAC) traverses the petrous apex from the opening of the porus acousticus in the posterior fossa. The abducens nerve is located within the bony Dorello's canal at the petrous apex.[7] Extension of COM to the petrous apex can produce inflammation of adjacent structures, causing the symptom triad of abducens palsy, retro-orbital pain, and otorrhea, known as Gradenigo's syndrome. The lateral sinus becomes the sigmoid sinus within the bony sulcus on the medial posterior surface of the temporal bone and exits the cranium through the jugular foramen located at the junction of the petrous and occipital bones.[3,4,6] Lateral to this foramen, the dome of the jugular fossa forms the floor of the hypotympanum.

7.3 The Tympanic Membrane and Middle Ear

The TM is a translucent window to the mesotympanum of the middle ear and the input for sound conduction to the middle ear transduction mechanism. Whereas the diminutive pars flaccida occupies the notch of Rivinus superior to the lateral process of the malleus, the pars tensa makes up the remainder of the TM (▶ Fig. 7.4). Both parts of the TM are lined by cuboidal middle ear epithelium medially and keratinized epithelium laterally.[2,8,9] The pars tensa, however, has an intervening fibrous layer that attaches the TM onto the manubrium of the malleus centrally and the tympanic ring peripherally. The annular ligament is continuous with the fibrous layer, which consists of radial and circumferential fibers, and occupies a groove within the tympanic bone from the anterior to posterior spines.

The middle ear contains the ossicular chain, its ligamentous attachments, and the tendons of the tensor tympani and stapedius muscles and is traversed by the chorda tympani.[8,10] The bony confines of the middle ear consist of the tympanic ring circumferentially and the labyrinth and facial nerve medially. Other fixed anatomic landmarks of the tympanic cavity include the cog, the cochleariform process, and the pyramidal process as well as intervening recesses, all of which have surgical relevance. Connected to the ossicular chain, mucosal folds arise, creating different middle ear compartments that shape the mucosal physiology and ventilation pathways of the middle ear.[8,10] The advent of middle ear endoscopy and its increasing use as a surgical tool in cholesteatoma surgery has led to a greater awareness of the intricacies of bony and membranous anatomy of the middle ear and its importance in the pathogenesis and treatment of cholesteatoma.

The middle ear can be divided into subspaces, based on their relationship with the tympanic rim. The central middle ear space is designated the mesotympanum and is contained

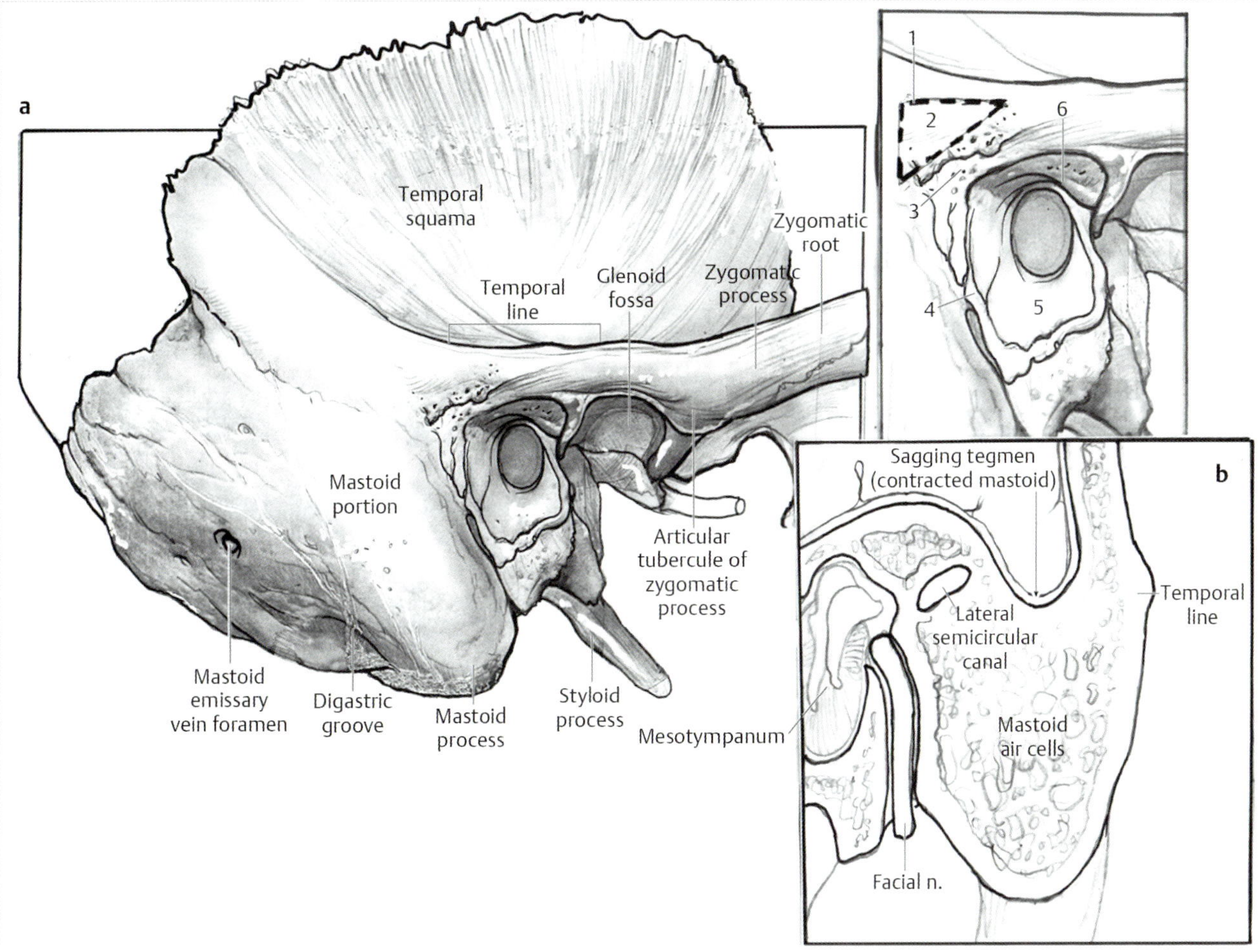

Fig. 7.2 (a) Lateral view of the temporal bone showing relevant bony landmarks of the mastoid operation and suture lines within the bony external auditory canal (inset; 1, Macewen's triangle; 2, cribriform area; 3, spine of Henle; 4, tympano-mastoid suture line; 5, external auditory canal; 6, tympano-squamous suture line). (b) Coronal section through mastoid showing low hanging tegmen in contracted mastoid and the increased vulnerabilty of the labyrinth and facial nerve if not carefully sculpted as the antrum is opened. Laterally, the tegmen is best found superior to the temporal line where it is most superficial.

within the limits of the tympanic annulus. Inferior to the tympanic annulus lies the hypotympanum; anterior to the hypotympanum is the protympanum; posterior to the mesotympanum is the retrotympanum; and superior to the lateral process of the malleus is the epitympanum.

7.3.1 Retrotympanum

The retrotympanum is an important middle ear location that encompasses different ridges and spaces lying in the posterior aspect of the tympanic cavity. The anterior limits of the retrotympanum include the tympanic segment of the facial nerve and the stapes posterior crura superiorly and the promontory inferiorly. Several authors have studied this region and have proposed different anatomic names over the years.[8,10,11] An understanding of the retrotympanic anatomy is crucial for the effective use of middle ear endoscopy given that this is the most frequent location for recurrence of cholesteatoma.

The pyramidal process is a consistent bony eminence from which two bony ridges arise. First is the ridge of the chorda tympani, which separates the lateral retrotympanum into the facial recess superiorly and the lateral tympanic sinus inferiorly. The second bony ridge, in the medial retrotympanum, is the ponticulus ridge, which extends from the promontory to the pyramidal process and divides the medial spaces into the sinus tympani inferiorly and the posterior tympanic sinus superiorly. The posterior sinus is limited anteriorly by the posterior stapes cura, superiorly by the horizontal segment of the facial nerve, inferiorly by the ponticulum, posteriorly by the pyramidal process and subpyramidal space, and laterally by the stapedius tendon (▶ Fig. 7.5).

The sinus tympani is a frequent location for recurrence of cholesteatoma. It is a space that lies medial to the vertical segment of the facial nerve, the stapedius muscle, tendon, and the pyramidal process. It lies lateral to the vestibule and posterior semicircular canal (SCC). The limits of the sinus tympani include the ponticulum superiorly, the subiculum inferiorly (which is a ridge of bone that extends from the styloid eminence to the posterior pillar of the round window niche), and the promontory anteriorly (▶ Fig. 7.5). Several authors have described the high variability of the sinus tympani configuration.[12,13,14] More recently, Marchioni, Mattioli, Alicandri-Ciufelli,

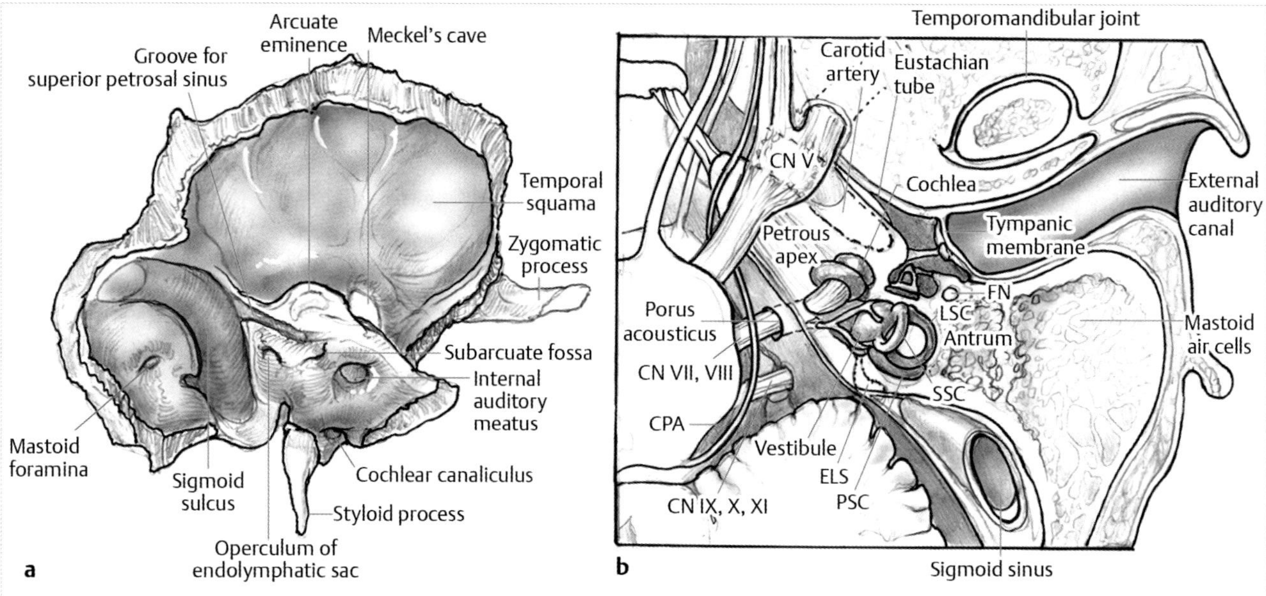

Fig. 7.3 (a) Postero-medial view of the temporal bone showing posterior and middle fossa surfaces and their bony features. (b) Axial section through well-developed temporal bone showing mastoid air cells. CN, cranial nerve; CPA, cerebellopontine angle; ELS, endolymphatic sac; FN, facial nerve; LSC, lateral semicircular canal; PSC, posterior semicircular canal; SSC, superior semicircular canal.

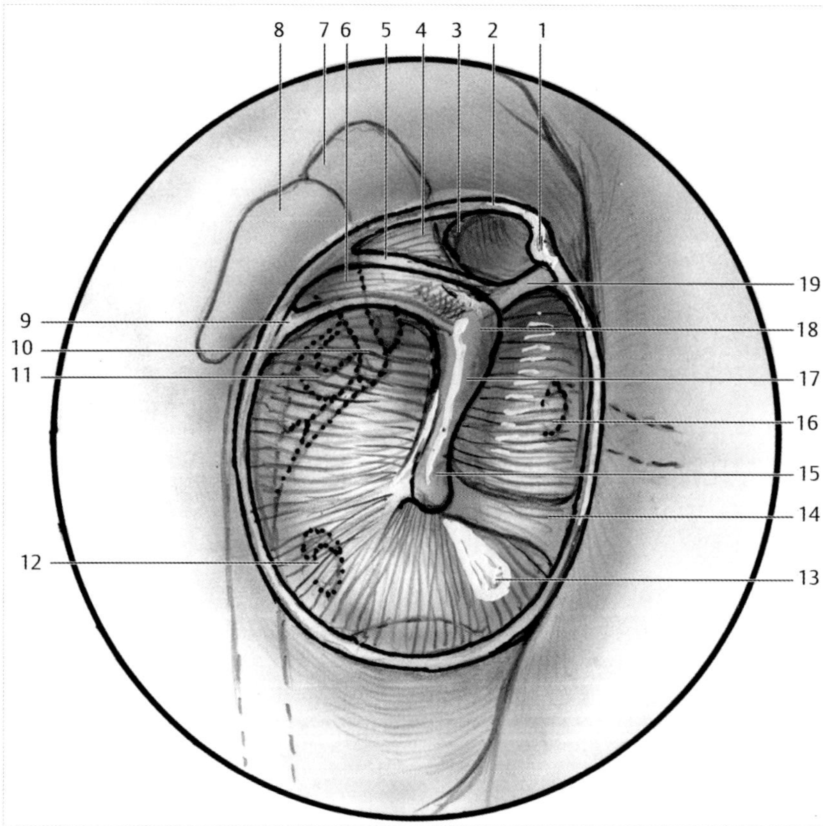

Fig. 7.4 Relationship of pars tensa and pars flaccida (removed) portions of the tympanic membrane and deeper ligamentous and ossicular anatomy. 1, anterior tympanic spine; 2, notch of Rivinus (pars flaccida removed); 3, anterior malleal fold; 4, lateral malleal fold; 5, posterior stria; 6, posterior malleal fold; 7, head of malleus; 8, body of incus; 9, posterior malleal ligament; 10, long process of incus; 11, stapes; 12, round window; 13, cone of light; 14, pars tensa; 15, umbo; 16, Eustachian tube; 17, manubrium of malleus; 18, lateral process of malleus; 19, anterior malleal ligament.

and Presutti classified the morphology of the sinus tympani based on intraoperative anatomic variations of the ponticulus during endoscopic cholesteatoma surgery.[15] Four major variations of the sinus tympani have been described:

- Classical shape. The sinus tympani is limited by the ponticulum superiorly, the subiculum inferiorly, and lies medial to the vertical segment of the facial nerve and the pyramidal process.

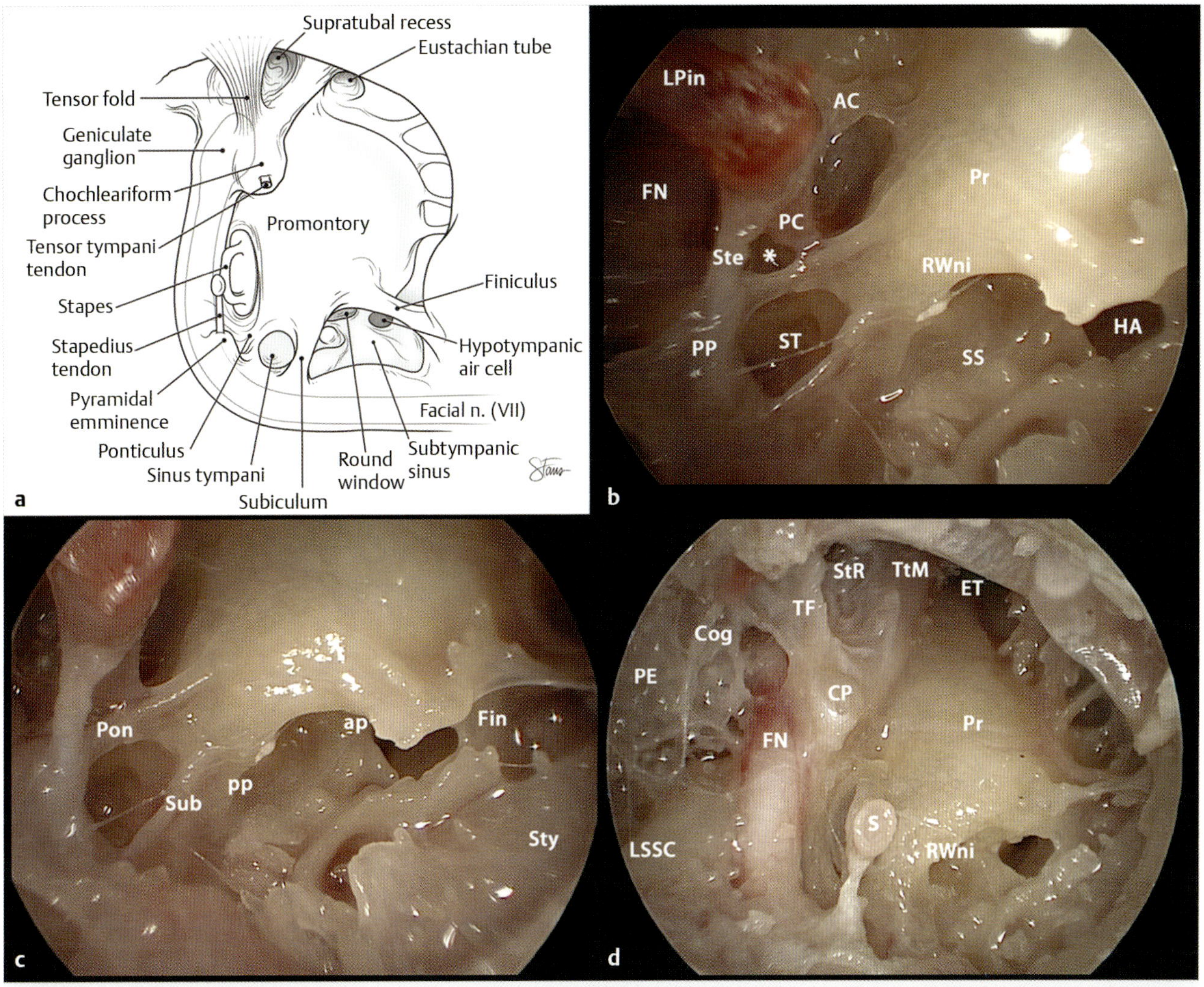

Fig. 7.5 Retrotympanum. (a) Schematic view of the medial surface of the right tympanic cavity. (b) Endoscopic photograph showing the structures of the superior retrotympanum. (c) View of the inferior retrotympanum. (d) Panoramic view of the medial surface of the tympanic cavity, where the scutum, tympanic membrane, malleus and incus have been removed, demonstrating the epi, meso, retro, hypo and protympanum. LPin, long process of the incus; FN, facial nerve; AC, anterior cura; PC, posterior crura; (*), Posterior sinus; Ste, stapedious tendon; PP, pyramidal process; ST, sinus tympani; Pr, promontory; RWni, round window niche; SS, subtympanic sinus; HA, hypotympanic aircell; Pon, ponticulus; Sub, subiculum; pp, posterior pillar of the round window niche; ap, anterior pillar of the round window niche; Fin, finiculus; Sty, styloid eminence; LSSC, lateral semicircular canal; PE, posterior epitympanum; TF, remnant of the tensor fold; StR, Supratubal recess; TtM, Tensor tympani muscle; ET, Eustachian tube; CP, cochleariform process; S, Stapes; Cog, cog, divides the epitympanum into anterior and posterior divisions.

- Confluent shape. The ponticulum is absent, and the tympanic sinus is confluent with the posterior sinus.
- Partitioned shape. A third ridge of bone between the ponticulum and subiculum is present, extending from the vertical segment of the facial nerve to the promontory and separating the sinus tympani into two portions (superior and inferior).
- Restricted shape. A high jugular bulb is present, reducing the inferior limit of the sinus tympani.

Like the sinus tympani, the ponticulum can be highly variable. These variations give an additional level of complexity when cholesteatoma is present in the sinus tympani. Three different ponticulum configurations have been described:[16]

- Classical morphology. The ponticulum is a completely formed bony ridge extending from the pyramidal process to the promontory.
- Incomplete ponticulum. The ponticulum is absent, making the sinus tympani and posterior sinus confluent. In these cases, removal of cholesteatoma from this configuration needs to be done under direct visualization with extreme care as mobilization and dislocation of the stapes can occur.
- Communicating ponticulum. The ponticulum has an incomplete partition, present laterally but absent medially, creating a communication between the sinus tympani and the posterior sinus under the ridge. In these cases, cholesteatoma can track under the ridge and involve the posterior crura and subpyramidal space. Curetting of the communicating ponticulum is recommended in these cases prior to cholesteatoma removal to improve visibility and prevent stapes trauma.

Several anatomical studies have focused on the depth of the sinus tympani.[12,14,17,18] It is important to analyze these

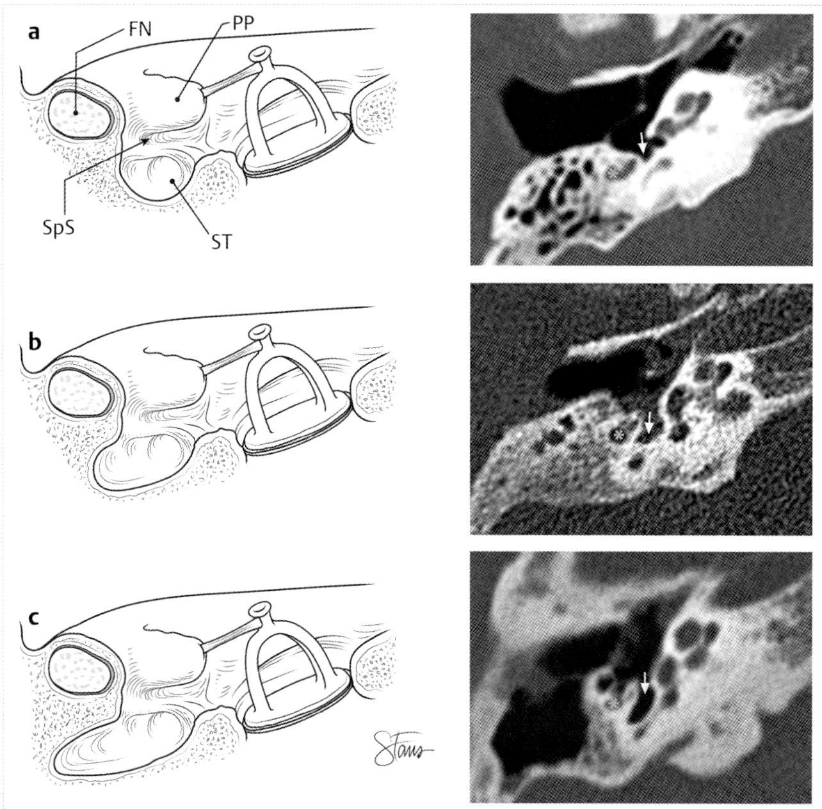

Fig. 7.6 Classification of the depth of sinus tympani (ST) aligned with corresponding axial CT images. Type A: Small sinus tympani. The sinus tympani extends no further than the anterior edge of the vertical segment of the facial nerve (FN). Type B: Deep sinus tympani. The sinus tympani extends medial to the vertical segment of the facial nerve but does not extend past the posterior edge of the nerve. Type C: Deep sinus tympani with posterior extension. The sinus tympani surpasses the posterior edge the facial nerve. Notice the corresponding CT images of the sinus tympani (arrows) with reference to the facial nerve (asterisk). PP, pyramidal process; SpS, Subpyramidal space.

variations in depth preoperatively when performing cholesteatoma surgery given that this might influence the surgical approach used to achieve complete excision of the disease. Marchioni, Mattioli, Alicandri-Ciufelli, and Presutti assessed the variations in depth of the sinus tympani, analyzing its posterior and medial extension based on CT axial slices.[15] This classification could be useful in preoperative planning for the optimal approach to the sinus tympani. The depth of the sinus tympani is classified into three categories as follows:

- Type A. Small sinus tympani. The posterior and medial boundaries of the sinus tympani extend no further than the anterior edge of the vertical segment of the facial nerve (▶ Fig. 7.6a). In this case, cholesteatoma may be removed through the facial recess, with a large canalplasty, or by using an endoscopic approach.
- Type B. Deep sinus tympani. The posterior and medial limits of the sinus tympani lie medial to the vertical segment of the facial nerve and do not extend past the posterior edge of the nerve (▶ Fig. 7.6b). In this instance, cholesteatoma may be removed using angled instruments with an endoscopic technique or through a transmastoid facial recess approach with close skeletonization of the anterior facial nerve.
- Type C. Deep sinus tympani with posterior extension. The posterior and medial limits of the sinus tympani surpass the posterior edge of the vertical segment of the facial nerve (▶ Fig. 7.6c). In these cases, the sinus tympani is very large and found frequently in well-developed mastoids. To access this space, a retrofacial approach is needed.[18]

Depending on the retrotympanum pneumatization, variations exist between the sinus tympani, posterior sinus, and the pyramidal process. A well-formed air space can exist medial and posterior to the pyramidal process. Marchioni, Alicandri-Ciufelli, Grammatica, Mattioli, and Presutti describe this space as the subpyramidal space.[19] The boundaries of this space include the Fallopian canal posteriorly and superiorly, the ponticulum inferiorly, and the medial aspect of the pyramidal process laterally; it is in direct continuity with the posterior sinus anteriorly (▶ Fig. 7.6). Depending on the variations of the ponticulum, it can also be in continuity with the sinus tympani. When present, a deep subpyramidal space carries an increased risk of recurrence of cholesteatoma.

The inferior retrotympanum was first described and characterized by Proctor.[20] He describes a constant and reliable bony ridge that joins the posterior hypotympanic rim to the promontory at the level of the basal turn of the cochlea. More recently, this ridge of bone was renamed the finiculus (from the Latin *finis* for "borderline") to delineate the separation between the inferior retrotympanum and the hypotympanum.[21] A third retrotympanic space has been described as the subtympanic sinus or area concamerata, as named by Proctor.[10] The name of this sinus reflects its location inferior to the sinus tympani. Its boundaries include the subiculum superiorly, the finiculus inferiorly, the styloid eminence posteriorly, and the round window niche and hypotympanic air cell (or tunnel) anteriorly. In cases of hypotympanic and inferior retrotympanic cholesteatomas, skin debris can extend through this air cell tract to the petrous apex (▶ Fig. 7.5).

7.3.2 Epitympanic Spaces and Ventilation System

The epitympanic space is the region of the tympanic cavity located medial and superior to the tympanic rim. The mesotympanum lies inferior to it. Several authors have studied the anatomy of the epitympanic compartments, the middle ear folds, and their role in establishing ventilation pathways, including Prussak in 1867,[22] Von Tröltsch in 1881,[23] Proctor in 1964,[10] and more recently Palva in 1996,[25] among others. Palva describes three malleal ligamental folds (the anterior malleal fold, the posterior malleal fold, and the lateral malleal fold), one incudal ligamental fold (the posterior incudal ligament), and two membranous folds (the tensor fold and the lateral incudomalleal fold).[25] Together with the malleus and incus, they form the epitympanic diaphragm.

The epitympanum is divided by the cog into the posterior epitympanum and anterior epitympanum. The cog is a bony septum that arises from the tegmen tympani and is oriented vertically toward the cochleariform process anterior to the head of the malleus. The posterior epitympanum is occupied primarily by the head of the malleus, the body of the incus, and the short process of the incus. Anterior to the cog and cochleariform process, the anterior epitympanum is located immediately superior to the Eustachian tube opening. The geniculate ganglion is located medial to this space, where it can be dehiscent in some cases, and the middle fossa is similarly in close proximity, raising the risk of complications due to cholesteatoma or its removal from this region (▶ Fig. 7.5a,d).[26]

The lateral incudomalleal fold (LIMF) separates the lateral posterior epitympanum into two portions, the superior and inferior lateral attic. The LIMF originates at the posterior end of the short process of the incus and projects anteriorly between the body and the proximal third of the long process of the incus, the head of the malleus, and the lateral aspect of the attic. The fold then bends inferiorly to join the posterior and lateral malleal ligament folds (▶ Fig. 7.7).

Ventilation of the attic and mastoid antrum occurs via apertures formed between adjacent ligaments, folds, and the ossicular mass, particularly those that partition the posterior attic

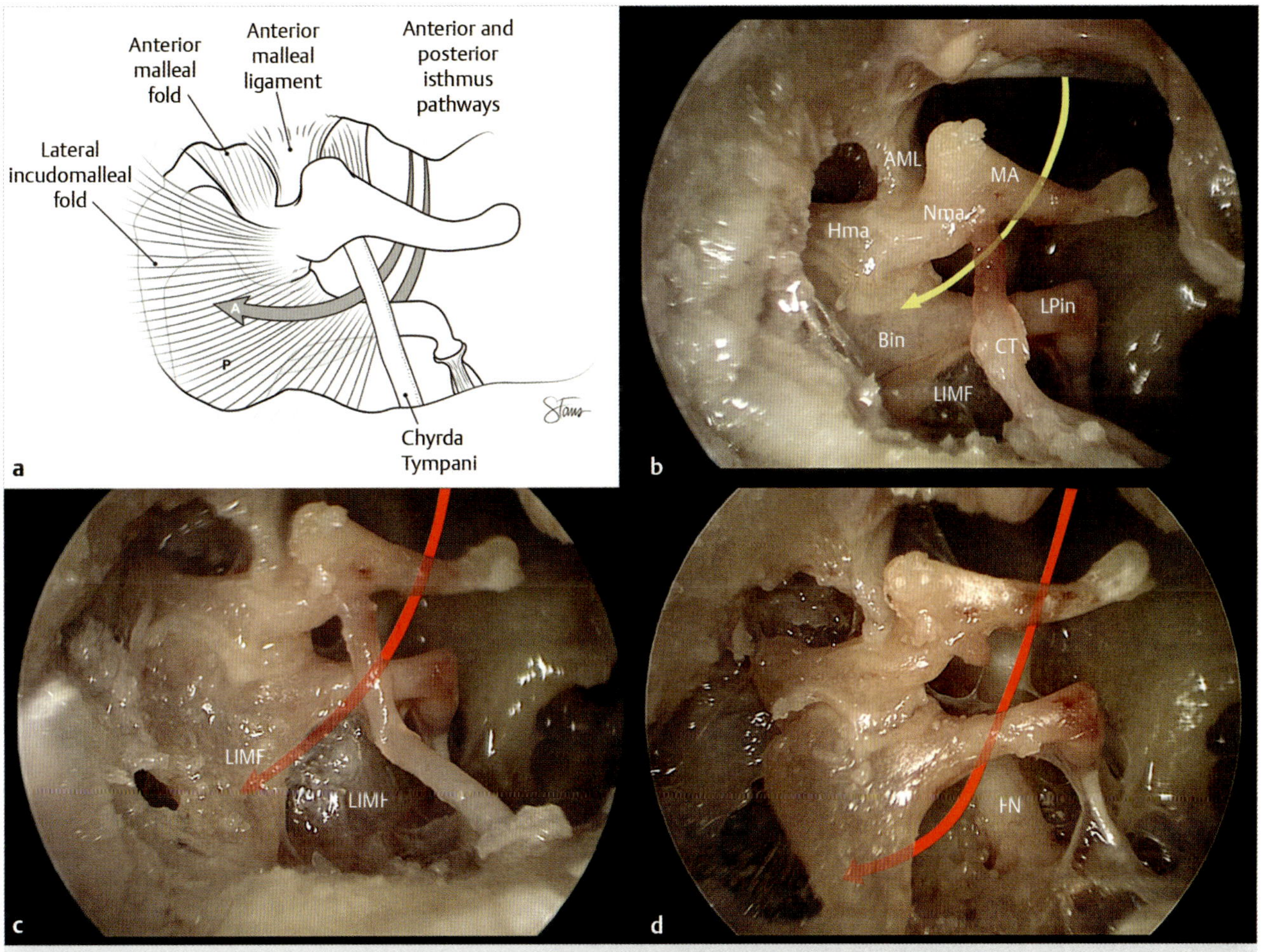

Fig. 7.7 Ventilation pathways. (a) Schematic view of the anterior (arrow A) and posterior (arrow P) isthmuses. (b) The anterior isthmus (yellow arrow), moves air from the Eustachian tube, under the malleus (MA), over the incus and lateral incudomalleal fold (LIMF) to ventilate the lateral posterior epitympanum. (c) The posterior isthmus (red arrow) moves air from the Eustachian tube, medial to the malleus, the LIMF and the incus to ventilate the mastoid, the posterior and anterior epitympanum. (d) Endoscopic photograph of the posterior isthmus after the LIMF has been resected. AML, anterior malleolal ligament; Nma, neck of the malleus; Hma, head of the malleus; Bin, body of the incus; CT, chorda tympani; LPin, lateral process of the incus; FN, facial nerve.

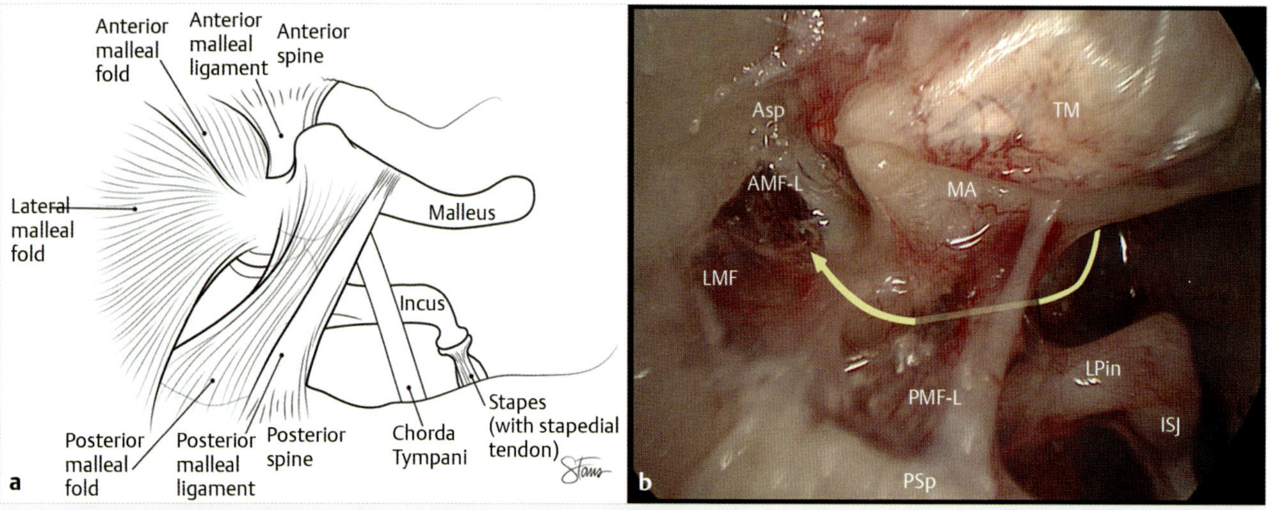

Fig. 7.8 Prussak's space. (a) Schematic representation of Prussak's space, showing its medial limits including the anterior malleal fold and ligament (AMF-L), the lateral malleal fold (LMF), and the posterior malleal fold and ligament (PMF-L). (b) Endoscopic photograph showing the ventilation pathway (yellow arrow) of Prussak Space. ASp, anterior spine; MA, malleus; PSp, posterior spine; LPin, long process of incus; ISJ, incudostapedial joint; TM, tympanic membrane (medial surface of reflected membrane).

into superior and inferior compartments. The inferior lateral attic is limited superiorly by the LIMF, laterally by the medial aspect of the scutum, and medially by the short process and body of the incus. This space communicates inferiorly with the mesotympanum. The ventilation pathway occurs through direct communication with the mesotympanum as well as through the anterior isthmus. In this pathway, air moves from the Eustachian tube into the mesotympanum, then moves medial to the manubrium and lateral to the long process of the incus into the inferior lateral attic (▶ Fig. 7.7b,c).

The superior lateral attic is bounded inferiorly by the LIMF, superiorly by the tegmen tympani, laterally and inferiorly by the body of the incus and the LIMF, and medially and inferiorly by the tympanic segment of the facial nerve. Posteriorly it communicates directly with the aditus ad antrum. Its aeration occurs primarily through the posterior isthmus. In this pathway, the air moves from the Eustachian tube into the mesotympanum, medial to the manubrium and long process of the incus, medial to the LIMF, and into the superior attic and antrum (▶ Fig. 7.7c,d).

Prussak's space is the most lateral of the posterior epitympanic compartments. It is anatomically and functionally independent from the rest of the posterior epitympanum. Medially, its limits include the posterior malleal fold inferiorly, the anterior malleal fold anteriorly, and the lateral malleal fold superiorly. The lateral boundary is the pars flaccida of the TM. Ventilation of this space comes from the mesotympanum through an opening between the posterior malleal fold and the lateral malleal fold (▶ Fig. 7.8).[27]

The limits of the anterior epitympanum include the tegmen tympani superiorly, the root of the zygoma anteriorly, the anterior tympanic rim and chorda tympani laterally, a bony plate overlying the geniculate ganglion medially, and an extension of the tensor tympani canal, the cochleariform process, and the tensor fold inferiorly. The tensor fold separates the anterior epitympanum from the supratubal recess, an anterior and superior extension of the mesotympanum, with significant variations in size and orientation (▶ Fig. 7.5a,d).[10,28] A vertical tensor fold creates a large and wide supratubal recess, whereas an almost horizontal tensor fold makes for a narrow and inferiorly displaced supratubal recess. The tensor fold is an important structure that can have direct influence on the aeration of the epitympanum. The tensor fold is incomplete in only 25% of cases,[29] which means that in 75% of the cases, the ventilation of the epitympanum can only occur through the posterior isthmus, preventing direct communication between the mesotympanum and the anterior epitympanum, which behaves as a blind sac in these instances (▶ Fig. 7.9). The negative pressure resulting from obstruction of posterior apertures leads to the retraction of the pars flaccida, leading to cholesteatoma. The tensor fold attaches to the anterior aspect of the cochleariform process and extends over the tensor tympani tendon to insert into the zygomatic root anteriorly. Opening of an uninterrupted tensor fold provides functional restoration of ventilation to the anterior epitympanum.

7.3.3 Protympanic Space

The protympanic space is the most anterior region of the tympanic cavity. Its boundaries include the promontory posteriorly; the Eustachian tube anteriorly; the cochleariform process, tensor fold, supratubal recess, and tensor tympani canal superiorly; the vertical segment and genu of the carotid canal inferiorly; and the anterior tympanic rim laterally (▶ Fig. 7.10). Although cholesteatoma rarely is found in this region, when present, it can uncover and surround the carotid artery or track into pneumatized protympanic and petrous apex air cells.

7.4 Pneumatization of the Temporal Bone

Primary regions of aeration, including the mastoid, petrous apex, and middle ear, are connected by air cell tracks that are

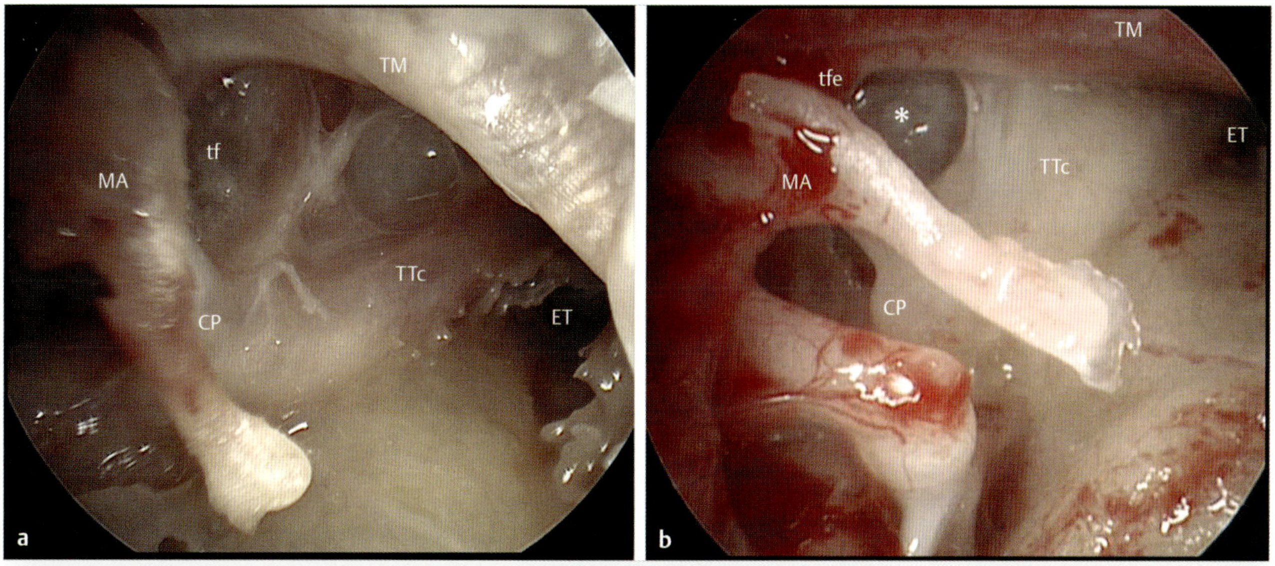

Fig. 7.9 Anatomic variations of the tensor fold. (a) Complete tensor fold (tf) that prevents direct ventilation into the anterior epitympanum. (b) Incomplete tensor fold. Notice the communication between the mesotympanum and the anterior epitympanum (asterisk). MA, malleus; CP, cochleariform process; TTc, tensor tympani canal; ET, Eustachian tube; TM, tympanic membrane; tf, tensor fold; tfe, tensor fold edge.

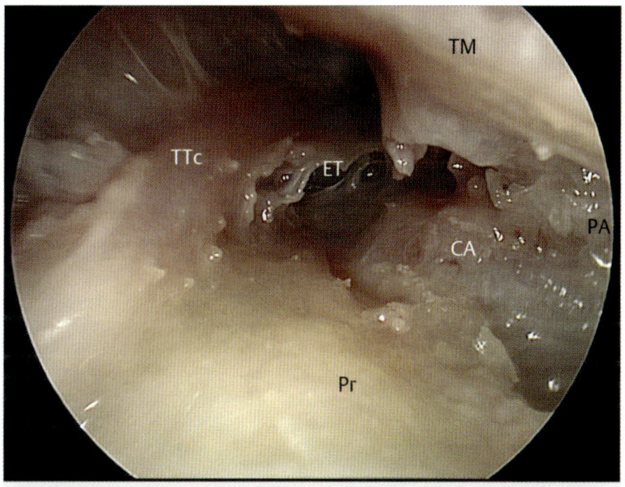

Fig. 7.10 Protympanic space. Its limits include the promontory (Pr) posteriorly; the Eustachian tube (ET) anteriorly; the tensor tympani canal (TTc) superiorly; the vertical segment and genu of the carotid canal (CA) inferiorly; and the anterior tympanic rim and tympanic membrane (TM) attachment laterally. PA, petrous apex aircells.

arranged between cortical plates of the middle and posterior fossae, the labyrinth, the facial nerve, and the sigmoid sinus. In addition to being paths of ventilation, they also serve as paths of disease spread and opportunities for surgical access to deeper regions of the temporal bone.[1,6] Some defined regions of pneumatization are[6,30] (1) the *mastoid*, consisting of the antrum, central mastoid tract, and peripheral mastoid cells (tegmental, sinodural, sinal, facial and tip cells); (2) *perilabyrinthine cells* (supralabyrinthine and infralabyrinthine cells); and (3) the *petrous apex* (peritubal area and apical area).

Air cell tracts connecting these regions include (1) the *posteromedial tract*, extending from the antrum along the posterior wall of the petrous pyramid superior to the IAC toward the apex; (2) a *superior tract*, extending from the epitympanum superior to the labyrinth toward the petrous apex; (3) a *subarcuate tract*, extending from the antrum through the center of the superior SCC toward the apex; (4) an *inferior tract*, extending from the hypotympanum underneath the cochlea toward the apex; and (5) an *anterolateral tract*, which includes the peritubal and pericarotid cells on its course toward the apex. These tracts serve as pathways by which cholesteatoma can extend from the middle ear or mastoid toward the petrous apex.

Poor pneumatization is associated with a greater likelihood of chronic ear disease[31] as it is a marker of reduced capacity to ventilate the middle ear and mastoid. The contracted size of the mastoid is often associated with a low-lying tegmen (▶ Fig. 7.2b) and anteriorly placed sigmoid sinus, which can limit surgical access to the attic and antrum. The low-lying or sagging tegmen can also disorient the surgeon, so that the vertical segment of the facial nerve and lateral SCC can be at risk when attempting a transmastoid approach to the attic.[32] Attention to the close delineation of the tegmen as it descends into the mastoid and then rises more medially toward the antrum is required for safe mastoid surgery in patients with COM.

7.5 Facial Nerve Anatomy

The facial nerve emerges from the geniculate fossa just medial to the anterior epitympanum and supratubal recess and projects posteriorly along the medial wall of the attic. In this location, the horizontal or tympanic segment of the nerve is found consistently adjacent and superior to the cochleariform process and the stapes (▶ Fig. 7.5).[26] The nerve makes a turn inferiorly to form the second genu at the pyramidal eminence just anterior to the lateral SCC. The vertical or mastoid segment of the facial nerve is oriented so that it approximately bisects the prominence of the lateral SCC in most ears.[33] The chorda tympani branch is oriented superior–anteriorly at varying locations between the second genu and stylomastoid foramen. The resulting triangle, known as the facial recess, formed by the chorda tympani nerve, the proximal segment of the mastoid division, and the inferior limit of the incudal fossa, provides a surgical conduit through which the retro- and mesotympanum can be accessed from the mastoid. The stapedial branch of the facial nerve innervates the stapedius muscle, which is located within a shelf of bone located medial and parallel to the facial nerve just distal to the second genu. The nerve exits the stylomastoid foramen, where it is surrounded by a sleeve of aponeurosis from the posterior belly of the digastric muscle.

The facial nerve is vulnerable to injury during cholesteatoma dissection in the anterior epitympanum and supratubal recess (▶ Fig. 7.5), where the geniculate may be dehiscent on the medial wall.[26] A low-hanging tegmen may cause the surgeon to dissect more inferiorly than anticipated at the opening to the attic, placing the facial nerve at risk in the region of the second genu.[32] In this area, the loss of usual landmarks, such as the ossicles and lateral SCC, can also disorient the surgeon. Dehiscence of the Fallopian canal further increases the risk of injury. The vertical segment is at risk when there is anomalous placement lateral to the horizontal SCC. Furthermore, inappropriate surgical technique, including inadequate thinning of the EAC cortex, can cause the surgeon to dissect too posteriorly in search of the facial nerve, which can lead to its inadvertent injury with the front of the bur. A thin EAC cortex, the lateral SCC, and the short process of the incus are important landmarks for the vertical segment of the facial nerve. The cephalic edge of the digastric muscle can be followed anteriorly to the stylomastoid foramen, where the aponeurosis can be followed superiorly to reveal the nerve sheath.[33]

References

[1] Nager GT. Pathology of the ear and temporal bone. Baltimore, MD: Williams and Wilkins; 1993.

[2] Schuknecht HF. Pathology of the ear. Philadelphia, PA: Lea and Febiger; 1993.

[3] Francis H, Niparko J. Temporal Bone Dissection Guide. New York, NY:Thieme: 2011.

[4] Anson B, Donaldson J. Surgical anatomy of the temporal bone. Philadelphia, PA: W.B. Saunders Company; 1981.

[5] Aslan A, Mutlu C, Celik O, Govsa F, Ozgur T, Egrilmez M. Surgical implications of anatomical landmarks on the lateral surface of the mastoid bone. Surg Radiol Anat. 2004;26(4):263–267.

[6] Schuknecht HF, Gulya AJ. Anatomy of the temporal bone with surgical implications. Philadelphia, PA:Lea and Febiger; 1986.

[7] Umansky F, Elidan J, Valarezo A. Dorello's canal: a microanatomical study. J Neurosurg. 1991;75(2):294–298.

[8] Isaacson G. Endoscopic anatomy of the pediatric middle ear. Otolaryngol Head Neck Surg. 2014;150(1):6–15.

[9] Lim DJ. Structure and function of the tympanic membrane: a review. Acta Otorhinolaryngol Belg. 1995;49(2):101–115.

[10] Proctor B. The development of the middle ear spaces and their surgical significance. J Laryngol Otol. 1964;78(7):631–648.

[11] Marchioni D, Molteni G, Presutti L. Endoscopic anatomy of the middle ear. Indian J Otolaryngol Head Neck Surg. 2011;63(2):101–113.

[12] Donaldson JA, Anson BJ, Warpeha RL, Rensink MJ. The surgical anatomy of the sinus tympani. Arch Otolaryngol. 1970;91(3):219–227.

[13] Holt JJ. The ponticulus: An anatomic study. Otol Neurotol. 2005;26(6):1122–1124.

[14] Steinbrugge H. On sinus tympani. Arch Otology. 1889;8:53–57.

[15] Marchioni D, Mattioli F, Alicandri-Ciufelli M, Presutti L. Transcanal endoscopic approach to the sinus tympani: A clinical report. Otol Neurotol. 2009;30 (6):758–765.

[16] Nogueira JF, Mattioli F, Presutti L, Marchioni D. Endoscopic anatomy of the retrotympanum. Otolaryngol Clin North Am. 2013;46(2):179–188.

[17] Abdel Baki F, El Dine MB, El Saiid I, Bakry M. Sinus tympani endoscopic anatomy. Otolaryngol Head Neck Surg. 2002;127(3):158–162.

[18] Ozturan O, Bauer CA, Miller CC III Jenkins HA. Dimensions of the sinus tympani and its surgical access via a retrofacial approach. Ann Otol Rhinol Laryngol. 1996;105(10):776–783.

[19] Marchioni D, Alicandri-Ciufelli M, Grammatica A, Mattioli F, Presutti L. Pyramidal eminence and subpyramidal space: An endoscopic anatomical study. Laryngoscope. 2010;120(3):557–564.

[20] Proctor B. Surgical anatomy of the posterior tympanum. Ann Otol Rhinol Laryngol. 1969;78(5):1026–1040.

[21] Marchioni D, Alicandri-Ciufelli M, Piccinini A, Genovese E, Presutti L. Inferior retrotympanum revisited: An endoscopic anatomic study. Laryngoscope. 2010;120(9):1880–1886.

[22] Palva T, Johnsson LG. Epitympanic compartment surgical considerations: reevaluation. Am J Otol. 1995;16(4):505–513.

[23] Prussak A. Zur Anatomie des Menschlichen Trommelfells. Arch Ohrenheilkunde. 1867;3:255–258.

[24] Von Tröltsch A. Lehrbuch der Ohrenheilkunde mit Einschluss der Anatomie des Ohres. Leipzig, Germany: Von F. C. W. Vogel; 1881.

[25] Palva T, Ramsay H. Incudal folds and epitympanic aeration. Am J Otol. 1996;17(5):700–708.

[26] Horn KL, Brackmann DE, Luxford WM, Shea JJ III. The supratubal recess in cholesteatoma surgery. Ann Otol Rhinol Laryngol. 1986;95(1 Pt 1):12–15.

[27] Palva T, Northrop C, Ramsay H. Aeration and drainage pathways of Prussak's space. Int J Pediatr Otorhinolaryngol. 2001;57(1):55–65.

[28] Inanli S, Oztürk O, Batman C, Tutkun A, Uneri C, Sehitoğlu MA. Clinical importance of supratubal recess in cholesteatoma surgery. Otol Neurotol. 2001;22 (6):754–760.

[29] Palva T, Ramsay H, Böhling T. Tensor fold and anterior epitympanum. Am J Otol. 1997;18(3):307–316.

[30] Allam AF. Pneumatization of the temporal bone. Ann Otol Rhinol Laryngol. 1969;78(1):49–64.

[31] Valtonen HJ, Dietz A, Qvarnberg YH, Nuutinen J. Development of mastoid air cell system in children treated with ventilation tubes for early-onset otitis media: A prospective radiographic 5-year follow-up study. Laryngoscope. 2005;115(2):268–273.

[32] Green JD, Jr, Shelton C, Brackmann DE. Surgical management of iatrogenic facial nerve injuries. Otolaryngol Head Neck Surg. 1994;111(5):606–610.

[33] Francis H. Facial nerve emergencies. In: Eisele D, McQuone S. eds. Emergencies of the head and neck. St. Louis, MO: Mosby; 2000:337–366.

8 Biomaterials in Tympanomastoid Surgery

Matthew Yung

Abbreviations used in this chapter:

ABG: air-bone gap
HA: hydroxyapatite
MRI: magnetic resonance imaging
PORP: partial ossicular replacement prosthesis
PTFE: polytetrafluorethylene
TORP: total ossicular replacement prosthesis

8.1 Introduction

The use of alloplastic materials in tympanomastoid surgery is well established. They are divided into three main types based on the tissue response. Bioinert materials elicit no tissue response, biodegradable materials dissolve over a period of time, and bioactive materials encourage a particular host tissue response (e.g., bonding to surrounding tissue, encouragement of bone in-growth, fibrosis). Alloplastic materials can be metals, polymers, ceramics, or a composite of these. Metals are typically bioinert, polymers could be bioinert or biodegradable, and ceramics could be bioinert, biodegradable, or bioactive. The advantages of using alloplastic materials in tympanomastoid surgery include general biocompatibility, lack of disease transmission, user-friendliness, and unlimited material supply. The typical disadvantages include additional surgical cost and risks of secondary infection or extrusion. Other specific advantages and disadvantages for each type of material and some common applications in tympanomastoid surgery are given in ▶ Table 8.1.

8.2 Types of Alloplastic Materials

8.2.1 Polymers

The commonly used polymers in middle ear surgery are Silastic® (Dow Corning Corp.), polyethylene, and polytetrafluorethylene (PTFE). The most well-known brand name of PTFE is Teflon™ (Chemours). The most popular polyethylene used in ossicular prostheses are Polycel (trademark refers to porous polyethylene) and Plastipore (trademark refers to high-density porous polyethylene). The main advantages of these polymers are a low production cost and the ease with which they can be easily trimmed by scalpel or scissors. Most tympanostomy tubes are made from polymers.

8.2.2 Metals

Because metals are typically strong and good conductors of sound, they are commonly used in middle ear prostheses; however, metals are also often used in the construction of tympanostomy tubes. Metallic strength enables very thin shafts, hooks, and claws to be engineered into a prosthetic design without the risk of breaking. This characteristic allows unique designs that can promote secure coupling between the prosthesis and the ossicular chain, and the thin shaft of the metal ossicular reconstruction prosthesis affords placement even through tiny gaps. The most common metals used in tympanomastoid surgery are titanium, platinum, and stainless steel. Titanium is particularly popular because of its outstanding biocompatibility, strength, low weight, and high resistance to corrosion. In addition to being used in middle ear prostheses, titanium mesh and plates are used by some surgeons to reconstruct bony defects in the mastoid cavity.

In recent years, Nitinol (Fort Wayne Metals), an alloy composed of titanium and nickel, has been used in the design of middle ear implants due to its unique property of shape memory. This material undergoes deformation at one temperature and then recovers its original shape when heated above its "transformation temperature." Nitinol is mainly used in the loop of stapes pistons because of this self-crimping property that can be initiated with heat application.

One concern raised by the use of metal is delayed hypersensitivity reaction. This is alleged to be extremely rare for titanium, gold, or stainless steel because they are noncorrosive. Although

Table 8.1 Types of alloplastic materials and their characteristics and applications in ear surgery

Materials	Advantages	Disadvantages	Applications in Ear Surgery
Polymers Silastic Teflon Polyethylene (Plastipore and Polycel) PTFE	Easy and relatively cheap to fabricate; easily trimmed	Not strong; deform with time; may degrade	Ventilation tubes; stapedotomy pistons; prosthetic ossicles; splints in middle ear
Metals Stainless steel Platinum Titanium Nitinol	Mechanical strength; versatility in prosthetic designs	Higher cost of fabrication; rigid	Prosthetic ossicles; stapedotomy pistons; mesh/plate for bony defect repair
Ceramics Bioglass Aluminium oxides Calcium phosphates/HA	Corrosion-resistant; low thermal and electrical conductivity	High cost of fabrication; brittle	Prosthetic ossicles; filler materials in mastoid obliteration

Nitinol is in part composed of nickel, which is known to be frequently involved with Type IV (delayed) hypersensitivity reactions, there is allegedly very little potential for a hypersensitivity reaction to Nitinol because a very stable protective titanium dioxide (TiO_2) layer forms that acts as a barrier against ion exchange. There presently is not a reliable diagnostic test available for the determination of hypersensitivity to implanted metallic devices, and the most common test for delayed hypersensitivity is still the skin patch test. As the amount of metal used in middle ear prostheses is tiny, it is difficult to separate clinically an allergic reaction from other inflammatory conditions.

8.2.3 Ceramics

Bioceramics include a variety of biomaterials, such as carbon, alumina, hydroxyapatite (HA), bioglass, and tricalcium phosphate. In general, they show high biocompatibility, high resistance to corrosion and compression, and low electrical and thermal conductivities.[1] Ceramics are mainly used as bone substitutes because the mineral component of bone is calcium phosphate micro-crystals, mainly as HA. Bioactive ceramics react with physiological fluids, forming bonds to bone through the formation of bone-like HA layers, leading to effective biological interaction.

The biological behavior of bioceramics depends on many factors, such as the chemical composition and microstructure pore size. Dense ceramics are more resistant than porous ceramics to infection and reabsorption and are mainly used in ossicular prostheses. With increasing porosity and pore interconnectivity, bone ingrowth becomes more effective. Porous ceramics are mainly used as filler materials for mastoid obliteration.

For ossicular reconstruction, the most popular bioceramic is HA. Although carbon, bioglass, and aluminium oxide middle ear prostheses have also been used, they are not as popular.[2] For mastoid obliteration, the most popular bioceramics are HA and bioglass. Hydroxyapatite has a chemical composition that includes calcium (Ca) and phosphate (PO_4). Bioglass has a chemical composition that includes silicon dioxide (SiO_2), calcium oxide (CaO), and sodium oxide (Na_2O). The bioactivity of these bioceramics, whether they are bioinert, biodegradable, or bioactive, depends on the ratio of their chemical components, degree of crystallinity, temperature, and surface area.[3] SerenoCem is a hybrid glass polymer composite consisting of an alkaline inorganic glass reacted with an organic polyacid. It chemically bonds to bone mineral and metals and does not undergo appreciable shrinkage. Its granular form is used for mastoid obliteration, and its cement form is used as bone cement in middle ear surgery. BonAlive (Boston Medical Products Inc., Westborough, Massachusetts) is a bioglass that can be utilized for mastoid obliteration that takes advantage of an osteo-inductive host interaction, thereby promoting new bone formation within the obliterated cavity.

8.3 Use of Alloplastic Materials

8.3.1 Ossicular Reconstruction

Most new-generation ossicular prostheses are made of HA and/or titanium, virtually all of which demonstrate magnetic resonance imaging (MRI) compatibility. The clinical outcomes for HA in middle ear reconstruction were first reported by Grote,[4] and so far it has stood the test of time. To make the HA prosthesis more user-friendly, various composite HA prostheses have been subsequently developed consisting of an HA head plate and shaft made from other materials, with advantages ranging from malleability or the potential to be trimmed easily with a scalpel. These materials include Plastipore, PTFE, FLEX HA (HA and silicone composites), and HAPEX (HA-reinforced polyethylene composites). Some prostheses even incorporate a stainless steel core in the shaft to aid sound conduction,[5] whereas others have been designed with a pure titanium shaft.

Hydroxyapatite and SerenoCem in cement form are also being used in middle ear surgery, mainly to repair the long process of the incus[6,7] or to reinforce placement of an ossicular prosthesis in challenging cases. Whereas the short-term results are promising, there are still doubts over their long-term benefits[8] and a need for further long-term studies.

Titanium was first introduced as an alloplastic material for ossiculoplasty in 1993.[9] Modern engineering techniques enable many innovative designs to be incorporated to make the prosthesis more user-friendly and secure within the middle ear. For example, an open head plate allows the surgeon to observe the position of the bottom end during the placement of the prosthesis. The bottom end of the titanium partial ossicular replacement prosthesis (PORP) can take the shape of a cup, a clip, or claws to accommodate the stapes head. The design of a separate shoe helps to stabilize the distal end of the titanium total ossicular replacement prosthesis (TORP) on the footplate.

There is currently a myriad of prosthetic designs used for ossicular reconstruction. The factors that influence choice are the user-friendliness of the design,[10] cost of the prosthesis, and the personal preference of the surgeon. Because new designs of HA and titanium prostheses are being introduced all the time, direct comparison of clinical results reported in the literature are difficult. In particular, some manufacturers are producing composite prostheses using one material desirable for the head plate and another material desirable for the shaft. Even though HA has been alleged to be compatible for direct interface with the tympanic membrane and because all ceramic and metal prostheses are rigid compared with the thin tympanic membrane, they are all at risk of extrusion, unless there is a cartilage buffer between the head plate and the undersurface of the drumhead,[11] especially in the setting of negative middle ear pressure and tympanic membrane retraction.

There is no evidence to date showing that alloplastic material is better than autologous bone or sculpted native ossicles in ossicular reconstruction. Even though computer model experiments of ossicular reconstruction with PORPs suggest a slight acoustic advantage in the speech frequencies with HA[12] compared with other alloplastic materials, including titanium, there is in fact very little comparative *in vivo* data showing one alloplastic material to be more successful than all others. However, certain alloplastic materials have already been found to be less favorable than others as middle ear implants for a variety of reasons. Reparative granuloma was reported when gold pistons were used in stapes surgery.[13] Multinucleated foreign body giant cells were present in large numbers in Plastipore and Proplast explants from the middle ear, and with histological evidence of the prostheses breaking down.[14] There is a high rate of

Table 8.2 Summary of the long-term outcome of ossiculoplasty

Author	Number of cases & prosthetic material	Follow-up period & rate	Success criteria	Extrusion %	Success rate
Vartiainen 1992[17]	277 autologous incus/ cortical bone	5 yr; 92%	ABG ≤ 20 dB	NA	POR: 59%; TOR: 30%
Hess-Erga 2013[18]	76 titanium	5 yr; 100%	ABG ≤ 20 dB	5%	POR: 82%; TOR: 63%
Shinohara 2000[19]	150 HA	5 yr; 67%	ABG ≤ 20 dB	16%	POR: 60%; TOR: 34%
Smyth 1982[20]	144 Plastipore with and without cartilage on top of head plate	5 yr; 97%	ABG ≤ 10 dB	11.8%	POR: 43%; TOR: 22%

POR, partial ossicular reconstruction when stapes superstructure is intact; ABG, air-bone gap; TOR, total ossicular reconstruction when stapes superstructure is absent; NA, not available

extrusion of the Plastipore prosthesis in long-term follow-up studies, even with the presence of cartilage between the implant and the tympanic membrane.[15]

Sometimes, unfavorable results only become apparent with time. Ceravital prostheses became resorbed over a long period, leading to poor long-term results in ossiculoplasty.[16] ▶ Table 8.2 provides a summary of the long-term outcome of ossiculoplasty. Only ossiculoplasty studies with 5-year follow-up or longer and a follow-up rate of at least 50% were included. For the purpose of comparison, the outcomes of autologous and homologous materials are also included. Few reports in the literature fulfill such strict criteria. The success rate of ossiculoplasty, if defined as an air-bone gap (ABG) closure to within 20 dB, was roughly 80% in cases where the stapes superstructure was present and about 60% when it was absent. There was no alloplastic material free from extrusion, even if the head plate was covered by a sheet of cartilage. Because the long-term success of ossiculoplasty is often more dependent on the middle ear pathology than the prosthesis biomaterials, it should also be noted that comparisons of one prosthesis material versus another require careful stratification of subjects according to middle ear risk factors to be meaningful.

As previously mentioned, Nitinol has become popular in recent years in the construction of "self-crimping" stapedotomy prostheses, as the Nitinol loop will close and crimp to the incus when it is heated by a laser or a hot wire. These self-crimping stapes pistons may make the surgery of stapedectomy easier from a technical standpoint, but there is no evidence that it gives a better hearing outcome than conventional prostheses.[21]

One problem of a medical implant is that it promotes the adherence of biofilms on its surface.[22] Biofilms have been implicated in persistent otorrhea following tympanostomy tube insertion. Surface modifications have been promoted as a means of reducing biofilm formation, such as coating the tympanostomy tubes with agents that reduce the surface adhesion of biofilms, such as polyvinylpyrrolidone, or antibacterial agents, such as silver oxide (e.g., Activent tube, Medtronic) and vancomycin.[23,24] Although the results from *in vitro* studies were encouraging, success has not been replicated in clinical studies. Biofilms are also observed on explants of ossicular prostheses; however, their role in ossiculoplasty failure is more uncertain. The interaction between biofilms and the host environment is complex, and many other factors may influence mucosal healing and hearing outcome in tympanomastoid surgery.[25] Further research in this area is needed.

8.3.2 Mastoid Cavity Reconstruction

Filler materials for mastoid obliteration should be biocompatible, able to maintain volume over time, resistant to infection, and easy to remove at revision surgery. Currently, the main alloplastic material used for obliteration is bioceramic granules. It is important that these granules are covered by a layer of soft tissue, ideally a vascularized rotational flap, to prevent exposure, infection, and leakage of these materials into the ear canal. Some surgeons prefer bio-absorbable ceramics to encourage bone regeneration to gradually replace the bioceramics in the mastoid cavity.[26] Others prefer that bioceramics remain permanently in the mastoid cavity.[27]

There is no evidence to date showing one particular filler material to be better than the other. The main bioceramics used for mastoid obliteration are HA, bioglass, and SerenoCem (Corinthian Surgical, 2 Church Lane, Brinsley, Nottingham).[27,28,29] The factors that are likely to influence the choice of the filler materials are cost and the personal preference of the surgeon. It is imperative that the granular instead of the cement form is used because there are reports of high infection rates when bioceramic cement was used for mastoid obliteration.[30,31] ▶ Table 8.3 is a summary of clinical reports on the outcome of mastoid obliteration using bioceramics. The outcomes of obliteration using autologous cartilage and bone are included in the table for the purpose of comparison. On the whole, the results of mastoid obliteration are very favorable, irrespective of whether the cavity was obliterated using alloplastic or autologous materials.

As an alternative to using autologous bony or cartilaginous plates, bioceramics and titanium mesh or plates have been used by some surgeons to repair bony defects of the mastoid cavity. Some of the indications and outcomes are given in ▶ Table 8.4. The results are generally favorable. For bony canal wall repair, it is essential that the alloplastic plates are well covered by soft tissue flaps to prevent exposure of the materials.

Table 8.3 Summary of the reports on mastoid obliteration

Authors	Cases	Filler materials	Follow-up period	Outcome
Edfeldt, Strömbäck, Kinnefors, and Rask-Andersen 2013[32]	330	Cartilage Bone paste	6 yr	recurrent chol 10%; residual chol 3%; dry ear rate 99%; water resistant 92%
Kang, Ahn, Gu, and Han 2009[33]	200	Cartilage Bone chip/paste	>5 yr	recurrent chol 0%; residual chol 5%;
Sarin, Grénman, Aitasalo, and Pulkkinen 2012[29]	23	Bioglass	Mean 34 mo	dry ear 96%; small cavity 92%
Silvola 2012[34]	14	Bioglass	Mean 26 mo	2 leakages of granules; 1 revision meatoplasty; others well
Punke, Goetz, Just, and Pau 2012[35]	20	NanoBone (HA in $SiO_{2)}$	Mean 29 mo	dry ear 90%; no leakage of granules
Minoda, Hayashida, Masuda, and Yumoto 2007[36]	12	Beta-tricalcium phosphate	1–5 yr	dry ear 100%; no leakage of granules
Clark and Bottrill 2007[28]	16	SerenoCem	2.5 yr	3 needed revisions
Takahashi 1991[37]	48	HA	2 yr	recurrent chol 0%; 1 residual chol; 2 cases of exposed granules
Mahendran and Yung 2004[30]	10	HA	1 yr	recurrent chol 0%; residual chol 0%; dry ear 100%; small cavity 100%
Yung 1996[27]	34	HA	>1 yr	dry ear 91%; fully re-epithelialized 94%

chol, cholesteatoma

Table 8.4 The use of alloplastic materials for repair of bony defects in mastoid surgery

Author	Cases	Material and indication	Outcome
Sudhoff, Brors, Al-Lawati, Gimenez, Dazert and Hildmann 2006[38]	14	Titanium mesh to repair canal wall	2 exposures of mesh, requiring revision
Kim and Wilson 2006[39]	99	Titanium mesh to repair mastoid cortex	1 exposure of mesh in canal; elimination of post-auricular pit in all
Deveze, Rameh, Puchol, Lafont, Lavieille, and Magnan2010[40]	113	Titanium plates to repair canal wall	Healed canal skin in 84%; dry ear in 88.5%
Grote 1998[41]	56	HA plate to repair canal wall	75% still have intact canal wall after 15 yrs
Magliulo and D'Amico, and Forino 2001[42]	8	HA-coated titanium mesh to repair canal wall	No exposure of alloplastic canal wall
Kveton Goravalingappa 2000[43]	13	HA cement to repair tegmen and CSF otorrhea	1 postoperative infection; successful repair in all cases
Zanetti and Nassif 2003[44]	7	HA/polymer composite plate to repair tegmen defect	No rejection or dislodge of implants in any cases

CSF, cerebrospinal fluid

8.4 Conclusion

Alloplastic materials have given otologists many options in tympanomastoid reconstruction. They are particularly beneficial when there is no other autologous alternative available, such as the stapes piston for stapedotomy or the ventilation tube for the middle ear. For ossicular and mastoid reconstruction, alloplastic implants offer convenience to the surgeon. The cost of the implants can be partially offset by the time saved in harvesting autologous materials; however, there is no evidence that alloplastic materials are better than autologous materials in tympanomastoid surgery for straightforward cases. The user-friendliness of alloplastic materials makes them popular among otologists. The strength of the metal allows many innovative designs to be incorporated into modern ossicular prostheses and may help to secure the prosthesis in the middle ear.

References

[1] Sáenz A, Rivera-Muñoz E, Brostow W, Castaño VM. Ceramic biomaterials: An introductory overview. Journal of Materials Education. 1999;21:267–276.

[2] Yung MW. Literature review of alloplastic materials in ossiculoplasty. J Laryngol Oto.l. 2003;117(6):431–436.

[3] Best SM, Porter AE, Thian ES, Huang J. Bioceramics: Past, present and for the future. J Eur Ceram Soc. 2008;28:1319–1327.

[4] Grote JJ. Tympanoplasty with calcium phosphate. Arch Otolaryngol. 1984;110 (3):197–199.

[5] Black B. Design and development of a contoured ossicular replacement prosthesis: clinical trials of 125 cases. Am J Otol. 1990;11(2):85–89.

[6] Tange RA. Repair of the ossicular chain with an ionomer cement by an inadequate incus after prior stapes surgery for otosclerosis. Eur Arch Otorhinolaryngol. 1996;253(4–5):313–315.

[7] Somers T, Van Rompaey V, Claes G, et al. Ossicular reconstruction: hydroxyapatite bone cement versus incus remodelling: how to manage incudostapedial discontinuity. Eur Arch Otorhinolaryngol. 2012;269(4):1095–1101.

[8] Kupperman D, Tange RA. Ionomeric cement in the human middle ear cavity: Long-term results of 23 cases. Laryngoscope. 2001;111(2):306–309.

[9] Dalchow CV, Grün D, Stupp HF. Reconstruction of the ossicular chain with titanium implants. Otolaryngol Head Neck Surg. 2001;125(6):628–630.

[10] Yung MW, Brewis C. A comparison of the user-friendliness of hydroxyapatite and titanium ossicular prostheses. J Laryngol Otol. 2002;116(2):97–102.

[11] Kobayashi T, Gyo K, Shinohara T, Yanagihara N. Ossicular reconstruction using hydroxyapatite prostheses with interposed cartilage. Am J Otolaryngol. 2002;23(4):222–227.

[12] Yao W, Guo C, Luo X. Study on effects of partial ossicular replacement prostheses with different materials on hearing restoration. J Mater Sci Mater Med. 2013;24(2):515–522.

[13] Tange RA, Schimanski G, van Lange JW, Grolman W, Zuur LC. Reparative granuloma seen in cases of gold piston implantation after stapes surgery for otosclerosis. Auris Nasus Larynx. 2002;29(1):7–10.

[14] Kerr AG. Proplast and Plastipore. Clin Otolaryngol Allied Sci. 1981;6(3):187–191.

[15] Colletti V, Fiorino FG, Sittoni V. Minisculptured ossicle grafts versus implants: long-term results. Am J Otol. 1987;8(6):553–559.

[16] Brewis C, Orrell J, Yung MW. Ceravital revisited: Lessons to be learned. Otol Neurotol. 2003;24(1):20–23.

[17] Vartiainen E, Nuutinen J. Long-term hearing results of one-stage tympanoplasty for chronic otitis media. Eur Arch Otorhinolaryngol. 1992;249(6):329–331.

[18] Hess-Erga J, Møller P, Vassbotn FS. Long-term hearing result using Kurz titanium ossicular implants. Eur Arch Otorhinolaryngol. 2013;270(6):1817–1821.

[19] Shinohara T, Gyo K, Saiki T, Yanagihara N. Ossiculoplasty using hydroxyapatite prostheses: long-term results. Clin Otolaryngol Allied Sci. 2000;25 (4):287–292.

[20] Smyth GDL. Five-year report on partial ossicular replacement prostheses and total ossicular replacement prostheses. Otolaryngol Head Neck Surg. 1982;90 (3 Pt 1):343–346.

[21] Van Rompaey V, Claes G, Potvin J, Wouters K, Van de Heyning PH. Systematic review of the literature on nitinol prostheses in surgery for otosclerosis: Assessment of the adequacy of statistical power. Otol Neurotol. 2011;32 (3):357–366.

[22] Costerton JW, Montanaro L, Arciola CR. Biofilm in implant infections: Its production and regulation. Int J Artif Organs. 2005;28(11):1062–1068.

[23] Ojano-Dirain CP, Silva RC, Antonelli PJ. Biofilm formation on coated silicone tympanostomy tubes. Int J Pediatr Otorhinolaryngol. 2013;77(2):223–227.

[24] Jang CH, Park H, Cho YB, Choi CH. Effect of vancomycin-coated tympanostomy tubes on methicillin-resistant Staphylococcus aureus biofilm formation: In vitro study. J Laryngol Otol. 2010;124(6):594–598.

[25] Jaryszak EM, Sampson EM, Antonelli PJ. Effect of ossicular prosthesis biofilms on middle ear scarring and hearing outcomes. Otol Neurotol. 2009;30 (8):1191–1195.

[26] Jang CH, Cho YB, Bae CS. Evaluation of bioactive glass for mastoid obliteration: A guinea pig model. In Vivo. 2007;21(4):651–655.

[27] Yung MW. The use of hydroxyapatite granules in mastoid obliteration. Clin Otolaryngol Allied Sci. 1996;21(6):480–484.

[28] Clark MP, Bottrill I. SerenoCem -glass ionomeric granules: a 3-year follow-up assessment of their effectiveness in mastoid obliteration. Clin Otolaryngol. 2007;32(4):287–290.

[29] Sarin J, Grénman R, Aitasalo K, Pulkkinen J. Bioactive glass S53P4 in mastoid obliteration surgery for chronic otitis media and cerebrospinal fluid leakage. Ann Otol Rhinol Laryngol. 2012;121(9):563–569.

[30] Mahendran S, Yung MW. Mastoid obliteration with hydroxyapatite cement: The Ipswich experience. Otol Neurotol. 2004;25(1):19–21.

[31] Ridenour JS, Poe DS, Roberson DW. Complications with hydroxyapatite cement in mastoid cavity obliteration. Otolaryngol Head Neck Surg. 2008;139 (5):641–645.

[32] Edfeldt L, Strömbäck K, Kinnefors A, Rask-Andersen H. Surgical treatment of adult cholesteatoma: long-term follow-up using total reconstruction procedure without staging. Acta Otolaryngol. 2013;133(1):28–34.

[33] Kang MK, Ahn JK, Gu TW, Han CS. Epitympanoplasty with mastoid obliteration technique: A long-term study of results. Otolaryngol Head Neck Surg. 2009;140(5):687–691.

[34] Silvola JT. Mastoidectomy cavity obliteration with bioactive glass: A pilot study. Otolaryngol Head Neck Surg. 2012;147(1):119–126.

[35] Punke C, Goetz W, Just T, Pau HW. [Mastoid obliteration with a highly porous bone grafting material in combination with cartilage] Laryngorhinootologie. 2012;91(9):566–570.

[36] Minoda R, Hayashida M, Masuda M, Yumoto E. Preliminary experience with beta-tricalcium phosphate for use in mastoid cavity obliteration after mastoidectomy. Otol Neurotol. 2007;28(8):1018–1021.

[37] Takahashi S. [Tympanoplasty with mastoid obliteration using hydroxyapatite granules for aural cholesteatoma—a clinical and experimental study] Nippon Jibiinkoka Gakkai Kaiho. 1991;94(6):833–842.

[38] Sudhoff H, Brors D, Al-Lawati A, Gimenez E, Dazert S, Hildmann H. Posterior canal wall reconstruction with a composite cartilage titanium mesh graft in canal wall down tympanoplasty and revision surgery for radical cavities. J Laryngol Otol. 2006;120(10):832–836.

[39] Kim HH, Wilson DF. Titanium mesh for functional reconstruction of the mastoid cortex after mastoidectomy. Otol Neurotol. 2006;27(1):33–36.

[40] Deveze A, Rameh C, Puchol MS, Lafont B, Lavieille JP, Magnan J. Rehabilitation of canal wall down mastoidectomy using a titanium ear canal implant. Otol Neurotol. 2010;31(2):220–224.

[41] Grote JJ. Results of cavity reconstruction with hydroxyapatite implants after 15 years. Am J Otol. 1998;19(5):565–568.

[42] Magliulo G, D'Amico R, Forino M. Reconstruction of the posterior auditory canal with hydroxyapatite-coated titanium. J Otolaryngol. 2001;30(6):330–333.

[43] Kveton JF, Goravalingappa R. Elimination of temporal bone cerebrospinal fluid otorrhea using hydroxyapatite cement. Laryngoscope. 2000;110(10 Pt 1):1655–1659.

[44] Zanetti D, Nassif N. Transmastoid Repair of Minor Skull Base Defects with Flexible Hydroxyapatite Sheets. Skull Base. 2003;13(1):1–11.

9 Middle Ear Mechanics in Hearing Reconstruction

Manohar Bance, John J. Rosowski, and Robert B. A. Adamson

Abbreviations used in this chapter:

ABG: air-bone gap
EAC: external auditory canal
FOM: footplate onto malleus
FOT: footplate onto TM
PGOW: pressure gain at the oval window
PORP: partial ossicular replacement prosthesis
RoWPOWA: round window protection with oval window access
SHOM: stapes head onto malleus
SHOT: stapes head onto TM
TM: tympanic membrane
TORP: total ossicular replacement prosthesis

9.1 Introduction

As every middle ear surgeon can attest, achieving good hearing results from middle ear reconstruction is difficult and unpredictable, with a myriad of factors impacting the outcomes. Published hearing results of middle ear reconstructions reveal an enormous range,[1] and in general are far from satisfactory. A weighted average calculated from a series totaling 4,389 partial ossicular replacement prosthesis (PORP) reconstructions and 1,413 total ossicular replacement prosthesis (TORP) reconstructions shows air-bone gap closure (ABG) to within 20 dB occurring on average in only 55% of the PORP reconstructions and in 43% of the TORP reconstructions.[1]

This variance is not unexpected; there are a host of patient factors, including differing residual middle ear anatomy, type and extent of pathology, and patient healing, that affect reconstruction success. This is well recognized by various middle ear risk indexes, such as the Ossiculoplasty Outcomes Parameter Staging (OOPS) index by Dornhoffer and Gardner, which assigns prognostic value to drainage, mucosal fibrosis, revision surgery, and type of surgery.[2] Variance in surgical factors, such as surgical techniques and philosophies, adds greatly to the diversity of outcomes. Finally, variability in prosthesis factors, such as its mechanical properties, compounds the diversity even further. There are literally hundreds of possible allograft and autograft prosthesis designs and shapes available, which compounds the spread in hearing results even further. Hence, even in the same ear with the same surgeon, different results may ensue due to differences in the original pathology, reconstruction technique, and the healing processes.

This chapter will focus on the mechanical principles of hearing reconstruction, rather than espousing one particular viewpoint, recognizing that surgeons will vary their technique to suit their own patient population and the individual ear they happen to be facing. Although we will focus on the issues of middle ear mechanics and the optimization of the transfer of sound power from air to the inner ear, it must be remembered that in the real world, stabilization of the reconstruction and other healing issues play an equal, if not greater, role in clinical hearing results. It is well known that long-term ossiculoplasty results decline with time due to a host of mechanisms, including scarring, resorption of ossicles, prosthesis displacement by trauma or eardrum movements, and extrusion due to biological processes.[3] Biocompatibility issues may dominate the inflammatory and scarring reaction around the prosthesis. Aeration of the middle ear air space is also a key issue given that decreased ventilation due to poor Eustachian tube function leads to fluid in the middle ear, retraction of the tympanic membrane (TM) onto the promontory, or abnormal static pressure within the middle ear, all of which reduce the middle ear movements produced by sound. In many ears, these factors will dominate the hearing results far more than the mechanical properties of the prosthesis used. None of these biological issues are addressed in this chapter.

Rather, because clinical studies can be difficult to interpret due to multiple confounding variables, in this chapter we focus on data from temporal bone studies, where individual mechanical factors within the middle ear can be more easily manipulated and measured. Unless otherwise stated, the illustrated results are from fresh cadaveric temporal bones. We also focus on reconstructive surgeries in which the normal ossicular structure cannot be maintained and some kind of prosthetic reconstruction is needed. This can involve allograft prostheses, such as titanium or hydroxyapatite variants, or a sculpted homograft, such as an ossicle, bone chip, or cartilage. In this context, "prosthesis" refers to any connector between residual or reconstructed middle ear structure, rather than only referring to an allograft commercial prosthesis. The surgical recommendations and reconstruction classifications, when alluded to, are from the clinical author (Bance). We will briefly review the normal physiology and pathophysiology of the external and middle ear, and then discuss the mechanical factors involved in surgical reconstruction options and techniques.

9.2 External Auditory Canal (EAC)

Sound first enters the auditory system at the pinna and propagates into the ear canal where it exerts dynamic pressure on the TM. The presence of the head, pinna, and ear canal all cause frequency-dependent changes to the amplitude and phase of the incident sound. Because the auditory system is insensitive to the absolute phase of the sound wave at either ear (although it is sensitive to phase differences between the two ears), it is customary to primarily emphasize the amplitude effects.

The presence of the head increases the sound pressure on the incident side and decreases it on the opposite side, producing a "head shadow." The degree of this effect is frequency-dependent. The wavelength is inversely proportional to the frequency, so higher frequencies have shorter wavelengths. When the head diameter is small compared with the sound wavelength (i.e., at lower frequencies), the sound wave moving towards one side of the head has time to pass around the head to the other side in a single half cycle without significant disturbance in the wave. As a result, the sound pressure seen on the two sides of the head is not much different. Hence, at low frequencies, both ears experience similar sound levels. As the wavelength

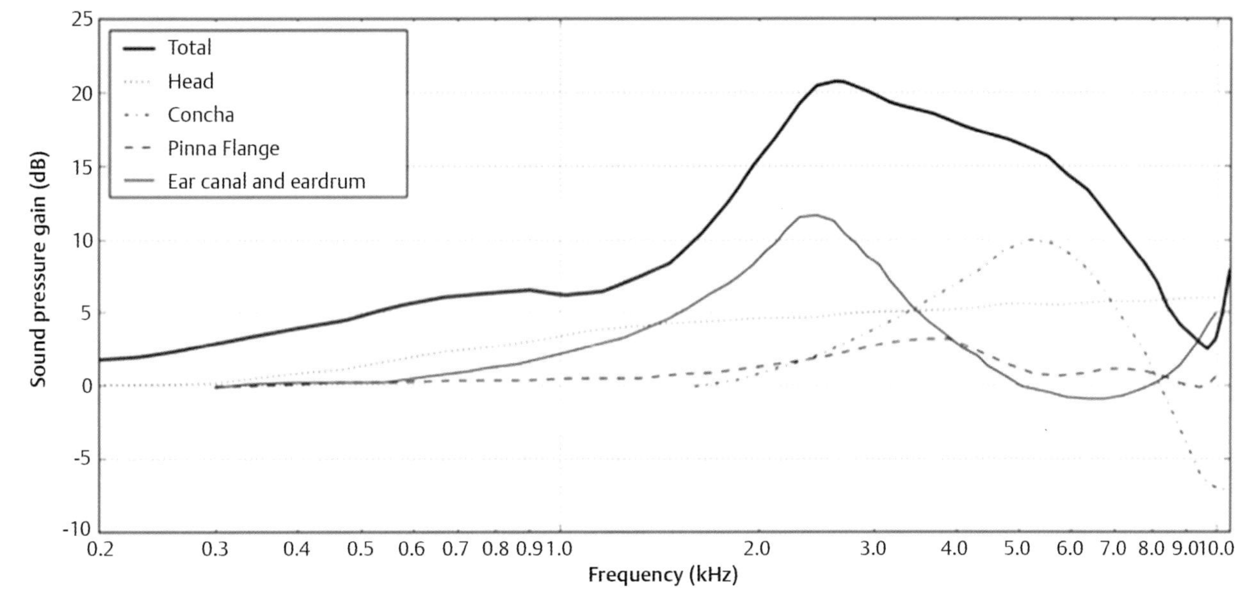

Fig. 9.1 Pressure gain for a 45-degree horizontal azimuth source. The gain due to the head is based on a spherical head model, that of the concha and pinna on experiments on blocked ear canals, and that of the ear canal and total gain on measurement at the TM. (Modified with permission from Shaw EAG. The External Ear. In: Kiedel WD, Neff WD, eds. Auditory System. Berlin: Springer-Verlag; 1974. p. 455-490.)

approaches the size of the head, the wave incident on one side of the head cannot travel around to the contralateral side within a single half cycle. This leads to a build-up of sound pressure on the incident side that, in the limit of high frequency, doubles the amplitude of the incident sound wave. At the same time, the pressure on the opposite side drops with increasing frequency. Although the sound pressure on the incident side of the head rises smoothly with frequency, there is little drop in sound pressure on the contralateral side until around 2000 Hz, where the wavelength is 17 cm, roughly the width of the human head. The drop in contralateral sound pressure reaches about -15 dB at 6000 Hz, compared with low frequencies.

Such behavior has been well studied by Teranishi and Shaw[4,5] who, in experiments on live human subjects and head models, demonstrated a steady increase in the sound pressure on the incident side of the head reaching about 6 dB at 10 kHz relative to that at low frequencies. This effect can be seen in the curve labeled "Head" in ▶ Fig. 9.1, which rises smoothly to about 6 dB at high frequencies. When the sound is directed at the incident ear, the ratio of sound pressure level between the incident and contralateral sides of the head is only a few dB at 200 Hz, rising to roughly 20 dB at 10–12 kHz.[6]

The pinna serves two main acoustical purposes. Given that it faces forward, it has a similar effect to the head in increasing the pressure of sound incident from the front and decreasing the pressure of sound incident from the back. Because it is much smaller than the head, the pinna's directionality only affects higher frequency (shorter wavelength) sounds. This can be seen in the curve labeled "Pinna Flange" in ▶ Fig. 9.1, which exhibits essentially no gain until about 3000 Hz. The other effect of the pinna is that the cavities of the pinna, and primarily the concha, act as resonators for sound. A resonator is a structure that stores acoustical energy of selected frequencies, termed the resonant frequencies, allowing the sound pressure at those frequencies to build up to a high amplitude. The resonant frequency depends on the dimensions of the elements that store energy. Teranishi and Shaw[5,7] showed that the response of the human concha and ear canal entrance can be approximated quite well by modeling a cylinder and surrounding flange, and that, when matched to the dimensions of the human ear, this model exhibits a resonant frequency that matches the average resonant frequency of human pinnas of 4700 Hz. This can be seen in the curve labeled "Concha" in ▶ Fig. 9.1. The typical gain in sound pressure from the concha as measured at the entrance of the external auditory meatus is approximately 10 dB, as shown in ▶ Fig. 9.2.

A second phenomenon associated with the concha is the pinna notch, a sharply tuned minimum in the response of the auditory system typically in the 9–11 kHz range. It arises due to the destructive interference between sound that directly enters the ear canal and sound that reflects off the concha before entering the ear canal. When these two pathways for sound differ in length by half a wavelength, they will destructively interfere with each other. This happens when the dimension of the concha is a quarter of a wavelength (because sound traverses it twice on reflection). The concha linear dimension is about 8–10 mm, resulting in destructive interference in the range of 8500–10,500 Hz. Five other weaker pinna resonances also occur in the range of 10–15 kHz. These pinna resonances play an essential role in sound localization in the elevation plane because their strength depends strongly on the elevation of the sound source. Temporarily and successively blocking the cavities of the pinna results in a decrease in elevation localization acuity, with the largest drop in acuity occurring when the concha is blocked and smaller drops occurring when the fossa and scaphae are blocked.[8]

The ear canal is a tube averaging 2.5 cm in length in adults, with an average diameter of 7 mm and an average volume of

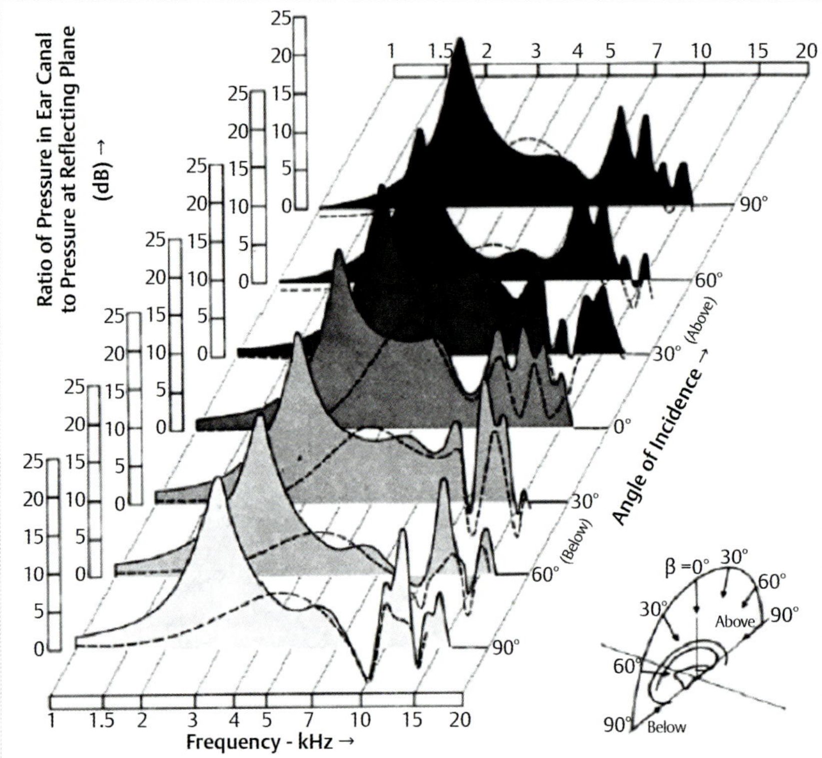

Fig. 9.2 Pressure at the TM compared with pressure seen at a reflecting plate at the same location in the absence of an external ear as a function of source elevation direction. The most significant spectral changes occur in the 9–15 kHz band, which is where most of the elevation pinna cues occur. (Used with permission from Shaw EA and Teranishi R. Sound pressure generated in an external-ear replica and real human ears by a nearby point source. The Journal of the Acoustical Society of America. 1968;44(1):240-249.)

1 cm^3. Acoustically it also forms a resonator. At specific frequencies, interference between the incoming sound and the waves reflected from the TM leads to an increase in the sound energy at the TM. This enhancement occurs when the length of the canal tube is 1/4, 3/4, 5/4, etc., of the wavelength of sound.

From this simple quarter wave resonator model, the 2.5-cm length of the ear canal should generate a resonance at 3400 Hz. In fact, the resonance is somewhat lower, typically closer to 2500 Hz, due to imperfect reflections at the TM and the influence of the wide opening of the concha around the lateral end of the canal. This wide opening effectively lengthens the canal and lowers the resonant frequency. The typical gain due to the ear canal with the characteristic resonance can be seen in the curve in ▶ Fig. 9.1 labeled "Ear canal and ear drum."

The imperfect reflection of the sound at the TM is essential to hearing: if the reflection were perfect, no sound would travel to the middle ear. The TM presents a high stiffness and, hence, a large impedance at low frequencies that results in a strong reflection, but the TM's impedance drops by a factor of four between 200 Hz and 2000 Hz. The reduced middle ear reflectance in the mid-range has the effect of reducing the ear canal pressure gain, lowering the resonance frequency and broadening the ear canal resonance. The TM impedance can be strongly affected by pathologies. Middle ear fluid creates a higher TM impedance by reducing the compliance of the middle ear cavity. This results in a stronger and more sharply tuned external ear resonance. Perforations in the middle ear reduce the impedance at the TM, allowing sound to travel directly into the middle ear. The resulting lower reflection reduces the ear canal gain and broadens the ear canal resonance.

In canal wall-down mastoidectomies, the ear canal is opened to the mastoid cavity, and so the ear canal length is effectively increased. Increasing the ear canal's length in this way measurably decreases the ear canal resonance frequency, and filling in the cavity can increase the resonance frequency to a value closer to that seen in the absence of a mastoid cavity. This effect was reported by Evans, Day and Browning who observed a 300-Hz decrease in ear canal resonance frequency after radical mastoidectomy in 12 patients.[9] More recently, Jang studied ear canal resonances in populations of 40 normal ears, 20 mastoid cavities, and 40 filled in or obliterated cavities, observing mean ear canal resonance frequencies at 2950 Hz, 2350 Hz, and 2750 Hz, respectively.[10] The measured acoustic response at the TM for the three populations is shown in ▶ Fig. 9.3.

Taken together, the effects of the head, pinna, ear canal, and TM act to increase the pressure seen at the TM by up to 22 dB compared with the pressure that would be seen at the same location if the head were not there (thick, solid curve in ▶ Fig. 9.1). The pressure enhancement peaks at about 2100 Hz and remains above 10 dB over a wide range, from 1500 Hz to 6000 Hz. It drops off slowly toward the lower frequencies, reaching 2 dB at 200 Hz. At higher frequencies, the response drops off sharply due to the pinna notch. Taken together, this means the EAC is a significant factor in generating pressure gain within the overall EAC/middle ear complex, and, at some frequencies, can provide more of the pressure gain than the middle ear does.

9.3 Normal Middle Ear Function

The middle ear is made up of the TM, ossicles, and the middle ear air spaces. The TM and ossicles move in response to sound pressure in the ear canal, while the high compressibility of the air within the middle ear permits these motions. At frequencies below 1–2 kHz, the TM and ossicles move almost as a unit, where all parts of the TM and ossicles move in phase. This in-phase motion suggests the entire middle ear approximates a single acoustico-mechanical device when responding to low-frequency sound. At frequencies above 2 kHz, parts of the TM surface move out of phase with each other,[11] the ossicles and their joints begin to bend,[12] and it becomes necessary to consider the mechanics of the individual components of the middle ear rather than to treat them as a single structure.

The difference between the low- and high-frequency action of the middle ear is schematized in ▶ Fig. 9.4, where the sizes of the different arrows indicate the magnitude of sound-driven motions and the directions of the arrows indicate in-phase or out-of-phase behavior. At frequencies less than 2 kHz (▶ Fig. 9.4a), the surface of the TM and the ossicles move with different magnitudes, but they all move in and out together. The different lengths of the arrows point out that the umbo moves less than the TM surface. At frequencies above 2 kHz, regions on the TM begin to move out of phase with each other as the TM surface appears to break up into different patterns of modal motions.[11,13] There is also a difference in phase in the motion of the umbo and the stapes as the ossicles bend and the ossicular joints allow relative motions between the components of the chain.

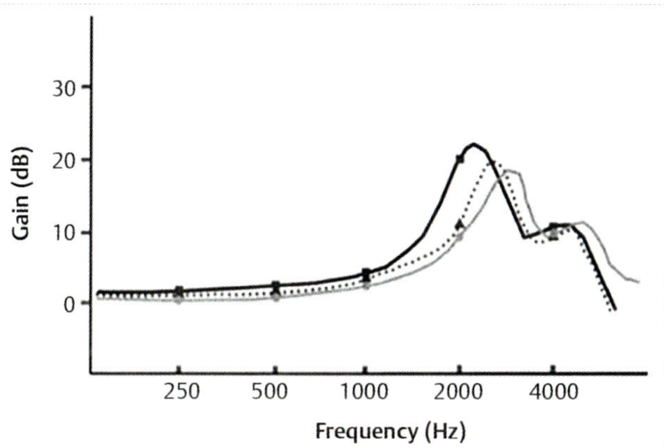

Fig. 9.3 Mean pressure gain at the eardrum for a population of normal patients (gray line), open mastoid patients (black line), and obliterated or filled mastoid patients (dotted line). (Used with permission from Jang CH. Changes in external ear resonance after mastoidectomy: open cavity mastoid versus obliterated mastoid cavity. Clinical otolaryngology and allied sciences. 2002;27(6):509-510.)

The function of the middle ear is to help match the difference in acoustic impedance between air and cochlear fluid, a process that provides a gain in sound pressure between the EAC and the oval window. This gain helps produce a sound pressure difference between the cochlear windows, which is the primary stimulus to the traveling wave and excitation of the cochlear partition.

9.3.1 The Tympanic Membrane

The TM is one of the primary elements in the transformation and coupling of sound energy from the ear canal to the oval window. The area of the TM is a primary determinant in its impedance transformation function,[14,15] and its mechanical properties help shape the frequency response of the middle ear. At frequencies below 1 kHz, the input impedance at the normal TM is dominated by the stiffness of the TM and ossicular ligaments[16]; at frequencies between 2 and 8 kHz, the impedance appears as a combination of resistance (from damping within the inner ear[17] and mass[18]). Therefore, in pathology and surgical reconstruction, changes in stiffness of the TM and oval window annular ligament primarily affect the transmission of low-frequency sounds, and alterations in ossicular mass should affect the high-frequency response of the ear.[19]

Some of these processes are observed in the sound-induced motion of the umbo. ▶ Fig. 9.5 illustrates the transfer function that describes the ratio of the velocity of the umbo to the sound pressure in the ear canal near the TM. At frequencies below 1 kHz, the increasing magnitude and ~ 0.2-period phase angle of the umbo motion is consistent with a stiffness-dominated impedance of the umbo. Between 2 and 4 kHz, the near-constant magnitude and phase between 0 and -0.2 is consistent with resistance and mass impedance effects. However, at higher frequencies, the phase angle drops and is more consistent with some kind of delay between the sound pressure and the resulting motion of the umbo, (e.g., from traveling waves or other sources).

While the TM moves in phase to sound at low frequencies, there are significant variations in the magnitude of motion across its surface, with the smallest motion occurring along the attachment of the malleus to the TM.[11,20] At frequencies above 2 kHz, different parts of the TM begin to move out of phase, and the increasingly complicated patterns of TM surface motion suggest that, at sound frequencies above 6 to 8 kHz, much of

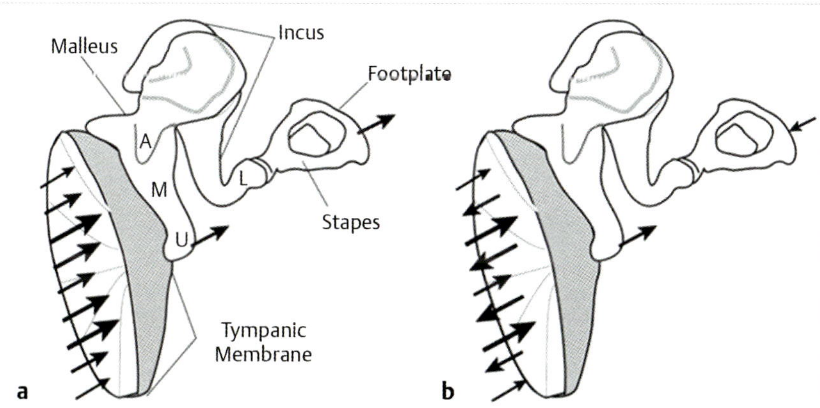

Fig. 9.4 (a,b) Schematics of the TM and ossicles illustrating the in-phase behavior of the middle ear at frequencies less than 2 kHz and the variations in phase that occur at higher frequencies.

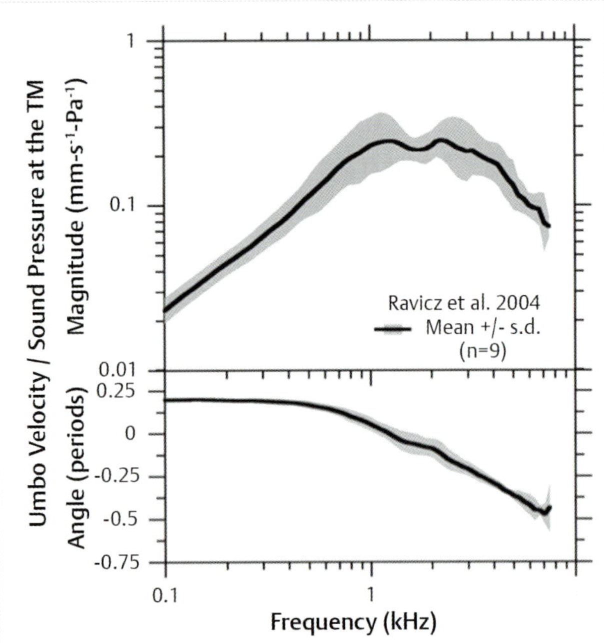

Fig. 9.5 Measurements of the sound-induced velocity of the umbo of the malleus normalized by the stimulus sound pressure within the ear canal near the TM made in fresh human temporal bones. The means ± the standard deviations from 9 ears are illustrated. (Data from Ravicz M, Rosowski J, Merchant S. Mechanisms of hearing loss resulting from middle-ear fluid. Hearing research. 2004;195:105-130.)

the eardrum may be decoupled from the ossicles.[21] However, others suggest tight coupling of the TM and malleus at high frequencies via the radial fibers within the TM.[22]

9.3.2 The Ossicular Chain

The three linked ossicles (the malleus, incus, and stapes) couple the TM to the oval window. At frequencies below 2 kHz, the ossicles act as a set of loosely coupled rigid bodies that rotate about an axis roughly passing through the posterior-incudal and anterior-malleal ligaments.[14,23] The loose coupling of the ossicles comes from the action of the incudomalleal joint, which allows relative motions of the incus and malleus at most acoustic frequencies, with this slippage increasing above 2 kHz.[24] Above 2 kHz, there is evidence of flexing of the ossicles themselves and more complicated motions of the ossicles.[12] Although it is generally assumed the piston-like motions of the stapes are the most relevant for sound transmission to the inner ear, there is some evidence that when piston-like movements are reduced, other modes of stapes motion, such as rocking motions, can contribute to inner ear stimulation. This can happen at high frequencies.[25] Such complicated motions of the footplate could also be excited by the eccentric forces that result from various ossicular reconstruction strategies.

9.3.3 The Middle Ear Air Spaces

Air is a compressible fluid, and according to the ideal gas law, the larger the volume of fluid, the lower the pressure needed to compress the fluid. The normal volume of the adult human middle ear air spaces varies from 2 mL to 20 mL, with estimates of mean volume near 6 mL.[26] The majority of this air is usually housed within the mastoid, with 1–2 mL in the tympanic cavity behind the TM.[16] Regardless of the location of the air, the total air volume determines the compressibility of the middle ear air spaces at low frequencies. In healthy ears with air volumes greater than 2 mL, the air is so compressible that it has little effect on the middle ear input impedance and plays nearly no role in determining the magnitude of the sound-induced motion of the TM. Mastoid obliteration will not change the volume of air in an otherwise well-ventilated middle ear sufficiently to have any mechanical impact on its input impedance; however, the compressibility of residual air within the cavity can become significant in diseased or reconstructed ears.[27,28] The air volume has to fall to very low levels (< 10% of normal volume) to have any significant effect on middle ear function.[27]

9.3.4 Middle Ear Pressure Gain

The main mechanism the middle ear uses in matching the impedance of air and cochlear fluid is its action as a hydraulic lever, in which the small area of the bony stapes footplate acts as a piston coupled to the larger area of the TM. The ratio of these areas is the primary determinant of how well airborne sound energy in the ear canal is transformed to sound energy at the oval window. Although the bony stapes footplate acts as a well-defined output piston, the TM is far from an ideal piston head: it fails to move in phase at frequencies greater than 2 kHz, and the growth of out-of-phase vibrations across its surface reduces the effective area of the piston. This non-piston-like behavior may be an immediate result of the light and flaccid construction required to minimize the mass of the TM and permit the relatively large TM motions produced by sound.

Associated with the transforming lever function is a middle ear gain, which in an ideal hydraulic level would be defined by the area of the input (TM) and output (stapes footplate) pistons.[14,29] In humans, the area of the TM is about 66 mm^2 and the area of the footplate is about 3.2 mm^2.[14] The resultant area ratio equals 20.6, which in dB is a ratio of 26.3 dB. To estimate this gain experimentally, Kurokawa and Goode[30] measured the stapes motions that resulted from a stimulus sound pressure in the ear canal and from acoustic stimulation of the isolated oval window (i.e., with the middle ear removed). The ratio of the pressures required with and without the middle ear to produce identical motions of the stapes is a measure of the pressure gain of the middle ear (▶ Fig. 9.6). The estimated middle ear pressure gain is within 6 dB of the 26.3 dB area ratio for sounds of frequencies less than 2 kHz (indicating an efficient hydraulic lever), but the gain falls as frequency is increased above 2 kHz and is effectively zero around 6 kHz.

If the middle ear were an ideal transformer, the measured gain would be close to the anatomical area ratio and frequency-independent. Deviations from this ideal state occur because of the action of nonideal processes within the middle ear, which include the effective loss of the TM area as it breaks up into out-of-phase segments at higher frequencies, the need to overcome stiffness in the TM and the ossicular supports, the masses of the ossicles and inner ear fluids, the damping within the cochlea, the losses of sound energy that occur with relative

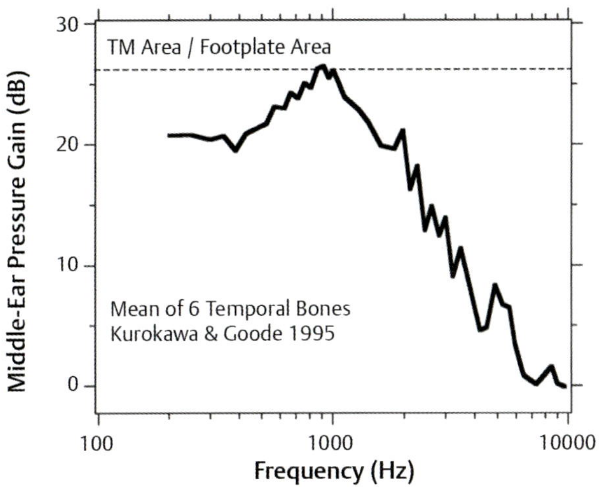

Fig. 9.6 The mean of measurements in 6 temporal bones of the ratio of the sound pressure produced at the oval window compared with the sound pressure input in the ear canal. This Middle Ear Pressure Gain is compared with the gain predicted by an anatomically realistic TM-to-footplate area ratio.

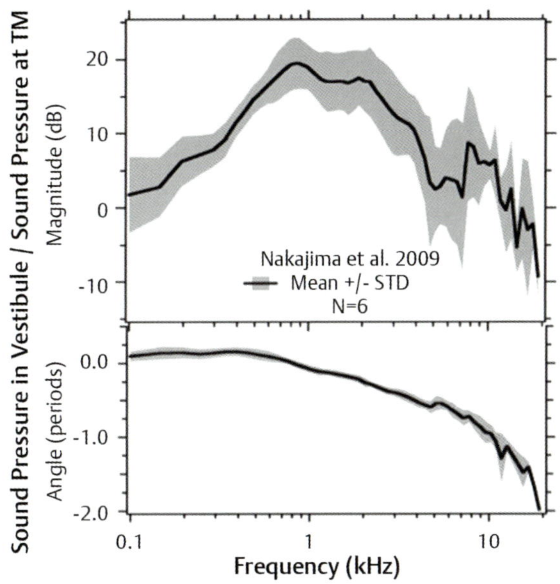

Fig. 9.7 Measures of the ratio of sound pressure in the vestibule to the sound pressure in the ear canal at the TM. The upper panel shows the magnitude of the pressure gain. The lower panel shows the difference in phase between the sound pressure in the vestibule and the sound pressure at the TM. (Data are from Nakajima HH, Dong W, Olson ES, Merchant SN, Ravicz ME, Rosowski JJ. Differential intracochlear sound pressure measurements in normal human temporal bones. Journal of the Association for Research in Otolaryngology: JARO. 2009;10(1):23-36.)

motion across the ossicular joints, and losses due to bending of the ossicles.

Although the middle ear pressure gain depends on the areas of the TM and the footplate, the relationship between this gain and the transfer of sound through the middle ear into the inner ear is complicated. Either a too-high gain or a too-low gain can lead to hearing loss. Consider what happens when replacing the stapes footplate with a piston of variable area: one can maximize the pressure gain at the interface of the replacement piston and the cochlear fluids by making the piston as small as possible; however, such a design would have two failings. First, as the piston area gets smaller, the volume displaced by motions of the replacement piston also decreases. Second, although the pressure at the interface point increases as the area decreases, the average pressure over the area of the whole oval window is unchanged. Indeed, estimates of the optimum piston area for stapes reconstruction suggest a piston area equal to the area of the normal footplate, with smaller and larger areas leading to decreases in middle ear sound transfer.[28]

The Kurokawa and Goode technique of comparing stapes motions produced by sound stimuli in the ear canal with those produced by sound stimuli presented directly to the lateral surface of the stapes after removing the TM, malleus, and incus gives one measure of middle ear gain. This estimate relates the sound pressure in the ear canal to the effective pressure that acts to move the stapes, the cochlear fluids, and the cochlear partition. However, some fraction of the pressure applied to the stapes is used to move the stapes and counteract the stiffness of the stapediovestibular joint, never reaching the inner ear. Another estimate of middle ear gain compares the sound pressure in the ear canal to the resultant sound pressure within the fluid of the cochlear vestibule. Such gain estimates exclude the stapes and its joint from the inner ear. Various authors have measured this pressure transfer function (Puria, Peake, and Rosowski,[31] Aibara, Welsh, Puria S, and Goode,[32] Nakajima, Dong, and Olson[33]). ▶ Fig. 9.7[33] shows that this sound pressure transfer ratio is bandpass and is of the largest magnitude between 1 and 3 kHz, with significant roll-offs above and below this range. It can also be noted that the primary differences between the data in ▶ Fig. 9.6 and ▶ Fig. 9.7 are at frequencies less than 0.5 kHz, the frequency range where the stiffness of the stapediovestibular joint most affects middle ear sound transfer.[16]

Protection of the Round Window by the TM

A minor effect of the presence of the TM in a normal ear is that it reduces the sound pressure within the middle ear spaces relative to the sound pressure in the ear canal. This leads to an attenuation of the sound pressure at the round window that occurs simultaneously with the gain in sound pressure at the oval window. Voss, Rosowski, Merchant, and Peake[34] have demonstrated that the pressure at the round window remains small compared with the oval window, even in ears with TM perforations, as long as the ossicular chain is normal and some contact exists between the ossicles and the remaining fraction of the TM.

Acoustic Coupling and Ossicular Coupling

An important concept is that of acoustic versus ossicular coupling, put forward by Peak, Rosowski, and Lynch.[35] The normal middle ear provides a pressure gain at the oval window of approximately 20 dB in the 0.1–3 kHz frequency band and partly shields the round window, producing a pressure difference between these two windows. Because the stimulus to the

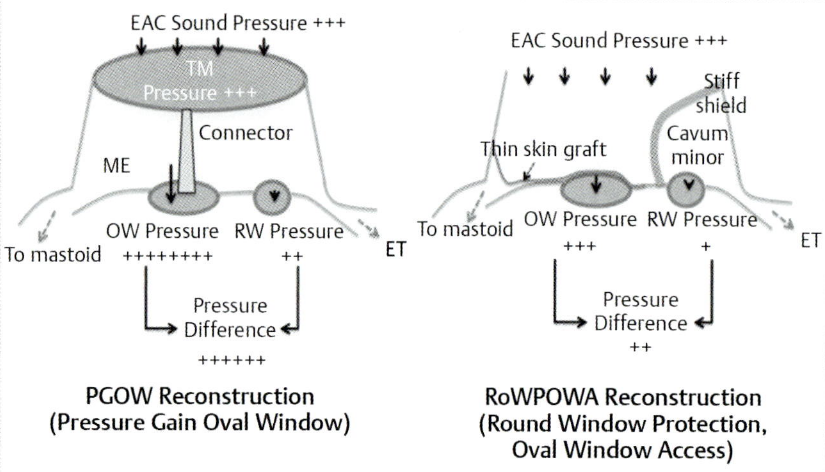

Fig. 9.8 The difference in anatomical construction between the PGOW-type and RoWPOWA-type reconstructions. All PGOW reconstructions require coupling of the large surface area of the TM to the smaller surface area of the oval window with some kind of stiff connector, typically an ossicular prosthesis or residual stapes superstructure. The "+" signs qualitatively signify pressure magnitude but are not meant to be numerically accurate. ET, Eustachian tube.

inner ear depends on the algebraic difference in sound pressure at the windows (not the dB difference), the attenuation of an already small sound pressure at the round window has little effect on the window-pressure difference in the normal ear. This route of coupling sound pressure to the inner ear has been termed ossicular coupling.[35]

If the middle ear is destroyed by disease, there is still a small pressure difference between the oval window and round window due to their spatial separation and protection of the round window, but this pressure difference is only about -40 dB of the EAC pressure. This can still drive the inner ear fluids, but at a much reduced level, about 50 dB or 60 dB below that of the ossicular coupling route. This method of hearing has been termed acoustic coupling[35] and is commonly seen with damaged middle ears. With acoustic coupling, hearing will actually improve slightly with a TM perforation, as the sound pressure at the two windows, and, hence, their pressure difference, is increased.[36]

9.4 Hearing Reconstruction of Diseased Middle Ears

Although the previous section has focused on normal middle ear physiology, in diseased ears, there are numerous factors that can lead to hearing loss. These include TM perforations, fixations of the ossicles (either bony or by soft tissue), missing ossicles, and footplate fixations. We will focus not on stapedotomy-type reconstructions, but, rather, reconstructions of remaining middle ear structures. Reconstruction of the middle ear for hearing gain attempts to maximize, again, the pressure difference between the oval window and the round window.

9.4.1 Classification of Hearing Reconstruction Surgeries

Practical ways to change the pressure differential between the oval window and round window and middle ear reconstruction with passive prostheses can essentially be divided into two groups. These are described below and illustrated in ▶ Fig. 9.8.

Pressure gain at the oval window (PGOW) reconstructions all attempt to reconstruct ossicular coupling by connecting a large-area TM to the smaller-area oval window to reconstitute the hydraulic lever pressure gain, and so they all require a vibrating TM. All the PGOW-type reconstructions require a structure to couple the TM to the oval window, either remaining ossicles (e.g., Wullstein type III) or, more commonly, some kind of connector such as an autograft or an artificial ossicular prosthesis. Therefore, in addition to the variability in the style of TM reconstruction, another source of variability in the PGOW-type reconstruction is the mechanical properties and placement of the ossicular prosthesis. Reconstruction mechanics research and clinical literature are easier to interpret and summarize if the specific contact points of the prosthesis within the middle ear, specifically the medial and lateral attachment points, are explicitly stated.

Round window protection with oval window access (RoWPOWA) reconstructions attempt to maximize acoustic coupling by allowing unimpeded acoustic access to the oval window while shielding the round window from sound, typically by covering it with a stiff shield such as cartilage. Because no attempt is made to couple a mobile inner ear window to a freely mobile TM by an ossicular replacement, a vibrating TM is not needed. Classically, these are the Wullstein Type IV and V tympanoplasties. Such approaches require that the round window area has some air as a buffer around it, so that it can move, and, therefore, require some ventilation pathway to the Eustachian tube, typically by constructing a small inferiorly ventilated segment from the Eustachian tube to the round window, a cavum minor. Lateral canal fenestration follows mechanics similar to RoWPOWA and are included with this group.

The Wullstein classifications[37] (mostly RoWPOWA reconstructions) are listed in ▶ Table 9.1. ▶ Table 9.2 shows a classification scheme for middle ear reconstruction adapted from one used by one of the authors,[38] the majority of which are PGOW-type reconstructions. The medial termination is specified first, as it is traditionally by the designation PORP and TORP, which implies reconstruction to the stapes head or to the footplate, respectively.

Table 9.1 Wullstein classifications of tympanoplasty

Type I	Essentially myringoplasty, with repair of perforation
Type II	Placing TM onto the remaining incus, in malleus necrosis; rarely used
Type III	Placing TM directly onto stapes superstructure
Type IV	Direct sound access to OW (usually grafted with split-thickness skin graft), round window protection with ventilated cavum minor
Type Vb	Open access to OW, footplate removed, round window protection with ventilated cavum minor
Type Va	Lateral canal fenestration, round window protection with ventilated cavum minor

Table 9.2 Classification of middle ear hearing reconstructiontechniques

A. PGOW reconstruction

In general, the lateral and medial and mid prosthesis interface/stabilizers should be specified, e.g., medial ± footplate shoe, lateral ± cartilage overlay, mid-shaft ± cartilage or other stabilizer. The most commonly used are in boldface.

***(I)* DirectConnection TM to residual ossicles**

a) Direct connection incus onto TM (D-IOT-Wullstein typeII)

b) Direct connection stapes head onto TM(D-SHOT-Wullstein type III)

***(II)* Connectorsbetween TM and residual ossicles**

Connecting	*Acronym*	*Current terminology orexamples*
Stapes Head onto TM	**SHOT**	**PORP**
Stapes Head onto Malleus	**SHOM**	**PORP**
Stapes Head onto Incus	SHOI	e.g., cement, Applebaum
Stapes Head onto both TM and Malleus	SHOTM	PORP
Stapes Head onto Artificial or relocated Malleus	SHOAM	PORP to relocated malleus
Stapes Footplate onto TM	**FOT**	**TORP**
Stapes Footplate onto Malleus	**FOM**	**TORP**
Stapes Footplate onto Incus	FOI	e.g., stapes piston on mobile footplate
Stapes Footplate onto both TM and Malleus	FOTM	TORP
Stapes Footplate onto Artificial or relocated Malleus	FOAM	e.g., TORP to relocated malleus
Vestibule onto TM	VOT	TORP with stapedotomy
Vestibule onto Malleus	VOM	Malleostapediopexy
Vestibule onto Incus	**VOI**	**Standard stapedotomy**
Vestibule onto Both TM and malleus	VOB	
Vestibule onto Artificial or relocated Malleus	VOAM	Rarely used
Incus onto TM	IOM	Rarely used
Incus onto Malleus	IOT	e.g., cementing IM joint, rarely used

B. RoWPOWA reconstruction

RoWPOWA-FP: Stapes footplate access (Wullstein type IV)

RoWPOWA-V: Inner ear access with removal of stapes footplate(Wullstein type Vb)

RoWPOWA-HC: Inner ear access with lateral canal fenestration(Wullstein type Va)

9.4.2 RoWPOWA Reconstruction: Reconstruction with Ossicular Function

Middle ear reconstructions that fall into the RoWPOWA classification (Wullstein's Type IV and V reconstructions[39] and Lempert's canal fenestration procedure[40]), make up a small part of the reconstructive surgeries performed today but were more numerous in the past. However, given the wide variety of results from PGOW procedures that reconstruct the TM and ossicles, these simpler procedures may be of use in selected circumstances. For example, the Type IV or V procedure may be useful in severely diseased ears where the ear canal wall has been taken down and the stapes superstructure has been compromised.[41]

With the Type IV and V reconstructions, the mobile footplate (Type IV) or fat graft (Type V) within the oval window is exteriorized to the ear canal whereas, in the fenestration procedure, a new window into the inner ear is exteriorized to the canal. When successful, these procedures isolate the mobile round window from sound pressure in the ear canal while maintaining aeration of the round window area by inclusion of the pro--tympanum behind the isolating graft shield in a ventilated cavum minor.

The basis for these procedures is the pressure difference theory noted above, where the fundamental stimulus to the inner ear is a difference in sound pressure at two cochlear windows that produces a net flow of incompressible fluid between them. In the Type IV and V procedures, the two windows are the oval window, which is filled with either a mobile stapes footplate or a loose graft, and the round window. The fenestration procedure was used as a treatment for otosclerosis, where the footplate is no longer mobile, and a new window is cut into the lateral semicircular canal and covered with a thin skin graft.[40,42]

For any of these RoWPOWA procedures an ideal reconstruction would include (1) a mobile input window to the cochlea exteriorized to the external ear, (2) a mobile round window that is protected or shielded from the sound pressure in the ear canal by a stiff graft, and (3) an air-filled space between the round window and the shield that is maintained by a working Eustachian tube.[43,44] If these three constraints are met, the sound pressure at the round window that results from ear canal sound stimulation is very small (approximately zero), and the window pressure difference then equals the ear canal stimulus pressure. However, all of these conditions can be difficult to meet. It is common to see scarring over the footplate after graft placement, and a very thin split-thickness skin graft is usually recommended. Providing ventilation to the cavum minor around the round window can also be a challenge in Eustachian tube dysfunction.

In RoWPOWA reconstructions, essentially the loss in pressure at the oval window is the loss of the middle ear transformer pressure gain and, because the round window is protected, the external canal pressure drives the inner ear. As we have seen, Kurokawa and Goode[45] estimated the middle ear gain to be 20–25 dB at frequencies less than 2 kHz (▶ Fig. 9.6), which is consistent with the observation of a residual 20–25 dB air-bone gap[46] in the best of these RoWPOWA reconstructions (▶ Fig. 9.9).[44]

Alternatives, such as increasing the pressure at the round window relative to the oval window, have been suggested ("sonoinversion"[47]). Such an increase is difficult with passive prostheses given the round window does not face the TM, but can be accomplished with active powered drivers.[48]

9.4.3 PGOW Reconstruction: Reconstruction of TM and Ossicular Function

Any PGOW reconstruction is predicated on a vibrating TM, which in turn relies on adequate ventilation and lack of middle ear or external ear scarring. There is evidence that pathology or reconstructive procedures (such as perforations of the TM, the placement of cartilage sheets on the TM surface, or repairing dimeric segments of the TM) can greatly alter the pattern of TM vibration produced by high frequencies but have little effect on the umbo or stapes vibrations.[11,49,50] Hence, it probably does not make much difference what material is used to repair small perforations as long as the repair restores the pressure difference across the TM that drives TM motion.[51] However, when nearly the entire TM is replaced, the stiffness of the eardrum reconstruction may come into play. For instance, cartilage is much stiffer than perichondrium or fascia, and thick cartilage is stiffer than thinned cartilage and displays lower amplitude vibrations for a given sound pressure.[52] Normally, we would expect this to result in low-frequency hearing loss if the whole TM was replaced.

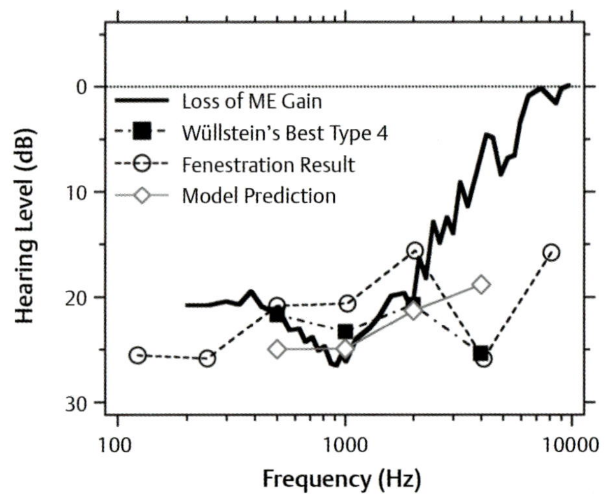

Fig. 9.9 A comparison of some of the best results of Type IV surgery. Shown are the mean of six cases.

Data from Wüllstein H. The restoration of the function of the middle ear in chronic otitis media. Ann Otol Rhinol Laryngol. 1956;65:1020–1041.

Wüllstein H. Results of tympanoplasty. Arch Otolaryng. 1960;71:478–485.

Lempert J. Endaural fenestration of external semicircular canal for restoration of hearing in cases of otosclerosis. Arch Otolaryng. 1940;31:711–779.

Lempert J. Fenestra non-ovalis: a new oval window for the improvement of hearing in cases of otosclerosis. Arch Otolaryng. 1941;34:880–912.

Merchant S, Rosowski J, Ravicz M. Middle-ear mechanics of type IV and type V tympanoplasty. II. Clinical analysis and surgical implications. Am J Otol. 1995;16:565–575.

Kurokawa H, Goode R. Sound pressure gain produced by the human middle ear. Am J Otol. 1995;113:349–355.

Despite these differences in TM stiffness when reconstructed with different materials, clinical studies suggest that cartilage and fascia result in similar air-bone gap closure,[53] with lower re-perforation rates obtained with cartilage.[54] There may be several reasons for this, including better coupling of the motions of the cartilage to the malleus or prosthesis,[55] lower re-perforation rates with cartilage, as well as the fact that cartilage is more often used in tympanoplasties for moderate and larger-sized perforations where the re-creation of a significant sound pressure difference across the TM is best aided by a stiffer graft material. Cartilage may also show in-phase motion extending to a higher frequency range than does fascia, resulting in a more efficient hydraulic lever in frequencies above 2 kHz, although there is no current data on this.

Simple mechanical models of the middle ear suggest that increases in mass of the TM and ossicles reduce the response of the ear to frequencies above 2 kHz. However, mass added to the TM does not seem to have a large effect on stapes vibrations. Nishihara, Aritomo, and Goode[56] loaded masses between 3 mg and 20 mg on various sites on the TM and saw narrow band decreases in the umbo velocity, which increased with the size of the mass. The effects were generally small, except in these narrow frequency bands, and stapes effects were even less marked.

Some authors have suggested that the cone shape of the TM, the relative asymmetry of the TM areas behind and in front of the malleus, the radial fibers of the TM, and the incudomalleolar joint[22,57] are important for transduction at frequencies above 4 kHz in the mammalian ear. Results at such high frequencies are rarely reported in hearing reconstruction literature, and the shape, microstructure, and 3-dimensional anatomy of the TM cannot be surgically reconstructed at present; however, these are interesting factors for future investigation, and, as ▶ Fig. 9.6 shows, there is little middle ear gain in the higher frequencies.

One of the most common defects repaired is a TM perforation. Well-conducted temporal bone studies[49,51] and clinical studies[58] show that the perforation size is the predominant determinant of the hearing loss. The primary effect of a perforation, at least up to the studied 7-mm diameter, is loss of the trans-TM pressure gradient that drives TM motion and not the loss of the hydraulic lever ratio. Hence, any baffle-like reconstruction that restores the protective function of the TM and reconstitutes a pressure gradient will restore hearing.

Furthermore, the location of the perforation is irrelevant, as a given perforation will have a similar effect on trans-TM pressure no matter where it is located on the TM. A common misconception is that the site of the perforation introduces a "phase effect," so that perforations over the round window are more deleterious than elsewhere. In fact, the wavelengths of audio frequency sounds are so large that both the oval window and round window experience almost equal pressure, with the very small difference only important in acoustic coupling when the ossicular pressure gain pathway is removed.

Hearing loss with a perforation is largest at low frequencies, with larger perforations causing larger hearing losses that spread to higher frequencies. Lerut, Pfammatter, Moons, and Linder[58] and Voss, Rosowski, Merchant, and Peake[49] also showed that, with larger perforations, the loss shows a notch around 2 kHz, where the loss is smaller than at higher and lower frequencies. This is matched by a larger trans-membrane pressure at this frequency in Voss's study, suggesting that it is due to middle ear resonance effects. The size of the mastoid/middle ear cavity also determines the hearing loss,[59] with smaller cavities associated with larger conductive losses.

Another set of experiments[11] has shown that the vibration patterns of the TM are primarily modal (i.e., with standing waves and fixed areas with nodes and antinodes of vibration amplitude) and are not dominated by traveling waves from the periphery of the TM to the umbo, as proposed by a competing theory.[60,61] The alternative traveling wave theory suggests there is an efficient transmission line between the periphery of the TM, which is well matched to acoustic impedance in air, and the central TM, which is well matched to the umbo. The traveling wave theory also suggests that changing any part of the TM would have repercussions on the traveling wave reaching the umbo. However, putting pieces of cartilage on the periphery changed the local vibration characteristics but not the overall modal pattern, umbo vibration, or stapes vibrations,[62] which runs counter to the traveling wave theory. Hence, for subtotal perforations, it really should not make too much difference what material (e.g., cartilage or fascia) is used to restore the baffle effect of an intact eardrum. This may be different for a total perforation, where the boundary "hinge" areas are also affected; without such a hinge, it may be more difficult to move the central portion of a TM graft.

The following sections all pertain to PGOW reconstructions.

9.4.4 Factors Affecting Transmission of Sound through the Middle Ear in Prosthetic Reconstruction

Because below 2 kHz, the TM and most of the middle ear move mostly in phase, the important determinant of vibration transmission in this frequency range is the coupling of the driven motions at the various structural interfaces (e.g., TM to prosthesis, prosthesis to stapes). Geometric considerations are also important, for example, to drive the stapes in and out of the oval window, in-line vibrations that are perpendicular to the footplate are best, whereas non-in-line motions will lead to rotation of the footplate or prosthesis. Other sources of loss are deformation of intervening structures that lead to dissipation. ▶ Fig. 9.10 shows some of the structural interfaces in a typical surgical reconstruction.

Global Factors Affecting Middle Ear Prosthetic Reconstruction

There are global factors that affect the structural interfaces in prosthetic reconstruction, including the angulation of the prosthesis relative to its connection at the TM and stapes, the tension it is placed under, mass of the prosthesis, and stiffness of the prosthesis. These are discussed below.

Angulation of the Prosthesis

As ▶ Fig. 9.11 shows, the latter end of the prosthesis can contact either the eardrum or the malleus, where the malleus is usually quite anterior to the stapes head or footplate. If we assume the

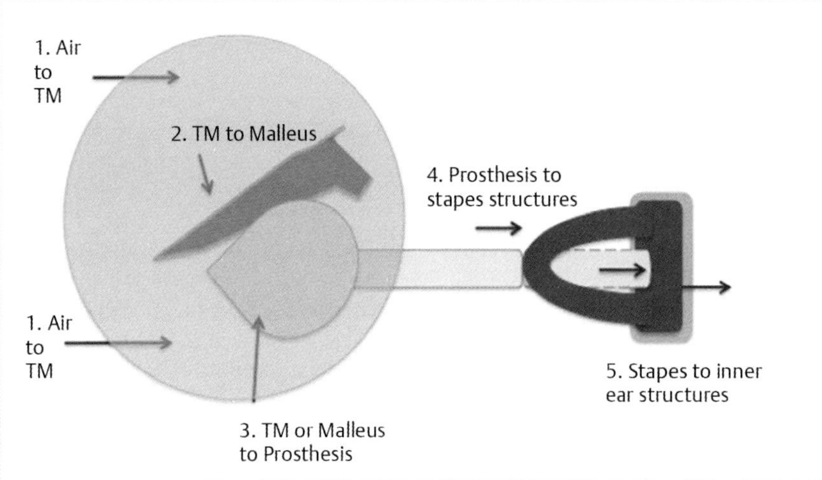

Fig. 9.10 Structural interfaces in a surgical reconstruction. This illustrates that forces have to be transmitted in-line to move the stapes footplate into the vestibule.

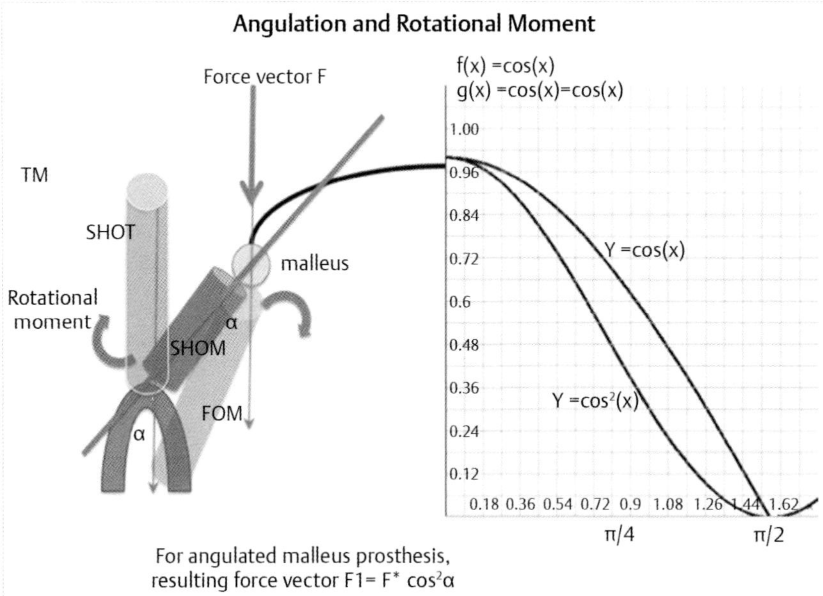

Fig. 9.11 How angulation of the prosthesis affects the force vectors in the "piston-like" axis of the stapes footplate and the rotational moments around the hinge joints. The translational vector follows the $\cos^2 x$ rule. A FOM-type prosthesis will have a more favorable angle than a SHOM-type prosthesis, and an anterior or medialized malleus will very much affect the angle of the prosthesis.

TM and the footplate parallel each other, for the angulated prosthesis, a force vector F generated by the umbo is transformed by the angulation of the prosthesis to a force actually in line with the piston-like vector for the stapes footplate of $F^*\cos^2\alpha$, where α is the angle between the prosthesis and the TM. At 45 degrees, the force is already reduced to 0.5 of its original value (a loss of 6 dB); this is the steep part of the function, so small changes in angle reduce transmitted force rapidly. Hence, if the malleus is very anterior, or medialized, then the force vector in the plane of the footplate is compromised, rotational moments of the prosthesis are increased, and the in-line orthogonal motions of the stapes are decreased. Because of the extra length of the prosthesis, connecting to the footplate from the malleus (footplate onto malleus, FOM, instead of to the footplate from the stapes head [stapes head onto malleus, SHOM]) will always result in a smaller contact angle and a better force vector (▶ Fig. 9.10). Mills[63] measured the angle between the malleus and stapes head in 31 cadaveric temporal bones and found the average to be 49 degrees, ranging from 14 degrees to 71 degrees. Todd[64] also measured this angle and found the median angle to be 64 degrees. In diseased ears, it is likely to be even more. Vlaming and Feenstra[65] nicely showed that larger angles to the stapes head in SHOM-type prostheses produced more tilting of the stapes footplate and less stapes footplate volume displacement.

Connecting to the TM (i.e., footplate onto TM [FOT] or stapes head onto TM [SHOT]) likely results in more favorable force and rotational vector directions than connections to the malleus (i.e., FOM or SHOM, respectively). There are other reasons to go to the malleus, however, including better stability, keeping away from the annulus to avoid adhesions to it, avoiding the fixed edges of the eardrum at the annulus, which will have decreased vibration amplitudes, and a possible advantage for transduction due to the special coupling of the malleus to the TM, which may result in a pressure gain at the malleus (catenary lever effect, see below).

Another equally important factor, illustrated in ▶ Fig. 9.11, is that, unless the joints between the TM and prosthesis and the prosthesis and stapes interfaces are completely fixed, angulation may result in rotation of the prosthesis around these points

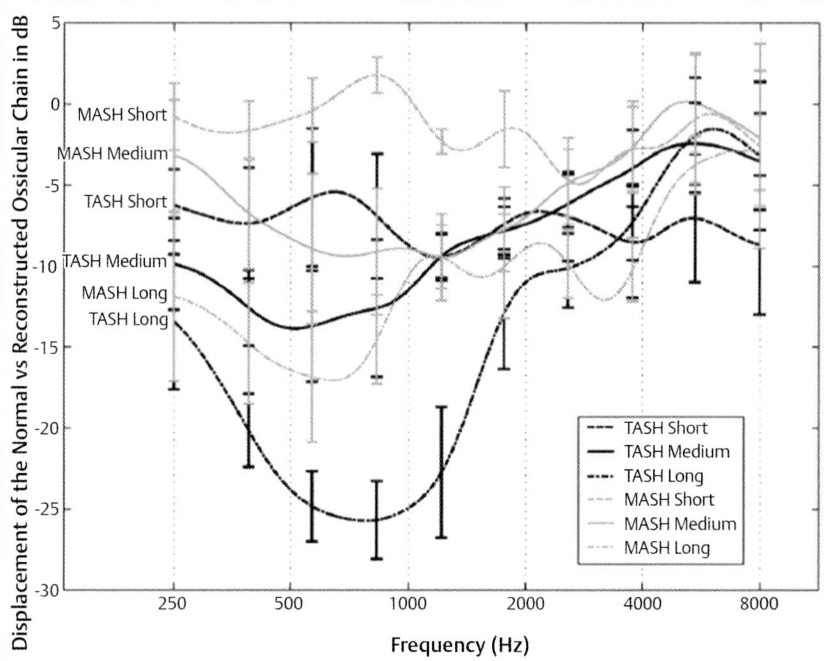

Fig. 9.12 Stapes displacement amplitudes for prostheses under different tensions from stapes head to malleus (formerly MASH, called SHOM in this chapter) or from stapes head to TM (called SHOT in this chapter). The y-axis shows the decrement in dB from intact ear of each of the reconstructions. long=tight; medium=medium; short=loose. (Used with permission from Bance M, Morris DP, Vanwijhe RG, Kiefte M, Funnell WR. Comparison of the mechanical performance of ossiculoplasty using a prosthetic malleus-to-stapes head with a TM-to-stapes head assembly in a human cadaveric middle ear model. Otology 25(6):903-909.)

of contact rather than a translation. Many factors determine how much rotation versus translation in line with the oval window is achieved, including how constrained from rotation is the lateral joint at the prosthesis-TM or prosthesis-malleus junction, as well as the medial joint at the prosthesis-stapes head or prosthesis-footplate junction. This is where stapes head (SHOT or SHOM) prostheses could be designed to have a distinct advantage over footplate-type (FOT or FOM) prostheses, because if the coupling to the stapes head is constrained by a deep clip or crimping, then it is likely to produce more translation. It is harder to constrain rotation at the footplate although designs such as footplate shoes attempt to do this.

In general, we would recommend keeping inclination minimal, hence avoiding the steep part of the cosine curve, and constraining the rotational moment around the medial end with a deep cup or other device on the stapes head or with some method to prevent hinge-like movements on the footplate if this is used.

Tension between the Prosthesis and the TM and the TM and Footplate

It is usually difficult to change the tension that the prosthesis is placed under during surgery because the TM is often grafted or raised and then laid back down over the prosthesis, and the final tension is unpredictable. However, in certain situations tension can be more carefully controlled. For instance, in second-stage surgery tension can be more easily predicted by raising only a small portion of the TM, by reconstructing through the facial recess, or by reconstructing to the malleus. Tension is often used to stabilize the prosthesis and is useful in this regard. However, results in cadaveric temporal bones from one of the authors (Morris, Bance, van Wijhe, Kiefte, and Smith[66]) showed that the looser the prosthesis (within the limits tested), the better the low-frequency transmission below 1 kHz and that higher tension markedly affects the low-frequency transmission to the stapes, with a difference of over 10 dB between the loosest and tightest SHOT prosthesis. The tighter prostheses produced a very slight (< 2 dB) improvement in transmission of the higher frequencies above 3 kHz. Yamada and Goode[67] and Vlaming and Feenstra[65] found very similar results. All showed a marked drop in sound transmission at frequencies below 1 kHz with increased tension. The region of decrease corresponds to the region where the normal middle ear is stiffness-controlled. The tension-induced decrease in this range is consistent with a tension-induced increase in the stiffness of the TM and ossicles. Such an increase could arise from increased tension on the annular ligament or on the TM, both of which contribute to the stiffness of the normal middle ear.[18]

Bance, Morris, Vanwijhe, Kiefte, and Funnell repeated this study,[38] shown in ▶ Fig. 9.12, with reconstruction to the malleus instead of the TM (SHOM rather than SHOT prostheses), and found a similar, if somewhat less marked, effect of decreasing transmission with increasing tension in these reconstructions. In the real world, this effect has to be balanced with the tension necessary to stabilize the prosthesis.

Another factor to consider is that a very loose prosthesis may lead to some distortion, particularly at high sound pressure levels. If the dynamic force generated is larger than the static pretension force on the prosthesis, the motions of the TM and the prosthesis are uncoupled over part of the sound stimulus, which could distort the transduced sound in a manner similar to the "loose wire" syndrome in stapedotomy.[68] Such stimulus-induced uncoupling has not been clinically or experimentally demonstrated. In an experiment with medium-tension prostheses, one of the authors found no evidence of non-linearity,[69] but this has not been performed with extremely loose prostheses.

In general, we would recommend the least amount of tension needed for stability but recognize that improved stability will often trump better sound transmission considerations.

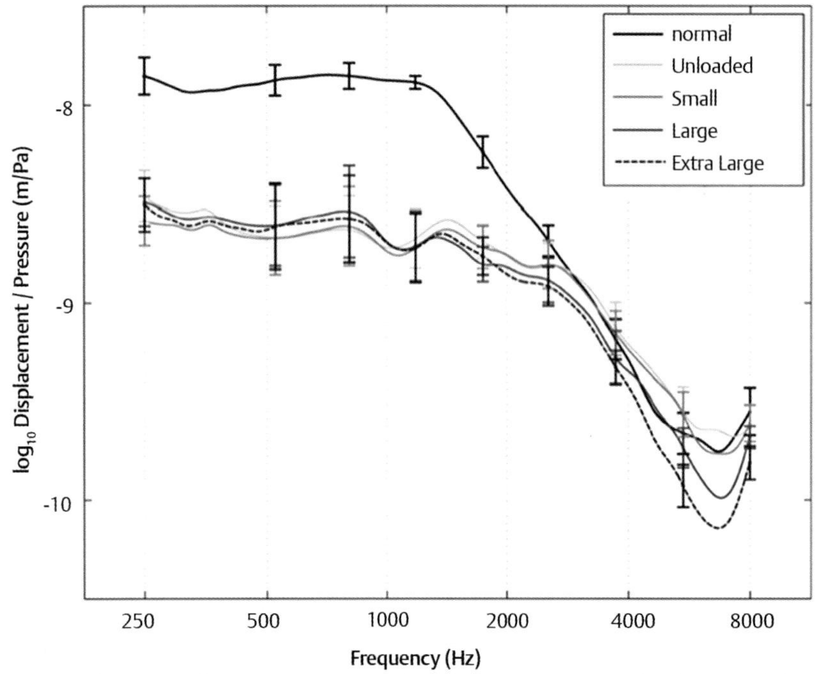

Fig. 9.13 Effects of mass-loading a SHOT-type prosthesis on its stem in 8 temporal bones. Normal=intact ear. Weights (small=27 mg; large=37 mg; and extra large=55 mg) were loaded on the stem, with the initial unloaded prosthesis mass of 25 mg. (Used with permission from Bance M, Morris DP, Van Wijhe R. Effects of ossicular prosthesis mass and section of the stapes tendon on middle ear transmission. The Journal of Otolaryngology. 2007;36(2):113-119.)

Prosthesis Mass

Prosthesis mass is one of the parameters that is easily controlled by choice of material or design. In general, the middle ear is stiffness-dominated in the lower frequencies, and simple mechanical models suggest the addition of mass alters the middle ear resonant frequency and reduces the response of the middle ear at frequencies above resonance.[19] However, more complicated circuit models of the middle ear (e.g., Rosowski and Merchant)[28] suggest that significant changes in ossicular mass have little effect on middle ear function. This result agrees with recent finite element models by Gan, Dai, Wang, Nakmali, and Wood,[70] who added the mass of an active driver to the incudostapedial joint and showed only a modest drop in stapes response and only in the frequencies above 1 kHz. Experimental data from mass-loading the normal middle ear supports this. Nishihara and Goode[56] added masses of 3–5 mg to the malleus head, stapes head, and long process of the incus, and found only minimal effects in two bones. On loading the TM at various sites, there was an increase in the depth of maxima and minima seen in the frequency response, which became more marked with masses up to 20 mg, but the overall average umbo vibrations seemed relatively little affected. Stapes vibrations were affected even less and then only in the higher frequencies.

Other data comes from physically constructed artificial models of the middle ear.

Meister, Walger, Mickenhagen, von Wedel, and Stennert,[71] using a simple artificial ear physical model, found only moderate changes (< 6 dB) only in the high frequencies (> 700 Hz), and Mojallal, Stieve M, Krueger I, Behrens P, Mueller PP, and Lenarz,[72] using a more complex artificial ear physical model, found no changes in vibration transmission caused by changing the mass of a FOT-type prosthesis.

Bance, Morris, and Van Wijhealso conducted prosthesis mass-addition experiments,[73] with results similar to those published (▶ Fig. 9.13). In this study, stapes head prostheses (SHOT-type) were loaded with masses of 2 mg, 12 mg, and 30 mg, and very little effect was found on stapes vibrations below 2 kHz, with only a limited drop (< 10 dB) above 3 kHz.

The only contrary data is from one temporal bone by Nishihara and Goode,[74] who used a SHOT-type rod. They reported similar small drops in high-frequency response with mass loading similar to the above reported studies, but also saw increased response at low frequencies with mass loading, not seen in the above studies. Nonetheless, the bulk of the data supports the view that mass mainly affects frequencies above 1 kHz and that this effect is small when mass is varied over the range common in clinical reconstruction. Some mass is needed to keep a low center of gravity during placement so that the prosthesis does not fall over when placed on the footplate, and a heavier prosthesis is not as likely to stick to blood or instruments when being placed; however, in general, a light prosthesis is most easily manipulated and may give slightly better high-frequency results.

Prosthesis Stiffness

Because acoustic dynamic pressures are small, most available prostheses are stiff enough, that is, they do not deform at pressures needed to drive the inner ear/stapes load or during acoustic stimulation, at least at frequencies below several kHz. Our own (Bance et al., unpublished) observations have shown that most artificial prostheses are essentially rigid at acoustic pressures and perform equally. This is similar to findings by Mojallal, Stieve, Krueger, Behrens, Mueller, and Lenarz in an artificial middle ear.[72] Prostheses made of less stiff materials, such as cartilage, may show bending modes that affect their transmission unless they are made quite thick in their cross-sectional area. This has not been directly tested, to our knowledge, but has been predicted by the finite element method of transfer function.[75] However, we would not recommend using compressible tissues to connect the ossicular structures.

Coupling Interfaces

TM-Prosthesis Interface

There are several factors at play at this interface, which is dominated by the physical characteristics of the TM or TM graft (e.g. cartilage or fascia). Of primary importance is whether the prosthesis couples to the malleus or the TM, and where on the malleus or TM the coupling takes place (variations in this placement effect the driving force acting on the prosthesis). Other factors are the surface area of the interface contact (e.g., prosthesis head size) and any material placed in the interface (e.g., the size and thickness of cartilage to cover the prosthesis). Experimental data is available on several aspects of this and is discussed below.

Whether to Reconstruct to the Malleus or to the TM

Although several clinical authors have claimed better results in reconstruction to the malleus than to the TM,[5,76,77] middle ear experiments have been few. One of the mechanisms of middle ear impedance matching proposed by Helmholtz in 1868 is the catenary lever.[78] Catenary describes the curvature of the TM between the fixed TM rim and the attachment to the relatively stiff manubrium of the malleus. In a catenary mechanism, the relatively small forces needed to move the loose free curved regions of the TM produce larger forces and smaller motions at the points that support the catenary region (the rim and the manubrium). The catenary mechanism is consistent with observations of the relative immobility of the umbo and manubrium compared with other locations on the TM surface.[11,79]

Elpern and Elbrond in 1966[80] observed that using a prosthesis as a SHOM rather than as a SHOT gave better high-frequency results, but only one bone was used and the measurement techniques were perhaps not as sensitive as the laser Doppler methods used today. Bance, Morris, Vanwijhe, Kiefte, and Funnell[38] compared reconstructions from the stapes head to the malleus (SHOM) and to the TM (SHOT) and also the varied tension of the SHOM and SHOT prostheses by using prostheses of different lengths. Results are shown in ▶ Fig. 9.12. Higher tension resulted in worse low- frequency responses, but it was found, for any given tension level, the SHOM outperformed the SHOT. This might be confounded by the fact that it is easier to put more tension on the TM in SHOT-type reconstructions, due to the in-line placement, than to the malleus in SHOM-type reconstructions, where the angulation results in the slippage of the prosthesis. However, even with the loosest prostheses, SHOM reconstructions were better by about 5 dB than SHOT prostheses across the frequency range.

Interestingly, Shimizu and Goode[81] interposed a sculpted incus between the stapes head and the malleus (SHOM). They then removed the malleus from the TM and reconstructed to a similar position on the TM. They found very little difference in stapes vibrations, on the order of a few dB, with a very slight advantage of SHOM or SHOT depending on the frequency range. Importantly, the angulation effects inherent in changing from the posterior TM to the malleus do not contaminate this study.

One consideration is that introducing a rigid structure, such as a prosthesis, to constrain the motion of the portion of the TM that it contacts might introduce a "pseudo-manubrium" that helps support the membrane. Such a new support point could be the focus of increased catenary forces although this is not proven.

In ears in which the malleus is very anterior or medialized, the angulation effects of going to the malleus should dominate the results, both in terms of poor transmission of force vectors and poor stability. On the other hand, if the malleus is favorably placed, there may be some advantage in a malleal attachment as the malleus may aid stabilization; however, the experimental data on the contribution of this reconstruction to sound coupling is not conclusive.

In general, the malleus can offer excellent stabilization opportunities; such a placement will keep the prosthesis head away from the annulus and prevent any scarring at the posterior aspect of the eardrum, but its mechanical advantages, although hinted at, have not been clearly demonstrated experimentally as of yet.

Site of Contact with the Malleus

Because the umbo is the site of the largest displacements on the malleus, it has been suggested to be the optimum contact point for reconstruction. Such arguments ignore the possibility of unfavorable geometry between the stapes and the umbo. The large displacements of the umbo come from the rotation of the malleus about a point near the anterior malleal ligament. However, the point of rotation moves with sound, and the location of the point of rotation changes with frequency.[83] The non-rotational modes result in motions of the point of rotation and the nearby malleus neck, which are translational, and so could drive translational movement of a prosthesis connected to the neck.

Goode, Killion M, Nakamura K, and Nishihara[82] report that the umbo vibrates with at least 10-dB greater amplitude than the short process of the malleus, but only below 1 kHz; above that, the displacement amplitudes become much more similar, so that there would be little advantage to the umbo. Goode and Nishihara[74] show results of placing a rod from the stapes head to the malleus at various points using two bones. Below 1 kHz, stapes vibrations for connections to the short process were worse than to the mid-manubrium or umbo, and, above this frequency, all contact points were within 5–7 dB of each other although the short process was still the worse. Interestingly, in this study, the results of choosing a TM contact point (i.e., SHOT versus SHOM) was similar to choosing the malleus as a contact point.

Zahnert and Huttenbrink,[83] in contrast, report similar results for contact to the short process, the mid-malleus, and the umbo at low frequencies, but worse results with contact to the umbo at high frequencies But, the differences were < 10 dB even at their most marked.

Overall, in practical terms, a good compromise would be attaching to the mid-manubrium if possible. Here, the angle is generally favorable, and there is likely to be significant motion below 1 kHz. It is possible that cutting the tensor tympani may also change some of the rotational mechanics.

Effect of Cartilage Overlay

Most otologists will cover the lateral surface of the prosthesis with cartilage, particularly if it is an allograft, such as titanium, to prevent extrusion of the prosthesis. The cartilage can vary in size and thickness. In a study performed by one of the authors,[84] the smaller the cartilage overlay for a SHOT-type prosthesis, the better the stapes response. Cartilage just bigger than the head of the prosthesis had little impact, and larger pieces caused low-frequency loss, probably by stiffening the eardrum directly and by changing tension in the non-contacted eardrum by forcing its conical shape to take on a flat shape.

This study also found that changing the SHOT-TM interface by putting something more rigid than cartilage (glass) in this interface made little difference to stapes vibrations, and, similarly, using a softer, spongier material also had little effect, except for some losses at the highest frequencies. Interestingly, Yamada and Goode[67] found that putting spongy material at the TM-prosthesis interface could act as a tension-regulating device because it mitigated the effects of longer prostheses.

Shimizu and Goode[81] also report on the effects of cartilage interposition over a SHOT-type prosthesis, with similar findings to that of Morris, Bance, and Van Wijhe[84] except in one respect: all cartilage interpositions resulted in some drop in stapes vibration at the low frequencies, this being about 17–18 dB for larger sizes and 5–10 dB for small and medium sizes of cartilage. The Morris, Bance, and Van Wijhe study did not find this drop, except in the very largest cartilage sizes tested, provided the length of the prosthesis was adjusted by shortening the thickness of the cartilage to avoid tension effects. Shimizu and Goode did not compensate for this increased tension. They also report better high-frequency responses with large cartilage, which is difficult to understand given that stiffness plays little part in this frequency range.

One of the authors (Bance) has also looked at cartilage thickness at this interface and found no difference in response for 0.2-, 0.4-, and 0.7-mm thickness cartilage interpositions (unpublished data).

In general, then, the literature seems divided. Published results from Morris, Bance, and Van Wijhe[84] show no difference from adding cartilage of similar size to the prosthesis head. Others who did not compensate for the added tension created show a decrease in transmission of 5–10 dB. Both the Morris, Bance, and Van Wijhe[84] and the Shimuzu and Goode[81] results suggest that larger cartilage pieces are worse, at least in the low frequencies, with an intact eardrum. This may be related to insertion-induced increases in tension in the TM. Such increases may be the major cause of the reported drops in low-frequency transmission with large cartilage overlays.

We support any thickness of cartilage cover, as long as it does not markedly increase tension at the TM, and suggest that any negative effects are likely to be only in the low frequencies and are likely to be small as long as the remaining eardrum is not put under undue tension. Often, however, larger cartilage pieces are needed to prevent retraction or increase stability.

Prosthesis Head Size

Prosthesis head size can have several practical implications. Large head sizes are unwieldy and may touch the annulus. However, they may collect energy from a larger surface and better couple sound to the prosthesis stem. Large head sizes may also deform the surface and increase the stiffness of the remaining TM.

One of the authors (Bance[85]) examined SHOT prosthesis head sizes, finding no differences in performance between 4 mm x 4 mm, 4 mm x 3 mm, and 3 mm x 2.3 mm sizes. Zahnert and Huttenbrink [83] compared prostheses with 1-mm, 3-mm, and 4-mm diameter head sizes. The 1-mm prosthesis was markedly worse than the 3-mm and 4-mm prostheses. The 3-mm and 4-mm head sizes were similar except for a mid-frequency drop in the 4-mm head prosthesis, which touched the annulus. Hence, their results reinforce the Bance study. The 1-mm prosthesis head may be affected by local nodes and antinodes in the vibrating TM, and also there may be difficulty coupling sound from the TM to such a small contact area. Mehta, Ravicz, Rosowski, and Merchant[55,86] comment on this possibility based on their work on Type III tympanoplasties. Adding a cartilage sheet on top of the stapes head seemed to improve results, perhaps by increasing the area over which motion was integrated at a small stapes head.

In general, we would suggest that for prostheses that couple to the TM, head sizes should be kept above 3 mm, but larger head diameters above 5 mm may touch the annulus, do not add much to performance, and may make the prosthesis more unwieldy.

Prosthesis to Stapes Superstructure Interface

An ongoing controversy revolves around whether it is best to reconstruct to the stapes head if it is available (i.e., SHOT or SHOM) or to the footplate (i.e., FOT or FOM). For FOM or SHOM reconstructions, going to the stapes head versus the footplate increases the angulation but may allow better constraint of rotation from the rotational moment by coupling the prosthesis to the stapes head with some kind of encasing mechanism. Clinically, it is often easier to reconstruct to the footplate if the superstructure is angulated inferiorly or, for SHOMs, if the malleus is anterior or medialized. The clinical literature is quite muddied in this regard, not offering a clear answer on the superiority of one type of reconstruction over the other.

For reconstructions to the TM, one of the authors compared SHOT and FOT reconstructions[87] and found a clinically negligible difference. The force vector is similar for the SHOT and FOT in these reconstructions. In this study, the stapes superstructure was left intact and may have added some stability to the FOT as well.

In comparing FOM- to SHOM-type reconstructions, Murugasu, Puria, and Roberson[88] found a consistent advantage of about 6.2 dB in reconstruction to the footplate compared with going to the stapes head, likely because of a better angulation vector for the FOM (▸ Fig. 9.11). However, their prosthesis design did not have any cup mechanism to engage the stapes head, and it is unclear if this would have made a difference in constraining any rotational movements at this interface.

In general, there appears to be little if any mechanical advantage of reconstruction to the stapes head compared with the footplate, but there may well be a stabilization advantage. And as always, the geometry of the middle ear dictates the most effective reconstruction in any one ear.

Prosthesis to Footplate Interface

The input impedance of the cochlear/oval window seems primarily resistive up to 10 kHz, with a fairly flat frequency response.[33] Where to place the prosthesis on the footplate is one of the more controllable factors in FOT-type reconstructions. Again, for FOM reconstruction, the angulation varies depending on where the prosthesis is placed, and the force vectors and rotational moments become an issue. The angulation will also change the tension on the reconstruction. The rotational moments are more of a factor in footplate prostheses given that the contact point on the footplate is difficult to constrain. Also, depending on where the prosthesis is placed and the angulation, it may cause tilting of the footplate rather than piston-like movement. The normal footplate mainly exhibits significant tilting movements only in the higher frequencies.[89]

Vlaming and Feenstra[65] compared FOM-type reconstruction onto the center of the footplate to reconstruction halfway between the center and anterior edge. They found some slight increase in tilting when the prosthesis was placed off-center, but overall the calculated footplate volume displacement was only slightly affected. Asai, Heiland, Huber, and Goode[90] used a custom-made cement rod-type FOM prosthesis, made in situ for each bone to avoid tension effects, and measured round window displacement. They found a clear advantage in all frequencies for contact at the stapes footplate center, minimal below 2 kHz, but found a more marked advantage to the stapes-center reconstructions above this frequency. At the higher frequencies, the center contact was better than the anterior, which was better than the posterior footplate, with a difference of 10–15 dB between the anterior and posterior footplate.

In an interesting 1966 cat experiment, using cochlear microphonics, Cottle and Tonndorf[20] found a wire strut between the lenticular process and the stapes footplate performed best at the stapes center, with a dropoff at frequencies above 2 kHz if placed anteriorly or posteriorly. In general, it makes theoretical sense to avoid tilting the footplate by reconstructing to its center. The work of Asai, Huber, and Goode[89], and Cottle and Tonndorf[20] supports this view.

The footplate shoe[91] has been advocated for stability of FOM/FOT-type prostheses. To our knowledge, this has not been tested in a temporal bone model. However, if the prosthesis is centered on the footplate, and does not itself form a hinge joint with the footplate, then rotational movements should be avoided and translational movements maximized.

Other Factors

Numerous other factors impact the mechanics of the reconstructed middle ear. A few, but by no means all, of them, are touched on below.

Scarring is one of the more significant factors that affects prosthesis movement. It is likely to add significant damping or resistance, as well as stiffness and mass loading. It is very commonly encountered clinically. Despite this, there is very little published data on the effects of scarring, and it is difficult to simulate realistically. One of the authors (Bance) has simulated scarring of the prosthesis to the posterior annulus with cyanoacrylates and noted drops of 10–15 dB in SHOT-type prostheses over a broad frequency range (unpublished data). Similarly, cementing the SHOT-type prosthesis to the promontory with slow-setting cement produced drops over a broad frequency range, which progressed over the setting time of the cement from minor to 10–20 dB.[92]

In other experiments, Bance (unpublished data) tried to simulate soft tissue scarring of the eardrum to the posterior canal using Steristrip (3 M, St. Paul, MN) to connect the posterior eardrum to the canal wall after SHOT reconstruction, which resulted in drops of 10 dB in vibration of the footplate, primarily in the low frequencies. Such results suggest that scarring could be one of the more potent factors affecting vibration transmission in the reconstructed ear.

Another underexplored factor is middle ear pressure. The effects of some interventions may depend on static middle ear pressure, which can affect the position of the eardrum or the contact area or properties of joints in the middle ear. There is very little data on this issue. A relevant publication is that of Offergeld, Hüttenbrink, Zahnert, and Hofmann,[93] who fixed the incudomalleolar and incudostapedial joints with cyanoacrylates and found only mild effects at ambient middle ear pressure but marked drops in vibration transmission at positive and negative middle ear pressures. This needs further exploration.

Other factors that could impact hearing results are the actions of the stapedius and tensor tympani. When they are active, they have a significant effect in the low frequencies (see Bance, Makki, Garland, Alian, van Wijhe, and Savage[94]), but their impact in reconstructed ears is unknown. The tendons of these muscles are routinely cut during reconstruction surgery. Temporal bone studies and measurements in deeply anesthetized animals suggest that the effect of these cuts on sound transmission is small[95,96]; however, whether static tension of these muscles plays a role in sound transmission in live conscious animals is not well known. In another study (Bance, Morris, and Van Wijhe[73]), the effects of cutting the stapedial tendon on SHOT-type reconstructions were minimal. Cutting the stapedial and tensor tympani tendons may change the tension on the prosthesis as well as the angulation.

The effects of fluid in the middle ear were explored in a study by Ravicz, Rosowski, and Merchant[27] in a temporal bone model. The authors showed that reductions in middle ear air volume were primarily responsible for the hearing loss at low frequencies and that mass-loading of the TM by the fluid contact was primarily responsible for the hearing loss seen at high frequencies. Viscosity of the fluid had little effect. These authors also point out that the low-frequency losses seen with reducing middle ear volume were minor compared with clinically reported hearing losses in low frequencies due to middle ear fluid. In addition, there may be other effects owing to the negative pressure that accompanies middle ear fluid that could change TM compliance in the low frequencies.

9.5 Conclusions

There are numerous factors that come into play in the ideal middle ear reconstruction. We have only briefly touched on many of the biocompatibility or adhesion issues or other biologic factors that affect middle ear function, although we have commented briefly on our observations on simulated scarring. Clearly, we recognize the importance of these issues, but they are beyond the scope of this chapter. It must be remembered that many of these factors interact with each other, so together their overall impact is larger than the sum of their individual effects.

There are many factors involved in a successful result. Pressure gain at the oval window can only be achieved if there is a vibrating TM. If this is not possible, RoWPOWA reconstructions are an option. Primarily for RoWPOWA reconstructions, achieving a low impedance access pathway to the oval window and adequate shielding of the round window with ventilation of the round window area are key factors. In PGOWA reconstructions, the key is first achieving a vibrating TM to drive the hydraulic lever pressure gain. This requires middle ear ventilation, a relatively thin membrane (i.e., not scarred over), and absence of perforations. Once this is achieved, the challenge is to couple it to the oval window in some way, usually with a connector of some short, although a direct TM-to-stapes head connection (D-SHOT) can also be a good option. (In designing the connector, it would appear that a rigid, light prosthesis with a head size of 3–5 mm, a clip to constrain rotational moments around the stapes head for SHOT or SHOM reconstructions, which is angulated minimally, not touching the annulus or promontory. Under little tension, it is placed on the stapes head or the footplate center, and would be most likely to result in efficient middle ear function.)

In practice, the anatomy and pathology a surgeon encounters will often limit the choices he or she faces, and passive prostheses have a limit to what they can overcome. When this limit is met, active middle ear implants (such as those discussed in Chapter 43) may become the preferred option.

References

[1] Merchant SN, Ravicz ME, Voss SE, Peake WT, Rosowski JJ. Toynbee Memorial Lecture 1997. Middle ear mechanics in normal, diseased and reconstructed ears. J Laryngol Otol. 1998;112(8):715–731.

[2] Dornhoffer JL, Gardner E. Prognostic factors in ossiculoplasty: A statistical staging system. Otol Neurotol. 2001;22(3):299–304.

[3] Mishiro Y, Sakagami M, Kitahara T, Kondoh K, Kubo T. Long-term hearing outcomes after ossiculoplasty in comparison to short-term outcomes. Otol Neurotol. 2008;29(3):326–329.

[4] Teranishi R, Shaw EA. External-ear acoustic models with simple geometry. J Acoust Soc Am. 1968;44(1):257–263.

[5] Shaw EA, Teranishi R. Sound pressure generated in an external-ear replica and real human ears by a nearby point source. J Acoust Soc Am. 1968;44 (1):240–249.

[6] Shaw EA. Transformation of sound pressure level from the free field to the eardrum in the horizontal plane. J Acoust Soc Am. 1974;56(6):1848–1861.

[7] Shaw EAG. The External Ear. In: Kiedel W.D NWD, editor. Handbook of Sensory Physiology. Berlin: Springer-Verlag; 1974. p. 455–90.

[8] Gardner MB, Gardner RS. Problem of localization in the median plane: Effect of pinnae cavity occlusion. J Acoust Soc Am. 1973;53(2):400–408.

[9] Evans RA, Day GA, Browning GG. Open-cavity mastoid surgery: its effect on the acoustics of the external ear canal. Clin Otolaryngol Allied Sci. 1989;14 (4):317–321.

[10] Jang CH. Changes in external ear resonance after mastoidectomy: open cavity mastoid versus obliterated mastoid cavity. Clin Otolaryngol Allied Sci. 2002;27(6):509–511.

[11] Cheng JT, Hamade M, Merchant SN, Rosowski JJ, Harrington E, Furlong C. Wave motion on the surface of the human tympanic membrane: Holographic measurement and modeling analysis. J Acoust Soc Am. 2013;133(2):918–937.

[12] Decraemer W, Khanna S. Measurement, visualization and quantitative analysis of complete three-dimensional kinematical data sets of human and cat middle ear. In: Gyo K, Wada H, Hato N, Koike T, editors. Middle Ear Mechanics in Research and Otology. Singapore: World Scientific; 2004. p. 3–10.

[13] Rosowski J, Cheng J, Merchant S. HArrington E, Furlong C. New data on the motion of the normal and reconstructed TM. Otol Neurotol. 2011;32 (9):1559–1567.

[14] Wever E, Lawrence M. Physiological Acoustics. Princeton: Princeton University Press; 1954.

[15] Rosowski JJ. Outer and middle ear. In: Popper A, Fay R, editors. Springer Handbook of Auditory Research: Comparative Hearing: Mammals. The Springer Series in Auditory Research. IV. New York: Springer-Verlag; 1994. p. 172–247.

[16] Zwislocki J. Analysis of the middle-ear function Part I: Input impedance. J Acoust Soc Am. 1962;34:1514–1523.

[17] Møller AR. Experimental study of the acoustic impedance of the middle ear and its transmission properties. Acta Otolaryngol. 1965;60:129–149.

[18] Rabinowitz WM. Measurement of the acoustic input immittance of the human ear. J Acoust Soc Am. 1981;70(4):1025–1035.

[19] Relkin E. Introduction to the analysis of middle-ear function. In: Jahn, Santos-Sacchi, editors. Physiology of the ear. New York: Raven Press; 1988.

[20] Cottle RD, Tonndorf J. Mechanical aspects of stapedial substitution. An experimental study. Arch Otolaryngol. 1966;83(6):547–553.

[21] Tonndorf J, Khanna SM. The tympanic membrane as a part of the middle ear transformer. Acta Otolaryngol. 1971;71(2):177–180.

[22] O'Connor KN, Tam M, Blevins NH, Puria S. Tympanic membrane collagen fibers: A key to high-frequency sound conduction. Laryngoscope. 2008;118 (3):483–490.

[23] Dahmann H. Zur Physiologie des Hörens: experimentelle Untersuchungen über die Mechanik der Gehörknöchelchenkette, sowie über deren Verhalten auf Ton und Luftdruck. Zeits. f. Hals- Nasen- Ohrenheilk. 1929;24:462–497.

[24] Willi UB, Ferrazzini MA, Huber AM. The incudo-malleolar joint and sound transmission losses. Hear Res. 2002;174(1–2):32–44.

[25] Eiber A, Huber AM, Lauxmann M, Chatzimichalis M, Sequeira D, Sim JH. Contribution of complex stapes motion to cochlea activation. Hear Res. 2012;284 (1–2):82–92.

[26] Molvaer OI, Vallersnes FM, Kringlebotn M. The size of the middle ear and the mastoid air cell. Acta Otolaryngol. 1978;85(1–2):24–32.

[27] Ravicz ME, Rosowski JJ, Merchant SN. Mechanisms of hearing loss resulting from middle-ear fluid. Hear Res. 2004;195(1–2):103–130.

[28] Rosowski JJ, Merchant SN. Mechanical and acoustic analysis of middle ear reconstruction. Am J Otol. 1995;16(4):486–497.

[29] Shera CA, Zweig G. Middle-ear phenomenology: The view from the three windows. J Acoust Soc Am. 1992;92(3):1356–1370.

[30] Kurokawa H, Goode RL. Sound pressure gain produced by the human middle ear. Otolaryngol Head Neck Surg. 1995;113(4):349–355.

[31] Puria S, Peake WT, Rosowski JJ. Sound-pressure measurements in the cochlear vestibule of human-cadaver ears. J Acoust Soc Am. 1997;101(5 Pt 1):2754–2770.

[32] Aibara R, Welsh JT, Puria S, Goode RL. Human middle-ear sound transfer function and cochlear input impedance. Hear Res. 2001;152(1–2):100–109.

[33] Nakajima HH, Dong W, Olson ES, Merchant SN, Ravicz ME, Rosowski JJ. Differential intracochlear sound pressure measurements in normal human temporal bones. J Assoc Res Otolaryngol. 2009;10(1):23–36.

[34] Voss SE, Rosowski JJ, Merchant SN, Peake WT. Non-ossicular signal transmission in human middle ears: Experimental assessment of the "acoustic route" with perforated tympanic membranes. J Acoust Soc Am. 2007;122(4):2135–2153.

[35] Peake WT, Rosowski JJ, Lynch TJ, III. Middle-ear transmission: Acoustic versus ossicular coupling in cat and human. Hear Res. 1992;57(2):245–268.

[36] Voss SE, Rosowski JJ, Peake WT. Is the pressure difference between the oval and round windows the effective acoustic stimulus for the cochlea? J Acoust Soc Am. 1996;100(3):1602–1616.

[37] Wüllstein H. The restoration of the function of the middle ear in chronic otitis media. Ann Otol Rhinol Laryngol. 1956;65:1020–1041.

[38] Bance M, Morris DP, Vanwijhe RG, Kiefte M, Funnell WR. Comparison of the mechanical performance of ossiculoplasty using a prosthetic malleus-to-stapes head with a tympanic membrane-to-stapes head assembly in a human cadaveric middle ear model. Otol Neurotol. 2004;25(6):903–909.

[39] Wullstein HL. The surgical restoration of hearing in chronic otitis media and its audiological basis. Ann Otol Rhinol Laryngol. 1958;67(4):952–963.

[40] Lempert J. Endaural fenestration of external semicircular canal for restoration of hearing in cases of otosclerosis. Arch Otolaryngol. 1940;31:711–779.

[41] Montandon P, Chatelain C. Restoration of hearing with type V tympanoplasty. ORL J Otorhinolaryngol Relat Spec. 1991;53(6):342–345.

[42] Lempert J. Fenestra non-ovalis: A new oval window for the improvement of hearing in cases of otosclerosis. Arch Otolaryngol. 1941;34:880–912.

[43] Merchant SN, Ravicz ME, Rosowski JJ. Mechanics of type IV tympanoplasty: Experimental findings and surgical implications. Ann Otol Rhinol Laryngol. 1997;106(1):49–60.

[44] Merchant SN, Rosowski JJ, Ravicz ME. Middle ear mechanics of type IV and type V tympanoplasty: II. Clinical analysis and surgical implications. Am J Otol. 1995;16(5):565–575.

[45] Kurokawa H, Goode RL. Sound pressure gain produced by the human middle ear. Otolaryngol Head Neck Surg. 1995;113(4):349–355.

[46] Wüllstein H. Results of tympanoplasty. AMA Arch Otolaryngol. 1960;71:478–485.

[47] Garcia-Ibanez L. Sonoinversion: A new audiosurgical system. Arch Otolaryngol. 1961;73:268–272.

[48] Colletti V, Soli SD, Carner M, Colletti L. Treatment of mixed hearing losses via implantation of a vibratory transducer on the round window. Int J Audiol. 2006;45(10):600–608.

[49] Voss SE, Rosowski JJ, Merchant SN, Peake WT. Middle-ear function with tympanic-membrane perforations. I. Measurements and mechanisms. J Acoust Soc Am. 2001;110(3 Pt 1):1432–1444.

[50] Morris DP, Bance M, Van Wijhe RG. Vibration characteristics and function of atelectatic segments in the tympanic membrane in fresh human cadaveric temporal bones. Clin Otolaryngol Allied Sci. 2004;29(2):133–137.

[51] Voss SE, Rosowski JJ, Merchant SN, Peake WT. Middle-ear function with tympanic-membrane perforations. II. A simple model. J Acoust Soc Am. 2001;110 (3 Pt 1):1445–1452.

[52] Mürbe D, Zahnert T, Bornitz M, Hüttenbrink KB. Acoustic properties of different cartilage reconstruction techniques of the tympanic membrane. Laryngoscope. 2002;112(10):1769–1776.

[53] Kim JY, Oh JH, Lee HH. Fascia versus cartilage graft in type I tympanoplasty: audiological outcome. J Craniofac Surg. 2012;23(6):e605–e608.

[54] Cayé-Thomasen P, Andersen J, Uzun C, Hansen S, Tos M. Ten-year results of cartilage palisades versus fascia in eardrum reconstruction after surgery for sinus or tensa retraction cholesteatoma in children. Laryngoscope. 2009;119 (5):944–952.

[55] Mehta RP, Ravicz ME, Rosowski JJ, Merchant SN. Middle-ear mechanics of Type III tympanoplasty (stapes columella): I. Experimental studies. Otol Neurotol. 2003;24(2):176–185.

[56] Nishihara S, Aritomo H, Goode RL. Effect of changes in mass on middle ear function. Otolaryngol Head Neck Surg. 1993;109(5):899–910.

[57] Puria S, Steele C. Tympanic-membrane and malleus-incus-complex co-adaptations for high-frequency hearing in mammals. Hear Res. 2010;263(1–2):183–190.

[58] Lerut B, Pfammatter A, Moons J, Linder T. Functional correlations of tympanic membrane perforation size. Otol Neurotol. 2012;33(3):379–386.

[59] Voss SE, Rosowski JJ, Merchant SN, Peake WT. How do tympanic-membrane perforations affect human middle-ear sound transmission? Acta Otolaryngol. 2001;121(2):169–173.

[60] Parent P, Allen JB. Time-domain "wave" model of the human tympanic membrane. Hear Res. 2010;263(1–2):152–167.

[61] Puria S, Allen JB. Measurements and model of the cat middle ear: Evidence of tympanic membrane acoustic delay. J Acoust Soc Am. 1998;104(6):3463–3481.

[62] Aarnisalo AA, Cheng JT, Ravicz ME, et al. Middle ear mechanics of cartilage tympanoplasty evaluated by laser holography and vibrometry. Otol Neurotol. 2009;30(8):1209–1214.

[63] Mills RP. Ossicular geometry and the choice of technique for ossiculoplasty. Clin Otolaryngol Allied Sci. 1991;16(5):476–479.

[64] Todd NW. The malleus-stapes offset. Laryngoscope. 2008;118(1):110–115.

[65] Vlaming MS, Feenstra L. Studies on the mechanics of the reconstructed human middle ear. Clin Otolaryngol Allied Sci. 1986;11(6):411–422.

[66] Morris DP, Bance M, van Wijhe RG, Kiefte M, Smith R. Optimum tension for partial ossicular replacement prosthesis reconstruction in the human middle ear. Laryngoscope. 2004;114(2):305–308.

[67] Yamada H, Goode RL. A self-adjusting ossicular prosthesis containing polyurethane sponge. Otol Neurotol. 2010;31(9):1404–1408.

[68] McGee TM. The loose wire syndrome. Laryngoscope. 1981;91(9 Pt 1):1478–1483.

[69] Majdalawieh OF, Alian WA, Katlai B, Van Wijhe RG, Bance ML. Linearity and lever ratio of the normal and reconstructed cadaveric human middle ear. Otol Neurotol. 2008;29(6):796–802.

[70] Gan RZ, Dai C, Wang X, Nakmali D, Wood MW. A totally implantable hearing system—design and function characterization in 3D computational model and temporal bones. Hear Res. 2010;263(1–2):138–144.

[71] Meister H, Walger M, Mickenhagen A, von Wedel H, Stennert E. Standardized measurements of the sound transmission of middle ear implants using a mechanical middle ear model. Eur Arch Otorhinolaryngol. 1999;25;6(3):122–127.

[72] Mojallal H, Stieve M, Krueger I, Behrens P, Mueller PP, Lenarz T. A biomechanical ear model to evaluate middle-ear reconstruction. Int J Audiol. 2009;48 (12):876–884.

[73] Bance M, Morris DP, Van Wijhe R. Effects of ossicular prosthesis mass and section of the stapes tendon on middle ear transmission. J Otolaryngol. 2007;36 (2):113–119.

[74] Nishihara S, Goode RL. Experimental study of the acoustic properties of incus replacement prostheses in a human temporal bone model. Am J Otol. 1994;15(4):485–494.

[75] Koike TWH, Toshimitsu K. Analysis of the finite element method of transfer function of reconstructed middle ear and their postoperative changes In: SN RJaM, editor. The Function and Mechanics of Norma, Diseased and Reconstructed Middle Ears. The Hague, Netherlands: Kugler Publications; 2000. p. 309–320.

[76] Goldenberg RA. Ossiculoplasty with composite prostheses. PORP and TORP. Otolaryngol Clin North Am. 1994;27(4):727–745.

[77] De Vos C, Gersdorff M, Gérard JM. Prognostic factors in ossiculoplasty. Otol Neurotol. 2007;28(1):61–67.

[78] Helmholtz HL. Die Mechanik der Gehörknöchelchen und des Trommelfells. Pflug Arch ges Physiol. 1868;1:1–60.

[79] Tonndorf J, Khanna SM. The role of the tympanic membrane in middle ear transmission. Ann Otol Rhinol Laryngol. 1970;79(4):743–753.

[80] Elpern BS, Elbrond O. Restoration of ossicular continuity with methyl methacrylate. Arch Otolaryngol. 1966;84(3):320–324.

[81] Shimizu Y, Goode RL. Effect of absence of malleus on ossiculoplasty in human temporal bones. Otolaryngol Head Neck Surg. 2008;139(2):301–306.

[82] Goode RL, Killion M, Nakamura K, Nishihara S. New knowledge about the function of the human middle ear: development of an improved analog model. Am J Otol. 1994;15(2):145–154.

[83] Zahnert TBM, Huttenbrink K-B, Eds. Calculations and experiments on the influence of prosthesis coupling to the middle ear transfer function. Middle ear mechanics in research and otology: Proceedings of the Third Symposium, Matsuyame, Ehime, Japan 9–12 July 2003; 2003 2004; World Scientific Publishing Co: World Scientific Publishing Co.

[84] Morris DP, Bance M, Van Wijhe RG. How do cartilage and other material overlay over a prosthesis affect its vibration transmission properties in ossiculoplasty? Otolaryngol Head Neck Surg. 2004;131(4):423–428.

[85] Bance M, Campos A, Wong L, Morris DP, van Wijhe R. How does prosthesis head size affect vibration transmission in ossiculoplasty? Otolaryngol Head Neck Surg. 2007;137(1):70–73.

[86] Merchant SN, McKenna MJ, Mehta RP, Ravicz ME, Rosowski JJ. Middle ear mechanics of Type III tympanoplasty (stapes columella): II. Clinical studies. Otol Neurotol. 2003;24(2):186–194.

[87] Alian WA, Majdalawieh OF, Van Wijhe RG, Ejnell H, Bance M. Prosthetic reconstruction from the tympanic membrane to the stapes head or to the stapes footplate? A laser Doppler study. J Otolaryngol Head Neck Surg. 2012;41(2):84–93.

[88] Murugasu E, Puria S, Roberson JB, Jr. Malleus-to-footplate versus malleus-to-stapes-head ossicular reconstruction prostheses: Temporal bone pressure gain measurements and clinical audiological data. Otol Neurotol. 2005;26 (4):572–582.

[89] Asai M, Huber AM, Goode RL. Analysis of the best site on the stapes footplate for ossicular chain reconstruction. Acta Otolaryngol. 1999;119(3):356–361.

[90] Asai M, Heiland KE, Huber AM, Goode RL. Evaluation of a cement incus replacement prosthesis in a temporal bone model. Acta Otolaryngol. 1999;119(5):573–576.

[91] Bremke M, Hüttenbrink KB, Beutner D. The sandwich cartilage shoe technique for ossicular reconstruction in a case of an unsecure stapes footplate. Laryngoscope. 2011;121(9):1950–1952.

[92] Morris DP, Wong L, van Wijhe RG, Bance ML. Effect of adhesion on the acoustic functioning of partial ossicular replacement prostheses in the cadaveric human ear. J Otolaryngol. 2006;35(1):22–25.

[93] Offergeld CFE, Hüttenbrink K-B, Zahnert T, and Hofmann G. Experimental investigations of ossicular joint ankylosis. In: JJ Rosowski SM, editor. The function and mechanics of normal, diseased and reconstructed middle ears. The Hague, Netherlands: Kugler Publications; 2000. p. 177–86.

[94] Bance M, Makki FM, Garland P, Alian WA, van Wijhe RG, Savage J. Effects of tensor tympani muscle contraction on the middle ear and markers of a contracted muscle. Laryngoscope. 2013;123(4):1021–1027.

[95] Voss SE, Rosowski JJ, Merchant SN, Peake WT. Acoustic responses of the human middle ear. Hear Res. 2000;150(1–2):43–69.

[96] Rosowski JJ, Ravicz ME, Songer JE. Structures that contribute to middle-ear admittance in chinchilla. J Comp Physiol A Neuroethol Sens Neural Behav Physiol. 2006;192(12):1287–1311.

Part 2

Clinical Evaluation and Office Management of Chronic Ear Disease

10 Pearls in Audiovestibular Assessment

John L. Dornhoffer, Samuel R. Atcherson, and Shane R. Anderson

Abbreviations used in the chapter:

ABG: air-bone gap
HL: hearing level
SDT: speech detection threshold
SRT: speech recognition threshold
VEMP: Vestibular Evoked Myogenic Potential

10.1 Introduction

The goal of surgery for the chronic ear is to create a safe, disease-free ear and improve the hearing as much as possible. With respect to the chronic ear, audiologists are tasked with providing valid and complete audiologic data that may determine a course of treatment and afterward be used to monitor treatment. Audiologists conduct a battery of physiologic and behavioral tests that can yield information with regard to how the chronic ear impacts hearing sensitivity and overall sound perception. This typically begins with an otoscopic examination, followed by physiologic assessments of the middle ear and pure-tone and speech audiometry. Otoscopy can help form some initial clues about how testing might go. The principle physiologic test is an immittance battery, which includes tympanometry, acoustic reflex testing, and, occasionally, Eustachian tube dysfunction testing.

From a surgical standpoint, the audiogram is arguably the most important functional tool in the preoperative assessment and the postoperative follow-up of patients. However, pure-tone audiometry should be considered as only part of the hearing evaluation, especially in difficult cases, and the surgeon should pay special attention to all aspects of the audiogram, including tympanometry, speech thresholds, and word recognition scores, all of which should be consistent with the pure-tone average. The tuning fork exam should be performed in all cases, and it should also support the findings on the audiogram. If there is disagreement, especially with the Weber portion of the exam, this should be reconciled before surgery is considered.

10.2 Pure-tone Audiometry

10.2.1 The Audiologist's Perspective

Pure-tone audiometry remains the unequivocal gold standard for the assessment of hearing sensitivity to identify thresholds across a range of test frequencies that generally encompass the speech range (250–8000 Hz, sometimes 125 Hz). Hearing loss is described primarily in terms of the magnitude of air conduction thresholds. The causes of hearing loss, however, have origins giving rise to the following terms: sensorineural (inner), conductive (outer and/or middle), or mixed (both).

During pure-tone audiometry, patients with chronic ear symptoms may exhibit reduced hearing sensitivity (i.e., poorer [elevated] thresholds) due to damping effects occurring within the middle ear; however, the effect across test frequencies may not be equally distributed. For example, significant negative pressure in the middle ear favors higher frequencies (stiffness tilt), resulting in a low-frequency hearing loss profile with air conduction testing (▶ Fig. 10.1). On the other hand, fluid in the middle ear results in the addition of mass, which impedes high-frequency signals and yields a high-frequency hearing loss profile with air conduction testing (mass tilt, ▶ Fig. 10.2). When

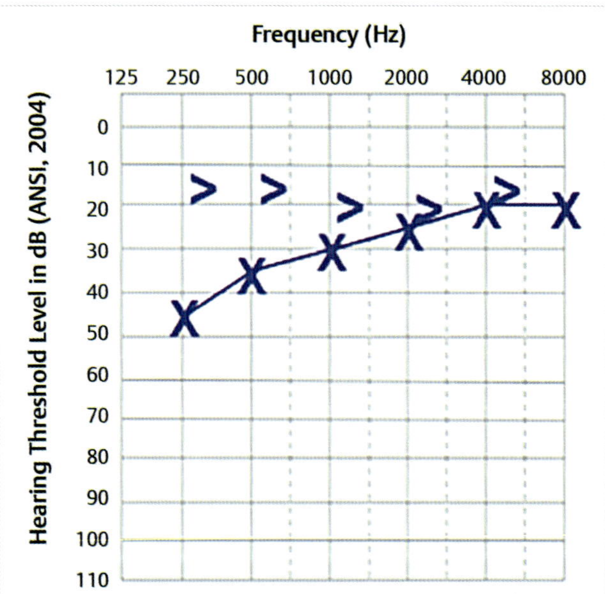

Fig. 10.1 Example of stiffness tilt. High-frequency air conduction is preserved, and there is an ABG in the low frequencies.

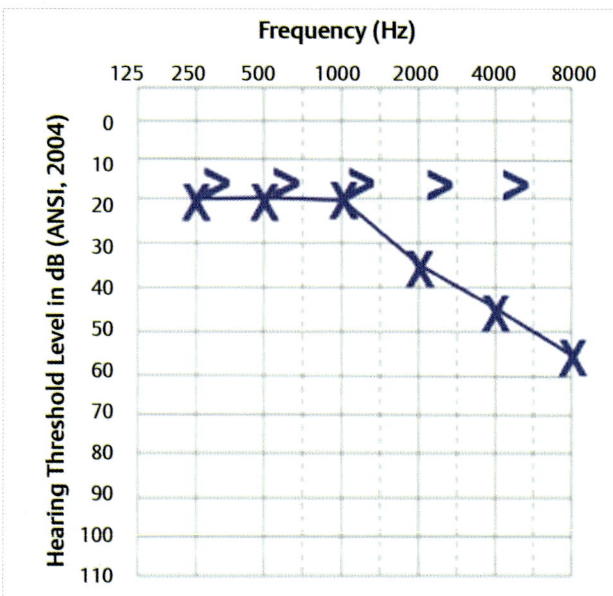

Fig. 10.2 Example of mass tilt. Low-frequency air conduction is preserved, and there is an ABG in the high frequencies.

negative pressure and fluid coexist in the middle ear, a flatter air conduction audiometric profile may be seen.

Bone conduction thresholds, on the other hand, will typically be better (lower) relative to air conduction thresholds, resulting in an air-bone gap (ABG). Middle ear diseases that decrease mobility of the ossicular chain and tympanic membrane (e.g., otosclerosis and lateral fixation) can also produce a stiffness tilt with a low-frequency air conduction hearing loss profile. A curious finding in otosclerosis involving stapes fixation is a reduction of bone conduction hearing sensitivity at 2000 Hz, called Carhart's notch or Carhart's effect.[1] The magnitude of this reduction is about 5 dB to 15 dB worse than at adjacent frequencies of 500, 1000, and 4000 Hz (▶ Fig. 10.3). Based on chief complaints, bone conduction thresholds may also be helpful with superior canal dehiscence, where ABGs of 10 dB or greater can exist in the lower frequencies (may be mild to moderate) and bone levels are better than expected (< 0 dB hearing level [HL]).[2]

Without bone conduction thresholds, the magnitude of a conductive hearing loss caused by middle ear diseases cannot be inferred. Large air conduction differences between ears (asymmetric hearing loss) may present a challenge, and audiometric testing will be influenced by interaural attenuation, which is on average around 60–65 dB for supra-aural earphones and about 20–30 dB higher for insert earphones with deep insertion. Supra-aural earphones have poorer interaural attenuation values because of their larger surface contact area with the skull and tissues, which can increase the probability of cross-hearing of high-intensity maskers via bone condition transmission. Conductive hearing losses can range to a maximum of 50–60 dB. Without the use of masking for the non-test ear, the test ear will essentially shadow the configuration of the better, non-test ear (▶ Fig. 10.4). Deep insertion of insert earphones can prevent shadow audiograms up to the limits of the interaural attenuation. Audiologists should be deliberate and diligent in obtaining valid bone conduction thresholds, especially when masking is used.

At least three issues come to mind. One, air conduction masking levels in one ear may be sufficiently loud to cross over to the non-test ear via the passage of vibration through the bones of the skull. Two, supra-aural earphones and shallow insert earphone placement can both produce an occlusion effect that falsely improves bone conduction thresholds. Finally, the audiologist should be wary of any measurement of a maximum conductive hearing loss that appears at only one test frequency but nowhere else on an audiogram.

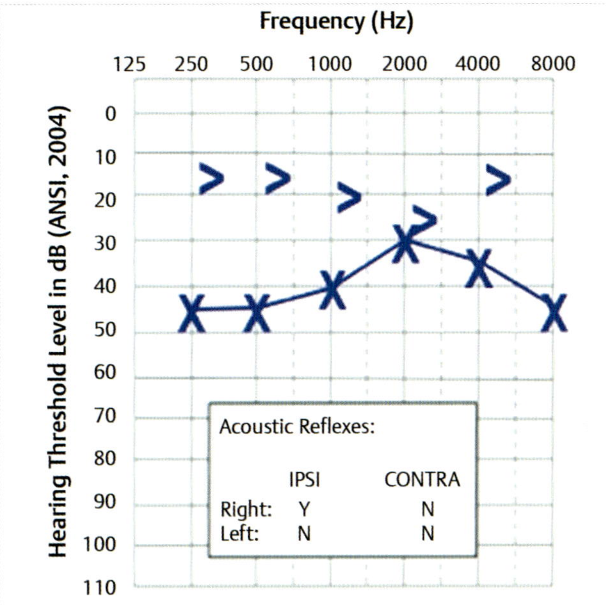

Fig. 10.3 Example of Carhart's notch. This is typically seen with a stapes fixation.

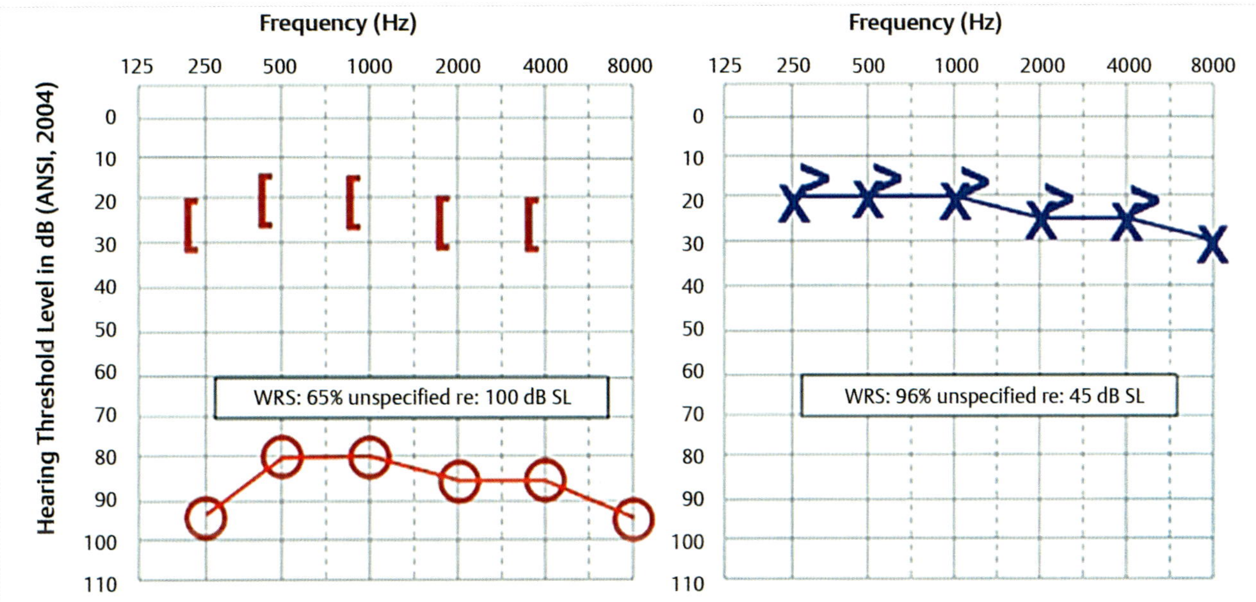

Fig. 10.4 Example of a shadow curve. The ABG exceeds what is physiologically possible. The gap is greater than interaural attenuation, and word recognition scores in the right ear are not typical of a conductive hearing loss.

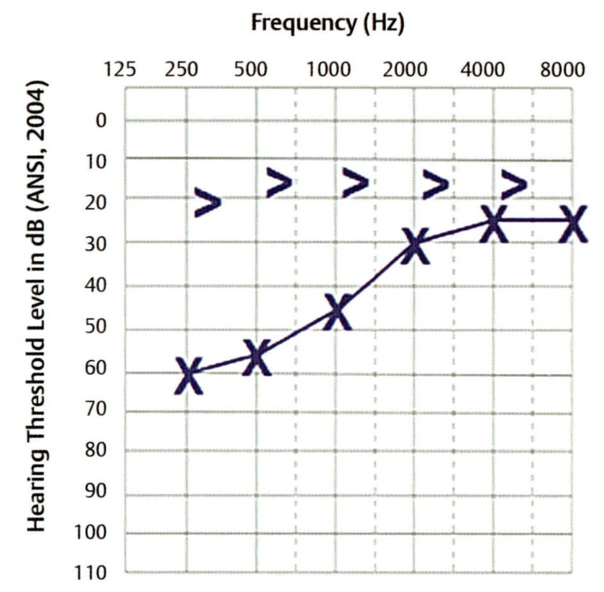

Fig. 10.5 Example of a hearing loss that would be considered out of proportion to a small anterior perforation.

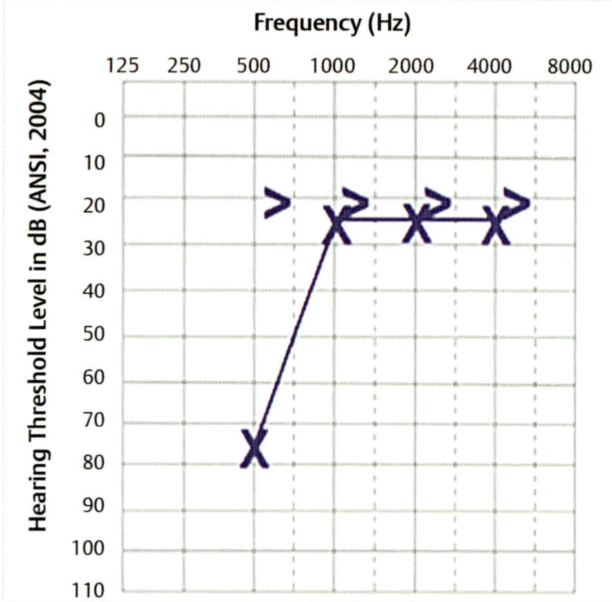

Fig. 10.6 Example of a wide ABG at a low frequency that is closed at 2000 Hz, suggesting vibrotactile feedback.

In cases of bilateral conductive hearing loss of at least 35 dB or more, audiologists may be confronted with a masking dilemma. This is a testing situation in which a masked threshold cannot be reached and the level of the masker crosses over to the non-test ear. A common solution to the masking dilemma is the use of insert earphones rather than supra-aural headphones due to slightly higher interaural attenuation. However, to achieve maximum benefit, deep insertion of insert earphones 2–3 mm inside the ear canal may allow the audiologist to reduce the overall effective masking level and avoid crossover hearing of the masker to the test ear. It is this audiologist's opinion that all air conduction testing should be performed using insert earphones unless supra-aural earphones are medically indicated.

10.2.2 The Otologist's Perspective

Preoperatively, the audiogram can give valuable insight, not only with regard to the magnitude of hearing impairment, but also with regard to the type of pathology, mechanism of involvement of the middle ear mechanism, and prognosis for improvement. The surgeon should be able to recognize the degree of conductive hearing loss to be expected for different pathologic processes as well as the pattern of loss on the audiogram specific for the condition.

If the degree of hearing loss is more than expected for a condition, then the surgeon should expect more than one point of involvement of the acoustic mechanism. An example would be an up-sloping 40-dB conductive loss at 500 Hz with a small anterior perforation (▶ Fig. 10.5). Knowing that a perforation in and of itself will cause a maximum 30-dB loss, one would anticipate concomitant fixation or erosion of the chain. The patient should be advised that a staged surgery might be necessary, especially if the stapes is fixed with tympanosclerosis.

Likewise, the hearing loss should be consistent with the pattern and degree of loss associated with a specific condition. For example, if an audiogram shows an ABG of 55 dB at 500 Hz but is closed at 2000 Hz, one would have to question the accuracy of the test (▶ Fig. 10.6). The gap of 55 dB would be suggestive of maximum conductive hearing loss associated with ossicular discontinuity, but if that were the case, there would almost certainly be a large gap at 2000 Hz. There is no condition that can result in both. In this situation, it is possible that the 500 Hz bone level was in part vibrotactile and not accurate. It is this otologist's experience that 500 Hz is the least accurate of the tested bone levels due to this possibility, and that 1000 Hz and 2000 Hz are more reliable.

In the postoperative period, the audiogram provides information on outcome, but it is also very important for follow-up in the eradication of disease. Especially in cases of cholesteatoma, where cartilage is often used in the eardrum reconstruction, potentially hiding recidivistic disease, a change in hearing is often the first sign of recurrence.

Hearing outcome is dictated to a large extent by the middle ear environment, so it is important for the otologic surgeon to consider the findings at the time of surgery in the evaluation of the postoperative audiogram. One should anticipate a specific hearing result based on the intraoperative findings. When these do not concur, it is important to use the frequency-specific information to determine where the problem lies. It is known that stiffness affects the low tones more (500 and 1000 Hz) and mass affects the high ones (4000 Hz). A tone of 2000 Hz, on the other hand, is relatively unaffected by either and is the most useful for follow-up in the otologist's experience.

Some complications following ear surgery are anatomical and are easy to diagnose by examination (recurrent perforation or cholesteatoma), whereas others are strictly functional (poor hearing). The latter cases involve an intact eardrum with a poorer-than-expected hearing outcome. These usually can be

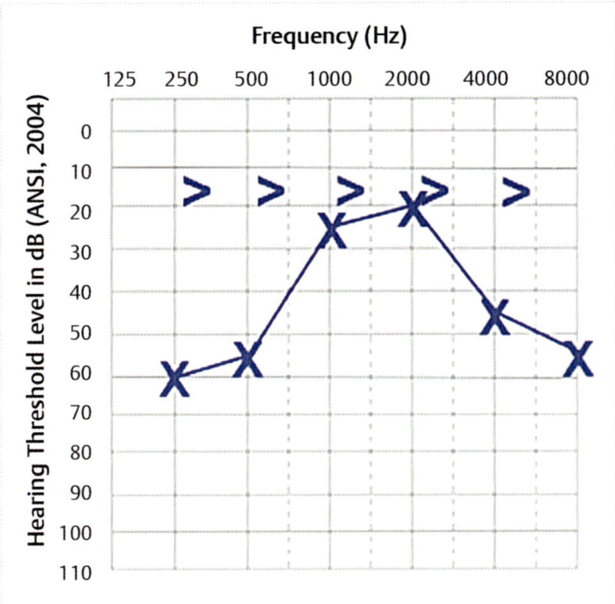

Fig. 10.7 Example of an inverted V loss. This is due to stiffening causing a low-tone loss and mass causing a high-tone loss, with preservation at 2000 Hz.

divided into effusion, fibrosis, bony fixation, recurrent cholesteatoma, and a slipped prosthesis, and this is where the pattern of loss shown on the postoperative audiogram is helpful.

If the conductive loss at 2000 Hz is > 15–20 dB, one should expect either effusion or a slipped prosthesis because fibrosis/fixation and cholesteatoma in and of themselves do not create much loss at 2000 Hz. Bony fixation of the stapes is the other condition that can cause a conductive loss at 2000 Hz if the stapes is fixed with hard tympanosclerosis, but this should have been obvious with palpation of the chain during the initial procedure. It should be noted that the level of the bony fixation is also frequency-specific. Medial fixation, at the level of the stapes, causes a conductive loss that is more prominent in the low tones but present at 2000 Hz and 4000 Hz as well. A Carhart's effect can be seen at 2000 Hz, as in otosclerosis (▶ Fig. 10.3). Lateral fixation, such as at the level of the malleus, will usually cause only low-tone conductive loss (stiffness tilt), with no losses at 2000 Hz and 4000 Hz (▶ Fig. 10.1). Fibrosis alone will usually show a conductive loss, primarily in the low tones, whereas cholesteatoma will often show an "inverted V" conductive loss (open in the low and high tones but closed at 2000 Hz). This is due to the fact that a growing cholesteatoma will stiffen the system by pressing against the reconstruction (low tones) and will show a mass effect due to its bulk (high tones) (▶ Fig. 10.7). When using the audiogram for cholesteatoma recurrence, it is this otologist's experience that a change at 4000 Hz in the post-operative period is the most sensitive. It should be kept in mind, however, that the 1995 American Academy of Otolaryngology criteria for guidelines in reporting interventions on conductive loss uses a pure-tone average of 500, 1000, 2000, and 3000 Hz, whereas 4000 Hz is not directly addressed in the outcome.[3]

Although the audiogram is very important in the management of the chronic ear, it is also very difficult to obtain in certain circumstances, and this fact must be considered in the interpretation of outcomes. The chronic ear offers several challenges when obtaining an audiogram. One is that the debris in the canal and eardrum as well as any granulations present can influence the results. The results may also fluctuate depending on the activity of the disease, further confusing the issue. The most significant problem, however, is that a conductive hearing loss is nearly always present and is frequently bilateral, making a masking dilemma a constant problem in the chronic ear. In addition, especially in cases of prolonged chronic otitis, a sensorineural loss may also be present; this is frequently asymmetrical, further compounding the masking dilemma.

In a child, especially due to the higher incidence of ongoing Eustachian tube dysfunction, a rule of three is advisable, especially when considering exploration for a conductive loss with an intact eardrum. In other words, is the audiogram consistent three times in a row over several visits? This otologist has experienced several situations in a child with a conductive hearing loss, especially in the low tones, with a totally normal eardrum who showed resolution in three months. Presumably the conductive loss was due to mucosal thickening or Eustachian tube dysfunction after a resolving ear infection that was not visible at the time of the exam, but resolved with time.

10.3 Tympanometry

10.3.1 The Audiologist's Perspective

Tympanometry is a useful test of middle ear function that may shed some light on how pure-tone audiometry may go if performed first. A 226 Hz tone is presented, while the ear canal pressure is changed from positive to negative (or vice-versa). It is important to note that neonates and infants 6 months and younger require the use of a 1000 Hz tone rather than, or in addition to, a 226 Hz tone due to anatomical and resonance differences.[4] A Type A tympanogram is normal and conveys ease of 226 Hz energy flow into the middle ear (high static admittance) when the ear canal pressure is at or near 0 daPa, with restriction of energy flow at high positive and high negative ear canal pressures. A Type B tympanogram suggests little to no mobility of the middle ear, which can be due to otitis media with effusion, tympanic atelectasis, or a perforation with large volume (measured volume of both ear canal and tympanic space). A Type C tympanogram indicates that the tympanic space is under negative pressure, usually due to chronic Eustachian tube blockage, and the static pressure peak is -200 daPa or more.

Subtypes As and Ad reflect ossicular chain restriction (e.g., significant tympanic scarring, otosclerosis, or lateral fixation) and hypermobility (e.g., tympanic membrane atrophy or ossicular discontinuity), respectively. The development of otitis media with effusion can show a progression of a series of Type A profiles, with increasing negative peak pressure, followed by Type C and Type B profiles when sufficient fluid is present. As otitis media with effusion resolves, it will reverse its tympanometric profiles. An audiologist may catch otitis media as it is developing or when it is resolving, and the results of a single test session do not necessitate a referral unless serial tympanograms are showing no improvement over time.

Tympanometric techniques to evaluate a patulous Eustachian tube may be possible, but these are often difficult to obtain if the ear canal cannot maintain a consistent pressure. In the chronic ear, acoustic reflexes will be elevated or absent anytime there is an ABG. Similar to patulous Eustachian tubes, it may be difficult to record acoustic reflexes in a middle ear with a Type *Ad* profile due to inability to maintain a constant ear canal pressure.[5]

Post-surgery, tympanometry and acoustic reflexes may or may not be useful depending on the physical status of the outer and middle ears and the type of surgery performed. Tympanometry is generally helpful for monitoring pressure equalization tubes. A Type B tympanogram with large volume will verify a patent tube whereas a Type A or C will indicate that the tube is blocked or has fallen out.

10.3.2 The Otologist's Perspective

Tympanometry may not be very helpful in the post-operative period, especially when cartilage is used in the eardrum reconstruction. In these cases a Type B or flat reading is usually present, even with no middle ear pathology, due to the non-distensible material used.

10.4 Speech Recognition Threshold and Word Recognition Testing

10.4.1 The Audiologist's Perspective

Speech thresholds can be captured in one of two ways. The speech recognition threshold (SRT) is the minimum hearing level at which recognition of speech material is achieved 50% of the time. The SRT is assessed using bisyllabic (spondee) words and is recorded in dB HL. For most patients, the SRT will be in fair agreement if within 7–12 dB (correlation: 0.95 to 0.98) with the pure-tone average at 500, 1000, and 2000 Hz. When an SRT cannot be obtained due to lack of speech recognition, a speech detection threshold (SDT) may be obtained. The SDT represents the patient's ability to detect the presence (awareness, not recognition) of speech material 50% of the time. The SDT is also recorded in dB HL.

Word recognition testing at a suprathreshold level (usually 30–40 dB above air conduction SRT) is performed using lists of monosyllabic words. Typically, lists of 25 or 50 words are commonly used (with a standard preference for the latter) and are recorded as the percentage of correct responses. Generally speaking, word recognition scores are of little use for differential diagnosis of conductive, sensorineural, and retrocochlear hearing loss due to wide variability among patients. However, word recognition scores tend to be least affected by conductive hearing loss and most affected by retrocochlear hearing loss. Even test-retest (or pre-test versus post-test) word recognition scores should be interpreted with some caution unless similar word lists are used with more or less the same testing conditions. In practice, word recognition scores are most consistently reliable with recorded speech materials compared with monitored live-voice, especially when different audiologists in a practice may see the same patient.

Similar to pure-tone audiometry, whenever there is risk for crossover of speech stimuli from a poorer test ear to a better non-test ear, masking will be required with a white noise or speech noise. The interaural attention for supra-aural headphones is about 45–50 dB; for insert earphones it will be 55 dB or higher.

10.4.2 The Otologist's Perspective

Word recognition scores can be extremely helpful for determining the degree of the sensorineural component of the hearing loss in a case of mixed loss. This can be especially helpful when there is bilateral mixed loss. In this situation, it might be impossible for the audiologist to accurately give bone levels for each ear, and it might be reported only as "at least one ear has a bone level at this level." This is by no means a reflection on the ability of the audiologist to accurately mask, but, rather, is an honest assessment of the limitations of the situation. This is another example of where word recognition scores can be very useful.

Generally, but not always, the word recognition correlates to the sensorineural hearing loss: the greater the sensorineural loss, the worse the recognition score. In a case of bilateral mixed loss, where it is not possible to separate the bone conduction for each ear adequately, a poor word recognition score in one ear would suggest poorer inner ear reserve in that ear. Likewise, it is unlikely in a case of purely conductive loss to have poor word recognition. Therefore, if a conductive loss is shown that does not agree with the fork exam, a poor word recognition score would indicate that there is a sensorineural loss instead.

A final note on word recognition scores is that the better-performing ear should be treated as the better-hearing ear during the preoperative planning for surgery, regardless of the hearing level.

Pearls and Pitfalls

Checklist for the audiometric assessment in the preoperative period:

1. Is the ear undergoing surgery the poorer-hearing ear?
2. Does the conductive hearing loss degree and pattern make sense based on the anticipated pathology?
3. Does the fork exam agree with the audiogram?
4. Does the speech recognition score correlate with the sensorineural level shown on the audiogram? If the answer is "no," then step back and reassess.

10.5 Supplemental Tests

10.5.1 The Audiologist's Perspective: Vestibular Testing

Middle ear disorders rarely warrant vestibular testing. However, serous and suppurative labyrinthitis may begin as bacterial infections within the middle ear that eventually invade the inner ear, resulting in both auditory and vestibular impairment.

More commonly, otitis media, endolymphatic hydrops, and trauma to the ear can result in transient symptoms of dizziness or vertigo. More long-term symptoms can arise from disorders of the inner ear, such as perilymph fistula and superior canal dehiscence. Not all cases of superior canal dehiscence have symptoms of vertigo, but a conductive hearing loss (ABG) for audiometric test frequencies < 1000 Hz may be present.[6] Whether or not vertigo is present, air conduction cervical (sternocleidomastoid) Vestibular Evoked Myogenic Potential (VEMP) testing exhibits abnormally low thresholds in patients with superior canal dehiscence. VEMPs may yield better clinical data for patients with significant ABGs compared with tympanometry and acoustic reflexes.[7]

10.5.2 The Otologist's Perspective: The Tuning Fork Exam

Although all three tuning forks are useful, the 512 Hz fork is most important for middle ear surgery. It is of sufficient acoustic energy to perform a reliable Weber exam, and for the Rinne exam, a negative result (bone louder than air) indicating approximately a 30 dB conductive loss, will suggest ossicular chain involvement. The Weber exam is very reliable for conductive loss and will nearly always lateralize to the impaired ear, unless there is a significant sensorineural loss as well. This exam is not as reliable for sensorineural loss, and with prolonged unilateral sensorineural loss, the results will often be midline. If the Weber exam does not agree with the audiogram for unilateral conductive loss, the audiogram should be repeated and the otologist should be suspicious of a shadow curve in an ear with sensorineural loss due to inadequate masking. Likewise, if a conductive hearing loss of less than 30 dB is present on the audiogram, and the 512 Hz fork shows bone conduction is greater than air conduction, then over-masking should be considered a cause of the discrepancy.

10.6 Conclusion

The otologist is in the privileged position of having both the audiologic data available as well as an intricate understanding of the physiological mechanism underlying this data and its limitations. It is important to correlate the objective findings of an audiogram and word recognition scores with subjective otologic findings. When audiologic data do not correspond to the otologist's findings, a degree of skepticism is required. In this scenario, the otologist should rely on the results of tuning fork examination. We have operated on more than one occasion based on audiologic data suggesting that a conductive loss was present when, in fact, the hearing loss proved to be sensorineural. It is important to have an open and frank relationship with the audiologist so that in circumstances where the audiologist is unsure of the hearing result, he or she can freely discuss this with the otologist.

References

[1] Carhart R. Clinical application of bone conduction audiometry. Arch Otolaryngol. 1950;51(6):798–808.

[2] Minor LB. Clinical manifestations of superior semicircular canal dehiscence. Laryngoscope. 2005;115(10):1717–1727.

[3] Committee on Hearing and Equilibrium guidelines for the evaluation of results of treatment of conductive hearing loss. American Academy of Otolaryngology-Head and Neck Surgery Foundation, Inc. Otolaryngol Head Neck Surg. 1995;113(3):186–187.

[4] Alaerts J, Luts H, Wouters J. Evaluation of middle ear function in young children: clinical guidelines for the use of 226- and 1,000-Hz tympanometry. Otol Neurotol. 2007;28(6):727–732.

[5] Atcherson SR, Stoody TM. Acoustic stapedial reflex test modification in ears with high static admittance and asymmetric hearing loss: A case study. Asia Pac J Speech Lang Hear. 2011;14(2):129–138.

[6] Mikulec AA, McKenna MJ, Ramsey MJ, et al. Superior semicircular canal dehiscence presenting as conductive hearing loss without vertigo. Otol Neurotol. 2004;25(2):121–129.

[7] Zhou G, Poe D, Gopen Q. Clinical use of vestibular evoked myogenic potentials in the evaluation of patients with air-bone gaps. Otol Neurotol. 2012;33 (8):1368–1374.

11 Radiographic Evaluation of Chronic Ear Disease

Richard K. Gurgel, Richard H. Wiggins, and Clough Shelton

Abbreviations used in this chapter:

ADC: apparent diffusion coefficient
CBCT: cone-beam CT
CSF: cerebrospinal fluid
CT: computed tomography
CTV: CT venography
DWI: diffusion-weighted imaging
EPI: echo planar imaging (also, non-EPI for non-echo planar imaging)
GRE: gradient recalled echo
IAC: internal auditory canal
MRI: magnetic resonance imaging
MRV: magnetic resonance venography
PORP: partial ossicular replacement prosthesis
SPGR: spoiled gradient recalled
SWI: susceptibility-weighted imaging
TOF: time of flight
TORP: total ossicular replacement prosthesis

11.1 Introduction

The role of preoperative imaging has been the subject of debate among those who perform chronic ear surgery. It has been argued that preoperative imaging of the chronic ear is beneficial because it provides a thorough understanding of the patient's anatomy and improves efficacy and safety of surgery.[1] Alternatively, others contend that routine imaging is not indicated because the diagnosis of chronic ear disease is made clinically, not radiographically, and the surgical management of chronic ear disease is mainly dictated by intraoperative landmark identification and decision-making.[2] Whereas there is controversy regarding the role of routine preoperative imaging for chronic ear disease, most agree that it is indicated for patients in whom a complication of chronic otitis media or a congenital malformation is suspected. Some also believe that routine imaging is also called for in the rare instance when surgery is indicated in an only-hearing ear.

What then, is the role for imaging in chronic ear disease? In this chapter, we will review the typical imaging characteristics of chronic ear disease, illustrate how imaging can aid in diagnosing many of the complications of chronic ear disease, and review how new imaging modalities can be useful for surveillance of chronic ear disease in the postoperative setting. For clarity in defining chronic otitis media, this chapter primarily deals with chronic suppurative otitis media caused by cholesteatoma.

11.2 Imaging Characteristics of Chronic Ear Disease

The diagnosis of chronic ear disease is primarily based on a comprehensive history and physical exam, including otomicroscopy and an audiogram. Despite the fact that the diagnosis is made based on this clinical information, imaging can provide useful adjunct information, such as anatomic information about the extent of disease for patients with cholesteatoma. There is a high reported correlation between temporal bone computed tomography (CT) findings in determining the presence, location, and extent of cholesteatoma, ossicular chain erosion, labyrinthine fistula, and intracranial complications.[3,4]

11.2.1 Extent of Disease and Degree of Pneumatization

Primary acquired cholesteatomas typically develop in the epitympanum from a posterior-superior retraction of the pars flaccida portion of the tympanic membrane.[5] As the cholesteatoma enlarges, the adjacent osseous structures become involved and are eroded. Cholesteatomas involving the epitympanum will often erode the scutum, the normally sharp bony overhang lateral to the head of the malleus (▶ Fig. 11.1). Epitympanic cholesteatomas will cause erosion or blunting of the scutum (▶ Fig. 11.2), which is best seen on a coronal CT scan.

Whereas there is not a strict correlation to the degree of mastoid pneumatization and severity of chronic ear disease or risk of developing a cholesteatoma, it is generally accepted that poor pneumatization is evidence of chronic ear disease. Poor pneumatization has been associated with pars flaccida cholesteatomas.[6] A spectrum of temporal bone pneumatization is illustrated in ▶ Fig. 11.3.

Preoperative imaging can influence a surgeon's choice of surgical approach. The more information the surgeon has to

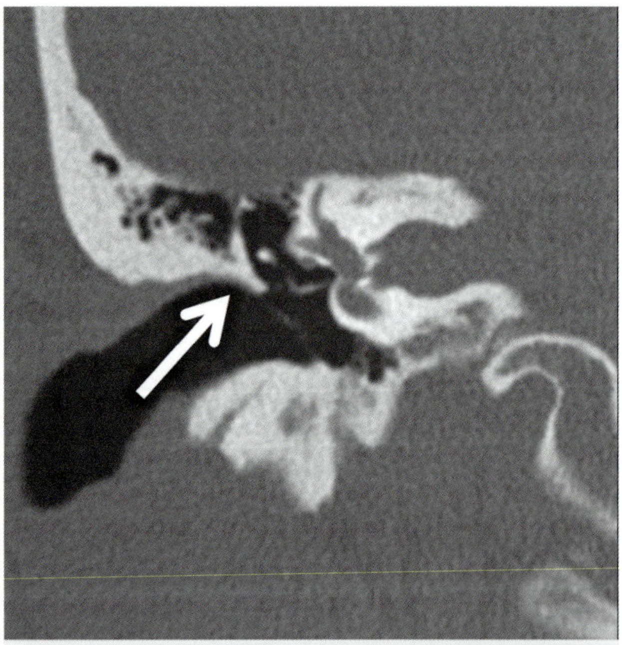

Fig. 11.1 Coronal bone algorithm CT through the right ear demonstrates a sharp scutum (arrow) at the superior attachment of the tympanic membrane.

augment the preoperative examination, the better he or she is able to plan what needs to be done surgically as well as to appropriately counsel the patient with regard to expectations and knowledge of risks.[1] For example, disease isolated to the epitympanum may only require a transcanal atticotomy. However, a preoperative scan that shows a poorly pneumatized mastoid with minimal disease may allow an otologic surgeon to prepare for and counsel the patient regarding a possible canal wall-down tympanomastoidectomy. This information may lead to shorter operating time given that an "inside out" mastoidectomy can be done at the outset, which involves lowering the posterior external auditory canal wall while the initial mastoidectomy is being performed. A canal wall-down tympanomastoidectomy in patients with contracted, sclerotic mastoids essentially creates an enlarged ear canal rather than a large mastoid bowl, which is found in patients with more extensive pneumatization.

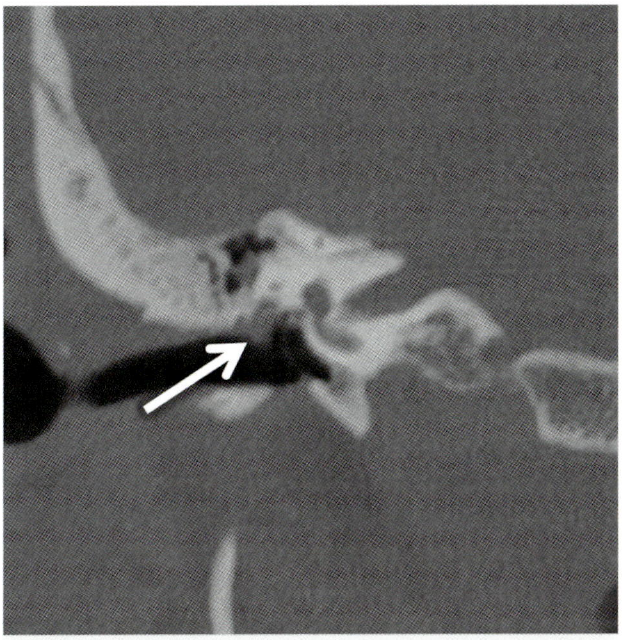

Fig. 11.2 Coronal bone algorithm CT through the right temporal bone shows a soft tissue mass (arrow) at the expected location of the pars flaccida portion of the tympanic membrane, found to be an epitympanic cholesteatoma eroding the scutum.

11.2.2 Anatomy of Critical Structures

Preoperative imaging in chronic ear disease allows the otologic surgeon to evaluate the location of certain critical landmarks, namely the tegmen, sigmoid sinus, and vascular structures as well as the course of the facial nerve. Whereas the temporal line is the typical external landmark used to identify the level of the tegmen and floor of the middle fossa, the true level can be quite variable. Coronal CT imaging will provide the best views of the tegmen (▶ Fig. 11.4). The tegmen is typically lower laterally and then rises in its more medial course. A low tegmen can have a significant effect on the exposure of the epitympanum and antrum in canal wall-up surgery.[1]

Imaging of the facial nerve in chronic otitis media can alert the surgeon about possible areas of dehiscence or an aberrant course of the nerve. This radiographic information can be especially useful when doing revision chronic ear surgery since the facial nerve can be exposed at the initial operation.[7] With regard to managing the facial nerve during chronic ear surgery, it is especially important to emphasize that a thorough knowledge of facial nerve anatomy, sound clinical judgment, careful surgical technique, and experience remain the cornerstones for avoiding facial nerve injury.[1] The majority of iatrogenic injuries result in failure to recognize key intraoperative landmarks.[8] Cholesteatoma can cause bony dehiscence adjacent to the facial nerve in the middle ear and mastoid (▶ Fig. 11.5). Cholesteatomas that form in the anterior epitympanum can erode bone adjacent to and exert pressure on or local irritation to the geniculate ganglion, which can result in facial paralysis.[9]

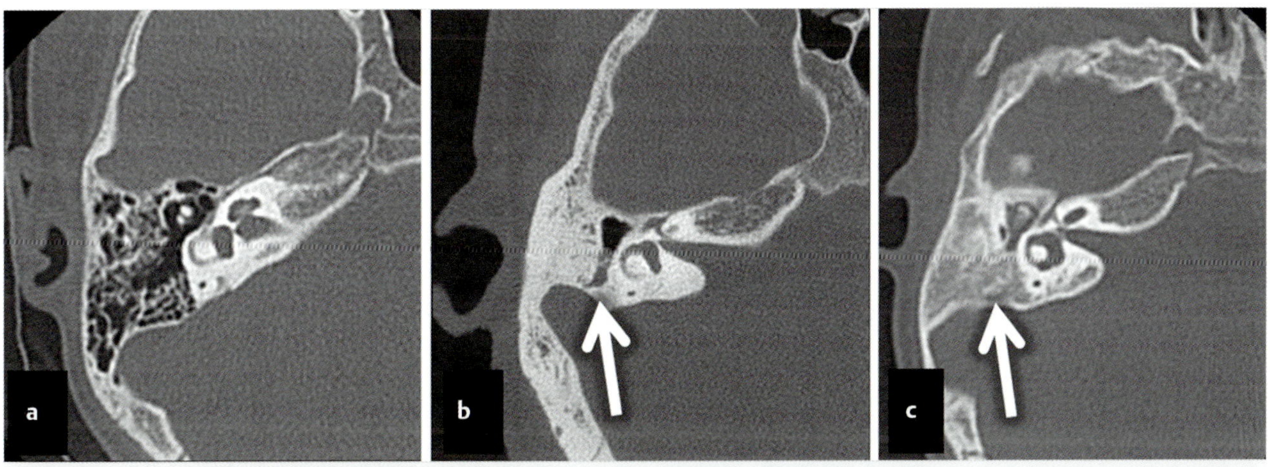

Fig. 11.3 Stage of pneumatization. Three axial CT images in three different patients. The first image (a) demonstrates well-pneumatized and well-aerated mastoid air cells in the middle ear of a normal healthy patient with normal hearing. The second image (b) shows a more poorly pneumatized mastoid bone compared to the example in (a) with dense cortical bone with aeration of only the mastoid antrum (arrow). The last image (c) shows no pneumatization, with a small opacified middle ear surrounding the ossicles. Bone density extends lateral to the lateral semicircular canals (arrow).

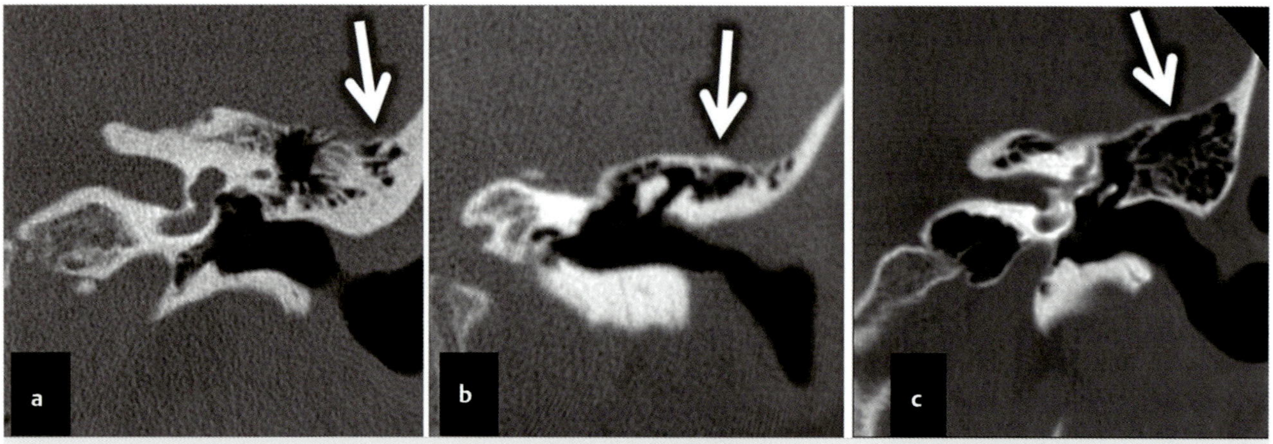

Fig. 11.4 Three coronal CT images from different patients all at the level of the external auditory canal. Various tegmen tympany configurations are shown, with a downward-sloping lateral portion (a, arrow), relatively flat tegmen (b, arrow), and an upward lateral sloping tegmen (c, arrow).

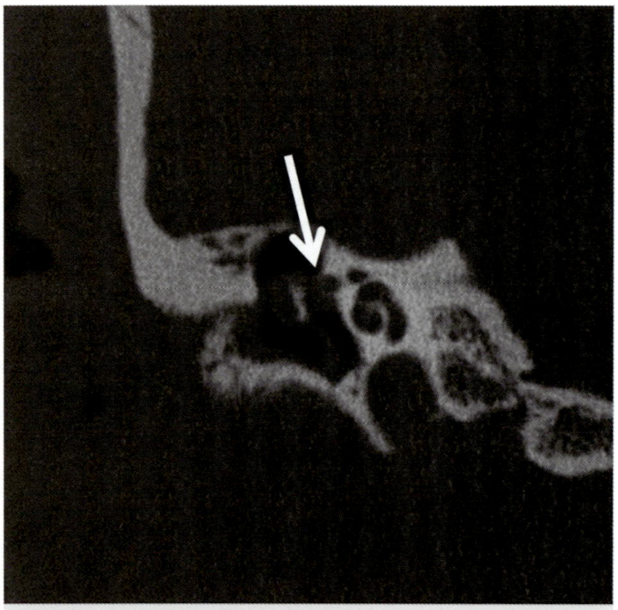

Fig. 11.5 Coronal CT through the right temporal bone showing a cholesteatoma as a soft tissue mass within the middle ear with erosion of the lateral wall of the proximal portion of the tympanic segment of the facial nerve (arrow).

11.2.3 Identifying Postoperative Features

When imaging patients with chronic ear disease who have had prior surgery, it is vital to recognize important postoperative features. One such feature is the appearance of various ossicular prostheses. Ossicular prostheses are commonly categorized based on their length, material, and whether or not they make contact with an intact and mobile stapes. The radiolucency of the material affects how well the prosthesis can be visualized radiographically (▶ Fig. 11.6). Prostheses that are placed on a mobile stapes are often referred to as partial ossicular replacement prostheses (PORPs). Prostheses that bridge the gap from the tympanic membrane to the footplate in the absence of a stapes superstructure are called total ossicular replacement prostheses (TORPs).

The postoperative hearing result following ossiculoplasty can be predicted with imaging. Postoperative imaging can precisely determine the position and angle of middle ear implants.[10] For example, in patients who have a significant persistent, postoperative conductive hearing loss, imaging may reveal a misplaced or dislocated prosthesis (▶ Fig. 11.7). Komori, Yanagihara, Hyodo, and Miuchi reported that volume-rendered 3-dimensional cone-beam CT (CBCT) images revealed TORP malpositioning or migration, which was not detected on 2-dimensional CBCT images.[11] In such cases, the TORP shaft was in contact with the wall of the oval window niche or the TORP had moved from the stapes footplate.

For patients who have postoperative complications following ossiculoplasty, imaging can often be helpful in making a diagnosis. For example, if a patient experiences postoperative sensorineural hearing loss or vertigo, the prosthesis may have been inserted too deeply and may have violated the inner ear (▶ Fig. 11.8).

11.3 Diagnosing Complications of Chronic Otitis Media

11.3.1 Intracranial

Sigmoid Sinus Thrombosis

Sigmoid sinus thrombosis occurs when inflammation from the mastoid, most often from infection, causes a thrombus formation in the sigmoid. Patients with sigmoid sinus thrombosis will often present with pain on the side of the sigmoid thrombosis or diffuse headache. Increased intracranial pressure may result from sigmoid thrombosis.

Dural venous sinus thrombosis is best seen radiographically on a CT venography (CTV) and magnetic resonance venography (MRV) (▶ Fig. 11.9). The preference for CTV or MRV is dependent on the radiologist's and clinician's experience interpreting these images and the availability of scanners to perform these different imaging modalities. A non-contrasted CT may demonstrate high density in the thrombosis sinus, greater in density

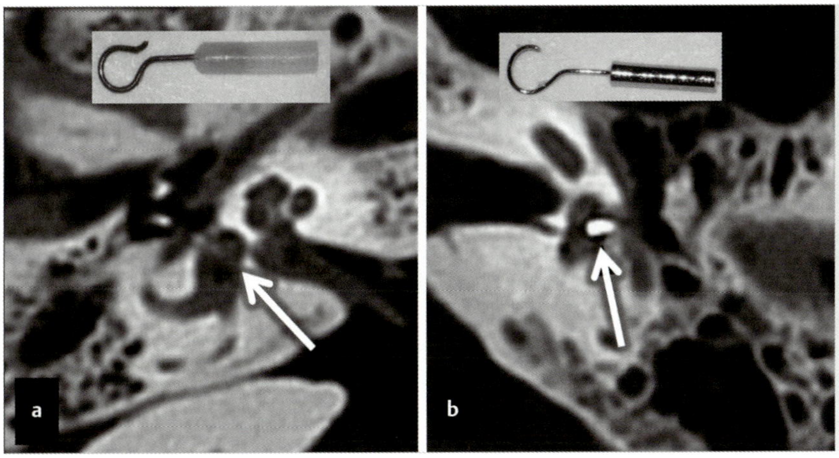

Fig. 11.6 Examples of stapes prostheses. Two axial temporal bone CT examinations showing different types of stapes prostheses, with a radiolucent (a, arrow) fluoroplastic prosthesis (a, insert), and a radiodense (b, arrow) stainless steel prosthesis (b, insert).

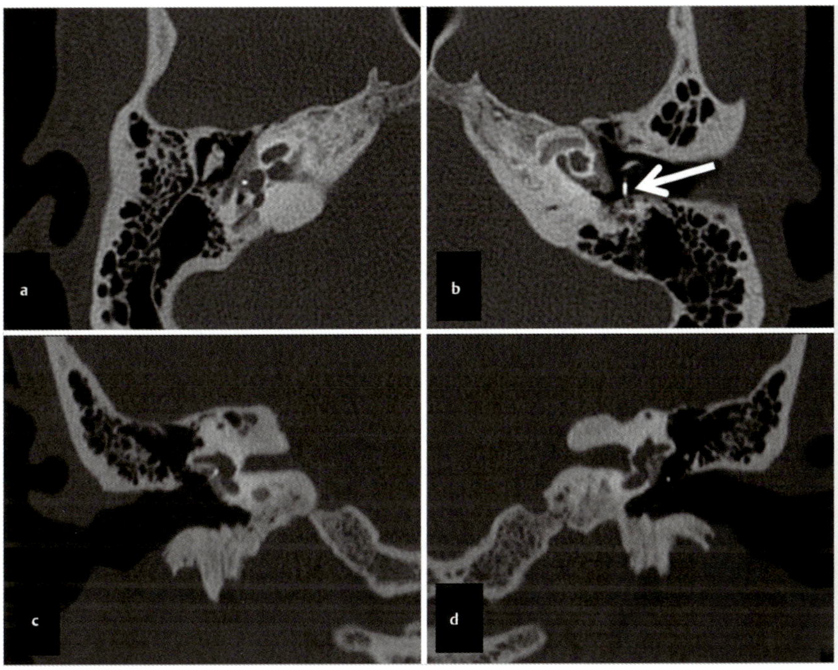

Fig. 11.7 Patient with bilateral stapes prostheses for bilateral cochlear otosclerosis (otospongiosis). The axial (a) and coronal (c) right-sided images show a normal right-sided prosthesis. The correlating left sided axial (b) and coronal (d) images show a misplaced left-sided prosthesis (arrow in panel b), extending posteriorly adjacent to the descending segment of the facial nerve.

than the remaining vessels. The CTV examination does require contrast as well as radiation, and, therefore, may not be favored in patients who have already received many CT studies in an effort to limit overall patient radiation dose. However, the CT modality is fast and less affected by artifacts, relying solely on the density of the object being imaged. Interpretation of CTV examinations is usually fairly obvious, with a clear-filling defect at the site of dural venous sinus thrombosis compared with other normal venous structures.

On a noncontrast magnetic resonance imaging (MRI) examination, the T1 series of images are helpful for visualizing the bright T1 signal within the blood clot, whereas the gradient recalled echo (GRE) sequence or the susceptibility-weighted imaging (SWI) sequences will show "blooming" with a hypointense thrombus within the affected sigmoid sinus. For a routine MRV study, a 2-dimensional time of flight (2D TOF) sequence is often initially performed, with a flow void present where the normal distribution of venous drainage through the sigmoid would be expected. A post-contrast 3-dimensional coronal acquisition spoiled gradient recalled (3D SPGR) image often nicely demonstrates the venous structures, and complex cases may require a catheter angiogram study.

Sigmoid sinus thrombosis is often managed with close surveillance. Anticoagulation may be beneficial if there is propagation of the clot or if a patient's clinical course deteriorates. Serial imaging may be of benefit to evaluate for propagation of the clot along the transverse or other intracranial sinuses.

Intracranial Abscess

Intracranial abscesses, either in the epidural space or within the brain parenchyma, are rare complications of chronic otitis media but can have serious neurologic sequelae. The abscess will often be located in the temporal lobe due to its proximity to the diseased middle ear and mastoid. Brain abscess develops from chronic otitis media via either direct extension of infection intracranially or via hematogenous spread of bacteria intracranially through bridging veins.

In patients with a brain abscess from chronic otitis media, the temporal bone will often show a dehiscent tegmen

(▶ Fig. 11.10). The abscess will often be well visualized on either CT or MRI, though MRI is preferable because it will better show the extent of brain reaction and vasogenic edema related to the infection. An intracranial brain abscess is typically characterized by rim-enhancement on post-contrast imaging and restricted diffusion (▶ Fig. 11.11).

11.3.2 Extracranial

Mastoiditis

Acute infection (otitis media or mastoiditis) can develop in the setting of chronic otitis media. It is critical for both clinicians and imagers to recognize that mastoiditis is a clinical diagnosis.

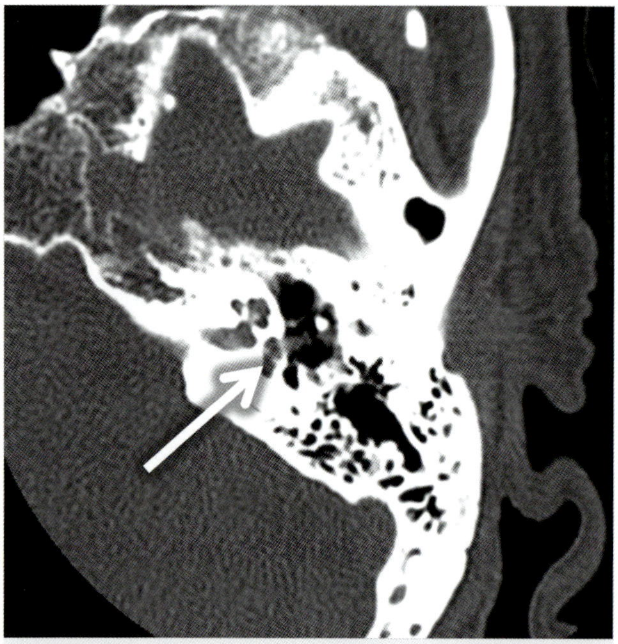

Fig. 11.8 Stapes within vestibule. Imaging can provide insight into postoperative complications with chronic ear surgery. This axial, temporal bone CT illustrates a PORP that has displaced the stapes into the vestibule (arrow), causing postoperative vertigo and sensorineural hearing loss.

The radiographic appearance of mastoid opacification does not equate to the diagnosis of mastoiditis. Rather, the diagnosis of mastoiditis suggests an infectious or inflammatory condition involving the mastoid. Mastoid opacification may occur in many settings that are neither inflammatory nor infectious, such as with serous otitis media, postoperative scarring, and/or neoplasm.

Imaging plays a critical role in differentiating non-coalescent mastoiditis from the more aggressive, osteolytic coalescent mastoiditis. Coalescent mastoiditis is best seen with a CT scan, which will show the breakdown of bony septae within the mastoid air cell system (▶ Fig. 11.12). As the infection breaks through bone, it can extend into the extratemporal soft tissue via the zygomatic root ("Luc's abscess")[12] or the digastric incisura into the soft tissue of the neck (Bezold's abscess). The imaging characteristics of a Bezold's abscess are similar to those of other abscesses. On CT imaging with contrast, the abscess will typically appear as a rim-enhancing lesion with central hypodensity and surrounding inflammatory changes. There will likely be adjacent radiographic signs of local infection, including fat-stranding and reactive lymphadenopathy. MRI imaging will often show a similarly ring-enhancing lesion, with central signal intensity similar to that of fluid, with central diffusion restriction.

Otic Capsule Erosion

Otic capsule bone is the densest bone of the body. Despite its relative resistance to erosion, an adjacent cholesteatoma can eventually create a fistula into the labyrinth, most often the lateral semicircular canal. Patients with a lateral semicircular canal dehiscence will often have disequilibrium. The "fistula sign" is a specific physical exam finding that suggests a "third window" into the inner ear due to a semicircular canal dehiscence.

Lateral canal fistulas are best seen on bone algorithm (maximum edge enhancement) CT imaging. An opacification will be apparent where the dense otic capsule bone would normally be expected (▶ Fig. 11.13). The facial nerve will be exposed in approximately 50% of lateral semicircular canal fistula cases.[13] Imaging is also useful to identify this finding (▶ Fig. 11.14).

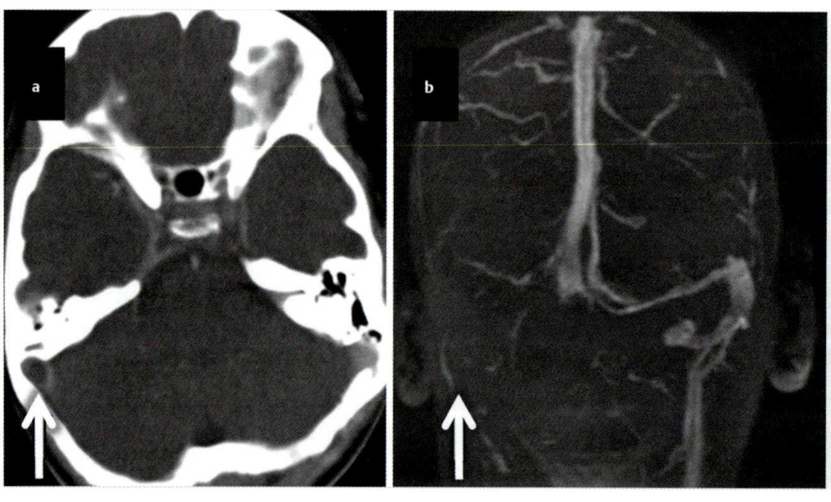

Fig. 11.9 Sigmoid sinus and jugular bulb thrombosis secondary to mastoiditis. This figure illustrates a poorly pneumatized right temporal bone with acute mastoiditis. There is an absence of contrast flow in the right sigmoid sinus seen on the axial, post-contrast head CT scan (a, arrow) and MRV (b, arrow). Used with permission from Diagnostic Imaging Techniques in Otology. In: Malekzadeh S, ed. Otolaryngology Lifelong Learning Manual. New York, NY: Thieme/American Academy of Otolaryngology-Head and Neck Surgery; 2014.

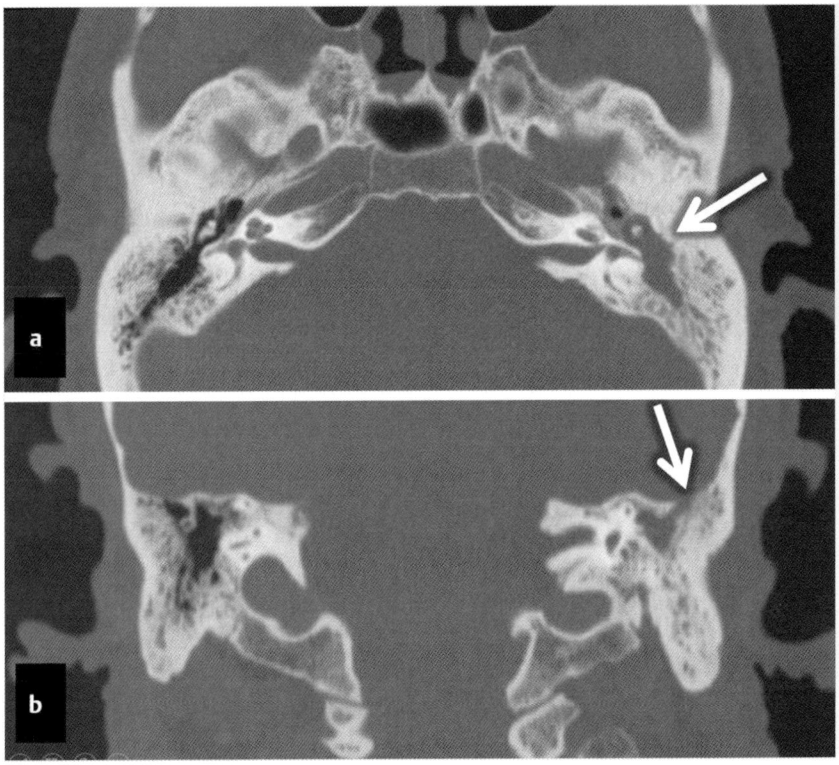

Fig. 11.10 Axial (a) and coronal (b) images thorough the temporal bones in a patient with mastoiditis. The axial bone algorithm images (a) show complete opacification of the left middle ear and mastoid air cells (arrow) with normally aerated right middle ear and mastoid air cells. The coronal (b) image shows the opacified left mastoid air cells with superior extension and osseous destruction extending toward the floor of the left middle cranial fossa (arrow).

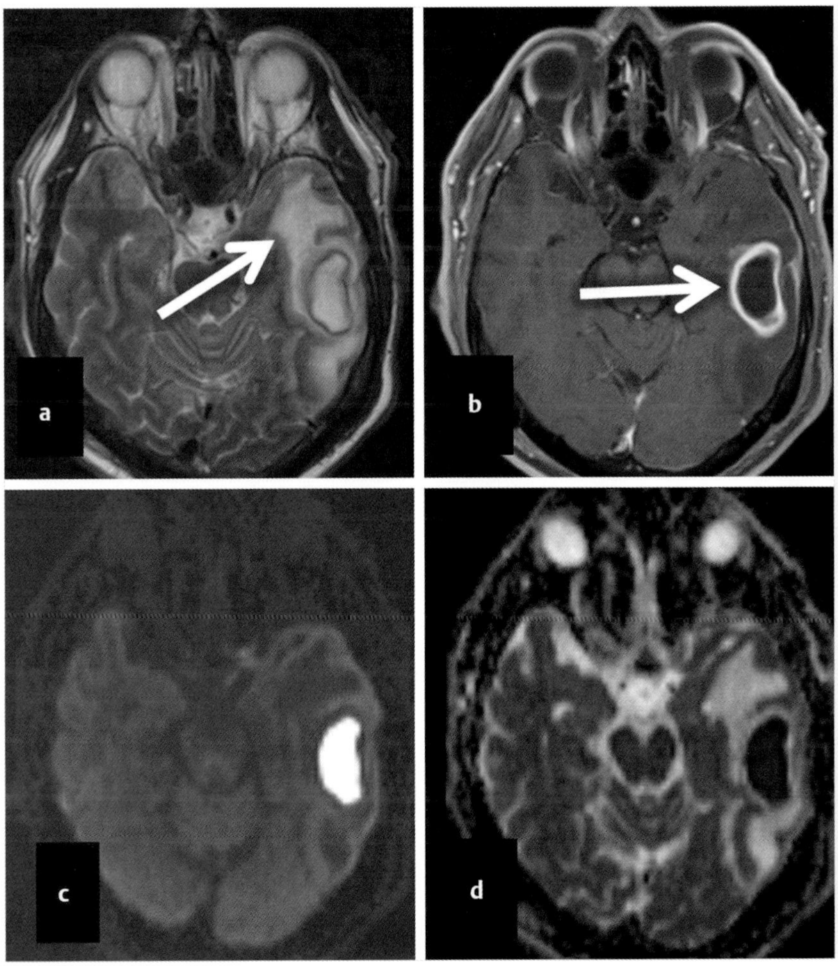

Fig. 11.11 Temporal lobe abscess MRI. Multiple sections from the same axial position from an MRI performed at the same time as the CT in the same patient as in ▶ Fig. 11.10. (a) Axial T2 image demonstrates vasogenic edema anterior (arrow) and posterior to a lesion within the left middle cranial fossa. (b) Correlating axial T1 postcontrast image shows peripheral enhancement (arrow) to the lesion with central low signal intensity, consistent with an abscess. (c) Axial diffusion shows bright signal intensity within the lesion centrally. (d) The correlating apparent diffusion coefficient (ADC) image demonstrates dark signal intensity, confirming the presence of an abscess at this location.

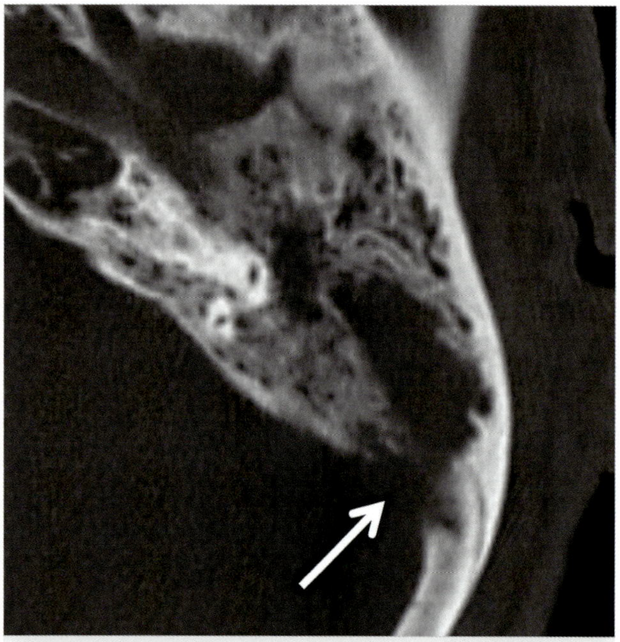

Fig. 11.12 Axial bone algorithm CT through the left temporal bone in a patient with ear pain demonstrates a large region of coalescent mastoid air cells with posterior osseous dehiscence (arrow).

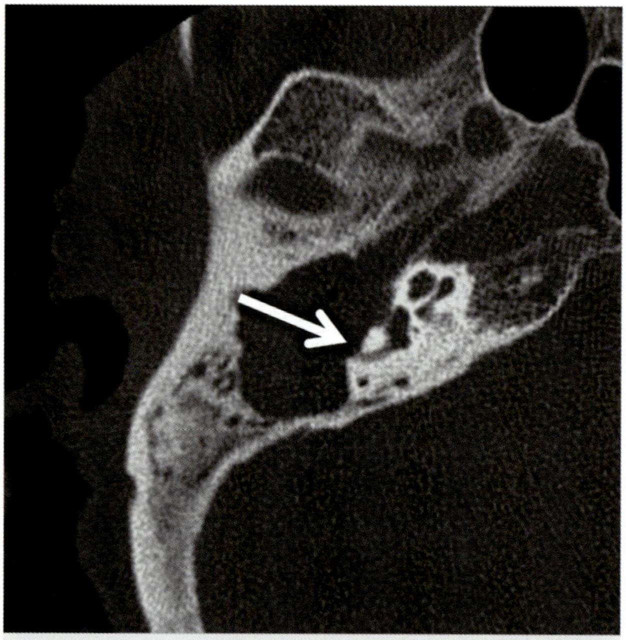

Fig. 11.13 Axial bone algorithm CT through the right temporal bone shows a soft tissue mass filling the middle ear and mastoid air cells with osseous erosion and destruction of the ossicles as well as erosion into the lateral semicircular canal (arrow).

11.4 Surveillance of Chronic Ear Disease

11.4.1 Residual and Recurrent Disease

Imaging has historically not played a significant role in the postoperative surveillance of cholesteatoma due to the inherent limitations of the various imaging modalities.[14] Whereas CT imaging can define the bony anatomy of the temporal bone, it cannot easily differentiate among types of similar soft tissue density pathologies in the absence of osseous erosion (e.g., scar, granulation tissue, fluid, inflamed mucosa, or recurrent cholesteatoma). Traditional MRI sequences have also lacked the ability to differentiate various forms of middle ear soft tissue and do not provide good anatomic resolution of fine structures. Newer MRI imaging modalities, such as diffusion-weighted imaging (DWI) techniques, however, have been shown to have high reliability for detecting cholesteatoma, with good inter-observer agreement.[15]

The DWI technique includes a preparation period before the image acquisition that enhances the signal intensity attenuation in response to diffusion and other spin motion.[16,17] Cholesteatomas and histologically similar epidermoid cysts are hyperintense on DW images compared with cerebrospinal fluid (CSF) and brain parenchyma (▸ Fig. 11.15; ▸ Fig. 11.16). Two variants of DWI are currently in use: echo planar imaging (EPI) and non-echo planar imaging (non-EPI). Non-EPI-based techniques, in the form of single-shot turbo-spin echo sequences (HASTE DWI) and multi-shot turbo-spin echo sequences (BLADE DWI and PROPELLER DWI), are preferred for imaging the temporal bone. These non-EPI techniques are less sensitive to magnetic susceptibility differences at air-tissue interfaces, which create significant distortion artifacts on EPI imaging, and show less anatomical distortion than images produced with EPI-based methods.[14] A meta-analysis of DW MRI sequences for detecting cholesteatoma showed that the overall sensitivity of DW MRI in detecting residual or recurrent cholesteatomas as small as 3 mm was 0.94 (confidence interval, 0.80–0.98), and the

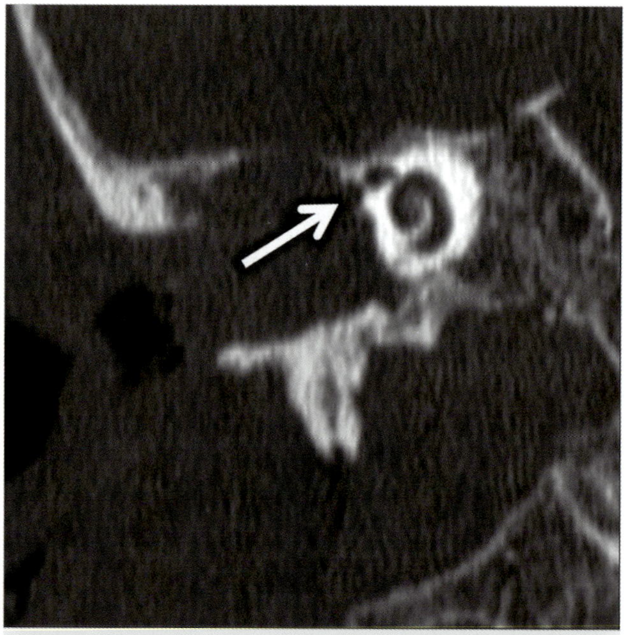

Fig. 11.14 Coronal CT through the right temporal bone demonstrates a soft tissue mass filling the middle ear cavity with destruction of the lateral wall of the proximal tympanic segment of the facial nerve (arrow).

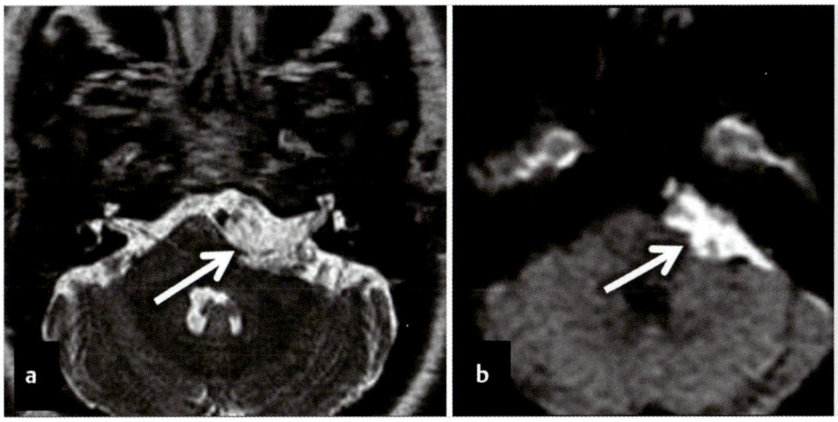

Fig. 11.15 Epidermoid cyst of the left cerebellopontine angle. (a) Axial T2-weighted MR image through the level of the left internal auditory canal (IAC) shows heterogeneous signal intensity and mild mass effect on the brain (arrow). (b) The correlating axial diffusion-weighted image shows bright signal intensity (arrow), significantly different than dark CSF, confirming the diagnosis of an epidermoid cyst.

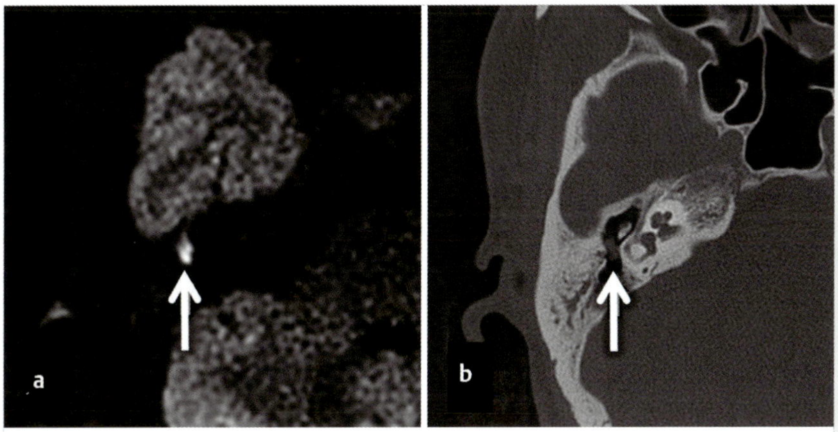

Fig. 11.16 Middle ear cavity cholesteatoma. (a) Non-echo planar diffusion-weighted (HASTE technique) MRI image with a bright area of signal intensity consistent with diffusion restriction, suggestive of cholesteatoma (arrow). (b) Correlating non-contrast temporal bone CT image of the same patient showing opacification in the antrum (arrow). The CT imaging alone would not allow a clinician to differentiate between residual disease versus postoperative fibrosis, mucosal edema, or fluid. Used with permission from Diagnostic Imaging Techniques in Otology. In: Malekzadeh S, ed. Otolaryngology Lifelong Learning Manual. New York, NY: Thieme/American Academy of Otolaryngology-Head and Neck Surgery; 2014.

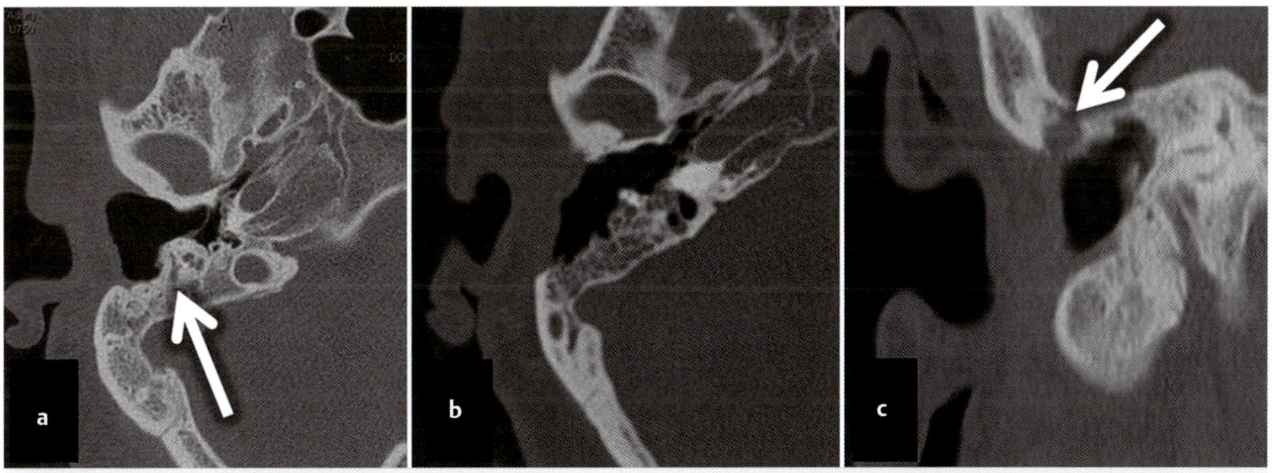

Fig. 11.17 Failed canal wall down procedure with unsaucerized edges, high facial ridge, retained air cells. These illustrate how imaging can provide information about sources of chronic otorrhea after a canal wall-down tympanomastoidectomy. (a) The first axial temporal bone CT image shows a high facial ridge with retained air cells lateral to the facial nerve (arrow). (b) The middle axial temporal bone CT image shows many retained mucosalized air cells that can drain and cause chronic otorrhea from the mastoid bowl. (c) The last coronal temporal bone CT illustrates poor saucerization of the tegmen with a large retained, mucosalized air cell (arrow).

specificity was 0.94 (confidence interval, 0.85–0.98).[18] Some feel that the inability to detect small residual cholesteatomas limits the clinical usefulness of DWI for routine postoperative surveillance at this time.

11.4.2 Persistent Otorrhea

Persistent postoperative otorrhea can be a challenging problem for both the patient and the practitioner. In addition to removing all diseased air cells, the principles of canal wall-down surgery dictate that the otologic surgeon adequately saucerize the mastoid cavity, lower the facial ridge, remove the mastoid tip and its dependent air cells, and create an adequate meatoplasty. When these principles are not followed, a chronically draining mastoid cavity can develop. Imaging is helpful to identify these areas and help guide surgical decision-making for revision canal wall-down surgery (▶ Fig. 11.17).

11.5 Conclusion

Whereas the routine use of imaging in chronic ear disease is debatable, there are undeniable advantages to imaging in certain clinical scenarios. Critical information can be obtained by imaging, including anatomic understanding of the extent of disease, degree of mastoid pneumatization, and anatomy of critical structures such as the facial nerve, otic capsule, tegmen, sigmoid sinus, and carotid artery. Imaging can also provide detailed information about complications of chronic otitis media. Newer imaging modalities, such as DW MRI scans, can also serve as a useful adjunct in surveillance of chronic ear disease and can successfully replace the postoperative evaluation of cholesteatoma cases, avoiding morbidity and mortality from second-look surgeries. Imaging can also be helpful prior to revision chronic ear surgery or to help identify causes of chronic otorrhea.

References

[1] Blevins NH, Carter BL. Routine preoperative imaging in chronic ear surgery. Am J Otol. 1998;19(4):527–535, discussion 535–538.

[2] Walshe P, McConn Walsh R, Brennan P, Walsh M. The role of computerized tomography in the preoperative assessment of chronic suppurative otitis media. Clin Otolaryngol Allied Sci. 2002;27(2):95–97.

[3] Gomaa MA, Abdel Karim AR, Abdel Ghany HS, Elhiny AA, Sadek AA. Evaluation of temporal bone cholesteatoma and the correlation between high resolution computed tomography and surgical finding. Clin Med Insights Ear Nose Throat. 2013;6:21–28.

[4] Mahmutoğlu AS, Celebi I, Sahinoğlu S, Cakmakçi E, Sözen E. Reliability of preoperative multidetector computed tomography scan in patients with chronic otitis media. J Craniofac Surg. 2013;24(4):1472–1476.

[5] Jackler RK. The surgical anatomy of cholesteatoma. Otolaryngol Clin North Am. 1989;22(5):883–896.

[6] Shinnabe A, Hara M, Hasegawa M, et al. Differences in middle ear ventilation disorders between pars flaccida and pars tensa cholesteatoma in sonotubometry and patterns of tympanic and mastoid pneumatization. Otol Neurotol. 2012;33(5):765–768.

[7] Sheehy JL, Brackmann DE, Graham MD. Cholesteatoma surgery: residual and recurrent disease. A review of 1,024 cases. Ann Otol Rhinol Laryngol. 1977;86 (4 Pt 1):451–462.

[8] Green JD, Jr, Shelton C, Brackmann DE. Iatrogenic facial nerve injury during otologic surgery. Laryngoscope. 1994;104(8 Pt 1):922–926.

[9] Chu FW, Jackler RK. Anterior epitympanic cholesteatoma with facial paralysis: A characteristic growth pattern. Laryngoscope. 1988;98(3):274–279.

[10] Offergeld C, Kromeier J, Merchant SN, et al. Experimental investigation of rotational tomography in reconstructed middle ears with clinical implications. Hear Res. 2010;263(1–2):191–197.

[11] Komori M, Yanagihara N, Hyodo J, Miuchi S. Position of TORP on the stapes footplate assessed with cone beam computed tomography. Otol Neurotol. 2012;33(8):1353–1356.

[12] Gurgel RK, Woodson EA, Lenkowski PW, Gubbels SP, Hansen MR. Zygomatic root abscess: A rare complication of otitis media. Otol Neurotol. 2010;31 (5):856–857.

[13] Sheehy JL, Brackmann DE. Cholesteatoma surgery: Management of the labyrinthine fistula—a report of 97 cases. Laryngoscope. 1979;89(1):78–87.

[14] Khemani S, Singh A, Lingam RK, Kalan A. Imaging of postoperative middle ear cholesteatoma. Clin Radiol. 2011;66(8):760–767.

[15] Jindal M, Riskalla A, Jiang D, Connor S, O'Connor AF. A systematic review of diffusion-weighted magnetic resonance imaging in the assessment of postoperative cholesteatoma. Otol Neurotol. 2011;32(8):1243–1249.

[16] Schwartz KM, Lane JI, Bolster BD, Jr, Neff BA. The utility of diffusion-weighted imaging for cholesteatoma evaluation. AJNR Am J Neuroradiol. 2011;32 (3):430–436.

[17] Le Bihan D, Breton E, Lallemand D, Grenier P, Cabanis E, Laval-Jeantet M. MR imaging of intravoxel incoherent motions: Application to diffusion and perfusion in neurologic disorders. Radiology. 1986;161(2):401–407.

[18] Li PM, Linos E, Gurgel RK, Fischbein NJ, Blevins NH. Evaluating the utility of non-echo-planar diffusion-weighted imaging in the preoperative evaluation of cholesteatoma: A meta-analysis. Laryngoscope. 2013;123(5):1247–1250.

12 Inflammatory Conditions and Systemic Diseases Affecting the Middle Ear

Shane R. Anderson

Abbreviations used in this chapter:

ACE: angiotensin-converting enzyme
ANCA: antibodies to neutrophil cytoplasmic antigens
c-ANCA: cytoplasmic-pattern ANCA
p-ANCA: perinuclear-pattern ANCA
COM: chronic otitis media
CSS: Churg-Strauss syndrome
CT: computed tomography
EOM: eosinophilic otitis media
GPA: granulomatosis with polyangitis
MPO: myeloperoxidase
OME: otitis media with effusion
RAST: Radioallergosorbant Test

12.1 Introduction

Diagnosis and management of chronic inflammatory conditions of the middle ear can be challenging. The spectrum of diseases that can present with otologic symptoms is broad, and common otological conditions may present in a similar manner, making a prompt diagnosis difficult. Having a high index of suspicion offers an opportunity to diagnose systemic conditions, some of which, if not detected, can be fatal.[1] Occasionally, there will be clues that an underlying systemic cause may be responsible for chronic otitis media (COM); however, it is resistance to standard treatment that usually raises a clinical suspicion.

A general clinical approach to this small group of patients who have treatment-resistant COM includes a thorough past medical history. Specific inquiry should be directed at rheumatologic conditions, other systemic illnesses, such as diabetes, and a medications history with specific questioning about immunosuppressive medications. An expanded clinical examination is undertaken that includes a thorough head-and-neck examination, including flexible nasoendoscopy looking for nasal polyposis, mucosal lesions, and mass lesions of the nasopharynx. Investigations are tailored to each individual disease process and will be outlined throughout this chapter. In general, a high-resolution computed tomography (CT) scan of the temporal bones is required to help exclude common conditions such as cholesteatoma.

In this chapter, we will discuss the inflammatory conditions that may present with chronic middle ear disease, the pathology behind these conditions, diagnosis, specific investigations, and management.

12.2 Eosinophilic Otitis Media

Eosinophilic otitis media (EOM) is a relatively new disease entity. EOM is characterized by a persistent otitis media, with or without suppuration, that is resistant to conventional treatment, in association with adult-onset bronchial asthma, often with nasal polyposis.[2]

Clinical suspicion should be raised by the discovery on myringotomy of a highly viscous middle ear effusion that is difficult to suction. The underlying middle ear mucosa is thickened and has eosinophil-rich granulation tissue that responds only to high-dose systemic steroids. This should prompt a biopsy. A characteristic of EOM is the high incidence of hearing loss, which is typically a progressive loss but can also be sudden.[3]

A significant number of patients with EOM have patulous Eustachian tubes, resulting in speculation that the pathological mechanism of EOM is due to the aspiration of antigenic material into the middle ear, causing a localized eosinophilic inflammatory reaction. Whether this is the cause or a sequelae of EOM remains to be established.[4]

Iino, Tomioka-Matsutani, Matsubara, Nakagawa, and Nonaka has published the largest cohort of EOM patients[2] and, with the EOM study group, proposed a diagnostic criteria system for this disease (▶ Table 12.1). In accordance with the diagnostic criteria, investigation mandates the histological examination of the middle ear contents and exclusion of hypereosinophilic syndrome and Churg-Strauss syndrome. Hypereosinophilic syndrome is diagnosed by the presence of a persistent eosinophil count $\geq 1.5 \times 10^9$/L for at least 6 months.[2] The diagnosis of Churg-Strauss syndrome will be discussed later. The mainstay of management is early recognition and the commencement of high-dose systemic steroids[2] and topical intratympanic steroids.[5] Rapid resolution of symptoms and reversal of sensorineural hearing loss has been reported.

12.3 Autoimmune Vasculitis

Churg-Strauss syndrome and granulomatosis with polyangitis are closely related autoimmune vasculitic syndromes that are characterized by granulomatous infiltration of small- to medium-sized vessels and are associated with antibodies to

Table 12.1 Unvalidated diagnostic criteria system established by the EOM study group

Major (Mandatory)
Otitis media with effusion with an eosinophil-dominant effusion
Minor (2/4 required)
1. Highly viscous middle ear effusion
2. Resistance to conventional treatment for otitis media
3. Association with bronchial asthma
4. Association with nasal polyposis
Exclusion Criteria
1. CSS
2. Hypereosinophilic Syndrome

neutrophil cytoplasmic antigens (ANCA). These autoimmune vasculitis commonly present with head and neck symptoms; rarely will they present with isolated otologic symptoms. Typical middle ear findings include a thick middle ear effusion on myringotomy, with middle ear granulation that is again resistant to typical treatment. Often, otalgia is significantly worse than would be expected due to middle ear involvement in the granulomatous process.

12.3.1 Granulomatosis with Polyangitis

Granulomatosis with polyangitis (GPA), previously known as Wegener's granulomatosis, is the most common autoimmune vasculitis to present with otologic symptoms. It can present either as a classic form with all components of the disease or a limited form. Classic GPA typically presents in young adult males and is characterized by a necrotizing, granulomatous vasculitis of the upper and lower respiratory tract, focal glomerulonephritis, and small vessel vasculitis. Because manifestations of GPA in the nose are typically more prominent than manifestations in the ear, the otologist should be alerted when typical GPA findings, such as nasal septal perforation, sinonasal synechiae, saddle nose deformity, friable sinonasal mucosa, and/or polypoid rhinosinusitis, are encountered alongside chronic ear disease. Symptoms of COM are reported in greater than 20% to 40% of patients, but in isolation are quite rare.[6,7] The expected conductive hearing loss may be associated with a sensorineural component and facial nerve palsy that is reversible with steroids.[8]

Diagnosis is based upon the criteria set forth in 1990 by the American College of Rheumatology (▶ Table 12.2) and laboratory investigations. Greater than 90% of GPA patients have been reported to have ANCA positivity during active disease,[9] specifically cytoplasmic-pattern ANCA (c-ANCA) directed against serine proteinase 3 antigen. Establishing a diagnosis of GPA can be difficult early in the disease process given that it is unusual to meet all the criteria shown in ▶ Table 12.2 and, although the c-ANCA is valuable, it is often normal during the early stages of the disease. Therefore, the most critical investigation for early diagnosis of GPA is histological examination of the middle ear contents for evidence of a perivasculitis of small vessels, infiltration of giant cells, and epithelioid cell granulomas.[10] However, histopathologic diagnosis is most often made based on a biopsy of an affected sinonasal site.

Table 12.2 1990 criteria for the classification of GPA.

• Nasal or oral inflammation - Mucosal ulceration with classical appearance of "saddle nose deformity"
• Abnormal chest radiography with pulmonary lesions
• Urinary Sediment - Microhematuria or red cast cells
• Histological - Vasculitis of small vessels, infiltration of giant cells and epithelioid granulomas
Note: A patient is said to have GPA if at least 2 of these 4 criteria are present. These criteria were established before the introduction of c-ANCA.

12.3.2 Churg-Strauss Syndrome

Like GPA, CSS is a granulomatous vasculitis associated with ANCA autoantibodies. Churg Straus Syndrome typically presents with adult-onset asthma, allergic rhinitis often associated with polyposis, a peripheral neuropathy, and systemic eosinophilia.[11] There are no reports of presentation with primary otologic symptoms. Excessive granulation tissue is present within the middle ear. Hearing loss generally involves a bilateral mixed loss but can be an isolated sensorineural hearing loss or unilateral in some cases.[12]

The natural history of the disease is that it mostly occurs in males and has three distinct phases. The first is characterized by a severe, steroid-dependent asthma, which commonly occurs in adulthood and is preceded by chronic recurrent rhinosinusitis. The second phase has a peripheral eosinophilia with eosinophilic organ infiltrates. The third phase is characterized by the appearance of a systemic vasculitis. During these later stages, the asthmatic symptoms generally resolve. It is later in the course of the illness that otologic symptoms present, hence the need for a thorough past medical history.[12]

Diagnosis is based on the criteria of the American College of Rheumatology, with four of six criteria required (▶ Table 12.3). Unlike GPA, CSS is more commonly associated with perinuclear-pattern ANCA (p-ANCA) directed against myeloperoxidase (MPO) although this is a less reliable test than for GPA.[13]

The suspicion of an autoimmune vascular disease should be raised by a rapid onset of disease in an adult with no past history of ear disease, clinical findings suggestive of systemic illness, or lack of response to typical therapy. Initial investigation should include a biopsy of inflamed mucosa and ANCA. Depending on results, this should also be supplemented by a CT of the chest looking for pulmonary infiltrates, erythrocyte sedimentation rate to establish a baseline, and urinalysis looking for micro-hematuria and red cell casts. Urgent referral to a rheumatologist after the commencement of high-dose steroids is required. Typically, otologic symptoms will respond or stabilize.[14] Therapy may be changed to steroid-sparing immunosuppressants, such as methotrexate or cyclophosphamide; however, this will be guided by a rheumatologist.[12]

The role for surgery in autoimmune vasculitis associated with middle ear disease is limited to tympanostomy tube insertion to expedite the resolution of middle ear symptoms and the treatment of abscess formation due to antrum blockage.

Table 12.3 Criteria for diagnosis of Churg-Strauss Syndrome.

• Asthma
• Eosinophilia (> 10% On white blood cell differential)
• Migratory Pulmonary infiltrates
• Neuropathy (Mono/Polyneuritis)
• Clinical/Radiological Evidence of Sinusitis
• Biopsy demonstrating extravascular eosinophils
Note: Diagnosis is based on the criteria of the American College of Rheumatology, with 4 of 6 criteria required to achieve sensitivity of 85% and specificity of 99.7%. Data from Masi T, Hunder G, Lie J, et al. The American College of Rheumatology 1990 criteria for the classification of Churg-Strauss Syndrome. Arthritis Rheumatology. 1990; 33:1094–1100

Table 12.4 Diagnostic differences between CSS, EOM, and allergy. These can all present with an eosinophil-dominant picture.

	CSS	EOM	Allergy
Peripheral Eosinophilia	yes	No	variable
Male: Female	Male > Female		Female < Male
Steroid dose	high	high	low
Histological feature of mucosal biopsy	Vasculitis	Eosinophilic infiltrates	Mixed inflammatory response, may be eosinophil-rich
Asthma Onset	Adult	Adult	Childhood
ANCA	+ve	-ve	-ve

12.4 Allergy

Allergy is a heterogeneous term that reflects reactivity to exogenous stimuli, resulting in the release of inflammatory mediators by one or a combination of inflammatory cascades. Hence, targeted therapy to a particular cascade may fail, making management challenging.[15] The middle ear cleft mucosa originates from the same ectoderm as the remainder of the upper respiratory tract epithelium and has the same intrinsic immunological responses to allergens as does the nasal, sinus, and bronchial epithelium, conforming with the unified airway theory.[16] The 2004 guidelines of the Academies of Pediatrics, Family Practice, and Otolaryngology–Head and Neck Surgery state that "the cellular response of the respiratory mucosa to allergens has been well studied. Therefore similar to other parts of respiratory mucosa, the mucosa lining of the middle ear cleft is capable of an allergic response." However, this goes on to say that "A linkage between allergy and otitis media with effusion (OME) has long been speculated but to date remains unqualified."[17] Epidemiological studies have demonstrated that allergy confers an increased incidence of OME in allergic versus non-allergic cohorts.[15]

Bluestone[18] and others have proposed several hypothetical mechanisms by which allergy may contribute to COM:

- Allergic reaction intrinsic to the mucosal membrane of the middle ear.
- Inflammation of the nasopharynx causing a direct mechanical obstruction of the Eustachian tube.
- Aspiration of allergen-laden mucous or cytokines from the nasopharynx into the Eustachian tube as part of the mucociliary transport to the Eustachian tube orifice or direct nasal expansion and obstruction of the Eustachian tube.

Diagnostic confirmation of allergy involvement in OME is difficult as, in practice, skin testing and Radioallergosorbant Test (RAST) detection of a specific IgE antibody systemically does not correspond to end-organ inflammation. In selected centers, the nasal provocation test in combination with the recording of parameters indicative of Eustachian tube dysfunction and middle ear effusion may help but are not readily available.[19]

In the setting of persistent, therapy-resistant otitis media, atopy must be taken into account. Management can be supportive to improve Eustachian tube function, such as adenoidectomy. Nasal steroids are the mainstay of inflammatory cascade suppression and may need to be augmented with septal and turbinate surgery to improve nasal airflow and steroid penetration. Other topical sprays that target specific arms of the inflammatory cascade, such as leukotriene antagonist, antihistamine, and mast cell stabilizing sprays, have also been proposed as treatment options but are not considered the mainstay of therapy.

Immunotherapy should be considered in resistant cases where the above measures have not proven effective. When a specific allergen can be identified, allergen avoidance counseling followed by targeted immunotherapy has demonstrated a significant improvement in COM in prospective cohort studies.[20]

In the setting of COM that is resistant to standard therapy, the finding of an eosinophil-rich middle ear effusion, respiratory symptoms, and nasal polyposis may correlate with several disease entities. ▶ Table 12.4 illustrates the key points of differentiation between CSS, EOM, and eosinophil-dominant allergy.

12.5 Sarcoidosis

This condition of unknown etiology is characterized by a bilateral hilar lymphadenopathy, pulmonary infiltrates, and ocular and skin lesions. It commonly affects young to middle-aged adults. Otological manifestations usually occur due to helical lesions.[21] Neurosarcoidosis occurs in 5% of patients with sarcoidosis[22] and can present with a sensorineural hearing loss but usually affects the facial nerve and is often associated with parotid swelling (Heerfordt's syndrome). Middle ear disease usually reflects Eustachian tube dysfunction secondary to nasal sarcoidosis although there are limited reports of direct middle ear involvement.

The diagnosis of sarcoidosis is confirmed when radiological and clinical findings of the above are supported by histological evidence of non-caseating epithelioid cell granulomas and any other cause of non-caseating granulomas has been excluded. Other causes of non-caseating granulomas can be excluded with ANCAs, fungal and atypical tuberculosis staining, along with syphilis serology. Serum angiotensin-converting enzyme (ACE) has been used for diagnosis; however, its role remains unclear and is more relevant to disease monitoring.[23]

The mainstay of treatment is steroid therapy, and, as directed by a rheumatologist, this may be changed to steroid-sparing immunosuppressives.

12.6 Immunosuppression

Recurrent otitis media is a hallmark of an immunodeficiency,[24] and, although this is a common presentation, suspicion should be raised in the context of otitis media when frequent and severe infections occur that are unresponsive to antibiotics or become associated with complications. Often these infections are caused by unusual organisms or organisms that would normally be considered of low virulence. Immunosuppression can be divided into primary and secondary categories.

Primary immunodeficiency is typically present in childhood due to a failure of maturation of the immune system. Presentation of this type of immunodeficiency is variable and dependent on the mechanism of immune failure. General features include failure to thrive, developmental delay, and opportunistic recurrent infections.

Secondary immunodeficiency can present at any age due to a suppression of a competent immune system. Causes of secondary immunosuppression include malignancy, immunosuppressive medication, malnutrition, diabetes, or infection (typically by HIV). General features of secondary immunodeficiency include unintentional weight loss, skin lesions, unexpected or particularly aggressive tumors, and reactivation of dormant infections, such as shingles, cytomegalovirus, Epstein-Barr virus, and tuberculosis.

Investigations to screen for an immunodeficiency include immunoglobulin subclass typing and a full blood count. Results need to be taken in context of the child; for instance, a low/normal neutrophil count or IgM level in the context of active acute infection should raise as much suspicion as an absolute result. Prompt immunologist referral and further provocation testing to assess humoral and innate immunity should be undertaken.[25] Management is directed by an immunologist and includes prolonged antibiotics[24] and either replacement immunoglobulin infusions or colony-stimulating factors at times of infection.[1]

In the setting of secondary immunosuppression, the otolaryngologist has an opportunity to detect a systemic condition that may be correctable or identify complications of treatment for a systemic condition. Symptomatic management of recurrent otitis media with ventilation tubes is not advisable given that the incidence of a persistent discharge after insertion is high, unless the underlying condition is managed.

12.7 Radiation-Induced Otitis Media

Radiation-induced injury to the temporal bone and nasopharynx can occur after life-saving treatment for malignancy of the head and neck. The underlying pathological process of endarteritis obliterans is progressive and long-lasting. Otitis media can occur due to direct osteoradionecrosis of the temporal bone or secondary to Eustachian tube dysfunction after nasopharyngeal malignancy. A common presentation is isolated otitis media and hearing loss. Often, this is quite bothersome to the patient and is escalated by the fear of tumor recurrence. Management requires a thorough head-and-neck examination, either by the clinician or by referral back to a head-and-neck specialist. It is tempting to place ventilation tubes in these patients for symptom relief, but often this will cause suppuration and should be avoided if possible. In the setting of suppuration, there are case reports of successful tympanoplasty[26] with reasonable results. This may be improved with the use of adjuvant hyperbaric oxygen. Although there is limited data to support this, it can be considered if available.

12.8 Conclusion

A high index of suspicion is required to establish the above diagnoses. Resistance to standard therapy for COM mandates a thorough history and systemic examination. In the setting of granulation, this requires biopsy. In doing so, the otolaryngologist has an opportunity to diagnose and alter potentially life-threatening conditions. This list is not exhaustive, however, and other conditions, such as cholesterol granuloma, Langerhans cell histiocytosis, and ciliary dyskinesia, need to be entertained. But their discussion is beyond the scope of this chapter.

References

[1] Otremba MD, Adam SI, Price CC, Hohuan D, Kveton JF. Use of intravenous immunoglobulin to treat chronic bilateral otomastoiditis in the setting of rituximab induced hypogammaglobulinemia. Am J Otolaryngol. 2012;33(5):619–622.

[2] Lino Y, Tomioka-Matsutani S, Matsubara A, Nakagawa T, Nonaka M. Diagnostic criteria of eosinophilic otitis media, a newly recognized middle ear disease. Auris Nasus Larynx. 2011;38(4):456–461.

[3] Lino Y, Usubuchi H, Kodama K, Takizawa K, Kanazawa T, Ohta Y. Bone conduction hearing level in patients with eosinophilic otitis media associated with bronchial asthma. Otol Neurotol. 2008;29(7):949–952.

[4] Chung WJ, Lee JH, Lim HK, Yoon TH, Cho KJ, Baek JH. Eosinophilic otitis media: CT and MRI findings and literature review. Korean J Radiol. 2012;13(3):363–367.

[5] Lino Y, Nagamine H, Kakizaki K. Effectiveness of instillation of triamcinolone into middle ear for EOM associated with bronchial asthma. Ann Allergy Asthma Immunol. 2006;97:761–766.

[6] Jennings CR, Jones NS, Dugar J, Powell RJ, Lowe J. Wegener's granulomatosis—a review of diagnosis and treatment in 53 subjects. Rhinology. 1998;36(4):188–191.

[7] Nicklasson B, Stangeland N. Wegener's granulomatosis presenting as otitis media. J Laryngol Otol. 1982;96(3):277–280.

[8] Wierzbicka M, Szyfter W. Puszczewicz, Borucki L, Bartochowska A. Otologic Sypmtoms as initial manifestation of Wegener Granulomatosis: Diagnositic Dilemma. Otol Neurotol. 2011;32:996–1000.

[9] Finkielman JD, Lee AS, Hummel AM, et al. WGET Research Group. ANCA are detectable in nearly all patients with active severe Wegener's granulomatosis. Am J Med. 2007;120(7):643.e9–643.e14.

[10] Tsuzuki K, Fukazawa K, Takebayashi H, Hashimoto K, Sakagami M. Difficulty of diagnosing Wegener's granulomatosis in the head and neck region. Auris Nasus Larynx. 2009;36(1):64–70.

[11] Martinez Del Pero M, Moffat D, Sudhoff H. Unusual presentation of temporal bone involvement in Churg-Strauss syndrome. J Laryngol Otol. 2008;122(4):425–427.

[12] Ishiyama A, Canalis RF. Otological manifestations of Churg-Strauss syndrome. Laryngoscope. 2001;111(9):1619–1624.

[13] Masi AT, Hunder GG, Lie JT, et al. The American College of Rheumatology 1990 criteria for the classification of Churg-Strauss syndrome (allergic granulomatosis and angiitis). Arthritis Rheum. 1990;33(8):1094–1100.

[14] Bacciu A, Bacciu S, Mercante G, et al. Ear, nose and throat manifestations of Churg-Strauss syndrome. Acta Otolaryngol. 2006;126(5):503–509.

[15] Hurst DS. The role of allergy in otitis media with effusion. Otolaryngol Clin North Am. 2011;44(3):637–654, viii–ix.

[16] Nguyen LH, Manoukian JJ, Sobol SE, et al. Similar allergic inflammation in the middle ear and the upper airway: evidence linking otitis media with effusion to the united airways concept. J Allergy Clin Immunol. 2004;114(5):1110–1115.

[17] American Academy of Family Physicians. American Academy of Otolaryngology-Head and Neck Surgery. American Academy of Pediatrics Subcommittee on Otitis Media With Effusion. Otitis media with effusion. Pediatrics. 2004;113(5):1412–1429.

[18] Bluestone CD. Eustachian tube function and allergy in otitis media. Pediatrics. 1978;61(5):753–760.
[19] Pelikan Z. Role of nasal allergy in chronic secretory otitis media. Curr Allergy Asthma Rep. 2009;9(2):107–113.
[20] Hurst DS. Efficacy of allergy immunotherapy as a treatment for patients with chronic otitis media with effusion. Int J Pediatr Otorhinolaryngol. 2008;72(8):1215–1223.
[21] Schwartzbauer HR, Tami TA. Ear, nose, and throat manifestations of sarcoidosis. Otolaryngol Clin North Am. 2003;36(4):673–684.
[22] Delaney P. Neurologic manifestations in sarcoidosis: Review of the literature, with a report of 23 cases. Ann Intern Med. 1977;87(3):336–345.
[23] Costabel U, Teschler H. Biochemical changes in sarcoidosis. Clin Chest Med. 1997;18(4):827–842.
[24] Wilson NW, Hogan MB. Otitis media as a presenting complaint in childhood immunodeficiency diseases. Curr Allergy Asthma Rep. 2008;8(6):519–524.
[25] Wiertsema SP, Veenhoven RH, Sanders EA, Rijkers GT. Immunologic screening of children with recurrent otitis media. Curr Allergy Asthma Rep. 2005;5(4):302–307.
[26] Hsu Y-C, Su CY. Tympanoplasty for chronic otitis media in post-irradiated nasopharyngeal carcinoma patients. Ann Otol Rhinol Laryngol. 2006;115(5):330–333.

13 Myringitis

Alexander G. Bien and Jason C. Goodwin

Abbreviations used in this chapter:

ABG: air-bone gap
CF-HC: chloramphenicol/fungizone–hydrocortisone
CSF-HC: chloramphenicol/sulfanilamide/fungizone–hydrocortisone
CT: computed tomography
5-FU: 5-fluorouracil

13.1 Introduction

Myringitis is a poorly understood inflammatory disease of the tympanic membrane and external auditory canal. It has been referred to by other names in the literature, including granular myringitis, chronic epithelitis, otitis externa with granulations, granulomatous otitis externa, myringitis granulosa, chronic myringitis, and myringitis chronica.[1,2] The disease involves a de-epithelialization of the tympanic membrane, with replacement by granulation tissue. Despite many historical descriptions of the disease, very little has been written on the topic. Toynbee first recorded a description of myringitis in his 1860 text, describing a method of treatment that involved irrigation of the ear canal followed by leeches to the affected area.[1] The next mention is by Politzer in his 1883 text.[1] He coined the term granular myringitis. It has since been mentioned sporadically in the literature.

13.2 Clinical Presentation

The true incidence of myringitis is unknown due to factors such as misdiagnosis, lack of knowledge of disease, and asymptomatic course in some patients.[1,2,3,4] Men and women are affected equally, and myringitis has been reported in all ages.[5] Although myringitis may affect both ears, most cases are unilateral.[6] Common misdiagnoses include cholesteatoma, chronic suppurative otitis media, or other chronic middle ear diseases.[1,2,4] Blevins and Neilson reported incidences of 1.2% and 1.7%, respectively, of all patients presenting to an otology-specific practice.[2,7] Stoney reported myringitis in 2% to 5% of all patients diagnosed with otitis externa.[1] El-Seifi and Fouad concluded that 1.8% of patients with otorrhea had myringitis.[4]

The presentation of myringitis is described in various ways in the literature. Otorrhea is the most common presenting symptom and is found in 75% to 86% of patients.[1,2,7,8] The drainage has been described as scant, weeping, mucopurulent, and/or foul-smelling. Other complaints include otalgia, itching, aural fullness, hearing loss, and tinnitus.[1,2,3,4,7,8] Some authors define myringitis as having an intact tympanic membrane with no hearing deficit[1,9] whereas others say that perforations are part of the natural history along with some degree of hearing loss.[2,3,4,7] Reported hearing loss associated with myringitis is both conductive and mixed, with an air-bone gap (ABG) of 10–20 dB.[2,6]

Imaging is not recommended for patients with myringitis. However, due to its frequent misdiagnosis as chronic middle ear disease, these patients may have obtained prior imaging. Imaging typically shows a diffusely thickened tympanic membrane with a normal-appearing external auditory canal and the absence of middle ear disease. ▶ Fig. 13.1 shows the typical findings on a computed tomography (CT) scan of myringitis.

13.3 Pathophysiology

The pathophysiology of myringitis is not completely understood. Normally, the tympanic membrane has a unique centrifugal epithelial migration pattern that acts as a self-cleaning mechanism. It is thought that this mechanism is altered in chronic myringitis, causing a buildup of keratin material and induction of a granulomatous response.[9]

Schuknecht was the first to describe the histopathology of the disease. He characterized the disorder as a focal or diffuse replacement of the tympanic membrane and adjacent external auditory canal wall with granulation tissue. The underlying lamina propria remains intact. Histologically, he showed a dense infiltrate of small round cells, polymorphonuclear leukocytes, edema, and vascular channels.[10]

Various authors have proposed mechanisms to explain the disease process, including trauma or infection to induce the granulation reaction. Several papers report an increased rate of myringitis among patients with a history of pressure equalization tube placement or tympanoplasty.[2,11,12] Blevins reported that 60% of patients in his series had a history of a previous

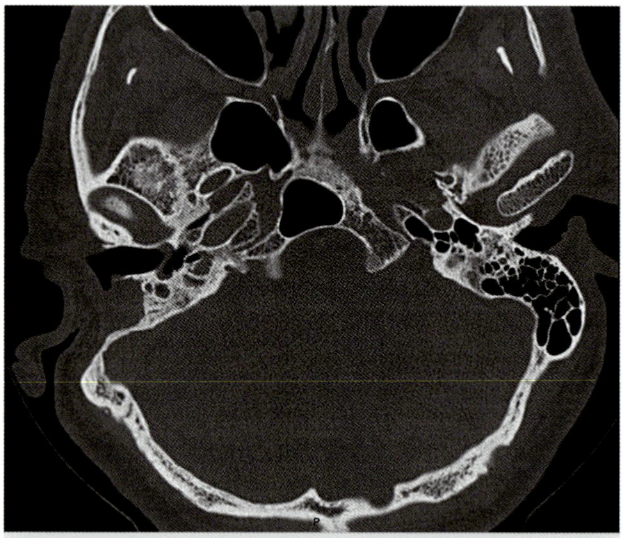

Fig. 13.1 CT scan of a right ear affected with myringitis. The tympanic membrane is diffusely thickened. There is no middle ear disease. The external auditory canal is normal. Interestingly, this patient had a history of a mastoidectomy on the right side for treatment of presumed cholesteatoma.

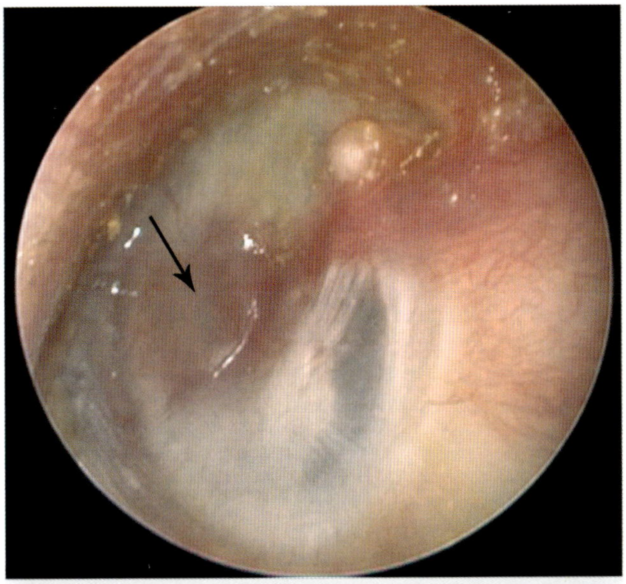

Fig. 13.2 Focal involvement of the tympanic membrane. An area of granular myringitis is present in the anterior portion of the tympanic membrane. The remainder of the tympanic membrane is normal.

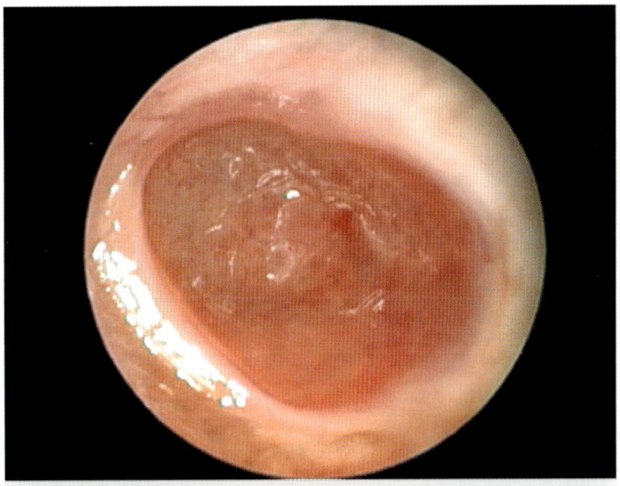

Fig. 13.3 A tympanic membrane severely affected with myringitis. The entire tympanic membrane is covered with granulation tissue, with extension onto the adjacent external auditory canal skin. The surface displays a glistening appearance.

otologic procedure, with most symptoms appearing within 1 year after surgery.[2] In a pediatric study, Levi et al showed that 87% of children had a history of pressure equalization tube placement and 53% had a history of myringoplasty.[11] As for possible infectious sources of chronic myringitis, several studies have cultured otorrhea for bacteriology. *Pseudomonas aeruginosa* has been the most common finding, with *Staphylococcus aureus* the second most common. Other bacteria found include *Staphylococcus epidermidis, Proteus, Cornybacterium, Providencia*, and *Enterobacter* species.[1,6,8,11] There is also an idiopathic form of chronic myringitis with which no inciting factors or comorbidities have been associated.[2]

13.4 Physical Examination

Otologic examination under binocular microscopy shows an inflamed tympanic membrane with or without involvement of the external auditory canal.[1,2,3,7] Otorrhea is typically present, and when present, is often scant. However, it can be thick and mucopurulent. Once the otorrhea is evacuated, the tympanic membrane may have yellow casts on its surface. After the removal of casts, the affected areas of the tympanic membrane show the beefy, red appearance typical of granulation tissue. Hypervascularity may be present. The granulations can be focal, involving a portion of the tympanic membrane, or diffuse, involving the entire tympanic membrane with extension to the adjacent external auditory canal skin. For focal lesions, the most commonly affected area is the posterior-superior quadrant.[2,4] The tympanic membrane is often diffusely thickened, with normal landmarks obscured; it is typically mobile although may show reduced mobility. In some instances, a camouflaged micro-perforation may be present. If there is involvement of the external auditory canal, it is often tender and painful. ▶ Fig. 13.2, ▶ Fig. 13.3, and ▶ Fig. 13.4 show the typical appearance of chronic myringitis.

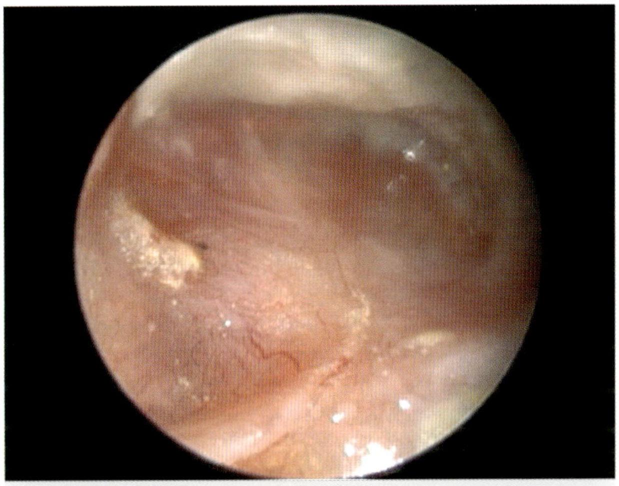

Fig. 13.4 Small yellow crusts seen on the surface of the tympanic membrane. Removal of these crusts revealed small areas of granulation tissue beneath.

13.5 Classification System

Wolf et al proposed a classification system based on presentation and the subsequent healing process. Grade I indicates a focal de-epithelialization of the tympanic membrane (▶ Fig. 13.2), characterized by a shallow, flat ulcer with granulation. Grade II lesions are focal lesions but exhibit raised, polypoid granulation tissue. Grade III myringitis presents as a diffuse involvement of the tympanic membrane (▶ Fig. 13.4). Grade IV myringitis involves raised, polypoid lesions covering the entire surface of the tympanic membrane and extending to the external auditory canal (▶ Fig. 13.3).[3]

El-Seifi and Fouad proposed an alternative classification system based on the location and degree of tympanic membrane involvement. They classified their patients into three groups: those with (1) a focal patch of less than one quarter of the tympanic membrane, (2) diffuse involvement of the tympanic membrane, and (3) segmental involvement, where triangular segments of the tympanic membrane are affected.[4]

13.6 Treatment

Treatment of chronic myringitis varies, and there is currently no widely accepted "standard" treatment regimen. The literature describes various treatment alternatives.

13.6.1 Medical Therapies

Topical preparations are the mainstay of medical treatment. In addition to topical steroid preparations, a myriad of other topical treatments have been described. Jung et al reported good resolution of granulations within 3 weeks using a solution of vinegar diluted with water instilled into the external auditory canal twice daily.[13] Another topical treatment is a douche of equal parts vinegar and alcohol. Application of gentian violet has also been described in a small series.[1]

Certain caustic agents have also been described for the treatment of chronic myringitis. Trichloracetic acid solution,[1] formalin,[14] and a carbol-fuchsin[15] solution have been described to be effective in the treatment of chronic myringitis. Silver nitrate has also been applied directly to granulations.[1]

In addition to therapy with a steroid-containing otic drop, lotion, or cream, certain otic powders may also be employed. A compounded mixture of chloramphenicol, sulfanilamide, fungizone (amphotericin B), and hydrocortisone, known as CSF-HC, is preferred by the authors. A similar compound for sulfa-allergic patients (CF-HC) eliminates the sulfanilamide component. A typical treatment regimen involves insufflator application once or twice a day for several weeks and then as needed for recurrences. Similar to the compounded otic powders, boric acid powder has also been described, either as a stand-alone treatment or in solution with alcohol.[2,7]

Regardless of the topical treatment used, most reports recommend a more prolonged course of treatment than is normally implemented for otitis externa. Treatment for chronic myringitis may last 3 to 4 weeks[1,7]; however, care should be taken when using the higher potency topical steroids for prolonged periods of time. Finally, an initial response to treatment may be followed by recurrences necessitating repeated treatment.

A newer treatment for myringitis refractory to topical steroids is the use of topical 5-fluorouracil (5-FU) applied directly to the external auditory canal and tympanic membrane. A single paper describes using 5-FU for treatment of granular myringitis. Atef et al showed significant improvement in otorrhea, granulation tissue, and recurrence rates with 5-FU treatment. Their method involved packing the ear with strip gauze impregnated with 5% 5-FU cream for two days, with subsequent removal in the office. Treatments were repeated at 2-week intervals for a total of three treatments.[16] The authors also use 5% 5-FU cream, but it is applied to plain strip gauze that is left in place for 30 minutes and removed by the patient. This process is repeated weekly for up to 3 weeks.

The authors also prefer a hierarchical, step-wise approach to topical treatment. This progressive approach is based on cost-effectiveness and simplicity for the patient. First-line treatment involves the use of topical steroid therapy. For mild cases, a combination steroid and antibiotic otic drop can be used. Ciprofloxacin/dexamethasone and neomycin/polymyxin B/hydrocortisone are two commonly used otic drops. More severe cases usually require a more potent topical steroid. The authors prefer using topical betamethasone lotion once or twice a day for several weeks. Other topical steroids include clobetasol and fluocinolone acetonide. If there is no response to these steroid preparations, then otic powder, with or without the concurrent use of a potent topical steroid, is employed. Finally, for difficult-to-treat cases, topical 5-FU is used.

13.6.2 Surgical Treatments

Despite medical therapy with topical treatments, some patients have recalcitrant disease. Surgical therapies have been instituted to treat these cases. Typically, these fall into two categories: laser resurfacing and tympanoplasty.

The CO_2 laser can be used on a low-power setting to ablate the affected areas of the tympanic membrane and external auditory canal, along with a small margin of normal tissue. Once the diseased area has been denuded, re-epithelialization can occur. Success rates ranging from 73% to 85% have been reported in both pediatric and adult populations.[17,18,19] Other lasers such as those having a wavelength in the 532 nm range (argon, potassium titanyl phosphate) can also be used with a handheld laser fiber positioned at a sufficient distance from the target so as to de-focus the applied energy.

Other authors prefer tympanoplasty. Zhang et al performed lateral graft tympanoplasty and achieved 100% success with no recurrences at follow-up times of 2–5 years. They concluded that for more severe forms (Wolf grades III and IV), tympanoplasty was preferable to more conventional treatments.[20] El-Seifi and Fouad performed cartilage graft tympanoplasty with skin grafting. In their series, they reported a 100% recurrence rate using limited topical treatment. With surgery, they had no recurrences, thus recommending surgical treatment for more advanced stage disease.[4]

13.7 Complications

Despite treatment, recurrence of myringitis is common. Recurrence rates vary widely in the literature, from 0% to 100%, with a mean recurrence rate of approximately 30%. Perforations can arise in the setting of chronic myringitis. These perforations can heal spontaneously if the underlying condition is treated and resolves. As with other causes of tympanic membrane perforations, tympanoplasty may be necessary although myringitis may reappear on the grafted tympanic membrane. Finally, and not uncommonly, chronic myringitis can incite fibrosis and stenosis of the external auditory canal.[7]

In cases of recalcitrant disease accompanied by hearing loss, hearing rehabilitation can be challenging. Often, patients with chronic myringitis are unable to wear a conventional hearing aid. If proper candidates, these patients are ideally suited for the placement of an osseointegrated auditory implant.

13.8 Future Directions

Chronic myringitis is a relatively uncommon disorder, but based on the incidence previously described, it is a disorder that the general otolaryngologist is likely to see and one an otologist is sure to see. Despite its infrequent mention in otolaryngology and otologic texts, myringitis can be quite troubling to the patient and difficult to treat. Consensus on a uniform name for the disorder and more research on treatment modalities will help further define the disease and its management.

References

[1] Stoney P, Kwok P, Hawke M. Granular myringitis: a review. J Otolaryngol. 1992;21(2):129–135.

[2] Blevins NH, Karmody CS. Chronic myringitis: prevalence, presentation, and natural history. Otol Neurotol. 2001;22(1):3–10.

[3] Wolf M, Primov-Fever A, Barshack I, Polack-Charcon S, Kronenberg J. Granular myringitis: Incidence and clinical characteristics. Otol Neurotol. 2006;27 (8):1094–1097.

[4] El-Seifi A, Fouad B. Granular myringitis: is it a surgical problem? Am J Otol. 2000;21(4):462–467.

[5] Wolf M, Primov-Fever A, Barshack I, Kronenberg J. Granular myringitis in children. Int J Pediatr Otorhinolaryngol. 2001;57(1):17–20.

[6] Hoshino T, Ueda Y, Mukohdaka H, Mizuta K. Acute granulomatous myringitis. J Laryngol Otol. 1998;112(2):150–153.

[7] Neilson LJ, Hussain SS. Management of granular myringitis: A systematic review. J Laryngol Otol. 2008;122(1):3–10.

[8] Kunachak S. Intractable granular myringitis: possible etiology and management. J Otolaryngol. 1992;21(4):297–298.

[9] Makino K, Amatsu M, Kinishi M, Mohri M. The clinical features and pathogenesis of myringitis granulosa. Arch Otorhinolaryngol. 1988;245(4):224–229.

[10] Schuknecht HF. Pathology of the Ear. Second Edition, 1993 194–196.

[11] Levi JR, Ames JA, Gitman L, Morlet T, O'Reilly RC. Clinical characteristics of pediatric granular myringitis. Otolaryngol Head Neck Surg. 2013;148 (2):291–296.

[12] Pulec JL, DeGuine C. Epithelitis of a tympanic membrane graft. Ear Nose Throat J. 1995;74(11):740.

[13] Jung HH, Cho SD, Yoo CK, Lim HH, Chae SW. Vinegar treatment in the management of granular myringitis. J Laryngol Otol. 2002;116(3):176–180.

[14] Yinglin Z. Three cases of chronic granular myringitis cured by formalin. J Otolaryngol. 1985;14(6):379–380.

[15] Kim YH. Clinical characteristics of granular myringitis treated with castellani solution. Eur Arch Otorhinolaryngol. 2011;268(8):1139–1146.

[16] Atef AM, Hamouda MM, Mohamed AH, Fattah AF. Topical 5-fluorouracil for granular myringitis: a double-blinded study. J Laryngol Otol. 2010;124 (3):279–284.

[17] Cheng YF, Shiao AS. Intractable chronic myringitis treated with carbon dioxide laser microsurgery. Arch Otolaryngol Head Neck Surg. 2008;134(2):152–156.

[18] Fechner FP, Cunningham MJ, Eavey RD. Laser therapy for refractory myringitis in children. Otolaryngol Head Neck Surg. 2002;127(3):163–168.

[19] Jang CH, Kim YH, Cho YB, Wang PC. Endoscopy-aided laser therapy for intractable granular myringitis. J Laryngol Otol. 2006;120(7):553–555.

[20] Zhang Z, Liu X, Chen S, Zheng Y. Combined tympanic epithelial layer avulsion and overlay myringoplasty for diffuse granular myringitis. J Laryngol Otol. 2010;124(8):842–845.

14 Office Evaluation and Management of a Canal Wall-Down Mastoid Cavity

Michael B. Gluth

Abbreviation used in this chapter:

CWD: canal wall-down

14.1 Introduction

The canal wall-down (CWD) tympanomastoid scenario poses several unique challenges in the practice of otology. Although the question of when to perform CWD mastoidectomy is somewhat controversial, all otologists are required to understand how to manage a CWD cavity in the office setting from time to time. Thus, this chapter will highlight the work-up and office management of patients presenting with a discharging open mastoid cavity. Particular attention is given to the pathophysiology associated with an unstable cavity and patterns of failure that will prompt consideration for revision surgery. This information is further complemented by Chapter 35 on CWD mastoidectomy surgical technique and Chapter 41 on mastoid cavity obliteration.

14.2 Pathophysiology and Theories of Mastoid Cavity Instability

A review of the literature projects a variable rate of open mastoid cavity instability ranging from 10% to 60% over the long term.[1,2,3,4,5] Several ideas have been proposed over the years to account for why some mastoid cavities will chronically discharge, whereas others are mostly dry and stable. In 1979 Rambo[6] put forth one of the first major theories on this topic that would eventually gain widespread popularity, some of which even continues today. Rambo's hypothesis was that chronic mastoid cavity instability is due to incomplete removal of diseased mastoid air cells that result in the production of moisture, as residual secretory mucosa remains present and active. This theory essentially ascribes mastoid cavity instability to untreated chronic mastoiditis, with the assumption that most ears should be dry if thoroughly drilled.

In 1982 Sade, Weinberg, Berco, Brown, and Halevy published a classic paper that further investigated mastoid cavity instability, wherein four predominant factors were identified among a large series of unstable ears, namely, an open Eustachian tube, a small meatoplasty, a large cavity, and a high facial ridge.[2] Interestingly, they noted that there was a cumulative effect of having multiple negative factors at once, to the point where a 100% chance of cavity instability was asserted if all four were in play. Consideration of these findings helped lead to the hypothesis that the shape and dimensions of the mastoid cavity may be the driving determinant of cavity stability as opposed to presence of residual secreting mucosa.

Youngs, who in 1992 published the histopathologic findings from 159 discharging mastoid cavities, explored this concept with further scrutiny.[5] His findings demonstrated a strong prominence of ulcerated squamous epithelium with acute and chronic inflammation as well as foreign body granulomas and aural polyp in response to retained keratin debris. Conspicuously uncommon among observed pathology was the presence of mucous cyst formation and secreting mucosa, which was seen in only a limited number of the examined specimens. As such, these findings seemed to reinforce the concept that cavity instability is predominantly a pathologic squamous epithelial response to retained keratin debris and associated infection as opposed to a mucosal secretory phenomenon as had been suggested previously by Rambo.

Wormald and Neilson examined this "retention theory" even further by studying the impact of various factors related to cavity shape and size on cavity stability.[4] In 1998, their publication included detailed mastoid cavity measurements from over 100 ears prospectively examined in a clinic over a one-year period of time. They determined that a high facial ridge, a "kidney-shaped" cavity, an open mastoid tip, an open Eustachian tube (typically in the form of a perforated tympanic membrane), and a small external auditory meatus would be expected to impart a negative effect on cavity stability. In particular, a high facial ridge and a kidney-shaped cavity, which relates to the contour of the inferior tympanic bone relative to the adjacent mastoid cavity, were noted to have particular impact from a statistical perspective. However, in contrast to Sade, they did not find the absolute volume of the cavity to be significant.

In addition to the contour of the mastoid cavity, the relative size of the meatus, and the status of the tympanic membrane, the presence of recurrent cholesteatoma has since been identified as an additional negative factor that is often found in unstable mastoid cavities.[7] Although residual and recurrent cholesteatoma rates should be low after CWD mastoidectomy, failures still can occur. It is a flawed notion that CWD surgery always alleviates the need for a second-look procedure. For example, this is certainly not the case if cholesteatoma extensively involved the mesotympanum because this area is not exteriorized during most CWD surgeries. Thus, chronic otorrhea should always prompt consideration that cholesteatoma may be present, even in the CWD setting.

14.3 Symptoms of an Unstable Mastoid Cavity

The hallmark of an unstable mastoid cavity is chronic otorrhea, which often can be quite foul smelling. Worsened hearing, otic fullness, and pain are possible but less common.[1] Vertigo is also possible due to caloric effects, even in a stable cavity, but may be more pronounced when the cavity requires treatment with otic drops or aural suctioning. An unstable cavity will not be compatible with an ear-level hearing aid. In some instances, a

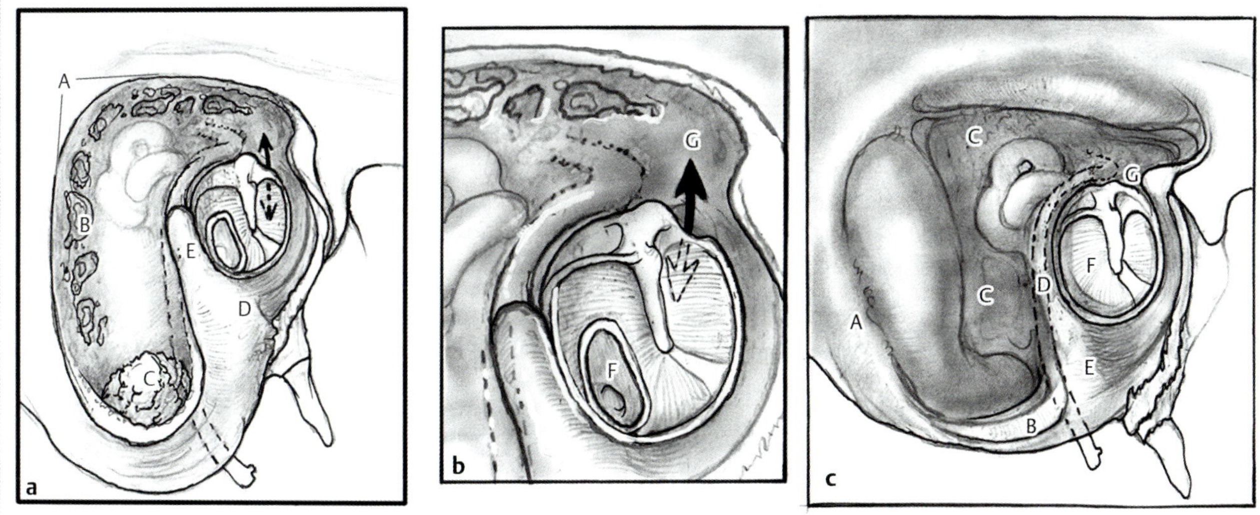

Fig. 14.1 An unfavorable versus a properly formed canal wall-down mastoidectomy. (a) In the unfavorable cavity note the steep non-saucerized edges, the potholes from residual air cells, the intact open mastoid tip with debris, the uncontoured tympanic bone forming a kidney-shaped cavity, the high facial ridge. A, steep non-saucerized edges; B, potholes from residual air cells; C, intact open mastoid tip with debris; D, uncontoured kidney-shaped tympanic bone; E, high facial ridge; (b) Also note the tympanic membrane perforation, and the unsealed communication between the mesotympanum and the exteriorized epitympanum. F, tympanic membrane perforation; G, unsealed communication with epitympanum. (c) In contrast, the properly formed canal wall-down mastoidectomy features saucerized edges, a mastoid tip that has been amputated from the digastric muscle, air cells that have been drilled away until the smooth posterior and middle fossa dural plates are exposed, a completely lowered facial ridge, an inferior tympanic bone that has been rendered concave having a smooth junction with the mastoid, an intact tympanic membrane, and an intact seal between the epitympanum and the mesotympanum. A, saucerized edges; B, mastoid tip amputated from digastric muscle; C, cells drilled away up to smooth dural plate; D, facial ridge lowered; E, tympanic bone smoothly fractured with junction of mastoid; F=intact tympanic membrane; G, middle ear sealed from epitympanum.

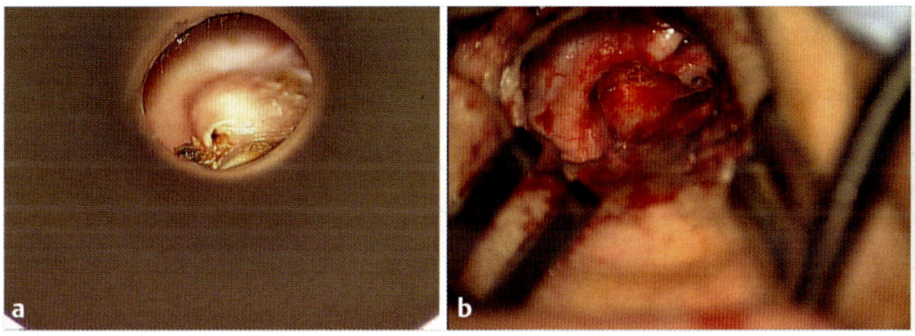

Fig. 14.2 High facial ridge. (a) Office view of a high facial ridge in a right ear. Note the presence of retained debris to the left of the ridge, which was extending into the mastoid tip. (b) Intraoperative view in the same patient with skin dissected off of the high facial ridge before drilling.

previously stable cavity will start to discharge after a hearing aid is fit, presumably due to the resultant increase in moisture and microbial load induced by canal occlusion.[8] In other ears, instability is brought about during periods of ongoing water exposure.

14.4 Examination and Assessment of a Mastoid Cavity

Microscopic examination of the ear should include inspection for the presence of pus, fungal elements, granulation tissue, aural polyp, cholesteatoma, and myringitis. Careful note is made of the status of the neotympanic membrane. Given our current evolved knowledge of open mastoid cavity pathophysiology, key factors that may contribute to chronic instability should be examined. These are portrayed in ▶ Fig. 14.1, and a brief description follows.

14.4.1 Mastoid Tip

If the mastoid tip is both present and open, it will possibly act as a gravity-dependent sewer or sump, with associated accumulation of moisture and debris. It may also be difficult in some cases to completely visualize and manipulate the entirety of an open tip in the office.

14.4.2 High Facial Ridge

A high facial ridge is defined as having > 2 mm of bone overlying the mastoid segment of the facial nerve, and it should be lowered at least to the level of the chorda tympani–facial nerve junction.[4,9] It has been found that surgeons tend to either lower the facial ridge completely or not at all. If high, the ridge of bone acts as a steep cliff that can impede epithelial migration (▶ Fig. 14.2). The determination of ridge height is made either by microscopic examination or by reviewing radiologic images.

14.4.3 Kidney Shape

The so-called kidney shape refers to the contour of the cavity as defined by the junction between the inferior tympanic bone and its transition into the mastoid cavity. If not properly lowered, there is a prominent convex corner in this area that can be perceived to define the hilum of an imaginary kidney. Similar to a high facial ridge, this will act to prevent epithelial migration from the inferior aspect of the mastoid cavity into the native external auditory canal.

14.4.4 Cavity Irregularities

Whereas some minor cavity irregularities may be unavoidable, especially in the perilabyrinthine area, excessive undrilled air cells cause widespread dimpling of the resultant cavity that may tend to retain debris. Drilling down to the smooth bone of the middle and posterior fossa dural plates and to the sigmoid sinus should minimize this. When inspected, a note is made as to whether these irregularities are observed to be involved with retention. Additionally, a severely atelectatic tympanic membrane may act in a similar matter.

14.4.5 Narrow External Auditory Meatus

The adequacy of the caliber of the eternal auditory meatus is judged against the dimensions of the underlying cavity. As such, there are not absolute size requirements for a meatus to be satisfactory. As a rule, the entirety of the cavity should be easily viewed and manipulated as needed. The most common area that cannot be adequately viewed is the posterior sulcus of the cavity, which is located adjacent to the sigmoid sinus and sinodural angle.

14.4.6 Open Eustachian Tube

There must be an intact barrier separating the epithelialized mastoid cavity and the mucosalized middle ear or Eustachian tube. An open Eustachian tube most commonly will take the form of a tympanic membrane perforation. However, if the epitympanum has been exteriorized without closure of the anterior communication to the mesotympanum and protympanum, a pseudoperforation will occur that acts in the same manner. If radical mastoidectomy has been performed and the tympanic membrane is thus absent, failure to plug the Eustachian tube orifice will have the same effect.

14.4.7 Non-saucerized Cavity

If the periphery of the cavity has not been widely beveled or saucerized, steep edges may prevent inward collapse of soft tissue that will otherwise act to auto-obliterate some of the cavity volume. This is particularly important with respect to removal of bone in the retrosigmoid region, which, when performed in combination with mastoid tip amputation, will have the effect of collapsing the lateral soft tissue in a way that establishes the anterior edge of the sigmoid sinus as the posterior boundary of the cavity. Even in a well-pneumatized temporal bone, the anterior edge of the sigmoid sinus is usually a mere 2 cm from the anterior wall of the native external auditory canal wall.

14.5 Office and Home Treatment

Given our understanding of the role that retention plays in cavity instability, it is understandable that by far the most important aspect of treatment involves meticulous evacuation of all debris and secretions. It is a common error to be overly reliant upon ototopical medication regimens while neglecting to completely assure thorough aural toilet. To achieve this, it is possible that a brief mask anesthesia may be required in children, but rarely in adults. When performing cavity debridement, it is important to systematically examine each region of the exteriorized tympanomastoid space in a stepwise manner, including the neotympanic membrane, epitympanum, tegmen, sinodural angle, and mastoid tip. It is also important to identify the facial nerve and the lateral semicircular canal and, when suctioning, to take into account the possibility of underlying dehiscence or fistula, respectively.

For cases where granulation tissue or myringitis are pronounced, application of a cauterizing agent is useful, typically phenol or silver nitrate. When doing so, extreme care must be made to avoid application onto the facial nerve and to prevent chemical access into the mesotympanum when the tympanic membrane is not intact. An aural polyp can usually be successfully debrided in the office with a cupped forceps. If the tympanic membrane is intact, it is also possible to irrigate the cavity using a bulb syringe with dilute hydrogen peroxide, saline, or a weak vinegar solution. Even if there is a tympanic membrane perforation, home irrigation with ½ strength vinegar solution (diluted with boiled tap water) is safe and typically well tolerated as a means of clearing secretions and acidifying a cavity. As a rule of thumb, vinegar irrigations typically do not cause pain at first, while the middle ear is acutely inflamed, but the ear will progressively become sensitive to pain during the irrigations as the middle ear mucosa becomes quiet; thus, the development of pain is a useful marker to discontinue the irrigations. Some otologists advocate the ongoing application of drying and acidifying agents at home, such as a combination of boric or acetic acid in ethanol. Although highly effective, ethanol application often results in severe pain and should not be utilized unless the tympanic membrane is definitively intact.

Although patch myringoplasty techniques are unlikely to be successful in closing a large chronic tympanic membrane perforation, using a patch consisting of paper or thin silastic to act as a temporary barrier may nonetheless be useful when managing a mastoid cavity. Doing so will temporarily act to reduce moisture within the cavity while it stabilizes. Another means of keeping the ear dry is to instruct patients to carefully apply air from a hairdryer twice daily.

14.6 Microbiology and Antimicrobial Therapy

It is useful to routinely obtain specimens for bacterial and fungal culturesto properly direct antimicrobial therapy. Although the same pathogens that affect any ear with chronic suppurative otitis media may be present, namely *Pseudomonas aeruginosa*, by far the most commonly encountered pathogen in an unstable open cavity is *Staphylococcus aureus*.[10] Fungus is also common, especially when the use of antibiotic- and steroid-containing otic drops has been long-standing.

The principles driving antimicrobial therapy for a chronically discharging mastoid cavity are similar to what has been thoroughly outlined for chronic suppurative otitis media in Chapter 5 and Chapter 16; thus, the reader is referred to those chapters for a discussion of specific antimicrobial agents. Fluoroquinolone-containing drops with or without a steroid are the mainstay of treatment, especially if there is a tympanic membrane perforation. However, there are a few unique aspects to consider when dealing with an open cavity. In particular, wide distribution of otic drops to reach the entire cavity may be problematic, especially if prescribed according to usual dosing for an intact canal wall. In general, at least 8–10 drops per application will be required to have any chance of reaching the entire surface area of a mastoid cavity. Also, chronic overuse of fluoroquinolone drops often leads to development of a secondary fungal infection, especially if debris remains within the cavity. One-percent clotrimazole solution is also safe to apply in the middle ear as an antifungal, but it tends to burn severely.

In refractory cases, alternative preparations, such as ointment or powder, may be preferred. Powders have the advantage of potential custom compounding to include various combinations of antibiotic, antifungal, acidifying, and corticosteroid agents per a particular patient's needs. These can be easily self-administered by patients at home using a powder insufflation applicator. Ointments have the advantage of completely filling a mastoid cavity and coating its entire surface area over a long period of time. These are usually applied in the office through a syringe and a large angiocath, with the expectation that it will take 1–2 weeks for ointment to fully clear. Mupirocin ointment is particularly useful in treating drug-resistant *S. aureus* infection in an open mastoid cavity, and this can be mixed in the office with steroid (triamcinolone) or antifungal (nystatin) ointments as needed.

14.7 Decision Making for Revision Surgery

When the cumulative burden of negative symptoms, frequent office visits, medication application, and hearing aid intolerance overwhelm a given patient's tolerance, revision surgery should be considered. Gluth, Metrailer, Dornhoffer, and Moore. have published a classification of factors that may help guide this decision that designates primary tympanomastoid pathology as Class 1, unfavorable aspects related to cavity contour as Class 2, and negative patient constitutional factors as Class 3.[7] When evaluating a patient, Class 1 factors may act as freestanding indications for revision surgery, as will the presence of multiple Class 2 factors acting together. However, when numerous Class 3 factors are present, cavity instability may be inevitable even after well-executed surgery.

The factors related to mastoid cavity instability follow:

Class 1: Primary Tympanomastoid Pathology
- Tympanic membrane perforation
- Tympanic membrane atelectasis
- Cholesteatoma
- Extruding/exposed ossicular replacement prosthesis

Class 2: Unfavorable Shape and Contour
- Intact open mastoid tip
- High facial ridge
- Poorly contoured inferior tympanic bone (kidney-shaped cavity)
- Small meatoplasty
- Numerous cavity irregular surfaces
- Non-saucerized cavity edges

Class 3: Unfavorable Patient Constitutional Factors
- Tobacco use
- Past radiation treatment
- Diabetes
- Poor hygiene
- Neglect of routine cavity care
- Malnutrition

In properly selected patients, revision CWD mastoidectomy is typically associated with a high rate of success, especially if performed by an otologist highly experienced with surgical management of chronic ear disease.[11] Proper execution of CWD mastoid surgery is described in Chapter 35. Furthermore, mastoid obliteration techniques (Chapter 41) are highly successful in reducing cavity volume and converting an ear to a state of sustained stability,[12,13] even to the point of newly afforded hearing aid tolerance.[8]

14.8 Conclusion

In summary, evaluation and management of a chronically discharging open mastoid cavity is founded upon an understanding that retention of keratin debris is the primary negative pathophysiologic factor that leads to cavity instability. When examining an unstable cavity, it is necessary to ascertain the contour and shape, with a potential view toward surgical revision. Although ototopical therapy is important, complete removal of secretions and retained debris is the most important aspect to keep in mind with respect to management in the office setting.

References

[1] Males AG, Gray RF. sade. Clin Otolaryngol Allied Sci. 1991;16(1):12–14.

[2] Sadé J, Weinberg J, Berco E, Brown M, Halevy A. The marsupialized (radical) mastoid. J Laryngol Otol. 1982,96(10).869–875.

[3] Smyth GD. Canal wall for cholesteatoma: up or down? Long-term results. Am J Otol. 1985;6(1):1–2.

[4] Wormald PJ, Nilssen EL. The facial ridge and the discharging mastoid cavity. Laryngoscope. 1998;108(1 Pt 1):92–96.

[5] Youngs R. The histopathology of mastoidectomy cavities, with particular reference to persistent disease leading to chronic otorrhoea. Clin Otolaryngol Allied Sci. 1992;17(6):505–510.

[6] Rambo JH. Mastoid surgery: effect of retained mucosa on healing. Ann Otol Rhinol Laryngol. 1979;88(5 Pt 1):701–707.

[7] Gluth MB, Metrailer AM, Dornhoffer JL, Moore PC. Patterns of failure in canal wall down mastoidectomy cavity instability. Otol Neurotol. 2012;33(6):998–1001.

[8] Gluth MB, Friedman AB, Atcherson SR, Dornhoffer JL. Hearing aid tolerance after revision and obliteration of canal wall down mastoidectomy cavities. Otol Neurotol. 2013;34(4):711–714.
[9] Wormald PJ, van Hasselt CA. A technique of mastoidectomy and meatoplasty that minimizes factors associated with a discharging mastoid cavity. Laryngoscope. 1999;109(3):478–482.
[10] Gluth MB, Tan BY, Santa Maria PL, Atlas MD. Unique microbiology of chronically unstable canal wall down tympanomastoid cavities: considerations for surgical revision. J Laryngol Otol. 2013;127(5):458–462.
[11] Dornhoffer JL. Surgical modification of the difficult mastoid cavity. Otolaryngol. Head Neck Surg. 1999;120(3):361–367.
[12] Black B. Mastoidectomy elimination. Laryngoscope. 1995;105(12 Pt 2) Suppl 76:1–30.
[13] Singh V, Atlas M. Obliteration of the persistently discharging mastoid cavity using the middle temporal artery flap. Otolaryngol Head Neck Surg. 2007;137(3):433–438.

15 Tubo-Tympanic Diseases: Retraction, Atelectasis, and Middle Ear Effusion

Stefan Volkenstein and Stefan Dazert

Abbreviations used in this chapter:

BET: balloon Eustachian tuboplasty
COME: chronic otitis media with effusion
CT: computed tomography
OME: otitis media with effusion
SPL: sound pressure level

15.1 Introduction

Dysfunction of the Eustachian tube may cause diseases that are reflected in alterations of the middle ear mucosa and in the appearance of the tympanic membrane. Details of the physiology related to negative middle ear pressure, mucosal gas exchange, and Eustachian tube dysfunction are covered in Chapter 2. This chapter deals with clinical assessment and medical decision making related to the so-called tubo-tympanic diseases: retraction, atelectasis, and effusion.

Otitis media with effusion (OME) describes the persistence of fluid or mucous (glue ear) behind an intact tympanic membrane, usually with no signs of inflammation. If this condition persists for more than three months, it is called chronic otitis media with effusion (COME). Chronic otitis media with effusion is considered to be the most common reason for hearing problems and the most common ear pathology in childhood in general. By the age of 10 years, 80% of all children have gone through at least one episode of COME.[1] Treatment options for these diseases vary widely, from watchful waiting to surgery.

Progressive Eustachian tube dysfunction may result in tympanic membrane atelectasis (also, adhesive otitis media), consistent with retractions or invaginations of the tympanic membrane into the middle ear that differ in size, localization, pathogenesis, and biological behavior. Treatment options for atelectasis vary from watchful waiting to small procedures (e.g., tympanostomy tube insertion or adenoidectomy) to intensive surgical procedures, including tympanoplasty and mastoidectomy. Some tympanic membrane retraction pockets resolve spontaneously over time, some remain stable for a long time period, and others develop into an aggressive cholesteatoma with potentially severe complications.

In the following chapter we will suggest a structured treatment guideline for the atelectatic ear with or without effusion according to its clinical presentation and diagnostic workup. However, we should point out that there is no consensus about the best treatment strategy in the literature.[2,3,4,5]

15.2 Clinical Presentation

Patients with COME and retraction pockets may be asymptomatic for a long time and may not complain about any symptoms in the beginning of the disease process. Adults usually present with a conductive hearing loss when sound-induced movement of the tympanic membrane is restricted due to effusion, adhesion of the tympanic membrane to the ossicles or promontory (▶ Fig. 15.1; ▶ Fig. 15.2; ▶ Fig. 15.3; ▶ Fig. 15.4; ▶ Fig. 15.5), or negative pressure. They will often complain about fullness in the ear. Children may be referred because of delayed speech development (due to a conductive hearing loss), snoring, or recurrent episodes of acute otitis media. An assessment should also be made of possible underlying speech delay or other developmental abnormalities as this may strongly impact decision-making. It should nonetheless be noted that during a routine check-up, deep retraction pockets may be discovered without any problems or complaints having been noted by the patient.

There are several classifications for retraction pockets, all of which aim to support the physician in giving the correct treatment advice depending on the retraction pocket subtype.[6,7,8,9,10,11] These classifications are based on the location of the invagination (pars tensa/pars flaccida), its history (age of the patient in combination with recurrent otitis media with or without otorrhea), its biological behavior (self-cleansing or retaining of epithelial debris; aggressively growing or not changing over several consultations), and the aeration of the middle ear cavity or pneumatization of the mastoid. The most widely accepted classifications are depicted in ▶ Table 15.1; ▶ Table 15.2; ▶ Table 15.3; and ▶ Table 15.4.

The proposed pathogenesis of atelectasis or adhesive otitis media is similar to that for the origin of COME.[1,12] It is based on the "*ex vacuo*" theory published by Politzer in 1867,[13] where a negative pressure in the middle ear cavity is induced by a dysfunction of the Eustachian tube and is followed by

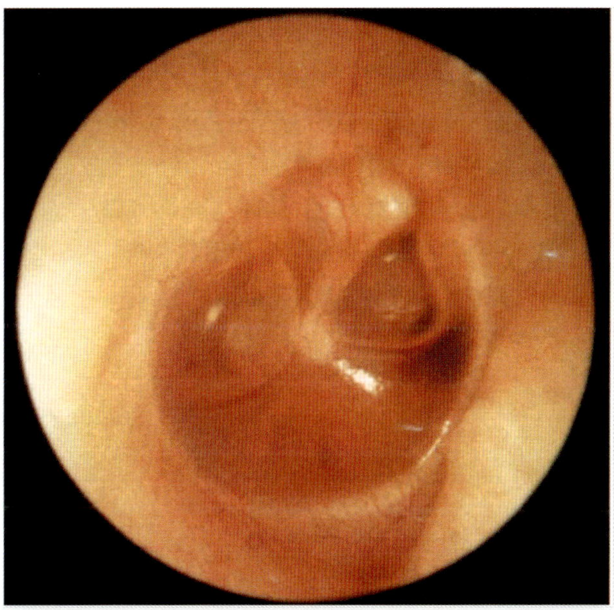

Fig. 15.1 Otitis media with effusion including air-fluid level in right ear.

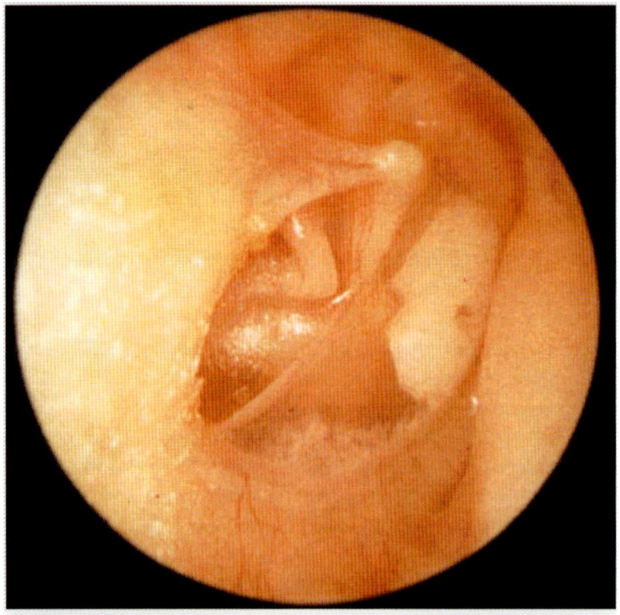

Fig. 15.2 Tympanosclerosis of the anterior pars tensa and fixed retraction of the posterior pars tensa onto the incudostapedial joint and promontory in a right ear.

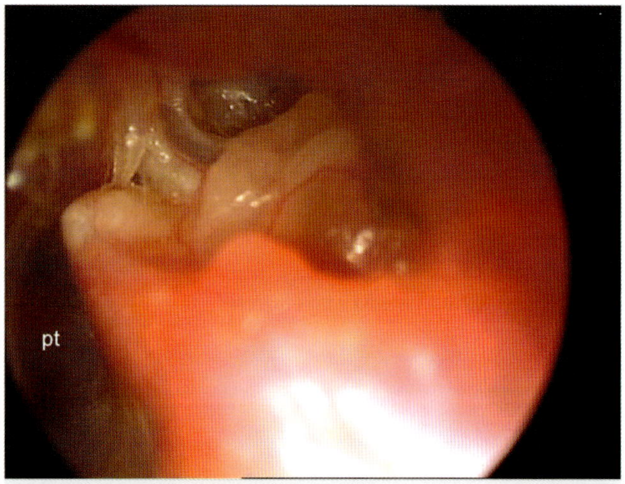

Fig. 15.3 Epitympanic retraction pocket (left ear). pt, pars tensa tympanic membrane

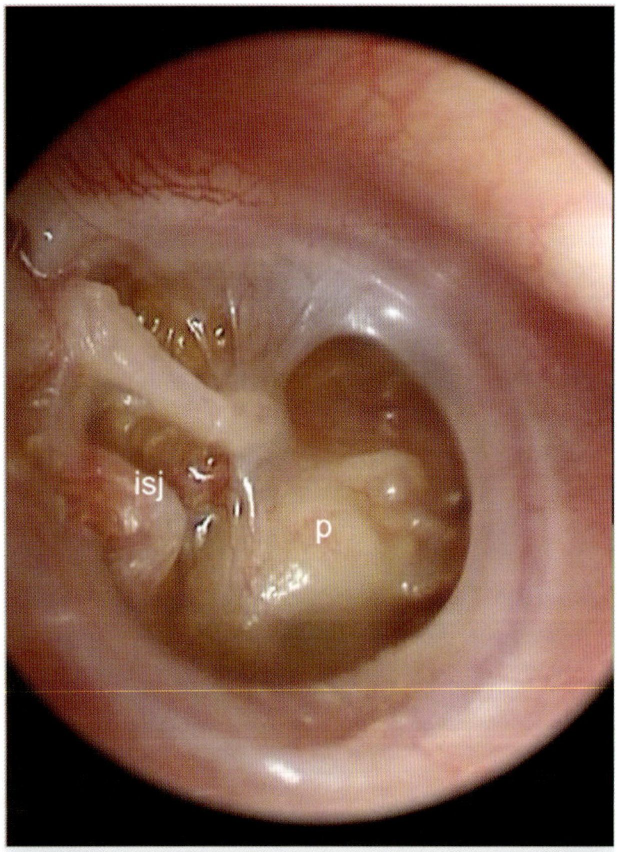

Fig. 15.5 Complete atelectasis of the tympanic membrane (right ear). p, promontory, isj, incudostapedial joint

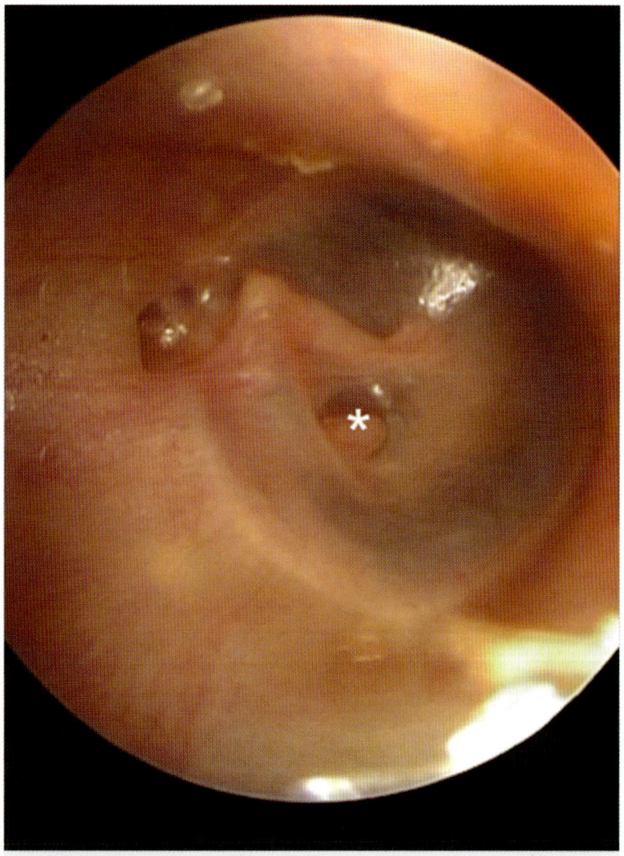

Fig. 15.4 Epitympanic retraction pocket and atelectasis of the pars tensa to the stapes (*) of a right ear.

inflammation and edema of the mucosal membranes of the Eustachian tube and middle ear cavity in combination with an epithelial proliferation as a reaction to the chronic inflammation.[14] The particular impact of the responsible preconditions is still under discussion, but the combination of retraction and proliferation for the development of cholesteatomas are the most accepted theories of pathogenesis to date.[14]

Table 15.1 Erasmus classification of pediatric atelectasis

Stage	Description
1	Tympanic membrane atrophic but not adherent to middle ear structures
2	Tympanic membrane adherent to the promontory only
3	Tympanic membrane adherent to incus and/or stapes
4	Tympanic membrane adherent to ossicles, with deep retraction pocket but without cholesteatoma
5	Retraction pocket with cholesteatoma and/or breakthrough

Used with permission from Borgstein J, Gerritsma TV, Wieringa MH, Bruce IA. The Erasmus atelectasis classification: proposal of a new classification for atelectasis of the middle ear in children. Laryngoscope. 2007; 117(7):12551259

Table 15.3 Black classification of pars tensa retraction

Grade	Description	Typical Treatment
1	Drum collapse without hearing loss	Observation or tympanostomy tube
2	Drum collapse with hearing loss but no ossicular dysfunction	Tympanoplasty
3	Drum collapse with hearing loss and ossicular dysfunction	Tympanoplasty with ossicular chain reconstruction
4	Deep retraction with hearing loss and cholesteatoma	Tympanomastoidectomy or epitympanectomy

Note: If an effusion is present, add an asterisk (*) to indicate a possible long term poor hearing prognosis: e.g., Stage II* for an severe collapse with an effusion. Data from Black B. Reporting Results in Ossiculoplasty. Otol Neurotol. 2003; 24 (4) 534-542.

Table 15.2 Sade classification of pars tensa atelectasis

Grade	Description
1	Retracted tympanic membrane which does not touch any middle ear structures
2	Retracted tympanic membrane touches the stapes or incus
3	Retracted tympanic membrane down to promontory
4	Retracted tympanic membrane into sinus tympani with collected keratin

Used with permission from Sadé J, Berco E. Atelectasis and secretory otitis media. Ann Otol Rhinol Laryngol. 1976; 85 Suppl 25:66–72.

Table 15.4 Tos classification of pars flaccida retraction

Grade	Description
1	Slight dimpling of the pars flaccida
2	Retraction to malleus neck; entire pocket is visible
3	Partly hidden retraction with possible erosion of the scutum
4	Deep retraction with definite scutal erosion; pocket is not entirely visualized

Used with permission from Tos M, Poulsen G. Attic retractions following secretory otitis. Acta Otolaryngol. 1980;89:479–486.

15.3 Diagnostic Tests

In addition to taking a specific medical history, the most important diagnostic tool is the microscopic examination of the tympanic membrane. In young children, cerumen or debris may sometimes not allow a reliable evaluation of the tympanic membrane; therefore, cleaning of the ears under general anesthesia may be required. In older children and adults, the entire tympanic membrane can usually be examined and evaluated with regard to retraction pocket size and location, whether the eardrum is fixed to the promontory/ossicles while performing the Valsalva maneuver, or if there is effusion.

Whereas otoacoustic emissions and tympanometry can be performed even in newborns, pure tone audiometry is usually not possible until the age of four years. Mild to severe conductive hearing loss can be observed in patients with atelectasis of the tympanic membrane, depending on retraction pocket size, effusion viscosity, or erosion of the ossicles. There is no reliable direct correlation of the conductive hearing loss and the severity of the disease. Especially in patients with mild hearing loss, the air conduction threshold may be less before removing the retraction pocket and scar tissue due to a sheeting effect, even for an eroded ossicular chain.

Tympanometry is routinely performed in a clinical workup of most otology patients. Whereas tympanometry is considered an easy method for measuring middle ear pressure, significant differences between the values read from the tympanogram and those measured by direct puncture of the tympanic membrane do exist. Tympanometry in ears with retracted or partially atelectatic tympanic membranes do not reflect the true middle ear pressure. The position of the tympanogram peak depends on the size of a retraction pocket and the remaining middle ear gas volume.[15] Nevertheless, if the tympanic membrane is not severely retracted, tympanometry is quite useful in the diagnosis of COME, with a sensitivity of about 93% and a specificity up to 70%.[16,17]

Dysfunction of the Eustachian tube can be caused by adenoid hypertrophy or nasal obstruction due to various underlying pathologic conditions (e.g., hyperplasia of the turbinates, retention cysts of the nasopharynx, nasopharyngeal tumors, etc.). Therefore, an endoscopic examination of the nose should be included at least once in routine workup when chronic ear problems are present.

Imaging is not necessarily required for routine cases of atelec tasis or COME. High-resolution computed tomography (CT) scan of the temporal bone is recommended in advanced cases where a cholesteatoma may be suspected or if there is any sign of an underlying chronic ear diseasecomplication.

There are high-risk groups of children with reduced Eustachian tube function for example, cleft palate patients, patients with Down syndrome or primary ciliary dyskinesia, as well as immunocompromised patients. These patients need a broader interdisciplinary workup involving pediatricians, oral surgeons, geneticists, and pediatric audiologists.

Table 15.5 Criteria to consider when deciding for or against surgical treatment

Watchful waiting	Surgical treatment
Entire retraction pocket can be visualized completely by microscopic examination	Entire retraction pocket cannot be visualized completely by microscopic examination
Conductive hearing loss < 20 dB SPL	Conductive hearing loss > 20 dB SPL
No otorrhea	Recurrent otorrhea
Good pneumatization	Poor pneumatization
Normal Eustachian tube function	Disturbed Eustachian tube function
Adult patient	Pediatric patient
Pars flaccida	Pars tensa
No progression	Progression
Poor medical conditions	Social criteria

SPL, sound pressure level

15.4 Treatment Decision-Making

In the following section, different clinical criteria are discussed with regard to their impact on whether or not to pursue a more conservative treatment or a surgical option. None of these criteria are a determining factor on their own, but each should be evaluated in the context of other findings (presented as a summary in ▶ Table 15.5).[18]

15.4.1 Microscopic Examination Findings

Microscopic examination of the tympanic membrane allows one of the most important decision-making criteria. In cases where the retraction pocket cannot be completely visualized through the microscope, the use of an angled endoscope can be helpful.[19,20] A self-cleansing retraction pocket without any noticeable or measurable symptoms usually does not need immediate surgical treatment. When a retraction pocket is filled with debris and/or cannot be completely visualized, a surgical treatment may be recommended. When examining tympanic membrane atelectasis, the presence of aeration within the protympanum may predict a good hearing result with tympanoplasty in that the tympanic membrane may be bound by adhesions to the underlying middle ear cleft in spite of subsequent recovery of Eustachian tube function (▶ Fig. 15.6).

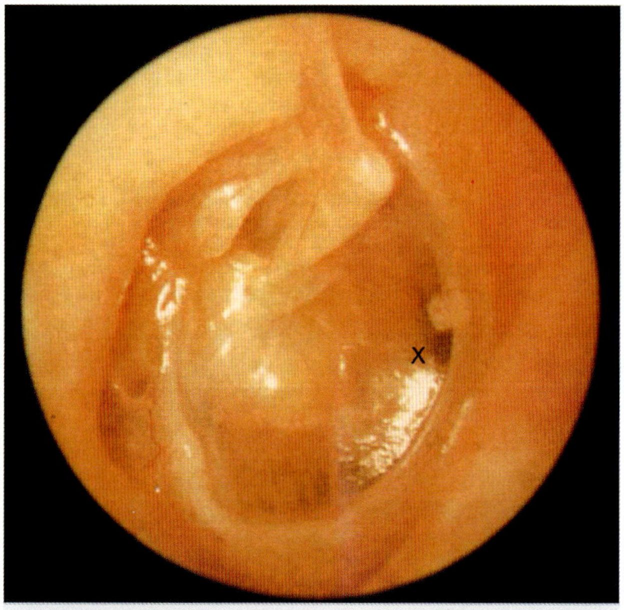

Fig. 15.6 Retraction of the posterior pars tensa of a right ear onto the incudostapedial articulation, which has been eroded and replaced by a fibrous band. Despite the retraction, note the presence of air in the anterior mesotympanum and protympanum (X), which suggests some degree of recovered Eustachian tube function.

15.4.2 Conductive Hearing Loss

A conductive hearing loss of more than 20 dB is often caused by restricted movement of the tympano-ossicular complex, erosion of the ossicles, or additional middle ear pathology and is considered to be an argument for a surgical treatment. However, there is a poor correlation between disease stage and audiometry.

15.4.3 Otorrhea

Chronic or recurrent otorrhea should be treated conservatively with intensive aural toilet and ototopical treatment, sometimes in combination with systemic antibiotics if there is concern for antimicrobial-resistant pathogens or if ototopical medications are not able to reach the target. In cases of persisting otorrhea and/or a growth in retraction pocket size, surgical treatment is favored.

15.4.4 Pneumatization of the Temporal Bone

Poor pneumatization of the temporal bone is often caused by disturbed Eustachian tube function during childhood, and, therefore, the same underlying pathogenic conditions are present that could lead to the development of retraction pockets. In a poorly pneumatized temporal bone, a retraction pocket may lead to the further reduction of mastoid aeration, resulting in cholesteatoma development in the future. Therefore, poor pneumatization is considered to be a "soft" argument for surgical intervention when a retraction pocket is present.[18]

15.4.5 Eustachian Tube Function

If a patient is judged to have pervasive underlying Eustachian tube dysfunction that is unlikely to spontaneously correct, such as seen in a patient with craniofacial abnormalities or cleft palate, more aggressive surgical management may be justified. Even temporary correction of Eustachian tube function may help to slow down or stop retraction pockets from developing into cholesteatomas. Obvious causes of Eustachian tube dysfunction, such as adenoid tissue, hyperplasia of the turbinates, etc., should be treated when possible.

15.4.6 Age

Retraction pockets display a higher proliferation rate in childhood compared with adolescence or adulthood.[21,22] Therefore, in young children, the presence of a cholesteatoma or its development has to be ruled out. A persistent conductive hearing loss of more than 20 dB can negatively influence children's hearing and speech development. Regular and repeated microscopic check-ups are difficult to perform in some children due to compliance issues and, when in doubt, we recommend surgical treatment as the safer option for these patients.

15.4.7 Localization

It is important to distinguish between retraction pockets of the pars tensa and the pars flaccida. Based on a different microanatomical structure (the pars flaccida is missing the fibrous stratum), a more intense underlying force has to be present to form retraction pockets of the pars tensa. In case of a persisting force (e.g., negative pressure), progression may be more likely. On the other hand, minor retractions of the pars flaccida may be difficult to visualize.

15.4.8 Time Course

Importance has to be attached to the time course of the presentation or for changes in retraction pockets. There is almost never an immediate indication for surgical treatment of asymptomatic retraction pockets at the first consultation. A patient with non-discharging retraction pockets completely visible under microscopic view without severe hearing loss may be followed for several years (first year at every four months, second year at every six months, than once a year thereafter).

15.4.9 Social Criteria

Social criteria have to be individually evaluated by the physician for each patient. A patient deemed unreliable to keep the required follow-up visits may be relatively more suited for surgical treatment over observation.

15.5 Treatment Options

There are no universally accepted treatment guidelines for OME/COME or tympanic membrane atelectasis. The need for therapy is widely discussed in the literature, but there is no consensus among different medical specialities involved in the treatment of these patients or within medical societies of different nations with regard to the intensity or accurate timing of treatment options. Due to a high spontaneous remission in OME/COME, patients suffering from these diseases should be treated conservatively within the first three months when they are not high-risk patients or when they have an underlying disease that can be treated effectively (▶ Fig. 15.7).[1,12,17]

15.5.1 Medications

In contrast to treatment guidelines for acute otitis media, the beneficial use of antibiotics in OME/COME is still unclear.[23] Whereas oral steroids, especially in combination with oral antibiotics, lead to a quicker resolution of OME in the short term, there is no evidence of long-term benefit and no evidence that they relieve symptoms of hearing loss. Neither is there any evidence of benefit from topical intranasal steroids, alone or in combination with an antibiotic, either at short- or long-term follow-up.[24,25] Antihistamines and decongestants have not shown benefit for the treatment of OME and are generally not recommended.[23]

15.5.2 Eustachian Tube Treatment

Different procedures can be performed to improve Eustachian tube function and increase middle ear pressure when indicated (e.g., Valsalva maneuver, use of an Otovent balloon (ABIGO Medical AB, Sweden), balloon dilatation of the Eustachian tube).[26,27,28,29] Transnasal balloon Eustachian tuboplasty (BET) is a new method where a balloon catheter is transnasally

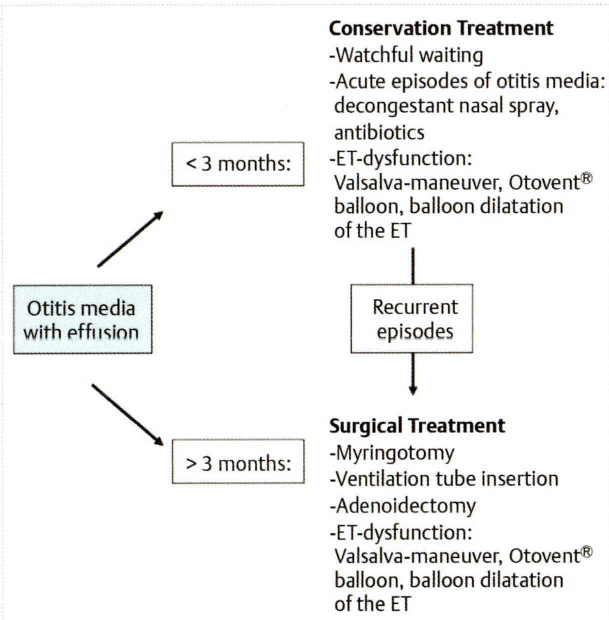

Fig. 15.7 Treatment algorithm for otitis media with effusion.

inserted via the pharyngeal ostium into the cartilaginous portion of the Eustachian tube and is then dilated to a pressure of 10 Bar for 2 minutes. Early results demonstrate that BET is a safe and effective treatment for improving Eustachian tube function and ear ventilation.[29] Eustachian tuboplasty is discussed in further detail in Chapter 45.

15.5.3 Tympanostomy Tubes With or Without Adenoidectomy

A persisting OME associated with conductive hearing loss for more than three months may evoke the need for tympanostomy tube placement, with the main goal of hearing improvement,[30,31] especially in children with speech delay or learning disabilities. Tympanostomy tube insertion often clears secretory pathology or the initial retraction pocket. Low-grade retraction pockets can be treated tentatively with ventilation tube insertion, especially when a persisting effusion is detectable. In children, we recommend an adenoidectomy in combination with ventilation tube insertion if there are signs/symptoms of chronic nasopharyngitis, obstructive adenoid hypertrophy, or the need for recurrent tympanostomy tube placement. Children having adenoidectomy together with tympanostomy/tube insertion at the same time have a reduced need for repeated tube insertion, which may be the result of clearing an infectious source in the nasopharynx rather than the removal of a large mass.[27] Children with OME/COME and the need for repeated ventilation tube insertion are at increased risk for perforation, retraction, cholesteatoma, and hearing loss[32]; thus, these patients must be monitored closely after tube extrusion.

15.5.4 Tympanoplasty

The management algorithm for removal and reconstruction of retraction pockets via tympanoplasty that we propose primarily considers the risk of cholesteatoma development and the functional handicap of the patient rather than the topographic description of the tympanic membrane pathology as suggested elsewhere.[5] Functional handicap comprises the cumulative burden upon the patient that is caused by hearing loss, need for frequent office inspection, and need for ototopical medication application.

After electing to treat tympanic membrane atelectasis with tympanoplasty, the applied surgical technique and the appropriate selection of a tissue transplant for the reconstruction of the tympanic membrane are crucial for optimum long-term results. Tympanic membrane reconstruction has to be stiff enough to prevent the development of new retractions and should also allow membrane vibration to reduce the conductive hearing impairment postoperatively. Most common transplant materials are temporalis fascia, perichondrium, cartilage, or composite grafts (Part 4, Roundtable on Tympanic Membrane Reconstruction).

Definitive surgical treatment of a retraction pocket includes complete eversion, excision, and removal of squamous epithelium from the middle ear, analogous to the principles of cholesteatoma surgery. This removal often results in a large perforation in the tympanic membrane, which has to be reconstructed with fascia, perichondrium, or cartilage grafts. To remove the entire invagination, we follow the invagination of the eardrum in a retrograde fashion and partially remove the posterior wall of the external ear canal to follow and completely remove the epithelium.[33]

15.5.5 Mastoidectomy

Some surgeons have advocated mastoidectomy as a means of expanding the volume of the tympanomastoid space in an effort to create a volumetric pressure buffer that may prevent the development of future negative middle ear pressure according to Boyle's law. This concept is discussed in detail in Part 6, Roundtable on Tympanomastoidectomy.

15.6 Outcomes

It is difficult to evaluate or compare the results after tympanoplasty or other treatment strategies for retraction pockets due to the multitude of relevant risk factors. In two randomized controlled trials for surgical treatment of retraction pockets, there has been no statistically significant benefit of cartilage tympanoplasty over watchful waiting with respect to disease progression or hearing outcome.[34] The results may depend on variable factors like Eustachian tube function, age of the patient, performance of an adenoidectomy, etc., which are often not clearly pointed out in available studies due to the small numbers for comparable patient groups.

Recently, there have been several long-term follow-up studies examining the recurrence of retraction pockets and postoperative hearing results after surgical treatment. After a 3- to 8-year follow-up period, up to 80% of patients with posterior retraction pockets were free of recurrence, whereas in patients with a nearly completely collapsed tympanic membrane, recurrence rates of up to 50% were described.[35,36] Postoperative hearing results in these patients are worse compared with patients with just posterior retraction pockets. Therefore, patients with a progression in retraction pocket size or depth should be treated surgically early in their disease course to achieve a better long-term hearing result and a lower chance for recurrence. Borgstein, Gerritsma, Bruce, and Feenstra[4] demonstrated that surgical intervention had a favorable effect on hearing level across all stages in their group of pediatric patients, but hearing was markedly worse in later stages.

Despite the intellectually satisfying concept that underlies the proposal of mastoidectomy as a therapeutic means of expanding tympanomastoid volume and creating a volumetric pressure buffer, especially in a sclerotic temporal bone, there is no high level of evidence to support this practice as a means of improving long-term tympanoplasty success or hearing outcomes for routine uncomplicated cases.[37]

The deterioration of retraction pockets to cholesteatoma is reported in 2% to10% of ears in long-term follow-up studies,[38] and even up to 4% of the ears with a minor retraction pocket presented with a cholesteatoma over time.[4] The careful and reliable long-term follow-up of atelectatic ears is essential, and whenever this is not ensured, an early surgical treatment should be recommended for minimizing the risk of cholesteatoma development in the long run.

References

[1] Robb PJ. Otitis media with effusion. In: Graham J.M., Scadding G.K., Bull P.D., Hrsg. Pediatric ENT. Heidelberg: Springer; 2007:413–420.

[2] Sadé J. Treatment of cholesteatoma and retraction pockets. Eur Arch Otorhinolaryngol. 1993;250(4):193–199.

[3] Spielmann P, Mills R. Surgical management of retraction pockets of the pars tensa with cartilage and perichondrial grafts. J Laryngol Otol. 2006;120 (9):725–729.

[4] Borgstein J, Gerritsma T, Bruce I, Feenstra L. Atelectasis of the middle ear in pediatric patients: Safety of surgical intervention. Int J Pediatr Otorhinolaryngol. 2009;73(2):257–261.

[5] Alzahrani M, Saliba I. Tympanic membrane retraction pocket staging: is it worthwhile? Eur Arch Otorhinolaryngol. 2013 Jul:27.[Epub ahead of print].

[6] Sadé J, Berco E. Atelectasis and secretory otitis media. Ann Otol Rhinol Laryngol. 1976;85(2) Suppl 25 Pt 2:66–72.

[7] Black B. The collapsed pars tensa: surgical classification and management. In: Magnan J, Chays A, eds. Proceedings of the Sixth International Conference on Cholesteatoma and Ear Surgery. Marseille: Label Production, 2001:267–278.

[8] Tos M, Poulsen G. Attic retractions following secretory otitis. Acta Otolaryngol. 1980;89(5–6):479–486.

[9] Ohnishi T, Shirahata Y, Fukami M, Hongo S. The atelectatic ear and its classification. Auris Nasus Larynx. 1985;12 Suppl 1:S211–S213.

[10] Bours AF, Decat M, Gersdorff M. Our classification of tympanic retraction pockets. Acta Otorhinolaryngol Belg. 1998;52(1):25–28.

[11] Borgstein J, Gerritsma TV, Wieringa MH, Bruce IA. The Erasmus atelectasis classification: proposal of a new classification for atelectasis of the middle ear in children. Laryngoscope. 2007;117(7):1255–1259.

[12] Healy GB, Rosbe KW. Otitis media and middle ear effusions. In: Snow Jr. JB, Ballenger JJ, Hrsg. Ballenger's Otorhinolaryngology Head and Neck Surgery. Hamilton: BC Decker; 2003:249–260.

[13] Politzer A. Diagnose und Therapie der Ansammlung seroeser Fluessigkeit in der Trommelhoehle. Wien Med Wochenschr. 1867;17:244–247.

[14] Sudhoff H, Tos M. Pathogenesis of attic cholesteatoma: Clinical and immunohistochemical support for combination of retraction theory and proliferation theory. Am J Otol. 2000;21(6):786–792.

[15] Pau HW, Punke C, Just T. Tympanometric experiments on retracted ear drums—does tympanometry reflect the true middle ear pressure? Acta Otolaryngol. 2009;129(10):1080–1087.

[16] Sassen ML, van Aarem A, Grote JJ. Validity of tympanometry in the diagnosis of middle ear effusion. Clin Otolaryngol Allied Sci. 1994;19(3):185–189.

[17] NHS-Guidelines. National CollaboratingCentre for Women's and children's health. Surgical management of otitis media with effusion in children. London: RCOG Press; 2008.

[18] Neumann A, Dazert S. [Recommendations for treatment of retraction pockets] Laryngorhinootologie. 2007;86(2):92–94.

[19] Kakehata S, Hozawa K, Futai K, Shinkawa H. Evaluation of attic retraction pockets by microendoscopy. Otol Neurotol. 2005;26(5):834–837.

[20] Plontke SKR, Plinkert PK, Plinkert B, et al. Transtympanic endoscopy for drug delivery to the inner ear using a new microendoscope. In: Felix D, Oestreicher E (eds) Rational pharmacotherapy of the inner ear. Adv Otorhinolaryngol, Basel, Karger;2002:59:149–155.

[21] Cassano M, Cassano P. Retraction pockets of pars tensa in pediatric patients: Clinical evolution and treatment. Int J Pediatr Otorhinolaryngol. 2010;74 (2):178–182.

[22] Jesic SD, Dimitrijevic MV, Nesic VS, Jotic AD, Slijepcevic NA. Temporalis fascia graft perforation and retraction after tympanoplasty for chronic tubotympanic otitis and attic retraction pockets: Factors associated with recurrence. Arch Otolaryngol Head Neck Surg. 2011;137(2):139–143.

[23] American Academy of Family Physicians. American Academy of Otolaryngology-Head and Neck Surgery. American Academy of Pediatrics Subcommittee on Otitis Media With Effusion. Otitis media with effusion. Pediatrics. 2004;113(5):1412–1429.

[24] Gluth MB, McDonald DR, Weaver AL, Bauch CD, Beatty CW, Orvidas LJ. Management of eustachian tube dysfunction with nasal steroid spray: A prospective, randomized, placebo-controlled trial. Arch Otolaryngol Head Neck Surg. 2011;137(5):449–455.

[25] Simpson SA, Lewis R, van der Voort J, Butler CC. Oral or topical nasal steroids for hearing loss associated with otitis media with effusion in children. Cochrane Database Syst Rev. 2011(5):CD001935.

[26] Caffier PP, Sedlmaier B, Haupt H, Göktas O, Scherer H, Mazurek B. Impact of laser eustachian tuboplasty on middle ear ventilation, hearing, and tinnitus in chronic tube dysfunction. Ear Hear. 2011;32(1):132–139.

[27] Park K. Otitis media and tonsils—role of adenoidectomy in the treatment of chronic otitis media with effusion. Adv Otorhinolaryngol. 2011;72:160–163.

[28] Ockermann T, Reineke U, Upile T, Ebmeyer J, Sudhoff HH. Balloon dilation eustachian tuboplasty: A feasibility study. Otol Neurotol. 2010;31(7):1100–1103.

[29] Sudhoff H, Schröder S, Reineke U, Lehmann M, Korbmacher D, Ebmeyer J. [Therapy of chronic obstructive Eustachian tube dysfunction: evolution of applied therapies] HNO. 2013;61(6):477–482.

[30] Browning GG, Rovers MM, Williamson I, Lous J, Burton MJ. Grommets (ventilation tubes) for hearing loss associated with otitis media with effusion in children. Cochrane Database Syst Rev. 2010(10):CD001801

[31] Berkman ND, Wallace IF, Steiner MJ, et al. In Otitis media with effusion: Comparative Effectiveness of Treatments. Rockville(MD): 2013.

[32] Hartzell LD, Dornhoffer JL. Timing of tympanoplasty in children with chronic otitis media with effusion. Curr Opin Otolaryngol Head Neck Surg. 2010;18 (6):550–553.

[33] Minovi A, Venjacob J, Volkenstein S, Dornhoffer J, Dazert S. Functional results after cholesteatoma surgery in an adult population using the retrograde mastoidectomy technique. Eur Arch Otorhinolaryngol. 2013[Epub ahead of print].

[34] Nankivell PC, Pothier DD. Surgery for tympanic membrane retraction pockets. Cochrane Database Syst Rev. 2010(7):CD007943

[35] Yung MW. Retraction of the pars tensa—long-term results of surgical treatment. Clin Otolaryngol Allied Sci. 1997;22(4):323–326.

[36] Yung M, Neumann C, Vowler SL. A longitudinal study on pediatric myringoplasty. Otol Neurotol. 2007;28(3):353–355.

[37] Eliades SJ, Limb CJ. The role of mastoidectomy in outcomes following tympanic membrane repair: A review. Laryngoscope. 2013;123(7):1787–1802.

[38] Saunders JE. Does early surgical intervention of middle ear atelectasis improve long-term results and prevent cholesteatoma? Arch Otolaryngol Head Neck Surg. 2008;134(10):1040–1044.

16 Evaluation and Nonsurgical Management of Chronic Suppurative Otitis Media

James Lin and Hinrich Staecker

Abbreviations used in the chapter:

CSF: cerebrospinal fluid
CSOM: chronic suppurative otitis media
CT: computed tomography
MIC: minimal inhibitory concentration

16.1 Introduction

There are many ways to manage chronic suppurative otitis media (CSOM), but attempting to describe all of the nonsurgical techniques that exist will likely confuse the audience of this chapter. The concepts and methods described here are largely based on the authors' experience, but the budding otologist should develop his or her own management style for chronic otitis media. As such, although we are quite satisfied with the outlook toward chronic otitis media that is presented below, we are not dogmatic about every fine point we describe and assert that the modern otologist is best served by keeping an open mind that allows for constant innovation as our modern collective knowledge of chronic ear disease expands.

The technical definition of otitis media is inflammation of the middle ear space without any reference to etiology, and, in medical terms, a chronic condition typically persists at least 3 months. Although this definition of chronic otitis media is not dependent upon underlying pathophysiology, the primary cause for middle ear disease discussed in this chapter is a dysfunctional Eustachian tube. More in-depth discussion of Eustachian tube anatomy and physiology is found in Chapter 2. Furthermore, other factors relevant to chronic otitis media, such as middle ear inflammatory conditions, microbiology, and cholesteatoma pathophysiology are also discussed in Chapter 12, Chapter 5, and Chapter 4, respectively. Thus, for the sake of simplicity, this chapter will focus on the management of chronic otitis media in terms of a perforation with inflammation of the middle ear space, retraction of the eardrum, and/or cholesteatoma.

We view CSOM as an entity with variable expression of associated signs, including otic discharge, granulation tissue, diseased mucosa, myringitis, ossicular erosion, and tympanosclerosis. Typically, the initiating event in CSOM is an acute bout of otitis media, leading to perforation of the eardrum. Persistent Eustachian tube dysfunction then allows the perforation to persist and the infection to flare up, particularly during upper respiratory tract infections or with excessive external contamination. Over time, the collective impact of pathogenic microbial colonization, reactive middle ear inflammatory mediators, and middle ear remodeling will result in a dysfunctional ear. ▸ Fig. 16.1 depicts the complex contribution of various pathophysiologic entities that lead to CSOM.

16.2 Clinical Evaluation

Whatever the cause, patients with CSOM usually present with hearing loss and foul otic drainage, with the possibility of pain, tinnitus, and/or vertigo, all of which follow a repetitive course of acute exacerbation and remission. Initial examination should include a thorough microscopic examination that may demonstrate disease, ranging from an ear involved with copious pus to a dry perforation. The mucosal disease or inflamed tissue may range from an ear canal filled with an aural polyp to evidence of relatively quiescent chronic inflammation, such as tympanosclerosis, myringosclerosis, ossicular erosion, and/or middle ear fibrosis. Indicators of either current or intermittent middle ear inflammation should be present for the disease to be classified as chronic otitis media.

For patients with an actively draining ear, regardless of cause, the ear should be thoroughly cleaned such that excess drainage is removed and an unobstructed view of the ear is attained; this is typically accomplished by suctioning. On occasion, suctioning is problematic for the patient due to noise and/or caloric vestibular stimulation, and so a cotton-tipped applicator may be used to absorb excess discharge. Serial examination of ears affected by severe inflammation and mucosal disease will better delineate the nature of the underlying ear after treatment has been instituted and the ear has been rendered quiet. Should a patient continue to have infection despite medical treatment inclusive of topical and systemic antibiotics, we typically perform cultures and laboratory testing for autoimmune disease or immunodeficiency.

Careful binocular microscopy of both ears will give the clinician hints about the nature of the particular chronic ear pathologic disease process and the general subtype of chronic otitis media that is in play. For example, a unilaterally diseased ear comprising an intact and mobile pars tensa with associated epitympanic cholesteatoma and scutum bone erosion (▸ Fig. 16.2) suggests an isolated atticoantral disease process. In contrast, a

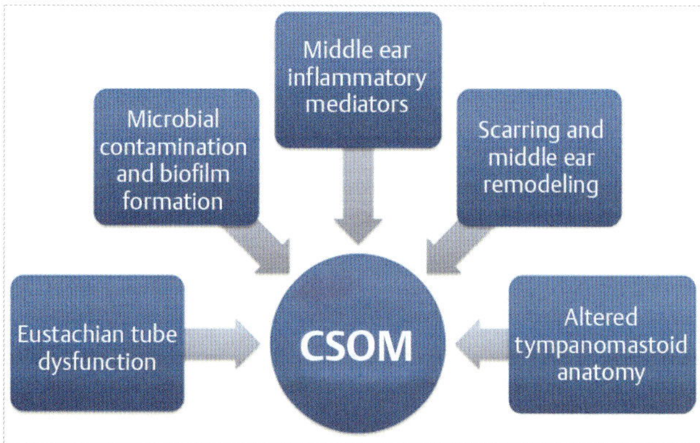

Fig. 16.1 Factors contributing to chronic ear disease.

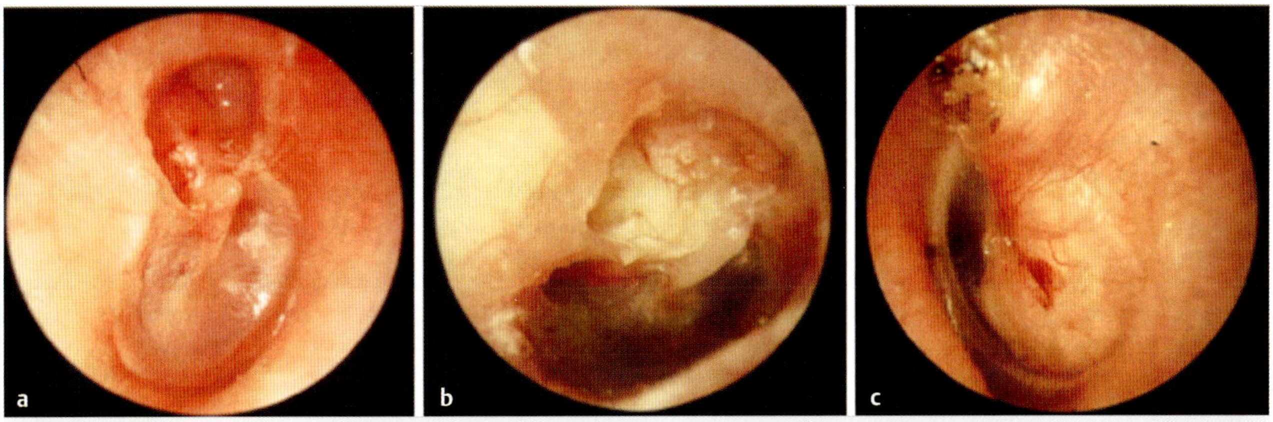

Fig. 16.2 The progressive stages of epitympanic cholesteatoma. (a) Right ear with epitympanic retraction and erosion of the scutum without debris accumulation. (b) Right epitympanic retraction with debris collection within the retraction pocket. (c) Left ear with epitympanic cholesteatoma that has expanded beyond the epitympanum into the posterior mesotympanum.

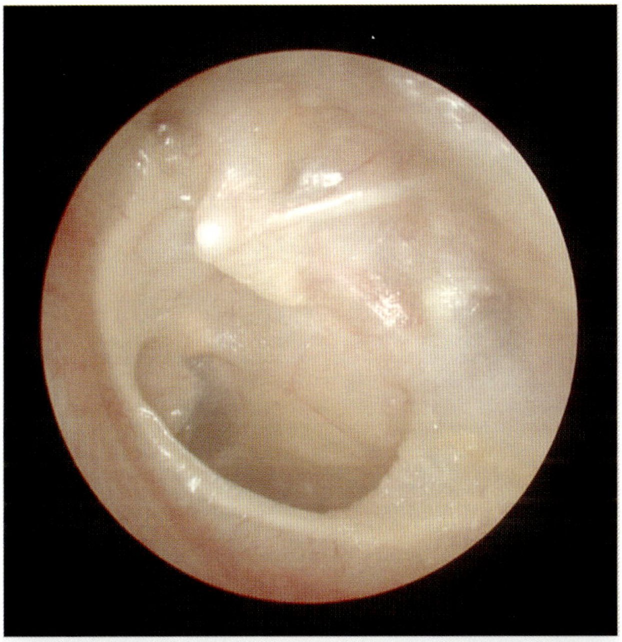

Fig. 16.3 Pars tensa retraction. Chronic retraction of the pars tensa of a left ear has led to a foreshortened malleus and middle ear adhesions.

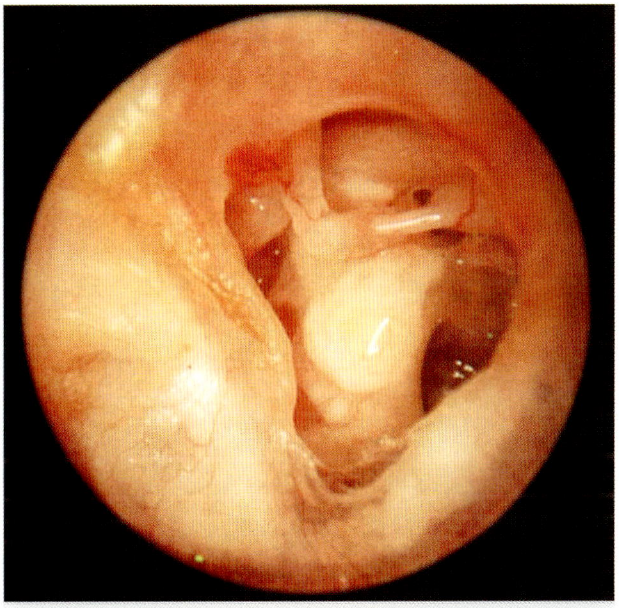

Fig. 16.4 Middle ear remodeling. Left chronic ear with extensive tympanosclerotic changes of the cochlear promontory, oval window niche, and ossicular chain.

severely retracted pars tensa (▶ Fig. 16.3) with an associated contralateral middle ear effusion signifies a more pervasive chronic tubotympanic condition. The presence of tympanosclerotic plaque and dry fibrotic mucosa depicts a relatively quiescent but long-standing remodeling process (▶ Fig. 16.4), whereas the presence of edematous middle ear mucosa and pus (▶ Fig. 16.5) portray an acute suppurative disease process. Notice should be made of any fungal element (▶ Fig. 16.6), which is often associated with retained debris, excessive moisture, and myringitis. Lastly, it is useful to note that an aural polyp (▶ Fig. 16.7) is typically generated by chronic mucosal irritation, most commonly in the form of a foreign body reaction to retained keratin debris; thus, the presence of polyp should heighten clinical suspicion for underlying cholesteatoma.

During the initial visit, we conduct a 512-Hz tuning fork examination in the form of the Weber and Rinne tests. If the patient is experiencing significant vertigo or if there is other concern about the status of the inner ear, pure tone audiometry is obtained during the initial assessment, but otherwise this may be done during the following visit once inflammatory effects have diminished. As a matter of good medical practice, we perform a thorough head and neck examination, paying close attention to the cranial nerves and potential underlying factors that may affect Eustachian tube function, such as craniofacial anomalies, rhinosinusitis, and adenoid disease. Additional effort is made to survey the patient for evidence of a complication, as outlined in Chapter 17.

The majority of patients we treat with chronic otitis media are shown pictures of their diseased ear(s) through video microscopy, and a rudimentary discussion of normal ear function and their pathology takes place. This way, the patient better understands why he or she has a hearing loss and the inherent dangers of ear disease. We believe this improves patient compliance with therapy and follow-up visits and also helps the patient better understand why surgery is being offered.

Radiologic evaluation of chronic otitis media is covered in detail in Chapter 11, but it should be noted that we have a lower threshold for obtaining radiologic imaging than what is taught in some textbooks. In particular, high-resolution computed tomography (CT) scanning is helpful in planning surgery, detecting underlying disease complications, and allowing us to more accurately counsel patients. Although imaging is not obtained in ears that are mildly diseased, we feel that it is quite important for particular situations, such as extensive mucosal disease, clinical findings suggestive of a complication, cholesteatoma of unclear extent, and persistent drainage despite medical therapy, or for patients who have had prior surgery elsewhere, syndromic patients, or patients who cannot provide a good otologic history.

Traditional arguments for not obtaining imaging of chronic ears include the idea that the surgeon should be well aware of his or her anatomy and that imaging is unlikely to change the course of surgical action. For comparison's sake, the most experienced and skilled rhinologist in the world would likely never perform sinus surgery without preoperative imaging, despite a similar risk profile. Knowledge of a potential encephalocele with or without a cerebrospinal fluid (CSF) leak in a young patient would change the management strategy to one in which neurosurgical standby is available if performing surgery in a potential inpatient setting (▶ Fig. 16.8). Knowledge of a potential labyrinthine fistula may lead the physician to recommend a canal wall-down mastoidectomy in advance, which has a risk of poor hearing outcome (▶ Fig. 16.9). A syndromic patient may have inner ear malformation, facial nerve abnormality, or even carotid abnormality (▶ Fig. 16.10).

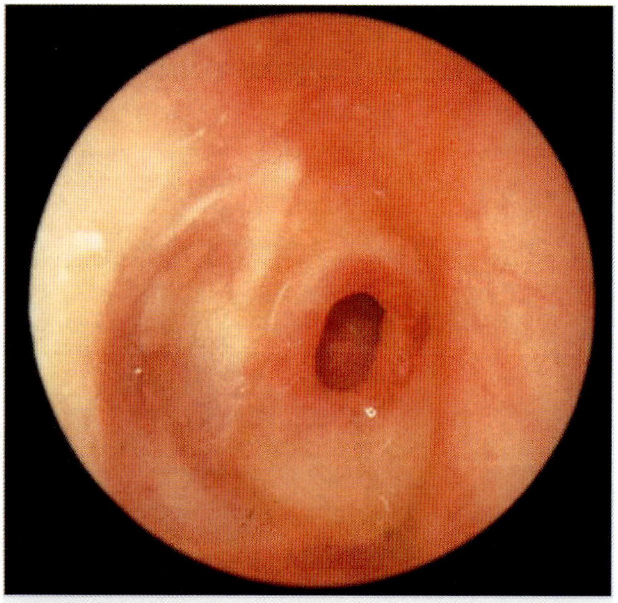

Fig. 16.5 Suppurating perforation. Right ear granulating anterior-superior pars tensa perforation with purulent drainage.

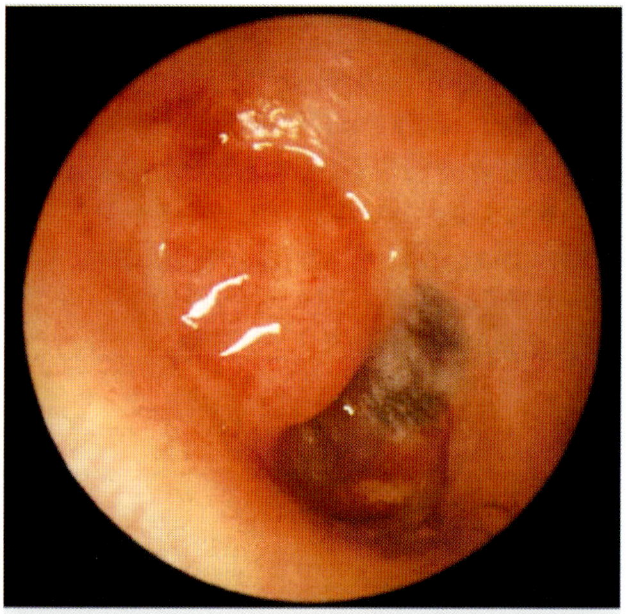

Fig. 16.7 Aural polyp. The presence of aural polyp should always heighten clinical suspicion for underlying cholesteatoma, especially when originating from the posterior-superior quadrant.

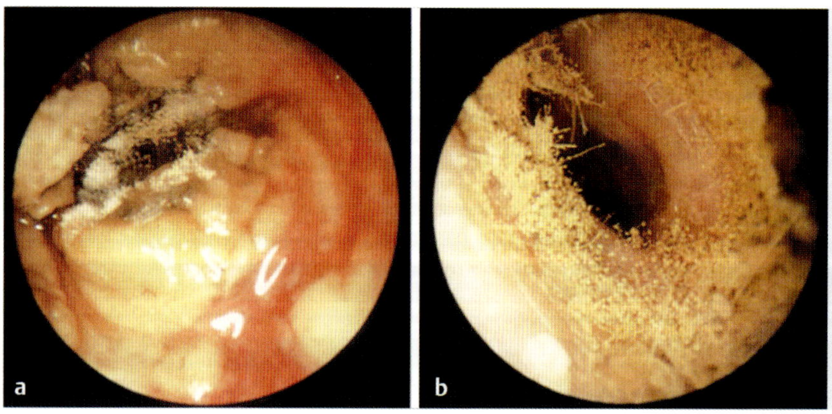

Fig. 16.6 Otomycosis. Ear canals with fungal debris. (a) Extensive pus and fungal debris. (b) Primary fungal colonization of the external auditory canal wall.

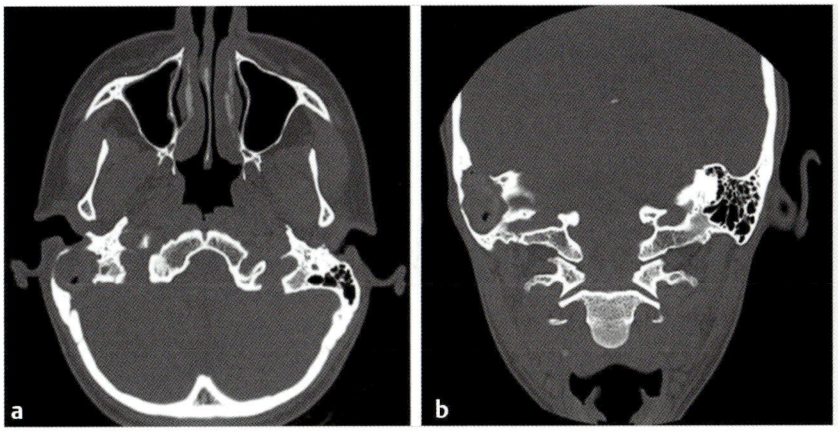

Fig. 16.8 Massive, erosive cholesteatoma. Imaging in cases such as these allows for improved surgical planning including planning and patient counseling. (a) displays the axial view with erosion of the mastoid cortex, ear canal, and posterior fossa plate. The coronal view in (b) reveals erosion of the tegmen mastoideum.

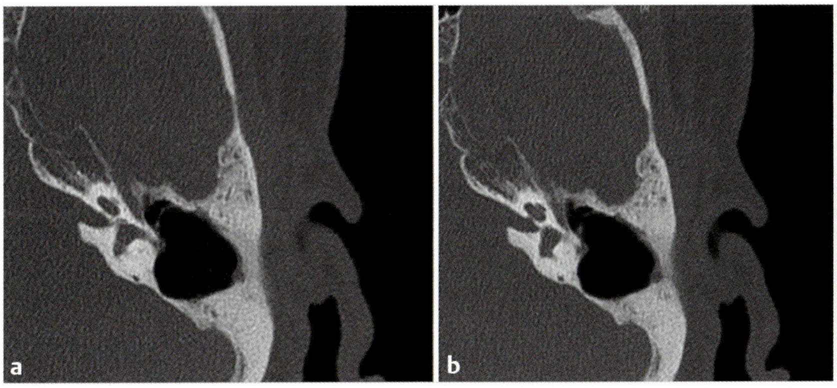

Fig. 16.9 This left ear underwent a canal wall-down mastoidectomy possibly because it was noted that he had a lateral canal fistula. Note the sequential axial CT scans (a; b) with bony erosion and small amount of opacification overlying the area of labyrinthine dehiscence; this opacification is on exam consistent with cholesteatoma matrix left over the fistula.

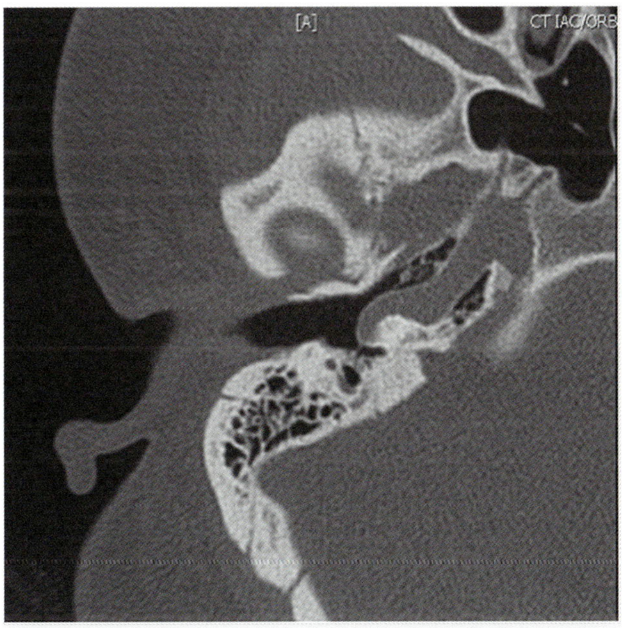

Fig. 16.10 CT scan of aberrant carotid artery. This patient with Down syndrome has an aberrant carotid artery seen in the left ear.

16.3 Medical Management of Routine Cases

After the ear is thoroughly cleaned in the office, we prefer to apply a topical antibacterial agent. If the medial portion of the ear canal is not accessible for eardrops, as in the case of an edematous ear canal and/or an aural polyp, an absorbent wick is placed into the ear canal followed by the ototopical agent. Without evidence of complication, a topical preparation of antibiotic alone is preferred, as the ototopical delivery of antibiotic will afford a drug concentration that will likely far exceed the minimal inhibitory concentration (MIC) of any pathogenic bacteria causing the infection.[1]

Antibiotic powder ingredients

— Boric Acid	16 mg
— Ciprofloxacin	36 mg
— Clotrimazole	36 mg
— Dexamethasone	3.6 mg

Fig. 16.11 Antibiotic powder.

The type of ototopical agent applied varies depending on clinical findings and patient disease manifestations; however, the balance of evidence within the medical literature appears to support the use of quinolones as the primary agent in most cases of CSOM.[2]

In the office, we will often use a powder comprising ciprofloxacin, clotrimazole, dexamethasone, and boric acid, which has antibiotic, antimycotic, anti-inflammatory, and desiccant effects, respectively (▶ Fig. 16.11). This mixture is prepared in #4 gelatin capsules for dispensing in a bulb powder insufflator. Application of the powder insufflator in the office will often dry up a draining perforation that has minimal granulation tissue and obviates patient compliance factors, such as affordability of ototopical drops and their daily use. As discussed below, it is also very effective in cases of primary otomycosis or otomycosis occurring secondarily as a result of prolonged antibiotic or antibiotic-steroid eardrop use.

If such a powder is not available, then twice daily application of topical quinolone-containing drops without a steroid is usually effective in routine cases for drying a minimally granulating ear without evidence of mycosis. In cases of moderate evidence of mucosal disease and granulation, the patient's ear is usually still treated with powder or the patient receives a prescription for a combination eardrop, with both antibiotic (typically a quinolone) and a steroid (typically dexamethasone), to be administered for at least 7–10 days to help decrease the body's overzealous inflammatory response. We typically start the antibiotic/steroid combination eardrops about 3–4 days after treating with powder.

16.4 Medical Management of Refractory Cases

Occasionally we encounter patients who have otorrhea of such severity that the drainage reaccumulates within a minute or two after initial suctioning. Because these patients have often sought treatment from other otolaryngologists and are referred for persistent drainage despite long-term oral and topical antibiotic therapy, they are advised that diligence will be required to dry the ear. Initial management involves vigorous suctioning of the fluid to decrease its reservoir, followed by a generous treatment with powder. We then direct patients to begin a twice daily regimen of rinsing, drying, and powdering the ear, as follows.

Adequate rinsing of an open perforation that does not have excessive granulation tissue is achieved with application of a fluoroquinolone eardrop without steroid (steroid-containing suspensions are not ideal for rinsing because the steroid component has the tendency to build up and "cake" within the ear). However, if the copiously draining ear demonstrates an excess of mucosal disease or an egress of pus so severe that it may impede access for powder and eardrop application, patients are instructed to use a medicine dropper to rinse the ear with a 50:50 mixture of vinegar and distilled, filtered, or boiled water. Vinegar (acetic acid) has favorable antimicrobial properties, but its ototoxic profile is uncertain; therefore, it must be used with caution in the setting of a perforation and perhaps is best reserved for cases in which diffusion through the round or oval window is unlikely due to mucosal disease or granulation tissue. One useful clinical caveat is that patients typically begin to experience pain with application of the vinegar preparation once mucosal disease begins to subside; thus, patients may be instructed to rinse in this manner up until it starts to become painful.

After rinsing, a hair dryer set on a cool setting is used to dry the ear as thoroughly as possible. This is followed by the final step, which involves the application of 2 to 3 puffs of powder. This requires a prescription for a powder insufflator and the powder capsules (this typically must be filled by a compounding pharmacy). Powder application may require assistance from a friend or family member. We see these patients back in 1–2 weeks, and, almost without fail, the ear is dry if the instructions were followed.

Systemic antimicrobials are not recommended for routine use in the treatment of CSOM given that they do not appear to affect the rate of resolution of otorrhea compared with ototopical therapy alone or a combined ototopical and systemic antimicrobial regimen.[3,4] However, there may be unique instances where oral or intravenous antibiotics may be required, such as refractory infection with a unique pathogen, complicated CSOM, risk of complications of bacteremia (immunocompromised or implanted central nervous system hardware), or an excessively narrowed external auditory canal.

16.5 Surgical Decision Making

For each diseased ear, we consider the individual suitability of the following options:

1. Observation with ongoing medical management.
2. Surgery to provide a dry/safe ear and to seek hearing improvement (when applicable).
3. Amplification with a traditional hearing aid or bone-conduction system.

To simplify matters in making these determinations we consider both disease factors and patient factors. With regard to disease factors, we note that diseased ears very rarely lead to complications. Because a major goal of surgery in chronic ear disease is to render the ear safe and to prevent complications, risk stratification is undertaken based on the underlying condition of the ear. In general, a dry perforation or an atelectatic eardrum without cholesteatoma is very unlikely to become unsafe. In contrast, cholesteatoma is more prone to generate complications as it tends to expand and erode bone, thereby allowing disease involvement of the cranial vault, facial nerve, or labyrinth.

For the dry perforation without evidence of cholesteatoma, there are no absolutes for "needing" surgery (▶ Fig. 16.12). Patients are counseled regarding the potential for recurrent otic discharge in the event of an upper respiratory tract infection or exposure to moisture. If the ear cannot be rendered consistently dry over the long term, despite diligent attempts to do so, surgery is more strongly considered. Some patients are not healthy enough or willing to undergo surgery for repetitively draining ears; these patients are given multiple refills for ototopicals and office visits as frequently as every 1–2 months.

Patients with cholesteatoma are in a higher-risk category compared with those without; thus, for all patients with cholesteatoma who are suitable for general anesthesia, surgery is generally recommended. An upfront discussion is undertaken about the rationale for surgery, and patients are informed about the possibility of staged surgery, an open mastoidectomy cavity, and/or future assessments via office exam or radiologic imaging. Because cholesteatoma surgery is much more difficult in an ear that is "angry" as opposed to one that is quiet, effort is spent to dry the ear prior to surgery using the methods described above.

Another factor to consider is hearing because the majority of ears affected by CSOM will have a conductive hearing loss. Some diseased ears may also have a sensorineural loss, presumably due to factors such as the ototoxic effects of inflammatory mediators[5] or the iatrogenic effects of past treatment. An operation on the ear always carries with it a small risk of worsening hearing; therefore, the worse the hearing loss, the more strongly we tend to favor surgical management. If the hearing loss has a conductive component, we discuss the potential for surgical correction in light of the underlying tympano-ossicular status but with the caveat that hearing restoration is considered to be a secondary priority compared with the main goal of rendering the ear safe and dry. For patients with suitable word recognition capabilities, amplification is an option; however, conventional hearing aid use is often incompatible with a chronic ear, and surgery may be required to facilitate tolerance of a conventional hearing aid.

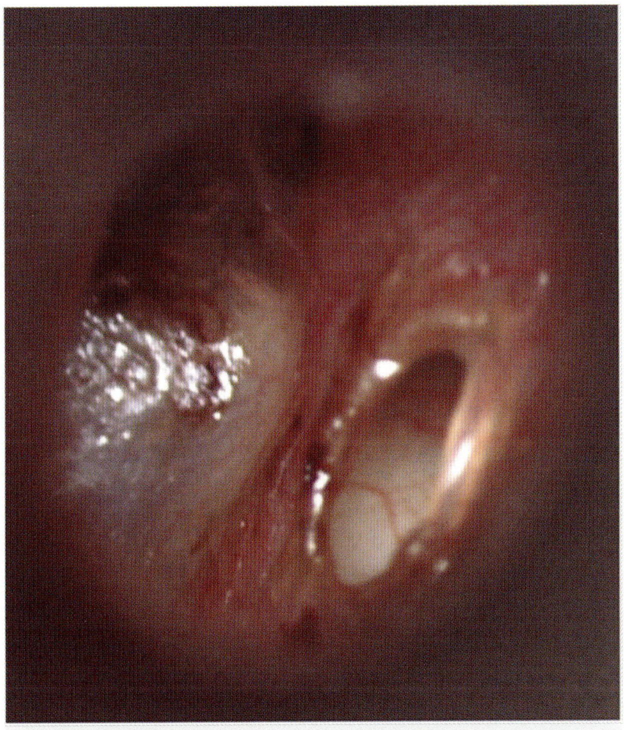

Fig. 16.12 Stable dry perforation. This left eardrum has a posterior pars tensa perforation without active drainage. Such perforations necessitate dry ear precautions and follow-up; however, if it remains dry, the ear can be considered to be relatively safe.

Timing, sequence, and laterality are considered in surgical decision-making with respect to hearing status. For example, if the diseased ear is the better-hearing ear, we usually discourage surgery if the perforation is dry and there is minimal history of infection. If the diseased ear is an only-hearing ear, surgery is only performed if severe infection persists despite medical management or if cholesteatoma is present. If both ears are diseased and require surgery, the worse-hearing ear is usually dealt with first in sequence.

For pediatric patients, repairing the tympanic membrane during the infection-prone years (≤3 years) is avoided when possible. Routine tympanoplasty is considered at age 4 years for an ear that is generally dry if the contralateral ear is normal. However, if the contralateral ear is diseased, adenoidectomy is considered and tympanoplasty is deferred until the contralateral ear reaches stable quiescence or the patient reaches 7 years of age.[6]

Patient characteristics are also important in the decision-making process. First, a healthy patient with a longer life expectancy is generally a more favorable surgical candidate because he or she has a longer period of time for the disease to progress and is healthy enough to undergo surgery and heal well. However, it is important to note that predicting the success of surgery should probably be impacted more by the underlying health of a patient than his or her age. Thus, factors such as suitability for general anesthesia, tobacco use, obstructive sleep apnea/continuous positive airway pressure therapy requirements, immunodeficiency, or other relevant systemic disease should be assessed. Second, consideration of the patient's personality type with respect to other factors, such as tolerance of manipulating the ear in the office and tolerance of the risk of a potential complication (either by the disease itself

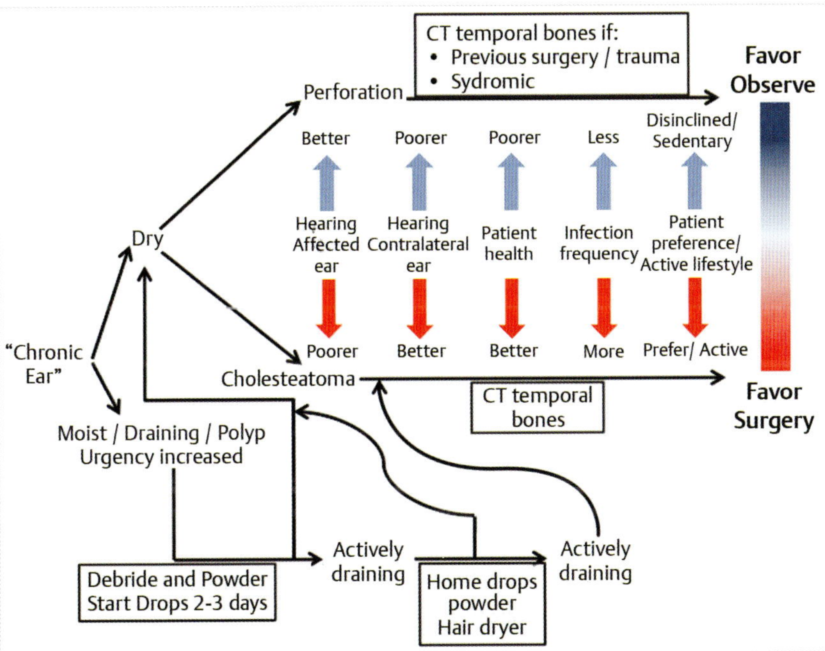

Fig. 16.13 Schema for clinical decision-making in chronic suppurative otitis media.

or by surgery), is useful to assess. Finally, a patient's professional life and lifestyle demands are also important. Active patients or those who enjoy aquatic activities may not only be at greater risk of ongoing ear contamination and otorrhea, but also may perceive a greater subjective benefit from successful surgery. A summary of disease and patient factors can be found in ▶ Fig. 16.13.

16.6 Conclusion

Despite this chapter's attempt at simplifying decision-making and therapy for chronic otitis media, much of patient outcome depends on the experienced judgment of the treating otologist. Otologists must have an open line of communication with patients who have chronic ear disease and gather knowledge of the patient's expectations and desires, while also providing the patient with educational time course estimates of their individual ear disease. In general, disease that has ability or evidence of progression despite medical therapy should likely undergo surgical intervention to decrease the risk of aforementioned complications. Stable disease with detrimental impact on quality of life should also undergo surgical therapy in a healthy patient with realistic expectations. Finally, patients who have medically controllable disease and are unhealthy should likely continue conservative therapy if at all possible. Further discussion regarding surgical philosophies and techniques are found elsewhere in this text.

References

[1] Roland PS, Wall M. Ciprofloxacin 0.3%/dexamethasone 0.1% topical drops for the management of otic infections. Expert Opin Pharmacother. 2008;9 (17):3129–3135.

[2] Daniel SJ. Topical treatment of chronic suppurative otitis media. Curr Infect Dis Rep. 2012;14(2):121–127.

[3] Hannley MT, Denneny JC, III, Holzer SS. Use of ototopical antibiotics in treating 3 common ear diseases. Otolaryngol Head Neck Surg. 2000;122(6):934–940.

[4] Macfadyen CA, Acuin JM, Gamble C. Systemic antibiotics versus topical treatments for chronically discharging ears with underlying eardrum perforations. Cochrane Database Syst Rev. 2006(1):CD005608.

[5] Cureoglu S, Schachern PA, Paparella MM, Lindgren BR. Cochlear changes in chronic otitis media. Laryngoscope. 2004;114(4):622–626.

[6] Friedman AB, Gluth MB, Moore PC, Dornhoffer JL. Outcomes of cartilage tympanoplasty in the pediatric population. Otolaryngol Head Neck Surg. 2013;148(2):297–301.

17 Intratemporal and Intracranial Complications of Otitis Media

Matthew L. Carlson, David S. Haynes, and George B. Wanna

Abbreviations used in this chapter:

AOM: acute otitis media
COM: chronic otitis media
CSF: cerebrospinal fluid
CT: computed tomography
FLAIR: fluid-attenuated inversion recovery
IL: interleukin
MRI: magnetic resonance imaging
TNF: tumor necrosis factor

17.1 Introduction

Prior to the commercial availability of antibiotics in the 1930s and 1940s, otologic surgeons were preoccupied with the treatment of life-threatening complications associated with acute and chronic ear disease. Mastoiditis with subperiosteal abscess was a common presentation of acute otitis media (AOM); approximately one in 20 patients with recurrent infection developed intracranial complications, and as many as 2.5% of hospital mortalities were attributed to advanced otitis.[1,2,3] Radical mastoid exenteration with mallet and chisel was commonly performed in order to halt advancing infection and marsupialize aural cholesteatoma. The discovery of antibiotics revolutionized the treatment of otitis media; disease-associated morbidity and mortality plummeted and, likewise, the need for surgical intervention significantly decreased. The debut of antibiotics, combined with adoption of the pneumatic dental drill and illuminated magnification, permitted early pioneering surgeons the unprecedented opportunity to focus on hearing restoration rather than disease eradication.

The modern era of otologic surgery welcomes a new set of challenges with regard to the management of complicated otitis media. Even at a tertiary referral center, the otolaryngologist may practice many years before encountering a patient with petrous apicitis, otogenic meningitis, or cerebral abscess. The low prevalence of advanced complications combined with the effectiveness of modern medical therapy may contribute to complacency, under-recognition of telling symptoms, delay in diagnosis, and unfamiliarity with treatment. Patients with recurrent acute or chronic otomastoiditis have often received dozens of treatments with ototopical and enteral antibiotics, selecting for greater pathogen virulence and increased antibiotic resistance. Finally, the mounting number of patients with compromised immunity from conditions such as advanced age, diabetes, chronic glucocorticoid use, and immunosuppressive drugs may lead to opportunistic infection and masked symptoms.

Whereas chronic ear disease is the primary focus of this book, the current chapter concentrates on intratemporal and intracranial complications of otitis media, which may result from acute or chronic infection. Following a general overview, a focused discussion of individual complications is presented, concentrating on disease presentation, diagnostic evaluation, treatment, and outcomes.

17.2 General Considerations

Complications of otitis media involve spread of disease beyond the confines of the pneumatized tympanomastoid space to adjacent structures. The development of one complication implies aggressive disease and warrants vigilance to rule out other concurrent or subsequent complications.[4,5] For example, the incidence of labyrinthine fistula is much higher in patients presenting with facial paralysis, and the finding of cerebritis may indicate antecedent epidural abscess or lateral sinus thrombosis.[4,5,6,7] Patterns of complication and pathogen involvement are often associated with the chronicity of disease.[8,9] AOM most commonly involves *Streptococcus pneumonia, Haemophilus influenza, and Moraxella catarrhalis* and is more likely to cause facial paralysis, labyrinthitis, and meningitis. Chronic otitis media (COM), on the other hand, is more commonly associated with labyrinthine fistula, encephalocele, lateral sinus thrombosis, subdural empyema, and cerebral abscess and more often involves combinations of *Pseudomonas aeruginosa, Staphylococcus aureus, Proteus mirabilis, Escherichia coli, and Klebsiella aeruginosa.*

There are three primary mechanisms by which infection may spread, including hematogenous seeding, retrograde thrombophlebitis, and direct extension through preformed pathways resulting from congenital or acquired defects.[2,4] Cadaveric studies have demonstrated that the facial nerve may lack circumferential bony encasement in more than 50% of temporal bones, most commonly within the tympanic segment.[10] Dural dehiscence of the tegmen, tympani and mastoideum can naturally result from congenital growth arrest and herniating aberrant arachnoid granulations.[11,12] Inner ear malformations may be associated with the development of perilymphatic fistulae involving the oval and round windows.[13,14] Anomalous temporal bone development can result in a dilated petromastoid (subarcuate) canal, persistent tympanomeningeal (Hyrtl's) fissure, or patent Fallopian canal, all of which are associated with an increased risk of cerebrospinal fluid (CSF) fistula and meningitis.[15] Similarly, acquired defects resulting from trauma or surgery, as well as bone erosion from acute coalescence mastoiditis or chronic ear disease, facilitate direct unimpeded spread of infection to important adjacent structures.[4]

Cholesteatoma is the most common cause of bone resorption from COM and therefore deserves special consideration (▶ Fig. 17.1). The pathophysiology of osseous erosion from cholesteatoma remains poorly defined but is theorized to result from several mechanisms.[16] Trapped squamous epithelium and keratin debris continue to expand in a rigidly confined space, exerting increasing pressure on surrounding bone. Cell cycle dysregulation results in accelerated cellular proliferation and hyperkeratosis. Additionally, the secretion of nitric oxide and chemotactic cytokines, such as tumor necrosis factor (TNF)-α,

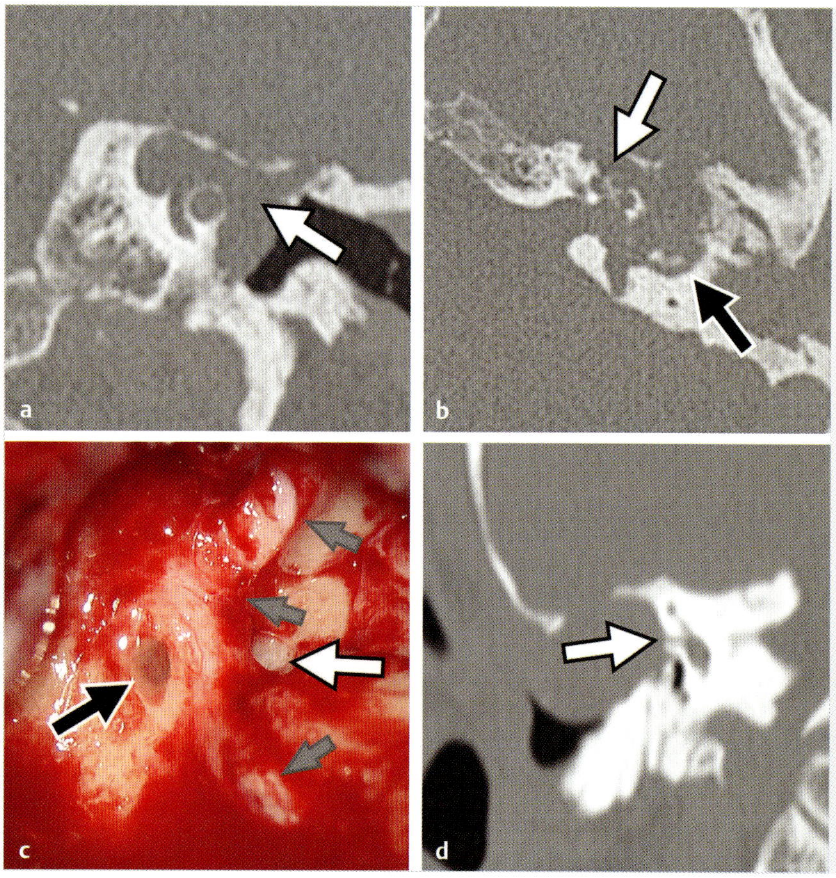

Fig. 17.1 Advanced aural cholesteatoma. (a) Coronal CT demonstrating extensive cochlear fistula (white arrow), invasion of the Fallopian canal, and tegmen erosion. (b) Axial CT revealing erosion of the carotid canal (white arrow) and inner ear (black arrow). (c) Intraoperative view of a right canal wall-down surgery demonstrating a large horizontal semicircular canal fistula (black arrow) and an extensively dehiscent facial nerve (small gray arrows); the oval window is labeled with a white arrow. (d) Coronal CT revealing a large fistula involving the lateral semicircular canal (white arrow).

interleukin (IL)-1, and IL-6, results in inflammatory cell recruitment and osteoclast activation.

Varying patterns of erosion are observed with different subtypes of disease. Classically, congenital cholesteatoma develops within the anterior-superior middle ear cleft, resulting in anterior tegmen tympani dural dehiscence, ossicular erosion, and involvement of peritubal air cells. Primary acquired cholesteatoma most commonly involves an atticoantral disease process, with resultant retraction of the pars flaccida that characteristically evolves into epitympanic cholesteatoma with associated scutal destruction and early erosion of the incus; however, severe posterior pars tensa retraction in the setting of chronic tubotympanic otitis media and severe tympanic membrane atelectasis is also a common pathway for acquired cholesteatoma that, in contrast to the classic pars flaccida version, originates within the mesotympanum. With progression of either version of acquired cholesteatoma, loss of the stapes superstructure, dehiscence of the tympanic segment of the facial nerve, and lateral semicircular canal fistula may occur. Finally, secondary acquired cholesteatoma, which is derived from squamous epithelial ingrowth into the middle ear from a pars tensa perforation, generally involves the mesotympanum, protympanum, and hypotympanum.

All patients suspected of having complicated otitis media should undergo a complete head-and-neck examination, including otomicroscopy and tuning fork testing. Close attention should be given to cranial nerve function, and a fundoscopic examination should be performed in patients with symptoms suggestive of elevated intracranial pressure. Audiometric evaluation should be obtained to evaluate for sensorineural hearing loss, which may occur with otogenic labyrinthitis, labyrinthine fistula, or meningitis. Contrast-enhanced computed tomography (CT) of the head and fine-cut temporal bone sequences should be considered in patients with an atypical presentation or concerning symptoms. Magnetic resonance imaging (MRI) and magnetic resonance venography may be particularly helpful in early detection of cerebritis, brain abscess, and lateral sinus thrombosis. In the absence of contraindications, lumbar puncture should be pursued in subjects with evidence of intracranial spread in order to evaluate opening pressure, cellular differential, protein level, gram stain, and bacterial culture. Early consultation with neurosurgery and infectious disease specialists should be considered.

The treatment paradigm for advanced otogenic complications has evolved considerably over the last century. Contemporary management has been significantly influenced by a combination of improved medical therapy, evolving surgical techniques, and advanced clinical imaging. Complications of AOM without coalescent infection are generally remedied by ventilation tube placement, aural toilet, and intravenous antibiotic therapy. Conversely, COM largely remains a surgical disease. Classically, canal wall-down surgery is performed in order to exteriorize cholesteatoma, permit unrestricted drainage, and offer easy in-office surveillance.[17] However, within the last several decades, the authors have favored canal wall-up surgery combined with aggressive medical therapy when feasible.

The management of otogenic intracranial infection remains highly controversial. Because the morbidity of intracranial surgery may be high in the setting of acute infection, the authors favor initial aggressive medical management of intracranial disease, combined with early surgical treatment of the ear once the patient is deemed neurologically stable. With this approach, craniotomy is often reserved for severe or recalcitrant disease. Regardless of treatment strategy, a multidisciplinary approach, including the otologist, neurosurgeon, neurologist, infectious disease subspecialist, and radiologist, is critical to optimize patient outcomes.

17.3 Intratemporal Complications

17.3.1 Acute Mastoiditis

The clinical distinction between otitis media and mastoiditis is somewhat nebulous because tympanic space infections invariably involve the mastoid air cells as a result of communication through the aditus ad antrum. Furthermore, asymptomatic mastoid air cell opacification is a common finding in patients with Eustachian tube dysfunction. To clarify, acute mastoiditis implies accumulation of walled-off purulence within the mastoid cavity or subperiosteum. Collecting granulation tissue results in antral block, inhibiting drainage of the growing suppurative process. Building pressure may cause the breakdown of bony trabeculae, manifesting the radiologic diagnosis of "coalescent mastoiditis." The presence of such coalescence is often used clinically as a threshold that designates a case of mastoiditis as being a complication of otitis media rather than routine disease extension. Septic thrombosis of the mastoid emissary vein or direct mastoid cortex erosion can result in postauricular swelling, posterior canal wall edema, otalgia, and proptosis of the auricle (▶ Fig. 17.2). Extratemporal spread, involving the various deep spaces of the neck and skull base, may also occur and is described by a myriad of eponyms including Bezold's abscess involving the sternocleidomastoid, Luc's abscess including the posterior canal wall, and Citelli's abscess invading the posterior digastric muscle. In contrast to acute infection, chronic mastoiditis commonly follows an indolent course, presenting with conductive hearing loss, otalgia, and persistent effusion or otorrhea.

The initial management of acute mastoiditis includes empiric antibiotic therapy, covering *Streptococcus pneumonia, Staphylococcus aureus,* and *Haemophilus influenzae*.[18,19] Early myringotomy with culture can assist with aural toilet and directed antibiotic therapy, which may hasten symptomatic improvement and time to resolution. Thin-slice CT of the temporal bones with and without contrast may be useful in guiding initial treatment and evaluating for associated complications. Cortical mastoidectomy should be considered for patients with radiographic coalescence, those who do not respond to initial medical therapy, subjects with evidence of complicated or progressing mastoiditis, and immunocompromised patients.

17.3.2 Petrous Apicitis

The petrous apex is continuous with the posterior petrous temporal bone and middle ear, and consequently apicitis may occur as an extension of tympanomastoid disease. As a result of the unique anatomic position of the petrous apex, several distinct signs and symptoms may arise with infection.[20,21] An envagination of the tentorium cerebelli at the trigeminal impression holds the gasserian ganglion, forming Meckel's cave. Additionally, the petrosphenoidal (Gruber's) ligament creates an inflexible fibrous band over the petroclival fissure and contributes to Dorello's canal, housing the sixth cranial nerve and the inferior petrosal venous network. Gradenigo's triad suggests the diagnosis of petrous apicitis and is described by the constellation of ipsilateral otorrhea, retro-orbital eye pain from trigeminal irritation, and abducens palsy from compression within Dorello's canal.[20,21]

Similar to the mastoid, anterior petrous air cell opacification must be carefully evaluated to distinguish simple effusion, infection, and diplopic bone.[22,23] Petrous apex development is variable; the majority of ears demonstrate poorly pneumatized bone with persisting marrow whereas up to one-third of petrous apices are found to have varying degrees of

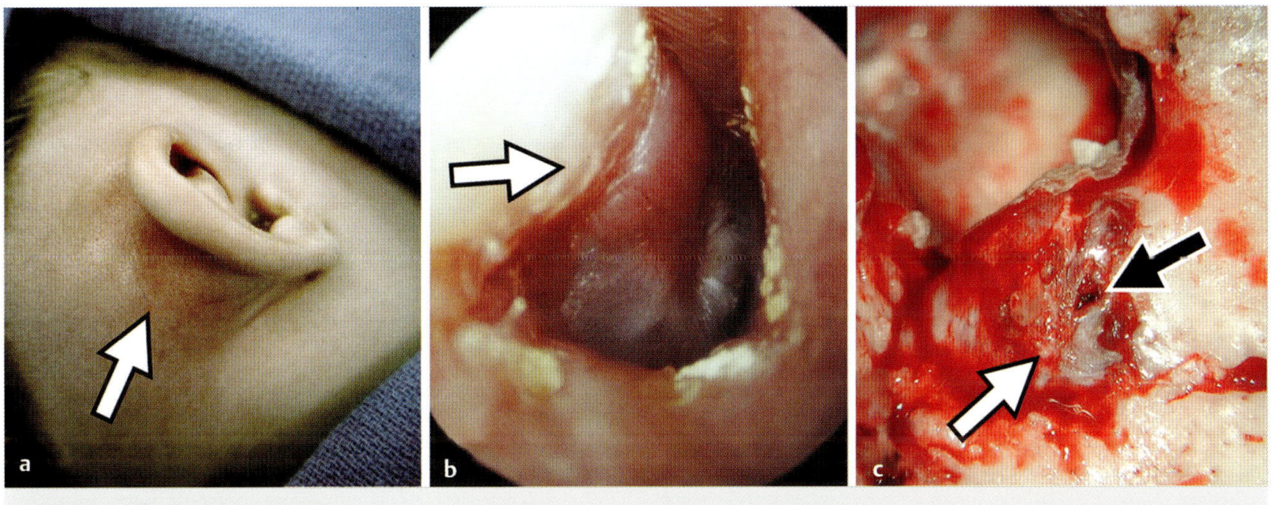

Fig. 17.2 Acute coalescent mastoiditis. (a) Pediatric patient with acute mastoiditis and subperiosteal abscess (white arrow). (b) Otomicroscopy reveals characteristic posterior canal wall erythema and edema (white arrow). (c) Intraoperative view demonstrating mastoid cortex erosion (white arrow) and emissary vein thrombosis (black arrow).

pneumatization, which may be asymmetric in approximately 5% of individuals. Magnetic resonance imaging with gadolinium is considered the workhorse for evaluating petrous apex lesions and is complemented by temporal bone CT. Heterogeneous enhancement on T1 post-contrast imaging and hyperintensity on T2-weighted MRI, combined with septal breakdown seen on CT, suggest the diagnosis of petrous apicitis.

Empiric intravenous antibiotics should be instituted and early surgical drainage should be strongly entertained. Several series have demonstrated successful treatment using directed intravenous antibiotics with or without mastoidectomy and ventilation tube insertion.[24] Depending on hearing status as well as the severity of disease, surgical drainage may be achieved through a variety of transtemporal approaches that either violate the inner ear with sacrifice of hearing and balance function (transcochlear or translabyrinthine approach) or spare the inner ear (infracochlear, retrolabyrinthine, and subarcuate approach). Rarely, if a surgeon desires to spare the inner ear but disease location and/or temporal bone pneumatization preclude one of the transtemporal approaches, a middle fossa craniotomy may be used to access disease; however, this approach does not readily establish a drainage pathway into the middle ear and adds the morbidity of temporal lobe retraction in the setting of infection and surrounding edema.

17.3.3 Labyrinthitis

Labyrinthitis may result from direct bacterial contamination (suppurative labyrinthitis) or from the diffusion of sterile inflammatory mediators across the oval window or round window membrane (serous labyrinthitis). Clinically, labyrinthitis manifests with sensorineural hearing loss, tinnitus, and severe vertigo. Physical examination yields spontaneous horizontal-jerk nystagmus with the fast phase directed toward the affected ear (irritative) in the immediate acute phase, but this usually will rapidly reverse direction away from the affected ear (hypofunctional) within 24–48 hours as vestibular neurosensory function declines. In addition to audiovestibular function, the labyrinth is important because it represents a critical anatomical barrier separating the middle ear and intracranial space. The inner ear communicates freely with the subarachnoid space via the cochlear aqueduct; therefore, otogenic labyrinthitis threatens to become ascending meningitis and, conversely, primary meningitis risks development of bilateral labyrinthitis.

Thin-cut CT of the temporal bones is helpful for evaluating predisposing conditions, such as Mondini malformations or labyrinthine fistula.[13,25] MRI will exhibit the sensitive but nonspecific findings of post-contrast T1 hyperintensity and increased fluid-attenuated inversion recovery (FLAIR) signal intensity within the labyrinth and, in addition, can help exclude other conditions such as vestibular schwannoma and stroke.[26] Patients with fever, headache, nuchal rigidity, and mental status changes should undergo lumbar puncture to evaluate for ascending meningitis.

The distinction between serous and suppurative labyrinthitis is purely based on patient history and convalescence since perilymph analysis is not performed. Therefore, practically speaking, all patients with suspected labyrinthitis should receive glucocorticoids and antibiotic therapy with favorable blood–brain barrier penetration. Early tympanomastoidectomy should be considered in the setting of acute coalescent disease. Patients with recurrent meningitis and congenital malformations of the inner ear may undergo vestibule obliteration.[14] All patients acquiring bilateral severe-to-profound sensorineural hearing loss following suppurative labyrinthitis or primary meningitis should be followed closely with T2-weighted MRI, with consideration for early cochlear implantation at the beginning signs of labyrinthitis ossificans.

17.3.4 Inner Ear Fistula

Inner ear fistula, most commonly involving the lateral semicircular canal, occurs in approximately 10% of aural cholesteatoma and is the second most frequent intratemporal complication of chronic ear disease behind ossicular erosion.[27] Labyrinthine fistula poses an imminent risk to inner ear function. Sensorineural hearing loss may result from labyrinthitis or mechanical injury to the membranous labyrinth during tympanomastoidectomy. Depressed bone conduction, a positive fistula test, and complaints of imbalance should raise concern over labyrinthine fistula and prompt temporal bone CT. However, because inner ear fistula may be present despite normal testing, the absence of concerning findings does not exclude the possibility of disease.[28] Intraoperative findings, including stapes superstructure erosion and facial nerve dehiscence, should indicate an increased possibility of fistula (▶ Fig. 17.1c).[29]

Management of labyrinthine fistula is complex and controversial. Traditionally, a canal wall-down procedure is performed, and the overlying cholesteatoma matrix is left undisturbed. This approach remains the preferred strategy when operating on an only-hearing ear with labyrinthine fistula.[30] Over the last three decades, several centers have reported good success with same-surgery fistula repair for small dehiscence or staged removal at a planned second-look procedure for a large, complex fistula or in the setting of acute inflammation.[27,31] With this strategy, a canal wall-up tympanomastoidectomy is performed, and the fistula is addressed in the final stages of cholesteatoma dissection. After delicately removing the opposing matrix, the fistula may be occluded with bone wax or resurfaced with bone paté or fascia.

17.3.5 Facial Paralysis

Facial paralysis in the setting of otitis media is a rare and distressing symptom for both the patient and clinician. The treatment and prognosis are strongly associated with onset, severity, and duration of weakness as well as underlying cause.[6,32,33,34] Whereas the mechanisms behind facial weakness with suppurative otitis remain speculative, most theorize that nerve irritation and edema result from surrounding osteitis or direct contact in natural areas of Fallopian canal dehiscence, most commonly in the horizontal segment near the oval window. Imposing granulation tissue and infection can result in tracking neural edema, which in turn can lead to vascular "choke" and ischemia.

Facial palsy with AOM commonly presents with an abrupt incomplete paralysis.[33] Thin-cut temporal bone CT should be obtained to evaluate for coalescence and associated complications. Initial management includes empiric antibiotic therapy and steroids. Additionally, myringotomy with pressure equalization tube placement will facilitate the culture and the administration of ototopical therapy. Patients who do not respond to initial conservative therapy or those with encapsulated infection may benefit from cortical mastoidectomy. Because the prognosis of facial neuropathy with AOM remains very favorable, electrodiagnostic testing and neural decompression is not advocated.

In contrast to AOM, the outcome of facial paralysis in the setting of COM with cholesteatoma is more variable.[6,32,34] Seventh nerve paralysis may result from local osteitis, direct neural invasion, and, potentially, from compression. Early treatment with antibiotics, steroids, and tympanomastoidectomy remains critical to a good outcome. Patients who undergo early surgical treatment are significantly more likely to recover normal facial motor function compared to those with long-standing neuropathy.[34] Facial nerve decompression of the adjacent proximal and distal segment may reduce ischemia with little added morbidity; however, opening of the epineurium raises the theoretical risk of introducing infection and is not recommended. Classically, a canal wall-down approach is utilized, and adherent granulation tissue and cholesteatoma matrix are left in place. The authors have increasingly employed canal wall-up techniques with upfront or staged removal of disease depending upon the degree of inflammation and ease of dissection.

17.3.6 Meningoencephalocele and Cerebrospinal Fistula

Meningoencephalocele and CSF leak may result from a variety of conditions, including trauma, prior surgery, and erosive processes such as cholesteatoma and tumor.[35] Over time, recurrent acute or chronic otomastoiditis may thin overlying tegmen, leading to dural exposure and weakening of the meninges. Repetitive dural pulsation, increased intracranial pressure, and age-related dural atrophy may lead to meningeal herniation and CSF fistulization.

Temporal bone encephalocele and CSF leak commonly present with symptoms of chronic ear disease, including conductive hearing loss and otorrhea; rarely does clear unilateral rhinorrhea, meningitis, or clinical pneumocephalus occur at disease presentation (▶ Fig. 17.3).[35,36] In patients with persistent clear otorrhea or effusion, a β-2-transferrin assay should be performed to confirm suspicion of an encephalocele, and a thin-cut CT of the entire skull base should be performed to diagnose and characterize tegmen dehiscence. Magnetic Resonance Imaging is a useful adjunct to distinguish encephalocele from other pathologies, including effusion, cholesterol granuloma, and cholesteatoma.

Unlike traumatic CSF leak, the chance of spontaneous resolution in the setting of chronic ear disease is low, and given the potential risk of intracranial infection, early surgical repair is generally pursued.[35,36] Small (< 1 cm) lateral defects may be addressed using a transmastoid approach, whereas a middle cranial fossa or combined mastoid–middle fossa repair is generally preferred for treating large, multifocal, medial or epitympanic defects. Regardless of surgical approach, an autologous multilayer repair is preferred to synthetic material.[35] Tympanomastoid fat obliteration with ear canal closure may be used in select patients with non-reconstructable defects or multiple-recurrent disease or in subjects who are poor candidates for craniotomy and temporal lobe retraction. Obliteration results in a maximal conductive hearing loss and risks the possibility of "buried disease" and is, therefore, less commonly used in the setting of COM within the authors' practices.

17.4 Intracranial Complications

17.4.1 Otogenic Meningitis

Meningitis is the most common intracranial complication of otitis media and occurs most frequently in the context of acute suppurative infection.[2,37,38,39] Direct extension through tegmen dehiscence and retrograde thrombophlebitis are common causes of otitic meningitis in adults, whereas repeated episodes in children should raise concern over inner ear malformations or other congenital defects.[25,39] Infections are generally monomicrobial, with *Streptococcus pneumonia* being the most commonly isolated organism from CSF culture.

Symptoms of meningitis include headache, pyrexia, phonophobia, photophobia, nuchal rigidity, vomiting, and altered mental status. Whereas Kernig's and Brudzinki's signs are often discussed, they significantly lack in sensitivity, only being present in a small fraction of patients with culture-positive meningitis.[40] A bulging fontanel, fever, and lethargy may be the only symptoms in infants. Computed Tomography of the head

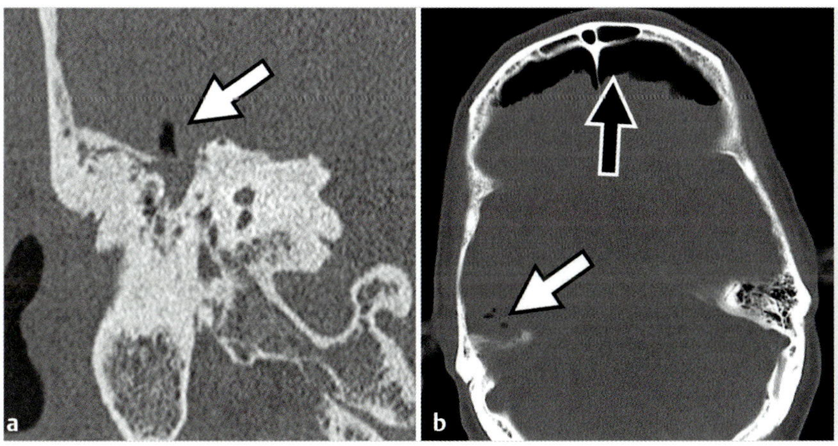

Fig. 17.3 Skull base erosion. Elderly patient with a history of COM presenting with acute mental status changes, fever, and otorrhea. (a) Coronal CT of the right temporal bone demonstrating a large defect in the tegmen mastoideum with intracranial air (white arrow). (b) Axial head CT revealing extensive pneumocephalus (black arrow) emanating from the right temporal bone defect (white arrow).

with thin-cut images of the skull base should be obtained, and lumbar puncture for opening pressure and CSF analysis should be performed. With bacterial meningitis, a negative gram stain and culture may occur in cases of focal meningeal involvement or if cultures are obtained after antibiotics have been administered.

Treatment consists of intravenous antibiotic therapy using agents with good blood-brain barrier penetration such as third-generation cephalosporins and vancomycin. Coadministration of glucocorticoids has demonstrated benefit in decreasing disease-associated mortality and long-term neurologic morbidity.[41] Myringotomy with ventilation tube placement should be performed in patients without tympanic membrane perforation to ensure drainage of aural infection, whereas mastoidectomy is generally considered for coalescent mastoiditis or refractory infection. Severe to profound hearing loss occurs in up to one-tenth of patients with bacterial meningitis, the majority of whom develop varying degrees of labyrinthitis ossificans.[42] Therefore, patients with binaural postmeningitic hearing loss should be followed closely, so that implantation can be pursued at the first signs of ossification.

17.4.2 Lateral Sinus Thrombosis

Suppurative thrombosis of the lateral dural sinuses can result from propagating thrombophlebitis originating within the mastoid or middle ear cavity or from erosion of the sigmoid bone plate. Patients frequently present with headache, fever, otalgia, and fetid otorrhea.[43,44] Edema and tenderness over the mastoid prominence often occurs from thrombophlebitis of the mastoid emissary vein, termed Griesinger's sign. Septic thrombi can become dislodged and shower downstream organs, resulting in "picket fence" fevers. Neurologic signs occur in approximately 50% of patients and commonly result from elevated intracranial pressure, a consequence of dominant sigmoid thrombosis, or involvement of the torcula or sagittal sinus system (▶ Fig. 17.4).[43] Diplopia, retro-orbital headache, proptosis, and chemosis herald involvement of the cavernous sinus.[4] Bacterial cultures in adults commonly reveal pathogens associated with COM, including *Proteus, Bacteroides, Pseudomonas,* and *Staphylococcus*, with a larger frequency of *Streptococcus* in the pediatric population.[43,44] The prevalence of prothrombotic conditions is higher among patients with lateral sinus thrombosis compared to the general population and warrants consideration.[43]

The diagnosis of lateral sinus thrombosis can be made using CT or MRI.[43,44] Contrast-enhanced imaging of the occluded sinus will reveal the empty delta sign, characterized by perisinus dural enhancement with a central-filling defect. Magnetic Resonance Imaging with venography remains the preferred test, revealing absent sinus flow (▶ Fig. 17.4b). Unless contraindicated, lumbar puncture with CSF analysis should be performed. Whereas no longer commonly utilized, the Queckenstedt-Stookey and Tobey-Ayer tests may be performed to evaluate for occlusive thrombosis. Following lumbar puncture, CSF pressures are obtained, first while occluding one internal jugular vein and then the other. Under normal circumstances, jugular vein occlusion should result in elevated intracranial pressure; however, in the setting of lateral sinus thrombosis, ipsilateral vein occlusion will not result in detectable changes whereas the contralateral side will.

Treatment requires prompt administration of intravenous antibiotics and consideration for early mastoidectomy and decompression of the involved sigmoid sinus. Venotomy and thrombectomy of the sigmoid sinus remains controversial; the limited available data suggests that thrombectomy is not superior to conservative sigmoid decompression.[43,44] If venotomy is performed, it is critical to avoid injury of the medial wall to prevent CSF fistula and intradural contamination. Distal ligation of the internal jugular vein may be considered with a rapidly propagating clot or showering septic emboli. The advantage of anticoagulation remains unclear, but several authors have reported benefit with inhibiting clot propagation, encouraging sinus recanalization, and lowering risk of long-term neurological morbidity.[43,45]

17.4.3 Otitic Hydrocephalus

Otitic hydrocephalus describes the condition of elevated intracranial pressure, normal CSF composition, and otitis media.[2,46] Whereas the exact cause remains unknown, it has been theorized to result from increased cerebral edema or venous sinus thrombosis. In the latter scenario, the passive process of CSF resorption through arachnoid granulations is compromised by dural sinus thrombosis. The mismatch between CSF production and uptake results in a net increase in intracranial pressure.

Patients with otitic hydrocephalus manifest symptoms similar to idiopathic intracranial hypertension syndrome (pseudotumor cerebri), with headache, nausea, and vision changes.

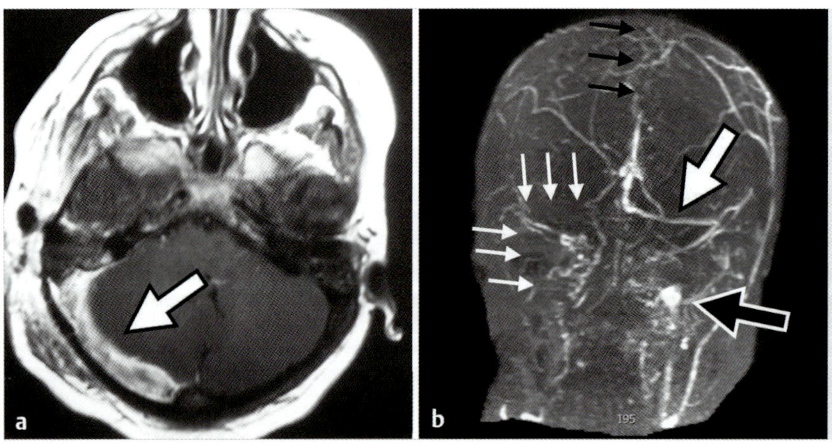

Fig. 17.4 Sigmoid sinus thrombosis. (a) Axial T1-weighted MRI of the head revealing complete thrombosis of the right transverse and sigmoid sinus (white arrow). (b) Magnetic resonance venography demonstrates compromised venous flow of the right sagittal (small black arrows), transverse, and sigmoid sinuses (small white arrows). By comparison, the contralateral left side demonstrates normal venous outflow of the transverse (large white arrow) and sigmoid sinus (large black arrow).

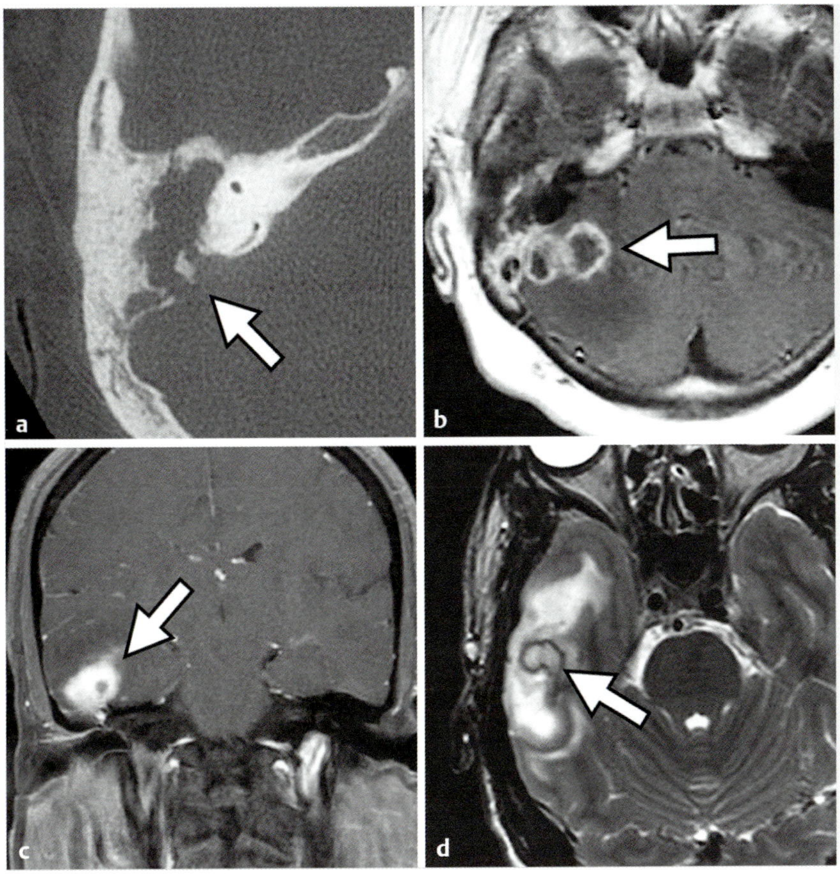

Fig. 17.5 Cerebellar abscess. (a) Axial CT of a right temporal bone demonstrating extensive osseous erosion and dehiscence of the posterior fossa bone plate (white arrow). (b) Axial T1-weighted post-contrast MRI revealing a multi-loculated cerebellar abscess (white arrow) in the same patient. (c) Coronal contrast-enhanced T1-weighted MRI and (d) Axial T2-weighted sequences demonstrating a temporal lobe abscess with surrounding vasogenic edema (c and d, white arrows).

Increased CSF pressures may cause optic neuropathy and cranial nerve six traction, resulting in diplopia.[43,46] Successful treatment requires cure of the underlying infection. For patients with persistently elevated pressure following disease eradication, medical therapy aimed at reducing intracranial pressure (acetazolamide, mannitol, and glucocorticoids) has been used with varying success.[46]

17.4.4 Epidural Abscess

Epidural abscess most commonly results from direct extension of infection through a tegmen defect in the setting of mastoiditis. Given an extradural location, even large epidural abscesses may cause few symptoms; however, progression to involvement of the subdural space, dural sinuses, or brain parenchyma remains a critical concern, warranting early aggressive treatment. Intravenous antibiotics with mastoidectomy should be considered. Once identified, the abscess may be opened from the mastoid vantage, taking care to avoid accidental durotomy.[2]

17.4.5 Cerebritis and Temporal Lobe Abscess

Whereas it was once considered a fatal diagnosis, the mortality from otogenic brain abscess has decreased substantially. However, in spite of such progress, cerebritis and brain abscess continue to carry a high risk of lasting neurological impairment. Localized phlegmon of the temporal lobe or cerebellum may result from hematogenous spread, propagating thrombophlebitis, or acquired tegmen defects associated with prior trauma, surgery, or cholesteatoma. Over time, suppurative inflammation causes focal parenchymal necrosis, giving way to abscess formation. Cultures commonly reveal polymicrobial infection involving *Streptococcus, Staphylococcus, Pseudomonas, Proteus,* and *Klebsiella*.[2,17,39]

Classically, the triad of headache, fever, and focal neurologic deficit suggests the diagnosis of brain abscess. Increasing mass effect results in nonspecific symptoms of elevated intracranial pressure, including headache and confusion, while focal neurologic signs, such as ataxia and nystagmus (with cerebellum abscess) or seizures (with temporal lobe disease), may occur. Such findings should prompt early imaging using contrast-enhanced CT and/or MRI in order to evaluate for a ring-enhancing lesion with surrounding vasogenic edema (▶ Fig. 17.5).

Initial neurological stabilization should take precedence. Aggressive medical therapy, including myringotomy, broad-spectrum intravenous antibiotics, and steroid therapy, should be instituted, and serial imaging should be employed to monitor for treatment response and abscess resolution.[39] Once deemed stable, any unresolved intratemporal infection should be managed with mastoidectomy. The treatment of intracranial abscess remains controversial, with options including upfront resection, repeated stereotactic aspiration, or initial observation with antibiotic therapy.[17,39] In most cases, the authors favor early surgical management of ear disease with an initial trial of medical therapy for parenchymal abscess, understanding that the morbidity of craniotomy in the setting of severe infection may be high, with questionable benefit.

17.5 Conclusion

In summary, the prevalence of advanced complications of otitis media continues to decline, and, with this, so does our experience and comfort evaluating and managing such conditions. The modern otologist faces a new set of challenges. The rising number of patients with compromised immune function and complex comorbidities, combined with growing antibiotic resistance, may select for more aggressive disease. The clinician must pay careful attention to telling symptoms, maintaining a high index of suspicion and a low threshold for evaluation, because a favorable outcome hinges upon early recognition and prompt treatment.

References

[1] Gower D, McGuirt WF. Intracranial complications of acute and chronic infectious ear disease: A problem still with us. Laryngoscope. 1983;93(8):1028–1033.

[2] Levine SC, De Souza C, Shinners MJ. Intracranial complications of otitis media. In: Gulya AJ, Minor LB, Poe DS, eds. Glasscock-Shambaugh Surgery of the Ear. 6th ed. Shelton, CT: People's Medical Publishing House; 2010:451.

[3] Kafka MM. Mortality of mastoiditis and cerebral complications with review of 3225 cases of mastoiditis, with complications. Laryngoscope. 1935;45:790–822.

[4] Dubey SP, Larawin V, Molumi CP. Intracranial spread of chronic middle ear suppuration. Am J Otolaryngol. 2010;31(2):73–77.

[5] Penido NdeO, Borin A, Iha LC, et al. Intracranial complications of otitis media: 15 years of experience in 33 patients. Otolaryngol Head Neck Surg. 2005;132 (1):37–42.

[6] Ikeda M, Nakazato H, Onoda K, Hirai R, Kida A. Facial nerve paralysis caused by middle ear cholesteatoma and effects of surgical intervention. Acta Otolaryngol. 2006;126(1):95–100.

[7] Manolidis S. Complications associated with labyrinthine fistula in surgery for chronic otitis media. Otolaryngol Head Neck Surg. 2000;123(6):733–737.

[8] Leskinen K, Jero J. Acute complications of otitis media in adults. Clin Otolaryngol. 2005;30(6):511–516.

[9] Barry B, Delattre J, Vié F, Bedos JP, Géhanno P. Otogenic intracranial infections in adults. Laryngoscope. 1999;109(3):483–487.

[10] Baxter A. Dehiscence of the Fallopian canal. An anatomical study. J Laryngol Otol. 1971;85(6):587–594.

[11] Rao AK, Merenda DM, Wetmore SJ. Diagnosis and management of spontaneous cerebrospinal fluid otorrhea. Otol Neurotol. 2005;26(6):1171–1175.

[12] Gacek RR, Gacek MR, Tart R. Adult spontaneous cerebrospinal fluid otorrhea: diagnosis and management. Am J Otol. 1999;20(6):770–776.

[13] Barcz DV, Wood RP, II, Stears J, Jafek BW, Shields M. Subarachnoid space: middle ear pathways and recurrent meningitis. Am J Otol. 1985;6(2):157–163.

[14] Desjardins R, Guerguerian AJ, Dube J, Deschamps N, Lavertu P. Meningitis and congenital fistula of the internal ear. J Otolaryngol. 1982;11(2):97–100.

[15] Jégoux F, Malard O, Gayet-Delacroix M, Bordure P, Legent F, Beauvillain de Montreuil C. Hyrtl's fissure: A case of spontaneous cerebrospinal fluid otorrhea. AJNR Am J Neuroradiol. 2005;26(4):963–966.

[16] Kumar A, Wiet R. Aural complications of otitis media. In: Gulya AJ, Minor LB, Poe DS, eds. Glasscock-Shambaugh Surgery of the Ear. 6th ed. Shelton, CT: People's Medical Publishing House;2010:437.

[17] Hafidh MA, Keogh I, Walsh RM, Walsh M, Rawluk D. Otogenic intracranial complications. A 7-year retrospective review. Am J Otolaryngol. 2006;27 (6):390–395.

[18] Anthonsen K, Høstmark K, Hansen S, et al. Acute mastoiditis in children: A 10-year retrospective and validated multicenter study. Pediatr Infect Dis J. 2013;32(5):436–440.

[19] Groth A, Enoksson F, Stalfors J, Stenfeldt K, Hultcrantz M, Hermansson A. Recurrent acute mastoiditis - a retrospective national study in Sweden. Acta Otolaryngol. 2012;132(12):1275–1281.

[20] Gillanders DA. Gradenigo's syndrome revisited. J Otolaryngol. 1983;12 (3):169–174.

[21] Chole RA. Petrous apicitis: surgical anatomy. Ann Otol Rhinol Laryngol. 1985;94(3):251–257.

[22] Moore KR, Harnsberger HR, Shelton C, Davidson HC. 'Leave me alone' lesions of the petrous apex. AJNR Am J Neuroradiol. 1998;19(4):733–738.

[23] Jackler RK, Parker DA. Radiographic differential diagnosis of petrous apex lesions. Am J Otol. 1992;13(6):561–574.

[24] Isaacson B, Mirabal C, Kutz JW, Jr, Lee KH, Roland PS. Pediatric otogenic intracranial abscesses. Otolaryngol Head Neck Surg. 2010;142(3):434–437.

[25] Lien TH, Fu CM, Hsu CJ, Lu L, Peng SS, Chang LY. Recurrent bacterial meningitis associated with Mondini dysplasia. Pediatr Neonatol. 2011;52(5):294–296.

[26] Petrovic BD, Futterer SF, Hijaz T, Russell EJ, Karagianis AG. Frequency and diagnostic utility of intralabyrinthine FLAIR hyperintensity in the evaluation of internal auditory canal and inner ear pathology. Acad Radiol. 2010;17 (8):992–1000.

[27] Sanna M, Zini C, Bacciu S, Scandellari R, Delogu P, Jemmi G. Management of the labyrinthine fistula in cholesteatoma surgery. ORL J Otorhinolaryngol Relat Spec. 1984;46(3):165–172.

[28] Kvestad E, Kvaerner KJ, Mair IW. Labyrinthine fistula detection: The predictive value of vestibular symptoms and computerized tomography. Acta Otolaryngol. 2001;121(5):622–626.

[29] Quaranta N, Liuzzi C, Zizzi S, Dicorato A, Quaranta A. Surgical treatment of labyrinthine fistula in cholesteatoma surgery. Otolaryngol Head Neck Surg. 2009;140(3):406–411.

[30] Carlson ML, Latuska RF, Pelosi S, et al. Evolving considerations in the surgical management of cholesteatoma in the only hearing ear. Otol Neurotol. 2014;35(1):84–90.

[31] Sheehy JL, Brackmann DE, Graham MD. Cholesteatoma surgery: Residual and recurrent disease. A review of 1,024 cases. Ann Otol Rhinol Laryngol. 1977;86 (4 Pt 1):451–462.

[32] Yetiser S, Tosun F, Kazkayasi M. Facial nerve paralysis due to chronic otitis media. Otol Neurotol. 2002;23(4):580–588.

[33] Redaelli de Zinis LO, Gamba P, Balzanelli C. Acute otitis media and facial nerve paralysis in adults. Otol Neurotol. 2003;24(1):113–117.

[34] Quaranta N, Cassano M, Quaranta A. Facial paralysis associated with cholesteatoma: a review of 13 cases. Otol Neurotol. 2007;28(3):405–407.

[35] Carlson ML, Copeland WR, III, Driscoll CL, et al. Temporal bone encephalocele and cerebrospinal fluid fistula repair utilizing the middle cranial fossa or combined mastoid-middle cranial fossa approach. J Neurosurg. 2013;119 (5):1314–1322.

[36] Sanna M, Fois P, Russo A, Falcioni M. Management of meningoencephalic herniation of the temporal bone: Personal experience and literature review. Laryngoscope. 2009;119(8):1579–1585.

[37] Dubey SP, Larawin V. Complications of chronic suppurative otitis media and their management. Laryngoscope. 2007;117(2):264–267.

[38] Migirov L, Duvdevani S, Kronenberg J. Otogenic intracranial complications: a review of 28 cases. Acta Otolaryngol. 2005;125(8):819–822.

[39] Wanna GB, Dharamsi LM, Moss JR, Bennett ML, Thompson RC, Haynes DS. Contemporary management of intracranial complications of otitis media. Otol Neurotol. 2010;31(1):111–117.

[40] Thomas KE, Hasbun R, Jekel J, Quagliarello VJ. The diagnostic accuracy of Kernig's sign, Brudzinski's sign, and nuchal rigidity in adults with suspected meningitis. Clin Infect Dis. 2002;35(1):46–52.

[41] de Gans J, van de Beek D European Dexamethasone in Adulthood Bacterial Meningitis Study Investigators. Dexamethasone in adults with bacterial meningitis. N Engl J Med. 2002;347(20):1549–1556.

[42] van Loon MC, Hensen EF, de Foer B, Smit CF, Witte B, Merkus P. Magnetic resonance imaging in the evaluation of patients with sensorineural hearing loss caused by meningitis: implications for cochlear implantation. Otol Neurotol. 2013;34(5):845–854.

[43] Novoa E, Podvinec M, Angst R, Gürtler N. Paediatric otogenic lateral sinus thrombosis: Therapeutic management, outcome and thrombophilic evaluation. Int J Pediatr Otorhinolaryngol. 2013;77(6):996–1001.

[44] Seven H, Ozbal AE, Turgut S. Management of otogenic lateral sinus thrombosis. Am J Otolaryngol. 2004;25(5):329–333.

[45] Bradley DT, Hashisaki GT, Mason JC. Otogenic sigmoid sinus thrombosis: What is the role of anticoagulation? Laryngoscope. 2002;112(10):1726–1729.

[46] Sadoghi M, Dabirmoghaddam P. Otitic hydrocephalus: case report and literature review. Am J Otolaryngol. 2007;28(3):187–190.

Part 3

Introduction to Surgical Management of Chronic Ear Disease

18 General Principles of Surgery for Chronic Ear Disease

Marcus D. Atlas and Paula Casserly

Abbreviations used in this chapter:

CT: computed tomography
CWD: canal wall-down
CWU: canal wall-up
MRI: magnetic resonance imaging
TIVA: total intravenous anesthesia
VTE: venous thromboembolism
WHO: World Health Organization

18.1 Introduction

This chapter provides an overview of several important general principles that are highly relevant to the safe and efficient surgical management of chronic ear disease. Although a diversity of opinion exists in the otologic surgical community regarding many of the fine points outlined here, it is critical for surgeons at all levels to consider the general themes discussed and to take primary responsibility for assuring a controlled surgical environment according to the existing evidence in the medical literature, official surgical practice standards, surgical experience, and general attention to detail. The author has published in-depth descriptions of the preferred techniques of middle ear and mastoid surgery outlined in this chapter.[1]

Temporal bone surgery is complex and challenging; therefore, it is imperative that a structured approach to each stage of surgery is adopted to optimize patient outcomes. Complications and difficulties that arise in temporal bone surgery can often relate to inadequate exposure or suboptimal operating conditions. Surgeons must recognize and minimize these conditions given that they could increase the risk of complications in advance. Many of these factors are outlined below. Correct patient positioning, local anesthesia infiltration for hemostasis, and correct surgical angles affording wide exposure, with identification and skeletonization of landmarks, are among some of the critical principles for performing effective and efficient microsurgery of the ear and skull base.

Factors that may contribute to a poor otologic surgical environment include the following:

- Malfunctioning operating room equipment
- Defective surgical instruments
- Disruptive noise or commotion
- Operating room staff and anesthesia colleagues unfamiliar with otologic surgery
- Excessively bloody surgical field
  - Insufficient hypotensive anesthesia
  - Poor preoperative local vasoconstrictor medication infiltration
  - Coagulopathy
  - Severe acute tympanomastoid inflammation
- Distorted tissue planes
  - Trauma
  - Prior surgery
  - Tumor
  - Infection
- Unfavorable patient anatomy
  - Large body habitus with prominent shoulder/chest
  - Poor neck flexibility
    - Sclerotic temporal bone
    - Congenital abnormalities
- Inadequate surgical exposure
  - Surgeon avoidance of identifying critical landmarks
  - Lack of canalplasty
  - Inadequate soft tissue (postauricular) exposure
  - Narrow mastoidectomy without saucerization

18.2 Operating Room Layout

The operating room is laid out as shown in ▶ Fig. 18.1. This is the positioning for a left ear. The surgeon sits to the patient's left, with the scrub nurse directly opposite. The microscope is at the cranial end of the table and is connected to a monitor. This must be at a comfortable viewing angle for the scrub nurse, whose role is as vital as that of the surgeon given that it will facilitate ease of instrument transfer and allow the nurse to anticipate what will be needed within the operative field. The anesthetist, anesthetic equipment, facial nerve monitoring equipment, and other space-occupying items (e.g., drip stands) are at the caudal end of the table. This minimizes the number of leads and wires around the surgeon's chair. The surgeon controls the drill foot pedal, and the scrub nurse or assistant controls the foot pedal for the bipolar diathermy.

18.3 Patient Positioning

The patient should be prone and the operating table tilted head up (reverse Trendelenburg). The head is flat on the table and turned to the opposite side, supported by a padded sandbag. The angle between the head and shoulder should be obtuse to allow enough space for the surgeon's hands to work comfortably. The patient is positioned so the shoulder is in line with the edge of the table, and the position is secured with three straps across the shoulders, abdomen, and feet, respectively. This facilitates changing the angle of view by moving the whole table up or down or by rotating the table to or away from the surgeon (▶ Fig. 18.2).

Certain patient factors can make optimal positioning difficult. Frequently encountered conditions include an immobile neck with a fixed flexion deformity, which can affect surgical lines of vision, or obesity, which can diminish the angle between the shoulder and neck and affect soft tissue and the parotid gland. To prevent patient injury and optimize operating conditions, a patient with an immobile neck may need a padded block or head ring under the head. The angle between neck and shoulder in an overweight patient can be increased by gently retracting the shoulder caudally and securing it with surgical adhesive tape.

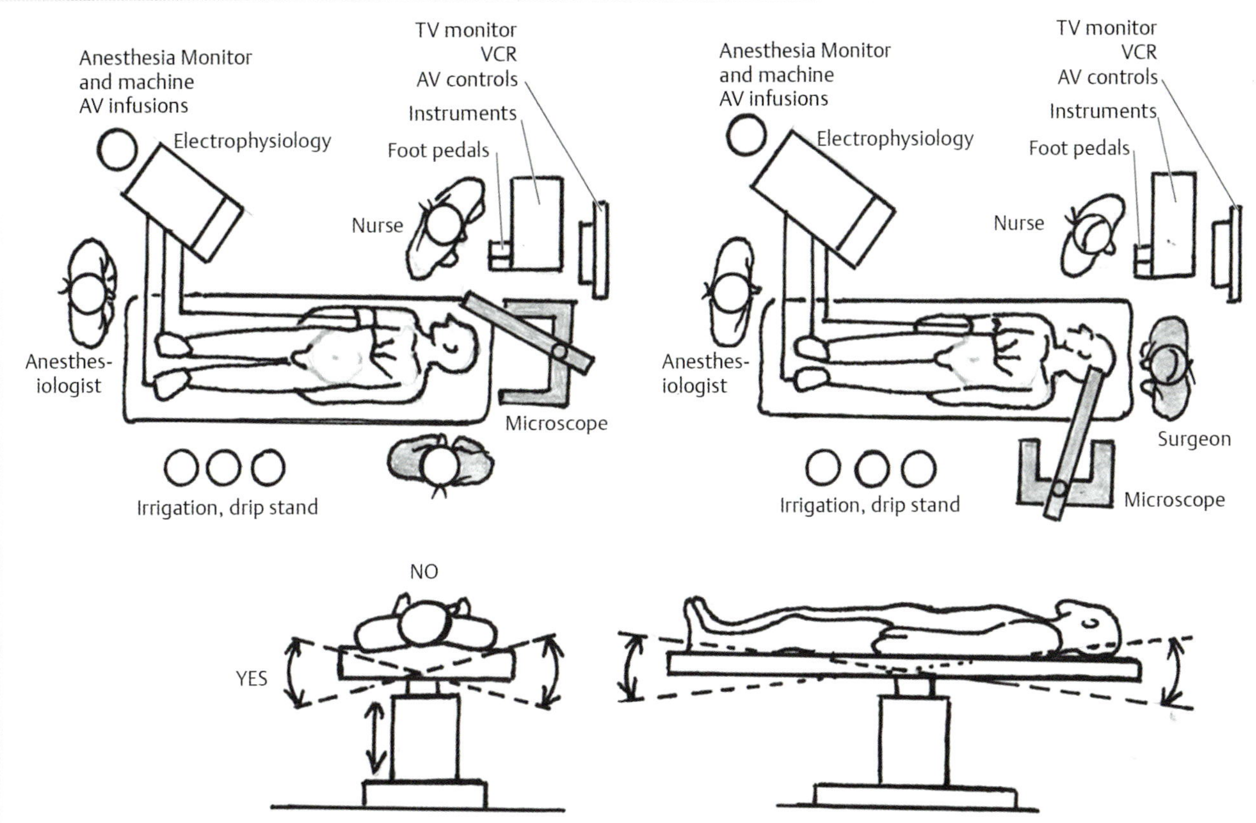

Fig. 18.1 Layout of operating room and personnel positioning for ear surgery. (Top Left) Standard layout for tympanomastoid surgery. (Top Right) Modified layout for middle cranial fossa approach. (Bottom left) The bed can be "airplaned" toward or away from the surgeon during tympanomastoid surgery to change the angle of view into the ear. (Bottom right) The incline of the bed is raised with "reverse Trendelenburg" positioning to increase the height of the head relative to the feet. The opposite "Trendelenburg" positioning may be undertaken during middle cranial fossa surgery to lower the head relative to the feet.

18.4 Surgeon Position

It is important to consider briefly the ergonomics of the surgeon's sitting position and his or her ability to carry out fine movements of the hand under the microscope without difficulty. The surgeon should be seated comfortably. Correct positioning of the operating table, chair, and microscope can facilitate this by enabling the surgeon to sit in the correct position with feet flat on the floor, back straight and supported, and hips at a 90-degree angle. The chair should have wheels and the armrests should be draped to decrease tension on the arms during prolonged periods operating through the microscope. The focal length (typically 240–260 cm) and microscope body size will determine the surgeon's distance from the operative field, and, therefore, will maintain the arms in the optimal position.

18.5 Preoperative Surgical Safety Protocol

In 2009 the World Health Organization (WHO) published guidelines for the provision of safe surgery ("Safe Surgery Saves Lives"). The first objective described in this guideline is the recommendation that all surgical operations are preceded by use of a universal protocol designed to ensure that the correct operation is carried out at the correct site on the correct patient. This protocol contains three steps:

Step 1. Verification. Identification of the correct procedure, site, and patient is checked and documented at every stage of the patient's preoperative assessment, including when the procedure is initially scheduled, at the time of the patient's entry to the operating room, at any stage when the patient's care is being transferred to another person, and before the patient leaves the operating room.

Step 2. Marking. The patient must be marked at the operative site with a clear unambiguous mark using a marking agent that will allow the mark to remain visible during the patient's preparation for surgery. The mark should be made by the surgeon performing the operation or a delegate who will be present during surgery.

Step 3. Time Out. A short pause, often referred to as a surgical pause or team time out, should take place immediately before the operation commences. All team members should be involved to allow any concerns or inconsistencies to be raised.

In our unit we follow a five-step process, similar to that described above, recommended by The Australian Commission on Safety and Quality in Healthcare[2] that also requires confirmation that appropriate and available diagnostic imaging is available in the operating theatre. This protocol has been shown

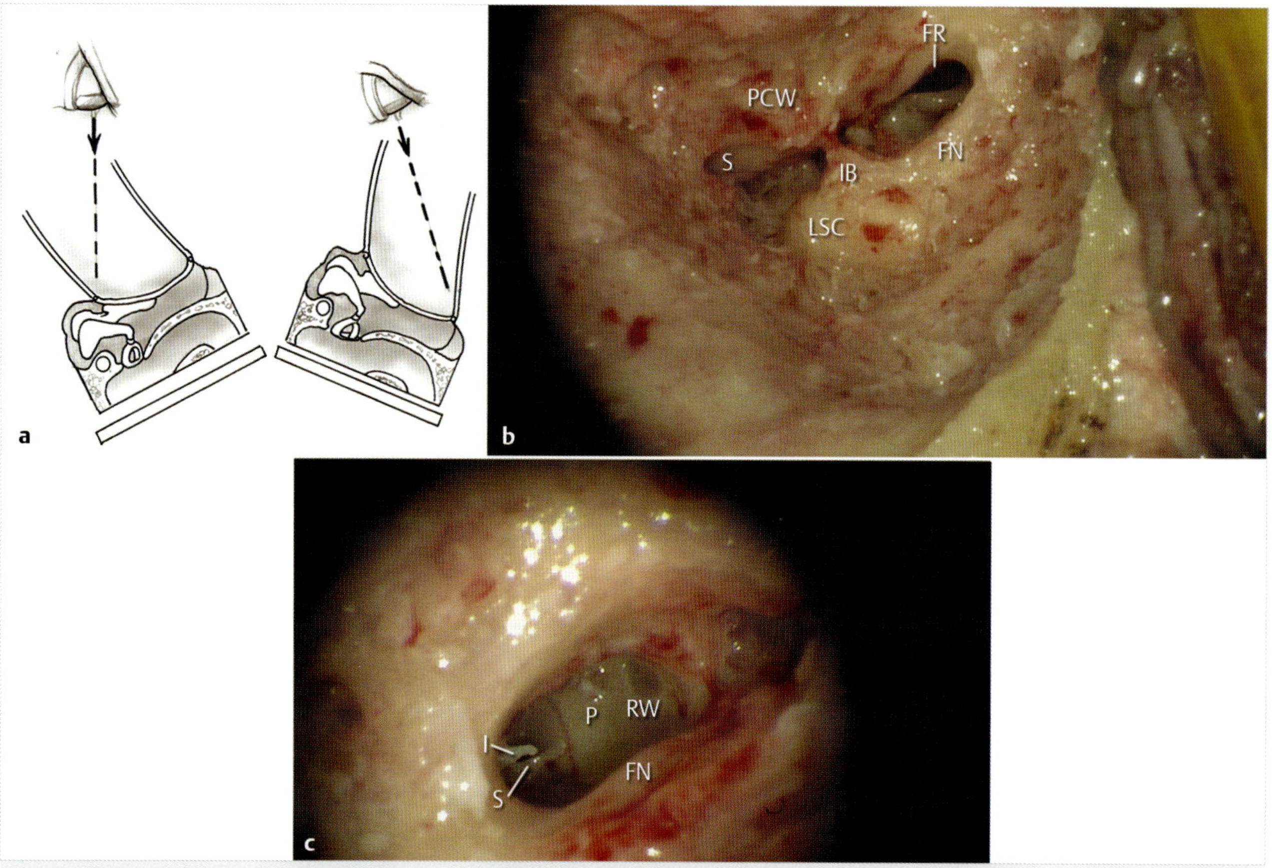

Fig. 18.2 (a) View down microscope with accompanying diagram of table position. The angle of rotation impacts the view into the (b) facial recess (S, short process of incus; PCW, posterior canal wall; IB, incus buttress; LSC, lateral semicircular canal; FN, facial nerve; FR, facial recess) and (c) round window niche (RW, round window; P, promontory; FN, facial nerve (in Fallopian canal); S, stapes; I, Incus (long crus)).

to reduce the incidence of wrong-site surgery in Western Australia.[3]

18.6 Preparation and Draping of Operative Site

A 10% povidone-iodine solution is used to prepare the surgical site. Judicious hair clipping is undertaken to prevent hair from interfering with the operation and is limited to the incision site. The remaining hair is brushed out of the surgical field. Hair removal preoperatively does not seem to reduce the rate of surgical site infection.[4] Specifically, a randomized controlled trial comparing the rate of surgical site infections in ear surgery between groups, with and without hair removal, has demonstrated that hair removal prior to surgery via a postauricular incision had no effect on the rate of surgical site infection.[5]

The surgical site is draped in layers, and measures are taken to ensure the drapes are effectively adherent to the skin to prevent irrigation fluid leaking into the non-sterile area. Four sterile absorbable cotton towels create an initial square drape. An otologic ENT split drape with adhesive edges forms the second layer. An irrigation pouch is secured to the split drape. The pinna is reflected forward and held in position with an adhesive antimicrobial incision drape. Once the initial skin flaps have been raised, they are retracted out of the surgical field with a posterior blanket suture through the drapes and skin (▶ Fig. 18.3).

18.7 Anesthesia

The type of anesthesia used depends on both patient factors and the type of surgery planned. The authors use general anesthesia for most ear surgery and consider it preferable for operations that include significant bone work. Local anesthesia can be used successfully in several areas of otology, particularly for stapes and middle ear surgery[6,7] and, more recently, for cochlear implantation.[8]

18.7.1 General Anesthesia

Traditionally, induction of general anesthesia involves use of both inhalational and intravenous agents; however, some inhalational drugs, particularly nitrous oxide, have been shown to alter middle ear pressure.[9] This may increase the risk of surgical complications during or after ear surgery by inflating the middle ear space and causing graft detachment. Avoidance of inhalation anesthetic agents is therefore preferable for otologic procedures, with the lone exception of temporary usage during induction specifically in cases with tympanic membrane

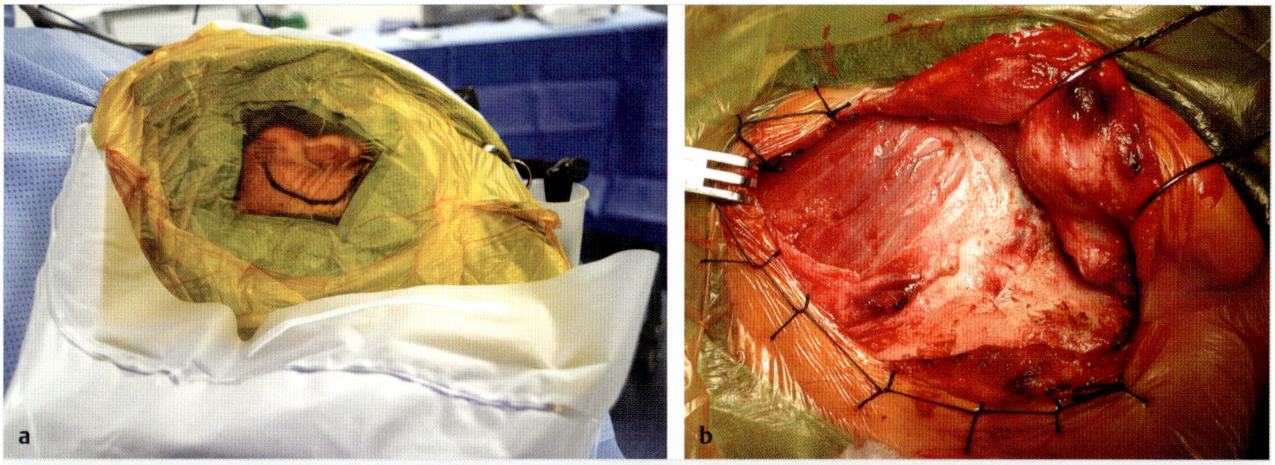

Fig. 18.3 Prepped and draped operative site. (a) As a final layer, an adhesive antimicrobial drape is placed to hold the pinna of a left ear forward and to expose the postauricular skin prior to incision. The adhesive drape passes into the irrigation pouch, thereby providing a watertight sealed junction so that irrigation fluid is properly contained. (b) A large piece of temporalis fascia has been harvested from this right ear prior to planned canal wall-down mastoid surgery. The soft tissues are held out of the surgical field with a running locking silk blanket suture and the pinna is reflected forward with the assistance of blunt hooked retractors.

atelectasis as a means of promoting outward eversion of the retracted drumhead.

At our institution, the combination of remifentanil and propofol is preferred for general anesthesia. Anesthesia is induced with propofol and remifentanil and maintained with 40% oxygen and 60% air, together with propofol and remifentanil. Total intravenous anesthesia (TIVA) not only avoids inducing pressure changes in the middle ear, but also facilitates maintenance of hypotensive anesthesia. The combined use of both a centrally-acting sedative (frequently a potent opiate, such as remifentanil, or a benzodiazepine, such as midazolam) with an intravenous anesthetic agent (such as propofol) allows for effective anesthesia to be achieved. Agents such as those highlighted above have desirable pharmacokinetic properties, with rapid onset and offset of effect, and a favorable adverse event risk, particularly in relation to optimizing the condition of the surgical field and minimizing nausea in the postoperative period.[10]

Hypotensive anesthesia, defined as the use of anesthetic agents to achieve a systolic blood pressure during surgery of 80–90 mm Hg or a mean arterial pressure of 50–65 mmHg, is often used in ear surgery with the aim of reducing bleeding during surgery to maintain a bloodless field.[11] Hypotensive anesthesia can be achieved with several different inhalational and intravenous agents. Cardiovascular active medications, such as sodium nitroprusside, clonidine, or nifedipine, or beta-adrenergic receptor antagonists, such as esmolol, can be used concurrently with anesthetic agents to achieve appropriate blood pressure and heart rate control. However, continuous monitoring of cardiovascular status and urine output intraoperatively and during the postoperative period is required with the use of these agents. This may involve use of central venous pressure catheters and intra-arterial catheters in some patient groups, including those undergoing surgical procedures with longer duration of anesthesia or those with additional comorbidities.

18.7.2 Local Anesthesia

Local anesthesia infiltration is undertaken for all otologic procedures. Local anesthetic agents produce a reversible block in the transmission of impulses along nerve fibers and, when used in combination with a vasoconstrictor, reduce the risk of systemic toxicity and intraoperative bleeding and prolong duration of action. Local anesthetic agents vary in terms of their potency and toxicity. Both lidocaine and bupivacaine are vasodilating amides available in injectable forms. Lidocaine can be administered to a maximum dose of 3 mg/kg or 7 mg/kg with adrenaline. The maximum dose of bupivacaine is 2 mg/kg or 3 mg/kg with adrenaline.

Complications are rare but may be potentially serious and are related either to toxicity or hypersensitivity. Manifestations of toxicity typically start as the drug is being administered or directly afterward and include cardiovascular complications, such as hypotension, bradycardia, or cardiac arrest, or neurological complications, such as seizures or coma. Recognition of impending toxicity requires immediate cessation of drug administration and may require monitoring in a High Dependency Unit in cases of severe, non-self-limiting reactions. For procedures carried out under general anesthetic, we use a solution of 0.5% lidocaine with 1:100,000 adrenaline. A higher concentration of 2% lidocaine is used when the procedure is carried out under local anesthesia.

Knowledge of the sensory innervation of the ear is necessary to achieve thorough local anesthesia. Four sensory nerves predominantly supply the external ear and external auditory canal: the greater auricular nerve, the auriculotemporal nerve, the lesser occipital nerve, and the auricular branch of the vagus nerve.

The greater auricular nerve (C2–3 branches of the cervical plexus) supplies the lower two-thirds of the anterior and posterior external ear. The auriculotemporal nerve (branch of V3) supplies the anterior superior one-third of the ear (tragus, crus

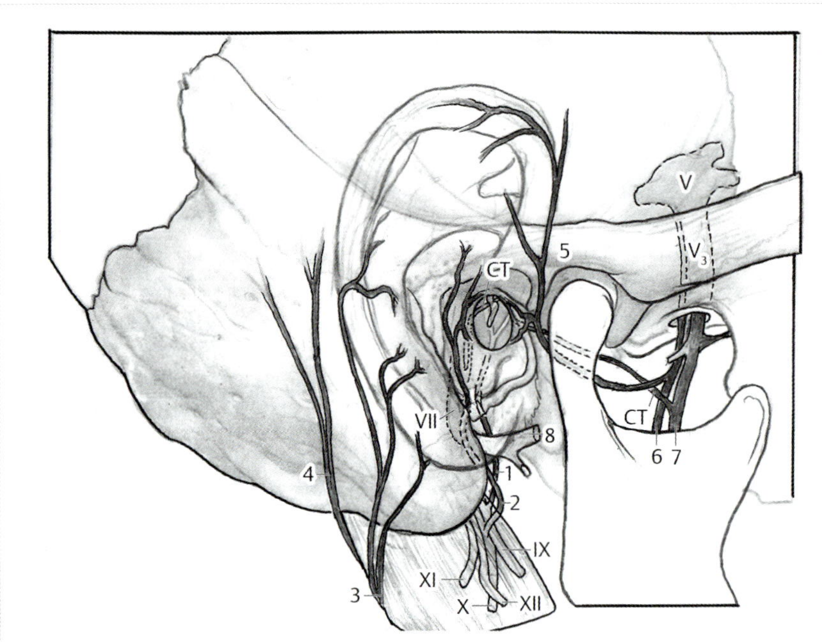

Fig. 18.4 Illustration of innervation of the ear. 1, auricular branch of CN IX; 2, auricular branch of CN X; 3, greater auricular n.; 4, lesser occipital n.; 5, auriculotemporal branch of CN V; 6, inferior alveolar n.; 7, lingual n. and chorda tympani n.; 8, CN VII (facial nerve).

helix, superior helix) and provides sensory information from the anterior wall and roof of the external auditory canal. The lesser occipital nerve (C2 branch of the cervical plexus) supplies sensory information from the posterior surface of the superior one-third of the external ear. The auricular branch of the vagus nerve (Arnold nerve) innervates the concha and posterior wall and floor of the external auditory canal. Small branches from the facial nerve contribute to the sensory innervation of the concha and the roof of the external auditory canal (▶ Fig. 18.4).

Effective anesthesia can be obtained by infiltrating the postauricular region and four-quadrant infiltration of the cartilaginous canal, with particular attention to the "vascular strip" of the posterior-superior aspect. Injection of local anesthetic is important for assisting in hemostasis during surgical dissection, and effective infiltration is vital (see "Control of the Surgical Field," below). The needle is advanced in an anterior direction from the level of the postauricular incision, and local anesthetic is administered by continuous infiltration at the level of the periosteum. This continues to the level of the posterior external auditory canal skin. Infiltration continues anterior-superiorly and anterior-inferiorly. Local anesthetic is also injected superiorly at the site of the temporalis muscle, inferior to the mastoid tip and anteriorly around the zygomatic arch.

18.8 Preoperative Imaging

Despite much clinical interest, development of new imaging techniques, accumulated clinical trial information, and consensus statements from national and international expert groups, there is still no universally accepted role for individual imaging modalities, nor indeed of imaging in general, prior to ear surgery. Radiologic imaging of the chronic ear is covered in detail in Chapter 11. We believe that present-day imaging techniques play a vital role in diagnosis and treatment planning. Although individual clinical trials have not been able to show a benefit for routine preoperative imaging, many expert bodies recommend it based on its usefulness for identifying complications of middle ear disease in some patients.[12] In addition, imaging techniques, such as magnetic resonance imaging (MRI), are increasingly used to refine clinical decision-making in selected cases, particularly in patients undergoing revision procedures for cholesteatoma.

High resolution computed tomography (CT) imaging prior to proposed ear surgery in patients with a clinical diagnosis of cholesteatoma should provide information on the degree of ventilation present in the middle ear and whether erosion of the ossicular chain or the labyrinth is present. The status of the facial nerve should be noted as well as any anatomical changes that are present due to previous surgery. Imaging before ear surgery is also carried out when there is a clinical suspicion of complications of middle ear disease. MRI scanning may be a necessary adjunct to CT scanning to identify complications of labyrinthine, facial nerve, and tegmen erosion seen on the CT scan (e.g., labyrinthitis, temporal bone meningocele, or encephalocele). MRI, often with magnetic resonance venography, is indicated if meningo-encephalitic complications are suspected or if sigmoid sinus thrombosis is suspected.

18.9 Facial Nerve Monitoring

There is no clear international consensus regarding the routine use of facial nerve monitoring during surgery for chronic ear disease.[13] The current evidence suggests that intraoperative facial nerve monitoring is of value for identifying the facial nerve, which is at surgical risk during middle ear and mastoid surgery, and that it is also cost-effective.[14,15]

Although systematic use of the facial nerve monitor is not current practice in our department, we generally recommend it for all trainee otologists and as a useful adjunct in complex or revision surgery. In particular, we recommend routine facial nerve monitoring in cases where significant abnormal anatomy is known to be present, in cases related to congenital abnormalities, and in all neurotologic skull base surgical cases.

18.10 Principles of Soft Tissue Exposure

18.10.1 The Postauricular Skin Incision

For the majority of tympanomastoid surgeries, we favor a postauricular skin incision. This is a C-shaped incision, just inside the hairline, extending from the mastoid tip inferiorly to a point superiorly, in line with the tragus. This posteriorly based incision keeps it behind the surgical cavity. It provides excellent exposure of the posterior soft tissues and structures of the middle ear and mastoid. Anterior extension of the incision is necessary to adequately expose the anterior canal wall and attic. Placement of the incision just behind the postauricular hairline results in the healed incision being mostly invisible and avoids postauricular contracture. The skin is incised to the level of the temporalis muscle, and the skin flaps are raised at this level and advanced anteriorly to the level of the external auditory canal.

The temporalis fascia is a commonly used autologous graft in surgery for chronic ear disease. Two layers of graft material can be harvested: the loose areolar tissue overlying the fascia and the fascia itself. The temporalis fascia is harvested from the surface of the temporalis muscle, avoiding the anterior area where fascia may be required for an endaural procedure for ossiculoplasty.

The middle temporal artery flap provides an excellent vascularized soft tissue flap for mastoid cavity obliteration (see Chapter 41). The middle temporal artery arises from a branch of the superficial temporal artery at the root of the zygoma. The temporalis muscle is reflected anteriorly to expose the underlying periosteum and artery. The periosteal flap is incised and elevated in an anterior and inferior direction. This axial flap is typically around 5 cm in length but can extended further superiorly if required.[16]

An inferior muscular and periosteal flap is also used in modified radical mastoidectomy surgery and is based on branches of the occipital artery and postauricular artery. The flap is inferiorly based and extends superiorly, posterior to the external auditory meatus, and inclines posteriorly along the border of the temporalis muscle, avoiding dissection of the muscle or middle temporal artery. The flap is created with a wide base that narrows superiorly and extends into the neck to allow placement into the mastoid cavity.[1]

18.10.2 The Endaural Incision

An endaural incision is used predominately when no extensive bone work is needed, such as when performing ossicular reconstruction, myringoplasty, stapes surgery, or second-stage ossiculoplasty after mastoid surgery. The body of the auricle is formed by elastic fibrocartilage, which forms a continuous plate, except for the area between the tragus and the anterior crux of the helix, where it is replaced by dense fibrous tissue. This is the site of the endaural incision (terminal incisure), where it will not damage the cartilage or perichondrium and will allow access to the medial component of the external auditory canal by splitting the soft tissue ring surrounding the bony canal. In most cases that require an endaural approach, it is not necessary to extend the external skin incision beyond the natural skin crease of the terminal incisure; thus, a conspicuous external scar is almost always avoided (▶ Fig. 18.5).

18.11 Principles of Bony Exposure

Written descriptions of the key principles that underlie safe and effective drilling cannot replace the accumulation of hands-on experience obtained by drilling in a temporal bone laboratory. However, a number of important factors that enhance drilling safety should remain uppermost in the otologist's mind when commencing temporal bone surgery.

Principles of modified radical mastoidectomy are complete elimination of all diseased air cell tracts, cavity obliteration with soft tissue flaps (when deemed safe due to lack of underlying cholesteatoma risk), and adequate contouring of the mastoid cavity. If all steps are properly performed, the resultant cavity should be small, dry, and well epithelialized. The steps of proper canal wall-down (CWD) mastoid surgery (Chapter 35) and mastoid cavity obliteration (Chapter 41) are described elsewhere in this textbook.

Canal wall-up (CWU) mastoidectomy (Chapter 33) likewise involves clearance of all diseased air cell tracts and wide lateral exposure of the entire epitympanum; however, the degree to which this is possible will be influenced by the degree of temporal bone pneumatization and whether or not the ossicular chain remains intact. Excessive thinning and burning of the intact posterior and superior canal wall bone must be avoided to prevent delayed canal wall bone loss. Canal Wall-Up mastoidectomy can be combined with a posterior tympanotomy via the facial recess when exposure to the mesotympanum is required, which will variably include sacrifice of the incus buttress and/or chorda tympani nerve depending on the status of the ossicular chain and degree of exposure required. Proper execution of CWU mastoid surgery will almost always require the extensive skeletonization of the middle cranial fossa dura

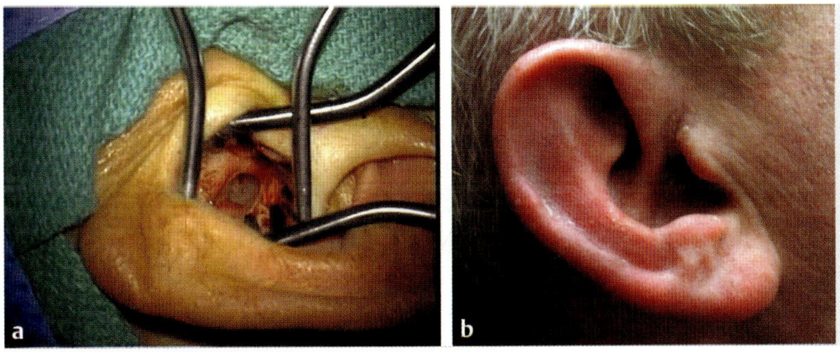

Fig. 18.5 Endaural approach. (a) Wide intraoperative exposure of the external auditory canal and tympanic membrane is afforded with a wide lateral angle for entrance of surgical instruments without the requirement of an aural speculum. (b) View of limited endaural incision only 3 weeks postoperative.

and the broad identification of the mastoid segment of the facial nerve to afford sufficiently wide exposure of the middle ear.

Canalplasty, the widening of the bony external auditory canal by drilling away bone, is a key and underutilized aspect of tympanomastoid surgery that is described in Chapter 20. It is most often carried out to facilitate exposure in tympanoplasty for anterior and subtotal perforations. Care must be taken during anterior exposure to avoid entering the temporomandibular joint. Care should also be taken to avoid damage to the mastoid segment of the facial nerve given that this may take a course lateral to the position of the tympanic ring in the inferior-posterior aspect of the medial canal wall. Canalplasty is complete when the entire annulus is exposed in one position of the microscope. Inadequate exposure to the entire annulus is a common mistake that may contribute to failed tympanic membrane repair, especially at the anterior drumhead.

The same principles of wide bony exposure underlie all mastoid and skull base procedures. A straight drill handpiece is preferentially used because it provides better fine motor control. However, the angled handpiece can be used in certain instances involving a narrow field, such as when performing canalplasty given that the hand that grips the straight handpiece may obstruct the surgeon's view. Cutting burs are used to remove bone quickly and are used with appropriate suction and irrigation to maintain a clear view of the operating field. This is important to prevent bone dust gathering on the sharp edges of the bur.

Use of wide burs initially allows for incremental exposure of a wider surgical field. Larger burs and wide skeletonization will help prevent injury to underlying structures because they are less likely to result in the dangerous practice of narrow deep penetration into poorly visualized underlying structures. Burs should be moved parallel to the structure being identified. Removal of the lateral cortical bone and skeletonization of the middle fossa dura and sigmoid sinus are primarily performed with large cutting burs, followed by contouring with a large coarse diamond bur. Wide saucerization of the cortical mastoidectomy aims to remove the mastoid cortex extensively, prior to deeper dissection, and to provide better exposure. Diamond burs are used when drilling directly on important structures, such as the dura, the jugular bulb, the sigmoid sinus, and the facial nerve, to allow safe skeletonization. No matter which type of bur is used, it is necessary to always drill under copious irrigation to prevent unwanted thermal injury to vital structures.

18.12 Control of the Surgical Field

The presence of significant bleeding in the operative field inhibits safe and successful otologic surgery. It is important to apply a multifaceted approach to attain satisfactory conditions. Preoperatively, any concomitant medical conditions that may cause hypertension or a hypercoagulable state should be managed appropriately. During microsurgery of the ear, the technique selected for anesthesia should help to provide good operative conditions for the surgeon. A 10- to 15-degree head-up tilt increases venous drainage, keeps venous pressure low, and decreases venous bleeding. The specific techniques to induce and maintain general anesthesia have already been described, and we have outlined how controlled hypotension is required for middle ear surgery to achieve a bloodless operative field. Different anesthetic agents will cause vasodilation to a varying degree, which should be minimized during ear surgery.[17,18]

It is vital to attain hemostasis of the soft tissues during the initial steps of the surgery, before the retractors are placed and bony work begins. Effective infiltration of the operative site with local anesthetic and adrenaline (described above) will greatly aid hemostasis. Soft tissue dissection is carried out with monopolar diathermy, which is also used to control troublesome bleeding and thus reduce the number of instrument changes, allowing the surgery to proceed in an efficient manner. Bleeding from bone can usually be controlled by drilling with a diamond bur and bone wax can also be applied to the area when there is more significant bleeding. Monopolar diathermy can be safely used to coagulate a bleeding emissary vein but is not advocated along the sigmoid sinus or dura given that it may easily perforate these structures. Careful bipolar coagulation is preferable. If the operative conditions are diminished and the above measures have not been successful, an adrenaline-soaked ribbon gauze can be placed in the surgical field and attention directed to another surgical step to minimize excessive delay. Bleeding from an exposed sigmoid sinus is controlled by applying a piece of gelatin sponge soaked in thrombin onto the affected area, followed by application of pressure with a cotton surgical patty. The cotton is removed after a few minutes and the thrombin-gelatin is left in place.

18.13 Venous Thromboembolism Prophylaxis after Ear Surgery

Although there is no clinical trial evidence specific to ear surgery to inform use of postoperative venous thromboembolism (VTE) prophylaxis, it is our practice to consider its use in appropriate cases. Venous thromboembolism prophylaxis after non-ear surgery is used in patients known to be at greater risk of VTE. This assessment is based on patient preoperative factors and the duration of anesthesia they will undergo. Our assessment takes into account the duration of anesthesia (> 60 minutes being supportive of VTE prophylaxis) and the following patient factors, one or more of which, if present, will support VTE prophylaxis: patient age > 60 years, body mass index > 30 kg/m^2, personal or family history of VTE, use of oral contraceptive agent or hormone replacement therapy, active cancer or cancer treatment, presence of significant medical comorbidity (e.g., ischemic heart disease).

In addition to the above, maintenance of adequate hydration and early mobilization during the postoperative period should be encouraged to reduce VTE risk. In our unit, VTE prophylaxis is provided with subcutaneous low-molecular-weight heparin and is continued until the patient is ambulating. Risk of postoperative hemorrhage needs to be considered in patients receiving VTE prophylaxis.

18.14 Antimicrobial Use in the Postoperative Period

Use of postoperative antibiotic therapy, or antimycotic therapy in patients with suspected fungal infection, is dependent upon the postoperative infection risk of the surgical procedure performed and the potential for postoperative infection to cause serious complications (e.g., tympanic membrane graft rejection). Antibiotic therapy is not recommended for otologic procedures with a low (<5%) postoperative infection risk. Operations in this category include tympanoplasty, stapedotomy, ossicular reconstruction, and cochlear implantation.[19] In our unit we administer systemic broad-spectrum antibiotic therapy empirically in such patients at induction of anesthesia and collect samples of abnormal mucosal tissue or cholesteatoma for intraoperative culture to refine antibiotic therapy in the postoperative period. Duration of antibiotic therapy is based on culture results and local microbiology guidance.

18.15 Conclusion

Deliberate control of the surgical field and operating room environment are some of the most fundamental responsibilities of a surgeon. The general principles outlined above have been formulated based on a combination of experience, published evidence, and official established practice guidelines, with a view toward optimizing patient safety and ensuring efficient surgical execution. Among these principles, consistent operating room set-up, wide deliberate surgical exposure, and controlled hemostasis are particularly key when executing otologic surgery for chronic ear disease.

References

[1] Marcus Atlas and Rob Eisenberg. A guide to temporal bone dissection. Ear Science Institute Australia. 2005.

[2] Department of Health. Correct patient, correct procedure and correct site policy and guidelines for Western Australian Health Services. Perth Government of Western Australia, 2006:1–26.

[3] Department of Health. Delivering safer healthcare in Western Australia: the second WA sentinel event report 2005–6. Perth, Government of Western Australia, 2006:1–25.

[4] WHO guidelines for safe surgery. Safe Surgery Saves Lives. 2009.

[5] Kattipattanapong W, Isaradisaikul S, Hanprasertpong C. Surgical site infections in ear surgery: Hair removal effect; a preliminary, randomized trial study. Otolaryngol Head Neck Surg. 2013;148(3):469–474.

[6] Wegner I, Bittermann AJ, Zinsmeester MM, van der Heijden GJ, Grolman W. Local versus general anesthesia in stapes surgery for otosclerosis: Aa systematic review of the evidence. Otolaryngol Head Neck Surg. 2013;149(3):360–365.

[7] Lavy JA, Powell HR. Stapes surgery under local anaesthesia. Ann R Coll Surg Engl. 2013;95(1):37–39.

[8] Hamerschmidt R, Moreira AT, Wiemes GR, Tenório SB, Tâmbara EM. Cochlear implant surgery with local anesthesia and sedation: Comparison with general anesthesia. Otol Neurotol. 2013;34(1):75–78.

[9] Nader ND, Simpson G, Reedy RL. Middle ear pressure changes after nitrous oxide anesthesia and its effect on postoperative nausea and vomiting. Laryngoscope. 2004;114(5):883–886.

[10] Mukherjee K, Seavell C, Rawlings E, Weiss A. A comparison of total intravenous with balanced anaesthesia for middle ear surgery: effects on postoperative nausea and vomiting, pain, and conditions of surgery. Aneasthesia. 2003;58(2):176–180.

[11] Degoute CS. Controlled hypotension: A guide to drug choice. Drugs. 2007;67 (7):1053–1076.

[12] Ayache D, Darrouzet V, Dubrulle F, et al. French Society of Otolaryngology Head and Neck Surgery (SFORL). Imaging of non-operated cholesteatoma: Clinical practice guidelines. Eur Ann Otorhinolaryngol Head Neck Dis. 2012;129(3):148–152.

[13] Greenberg JS, Manolidis S, Stewart MG, Kahn JB. Facial nerve monitoring in chronic ear surgery: US practice patterns. Otolaryngol Head Neck Surg. 2002;126(2):108–114.

[14] Heman-Ackah SE, Gupta S, Lalwani AK. Is facial nerve integrity monitoring of value in chronic ear surgery? Laryngoscope. 2013;123(1):2–3.

[15] Wilson L, Lin E, Lalwani A. Cost-effectiveness of intraoperative facial nerve monitoring in middle ear or mastoid surgery. Laryngoscope. 2003;113 (10):1736–1745.

[16] O'Sullivan PG, Atlas MD. Use of soft tissue vascular flaps for mastoid cavity obliteration. Laryngoscope. 2004;114(5):957–959.

[17] Hugo VA, Edward DM. Deliberate hypotension. In: Miller RD, ed. Anesthesia. Philadelphia: Churchill Livingstone, 2000;1473–1479.

[18] Degoute CS, Ray MJ, Manchon M, Dubreuil C, Banssillon V. Remifentanil and controlled hypotension; comparison with nitroprusside or esmolol during tympanoplasty. Can J Anaesth. 2001;48(1):20–27.

[19] Verschuur HP, de Wever WWH, van Benthem PPG. Antibiotic prophylaxis in clean and clean-contaminated ear surgery. Cochrane Database Syst Rev. 2004 (3):CD003996.

19 Tympanostomy Tubes

Shane R. Anderson

Abbreviations used in this chapter:

AOM: acute otitis media
AOMT: acute otitis media with tympanostomy
MRSA: methicillin-resistant *Staphylococcus aureus*
TT: tympanostomy tube(s)

19.1 Introduction

The placement of tympanostomy tubes (TT) is a well-established procedure in most otolaryngology practices. The relative indications, although still debated, are generally accepted to include recurrent acute otitis media affecting the quality of life of the patient and persistent hearing loss due to otitis media with effusion affecting development. Other considerations for the use of TT are the delivery of intratympanic medications, management of the complications of acute otitis media, and the relief of symptoms resulting from tympanic barotrauma (especially air travel).

Each year in the United States more than 600,000 children under the age of 15 years have TT inserted under a general anaesthesia.[1] This procedure has consistently been proven to be effective and safe. However, because of the frequency of TT insertion, complications of their use are encountered in most practices. The purpose of this chapter is to illustrate some key points regarding the choice of tube, special circumstances of use, and management of complications of TT insertion.

19.2 Materials, Tube Design, and Flange Design

The number and type of TT on the market is overwhelming, with a variety of manufacturers making multiple tubes with varying sizes and materials. A synopsis of all TT is beyond the scope of this chapter. Rather, an overview of the types of TT is provided so the otolaryngologist can make a more considered choice and tailor TT use to the specific clinical scenario.

19.2.1 Materials

TT materials can be divided into plastics and metals. All materials in TT have the common characteristics of being biocompatible and smooth, which reduces but does not prevent biofilm formation. The following section provides a brief description of the common materials used and the advantages of each product.

Plastics

Polyethylene

Polyethylene is a thermoplastic polymer consisting of long hydrocarbon chains. The density and melting point is dependent on the type of branching, crystal structure, and molecular weight. The most common type of polyethylene used in medical prosthetics is ultra-high-density polyethylene due to its rigidity and high melting point.

Fluoroplastics

These are a group of plastics that contain carbon and fluorine molecules. The most familiar of these is polytetrafluoroethylene (Teflon) by DuPont (Wilmington, Delaware). Like polyethylene, it is rigid and has a high melting point. It is also nonstick and is thought to help retard biofilm growth.

Silicone

Silicone is an inert polymer with a silicone backbone and organic side groups. It can be synthesized in a variety of consistencies or "durometers" for tubes, from soft to firm. Unlike the other plastics, it is soft. This elasticity makes it easy to compress for insertion and allows removal with minimal discomfort in the clinic setting.

Metals

Stainless Steel

This is a steel alloy with a minimum of 10.5% chromium that is resistant to oxygenation and corrosion. Its stiffness allows easy insertion. Stainless steel has a long history of reliability in medical prosthetics.

Titanium

Titanium is progressively becoming the more common choice for metal tubes given that it is durable, lightweight, corrosion-resistant, and MRI-compatible. Lightweight tubes have been shown to decrease tympanosclerosis.[2]

Each of the above materials can come with a bacteriostatic coating that is the intellectual property of the manufacturers of TT. Conclusive evidence is lacking regarding increased efficacy of any one coating.

19.2.2 Tube Design

Design is dictated by the internal and external diameter of the tube. Theoretically, the wider the internal diameter, the better the drainage of mucoid effusions and resistance to blockage. This is offset by the risk of contamination of the middle ear from external ear pathogens as the surface tension required to breach the middle ear is reduced. The outer diameter dictates the size of perforation that will remain post-extrusion. In the normal setting of short- to mid-term tube extrusion, even a large diameter will have little consequence; however, over the long term, a larger diameter tube will have a higher perforation rate.

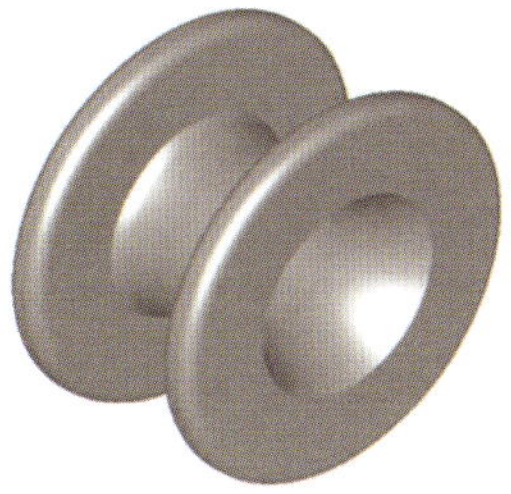

Fig. 19.1 Bobbin tympanostomy tube. This grommet-style tube has two collars that keep the tube in place over the short term. (Image courtesy of Grace Medical.)

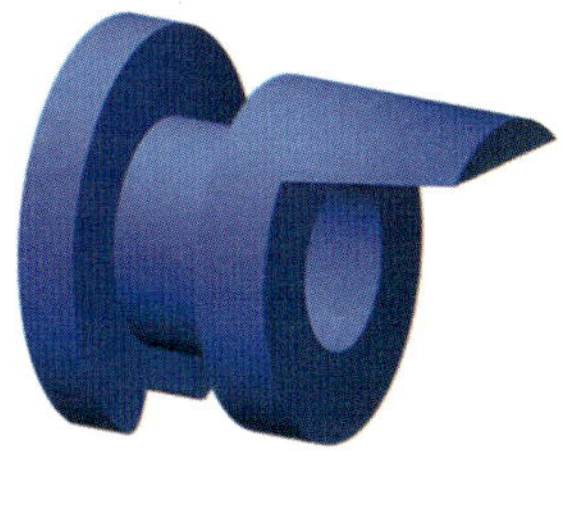

Fig. 19.2 Paparella tympanostomy tube. This short-term tube has two collars and a tab to facilitate removal. (Image courtesy of Grace Medical.)

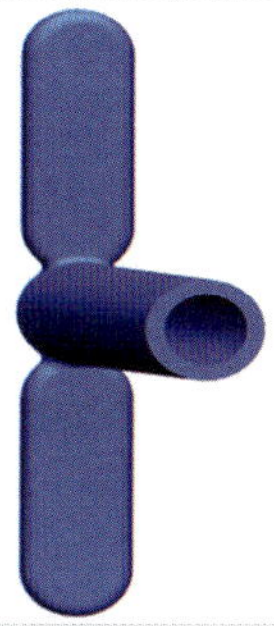

Fig. 19.3 T-Tube tympanostomy tube. This classic long-term tube has a long barrel and two flanges. (Image courtesy of Grace Medical.)

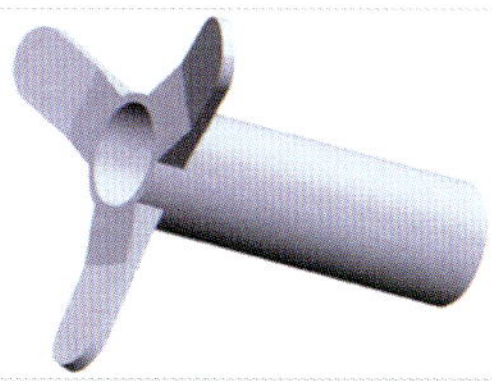

Fig. 19.4 Triune Tube tympanostomy tube. This T-style tube has a long barrel and three short flanges, which are designed to hold the tube in place from a medium to long term. (Image courtesy of Grace Medical.)

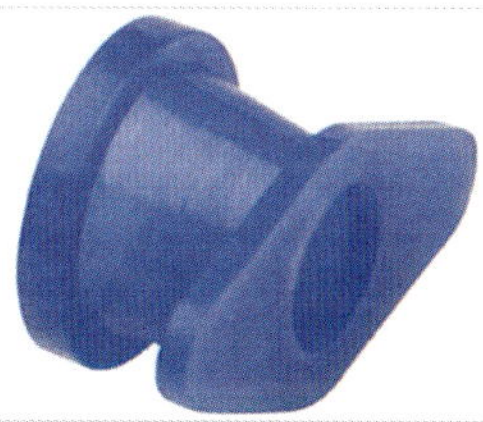

Fig. 19.5 Taper Vent tympanostomy tube. This tube has a short wide barrel and two short flanges, which will keep the tube in place for a medium term. This style of barrel better facilitates entry of ototopical medications compared with traditional T-style tubes. (Image courtesy of Grace Medical.)

19.2.3 Collar and Flange Design

Most TT feature a collar or a set of flanges that are designed to keep the tube from extruding. The wider the profile of the collar or flanges, the more probability that the TT will remain in situ for a longer period of time. In general, flanges are expected to keep a TT in place longer than a collar. A typical TT with a collar or flange diameter of ≤ 2.5 mm will, on average, extrude between 8 months and 24 months, whereas a T-shaped TT with wide flanges will typically not extrude before 2 years.[2] Using a double or triple flange design also reduces movement of the tube and prevents enlargement of the myringotomy.

19.3 Features of TT for Specific Purposes

Broadly, TT can be divided into short/medium-term tubes and long-term tubes. In general, short-term tubes tend to be smaller and have a collar, whereas long-term tubes are larger and have wide flanges. Because the collar of a short-term tube is only a modest barrier to extrusion, it can be used for temporary ventilation with a high degree of confidence that it will spontaneously extrude and heal. Examples of this include the Bobbin (▶ Fig. 19.1) by Grace Medical, Inc. (Memphis, Tennessee) and the Paparella (▶ Fig. 19.2), also by Grace Medical.

Long-term tubes featuring flanges can be divided into those with a long barrel and those with a short barrel. The disadvantages of long-term tubes are that biofilm formation can occur and the flange design can increase the risk of a permanent perforation once extrusion occurs. A common long-term tube with a long barrel that most otolaryngologists would be familiar with is the T-Tube by Grace Medical (▶ Fig. 19.3; ▶ Fig. 19.4). An advantage of the T-Tube is that it can be trimmed in length to the surgeon's desire. The longer barrel has a greater resistance to water intrusion but has the disadvantages of becoming blocked more frequently, having reduced otological drop penetration, and being more difficult to inspect through the tube into the middle ear. In addition, thick, mucoid effusions that are difficult to evacuate will often not drain effectively through a long-barrel tube, risking occlusion and early extrusion. Hence, short-barrel flanged tubes with a wider internal diameter are preferred if the need for ototopical medication administration or blockage is judged to be high (▶ Fig. 19.5).

Often the TT selected is based on the preference of the facility that the surgeon attends due to economic or historical reasons.

Unfortunately, there is no TT that caters to all scenarios and a one-size-fits-all approach to TT selection will result in inappropriate insertion of TT in specific patients, often with poor results.

19.4 Complications of TT

19.4.1 Early Extrusion/Retention of Tube

Tailoring the correct TT as described above to the correct clinical scenario will help prevent this complication from occurring frequently, but will not prevent it outright. Heaton, Bingham, and Osborne[3] demonstrated that tubes placed in the anterior pars tensor had a lower incidence of early extrusion. Bleeding has been shown to increase tube obstruction and extrusion.[4] Hence, making the radial incision between the vessels of the tympanic membrane is beneficial. The nature of the middle ear effusion and the number of previous tubes has been shown to influence early extrusion.[5] Anecdotally, making the myringotomy only long enough to just allow atraumatic insertion of the TT and avoiding an atrophic tympanic membrane may help to maximize the life of a TT.

19.4.2 Tube Removal

The decision that a TT has been retained for too long is based on the individual patient's clinical scenario. Traditionally, evidence suggests that a tube that has been in situ for more than 18 months has an increased risk of leaving a perforation.[6] In practice, the removal and replacement of a long-term tube is rarely performed on the basis of time alone. Often, a tube will be removed if it is thought to be the nidus of biofilms, myringitis, and recurrent TT otorrhea. More often than not, the decision to remove a TT is based on the fact that the patient no longer requires the tube. Typically, this only has to be carried out for long-term tubes, and the decision is based on symptom-free intervals, normal hearing, age, and the ability to perform the Valsalva maneuver. If the patient can demonstrate resolution of Eustachian tube dysfunction by performing the Valsalva, then the TT is removed.

19.4.3 Perforation

Tube placement can be associated with an inflammatory reaction and secondary development of a fibrous ring around the TT. After extrusion, epithelial cell hyperplasia and migration at the edge of a perforation allow for normal healing, often as a so-called "monomeric" tympanic membrane. Wilson[7] suggested that the ingrowth of squamous epithelium onto the undersurface of the tympanic membrane may cause contact inhibition and prevent epithelial hyperplasia and closure of the tympanic perforation. Bingham[8] noted the spontaneous closure of a perforation up to 12 months after extrusion and argued that the definition of post-extrusion perforation should be defined as one present at 12 months. Others have defined it as 6 months, making it difficult to quote the actual residual perforation rate. Yum[9] quotes a perforation rate of 2.8% at 6 months that can be as high as 16.6% in long-term tubes.[10] Apart from the use of long-term tubes, other risk factors for post-extrusion perforation include age > 7 years,[11] recurrent postoperative otorrhea,[12] atrophy of the tympanic membrane,[13] and spontaneous extrusion (as opposed to active removal as the edges are freshened in the latter). If the perforation is small, dry and the patient has no desire to dive or join the armed forces, then no intervention may be needed. Tympanoplasty for persistent tube perforations causing concern is covered in Part 4, Roundtable on Tympanic Membrane Reconstruction.

19.4.4 Acute Otitis Media with Tympanostomy (AOMT)

AOMT is a common and separate clinical and microbiological entity to acute otitis media (AOM). AOMT presents with a purulent otorrhea, in contrast to the otalgia, fever, and hearing loss that is expected with AOM without a tube. The microbiological cause of this is typically bacterial, with *Streptococcus pneumonia, Haemophilus influenza, Moraxella catarrhalis, Staphylococcus aureus,* and *Pseudomonas aeruginosa* most commonly cultured.[14] The mechanism of infection is caused by either influx of bacteria from the external auditory canal or by reflux of contaminated fluid from the nasopharynx up the Eustachian tube. The incidence of AOMT varies but is frequent and ranges from 0.36 to 3.6 episodes/child/year.[2] In a systematic review of the literature by Hellström, Groth, and Jörgensen,[2] there was no or only slight evidence that water exposure affects otorrhea, and for this reason we do not exclude our patients from water exposure on the basis of preventing AOMT.

The most effective management of AOMT is in the preoperative encounter, with appropriate consenting and education. The importance of educating the patient's caregiver that TT reduce the frequency, duration, and severity of otitis media but do not eliminate middle ear infections cannot be overstated. Tubes can reduce the duration of otitis media from months to days, allow for the use of topical antibiotics instead of systemic antibiotics,[15] and allow the administration of culture-directed antibiotics, if needed, without the need for tympanocentesis.[16] In a randomized trial of 270 patients between 1–10 years of age, antibiotics/steroid drops were compared with systemic antibiotics and observation. A significant reduction in time to resolution of otorrhea was observed in the antibiotic/steroid drops group.[15] An antibiotic/steroid combination has also been demonstrated to be superior to antibiotics alone.[17]

19.4.5 Special Circumstances in AOMT

Otorrhea Despite Appropriate Topical Drop Management

Occasional failure of treatment with appropriate ototopical therapy will occur. This most frequently is due to inadequate drop delivery. If the tube is observed to be blocked by keratin debris or crusting, some patients will tolerate clearance of this in the office setting using a micropick or suction. If excessive viscous secretions are the cause of blockage, careful aural toilet is required. Demonstration to parents on how to do this with tissue paper is instrumental. The instillation of drops followed by 5–10 minutes in an ear-dependent position and the use of tragal pumping to help the drops to penetrate may help. Occasionally, the patient will require regular aural toilet and irrigation with warmed sterile saline. At this point, the role that biofilms on the TT may be playing in the ongoing otorrhea needs to be discussed, and TT removal and replacement may need to be considered.

Methicillin-Resistant Staphylococcus Aureus (MRSA) Tube Otorrhea

Swab results showing MRSA are often discovered with trepidation. The most common cause of MRSA colonization of the middle ear is due to repeated use of systemic antibiotics. Hence, the use of further doses of systemic antibiotics in most circumstances is usually not indicated. It is difficult to treat MRSA with systemic antibiotics without also affecting normal flora, which may act as a competitor to MRSA growth. Therefore, the objective of management is control of MRSA, not eradication.

As a first-line treatment, the above advice for all tube otorrhea should be followed. Even in the setting of a report stating resistance to fluoroquinolones, it is this author's opinion that topical fluoroquinolones with steroid should be considered as first-line medical management.[18] Topical antibiotics can have a 1000-fold higher concentration within the middle ear cleft than systemic antibiotics,[16] and the minimum inhibitory levels reported do not reflect this high concentration. Often, conventional therapy with drops has already been attempted. If this is the case and proper technique is being demonstrated, then the topical use of mupirocin ointment around the perforation, the promontory, and the ear canal will result in the relief of otorrhea with no ototoxicity, as shown by Furukawa, Minekawa, Haruyama et al.[19] In these circumstances, we also recommend treating any other known nidus of MRSA colonization, such as in the nasal cavity, with mupirocin ointment, and to perform chlorhexidine body washing.

If this fails, systemic antibiotic therapy directed by culturing is mandated. Consideration needs to be given to the presence of silent mastoiditis or occult choleasteatoma. Special cultures for mycobacterium should be taken, and immunological screening investigation of systemic causes of middle ear disease and immunodeficiency need to be investigated, as outlined in Chapter 12.

19.5 Long-Term Consequences of Tubes

A 25-year follow-up of a cohort of patients who had a myringotomy in one ear and a tube in the opposite ear conducted by Cayé-Thomasen, Stangerup, Jørgensen, Drozdziewic, and Bonding, [20] demonstrated that myringosclerosis was more frequent (50%) in the tubed ear. Furthermore, it progressed well after the tube had extruded but did not have any clinical effect on audiologic outcomes. In this same study of ears treated for serous otitis media, there was no increase in the incidence of cholesteatoma or other adverse pathology. Retractions increased early but were observed to resolve over time.

19.6 Special Applications of Tympanostomy Tubes in Chronic Ear Disease

19.6.1 Primary T-Tube Cartilage Tympanoplasty

Primary intubation of a cartilage tympanoplasty in the setting of atelectasis was introduced by Hall[21] and promoted by Duckert, Makielski, and Helms.[22] The latter proposed, in a series of 40 patients, that the union of the cartilage graft and the ventilating tube "offered an attractive option when used simultaneously to reverse atelectasis, reconstruct the tympanic membrane and re-pneumatize the middle ear, so to eliminate recurrent effusion." We have modified this technique and use the same T-Tube tympanoplasty in a double-island composite graft, as described by Brackman, Shelton, and Arriaga (▶ Fig. 19.6).[23] In the experience of Duckert, Makielski, and Helms, they were able to reduce the air-bone gap to < 25 dB in > 80% of patients in the early stages of follow-up. They also experienced no post-extubation perforations and no epithelial ingrowth. Sixty-five percent of patients retained their T-Tube for over 4 years. They did report 7 out of 40 patients having tube otorrhea. Keeping in mind that this technique is reserved for those high-risk ears resistant to traditional therapy, we believe this to be a good result. We also experience episodic

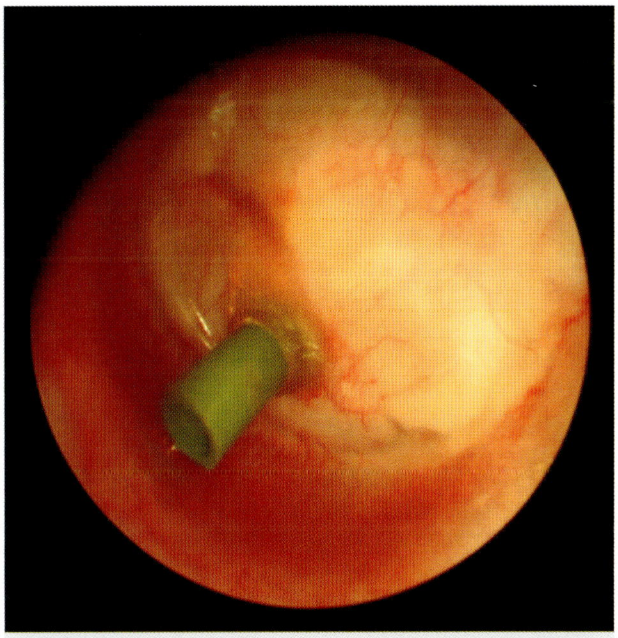

Fig. 19.6 Intubated cartilage graft. A cartilage graft can be intubated primarily during surgery if there is no ongoing infection or as part of a staged process. Secondary intubation of a cartilage graft can be facilitated by use of a laser.

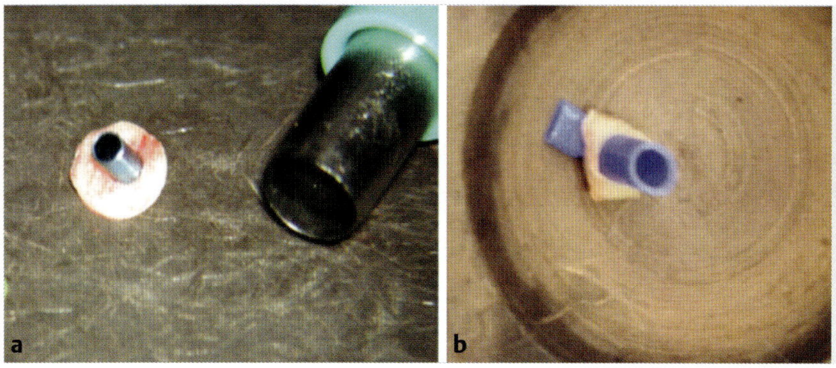

Fig. 19.7 Cartilage washer tube technique. (a) A 3- to 5-mm dermal punch may be useful for creating a small cartilage washer. A metallic tube can be passed through the cartilage, or a silicone tube can be used. (b) The cartilage acts to keep the tube in place over the long-term and prevents perforation after extrusion or removal.

otorrhea with this technique and address this in exactly the same manner as described for AOMT, with successful results. Rarely do the tubes need to be removed and replaced.

The indications for primary T-Tube tympanoplasty are relative and open to interpretation and are not reflected well in a treatment algorithm. Essentially this technique is reserved for patients who are likely to experience a postoperative effusion that will affect audiologic outcome, namely those that demonstrate ongoing Eustachian tube dysfunction and intraoperatively have a thick mucoid effusion.

Patients who do not experience improved hearing, even after addressing rhinological causes and performing the Valsalva maneuver, are offered secondary intubation. As outlined by Duckert, of Duckert, Makielski, and Helms.[22] The morbidity associated with T-Tube total cartilage tympanoplasty is negligible, but the benefits in audiologic outcomes are significant.

In this scenario, tympanostomy is performed under general anesthetic in the anterior-superior quadrant given that the space between the neotympanum and medial wall of the middle ear is greatest in this location. We use a sickle knife and an 0.2-mm hook to remove a small island of cartilage to allow TT placement.

19.6.2 Washer Tube Technique: A Novel Approach to Improve T-Tube Retention and Prevent Complications of Long-Term Intubation

Many methods have been described to prolong the function of long-term tubes. These include the use of a subannular and transosseous tympanostomy. We use a novel approach to help ensure tube retention in those that require long-term T-Tubes. Using cartilage of approximately 5 mm in diameter with perichondrium still attached, a size 5 sucker is used to punch a hole through the cartilage, allowing the T-Tube to be threaded over the cartilage. Once this is done, the tube and cartilage can be trimmed to ensure a good fit in the anterior tympanic membrane. A tympanostomy is performed in the anterior mesotympanum long enough to accommodate the cartilage (▶ Fig. 19.7).

Typically, this is performed at the time of a cartilage tympanostomy, where the contralateral ear has demonstrated a persistent effusion resistant to conservative measures. Anecdotally, the experience of the editors of this book has been that it allows good tube retention and prevents tube movement that can lead to widening of the tympanostomy. If the patient regains Eustachian tube function, indicated by the ability to perform the Valsalva maneuver, the tube can often be removed in the outpatient setting from the insensate cartilage. As the residual perforation is small, it typically heals, especially because the underlying perforation margins are reinforced with cartilage. Patients are allowed to swim with these tubes, but we restrict swimming to the surface and advocate against deep diving. We hypothesize that the long narrow T-Tube allows gases to diffuse, preventing negative pressure from forming in the middle ear, while at the same time providing enough surface tension to prevent water intrusion. As with all long-term tympanostomy tubes, occasionally otorrhea will occur and granulation will form around the tube, which we treat reliably with antibiotic/steroid drops.

References

[1] Rosenfeld RM, Schwartz SR, Pynnonen MA, et al. Clinical practice guideline: Tympanostomy tubes in children. Otolaryngol Head Neck Surg. 2013;149(1) Suppl:S1–S35.

[2] Hellström S, Groth A, Jörgensen F, et al. Ventilation tube treatment: a systematic review of the literature. Otolaryngol Head Neck Surg. 2011;145(3):383–395.

[3] Heaton JM, Bingham BJ, Osborne J. A comparison of performance of Shepard and Sheehy collar button ventilation tubes. J Laryngol Otol. 1991;105 (11):896–898.

[4] Altman JS, Haupert MS, Hamaker RA, Belenky WM. Phenylephrine and the prevention of postoperative tympanostomy tube obstruction. Arch Otolaryngol Head Neck Surg. 1998;124(11):1233–1236.

[5] Song CM, Park MH, Kim YH, Lee JH. Factors affecting the extrusion rate of ventilation tubes. Clin Exp Otorhinolaryngol. 2010;3(2):70–75.

[6] Moon IS, Kwon MO, Park CY, et al. When should retained Paparella type I tympanostomy tubes be removed in asymptomatic children? Auris Nasus Larynx. 2013;40(2):150–153.

[7] Wilson DF. Tympanic membrane perforations secondary to ventilation devices: special considerations. Laryngoscope. 1981;91(6):877–882.

[8] Bingham BJ, Gurr PA, Owen G. Tympanic membrane perforation following the removal of ventilation tubes in the presence of persistent aural discharge. Clin Otolaryngol Allied Sci. 1989;14(6):525–528.

[9] Yum JH, Park YS, Jeon EJ, Kim DH, Jung MK, Lee DH. Factors affecting the persistence of tympanic membrane perforation developed with the extubation of ventilation tube. Int J Pediatr Otorhinolaryngol. 2008;72(1):49–55.
[10] Kay DJ, Nelson M, Rosenfeld RM. Meta-analysis of tympanostomy tube sequelae. Otolaryngol Head Neck Surg. 2001;124(4):374–380.
[11] El-Bitar MA, Pena MT, Choi SS, Zalzal GH. Retained ventilation tubes: Should they be removed at 2 years? Arch Otolaryngol Head Neck Surg. 2002;128 (12):1357–1360.
[12] Liew L, Daudia A, Narula AA. Synchronous fat plug myringoplasty and tympanostomy tube removal in the management of refractory otorrhoea in younger patients. Int J Pediatr Otorhinolaryngol. 2002;66(3):291–296.
[13] Hydén D. Ear drum perforations in children after ventilation tube treatment. Int J Pediatr Otorhinolaryngol. 1994;29(2):93–100.
[14] Schmelzle J, Birtwhistle RV, Tan AK. Acute otitis media in children with tympanostomy tubes. Can Fam Physician. 2008;54(8):1123–1127.
[15] van Dongen TM, van der Heijden GJ, Venekamp RP, Rovers MM, Schilder AG. A trial of treatment for acute otorrhea in children with tympanostomy tubes. N Engl J Med. 2014;370(8):723–733.
[16] Dohar J. Tympanostomy Tubes: not the magic bullet for Acute Otitis Media. Medscape Education infectious disease. Medscape, 2010.
[17] Roland PS, Kreisler LS, Reese B, et al. Topical ciprofloxacin/dexamethasone otic suspension is superior to ofloxacin otic solution in the treatment of children with acute otitis media with otorrhea through tympanostomy tubes. Pediatrics. 2004;113(1 Pt 1):e40–e46.
[18] Dajcs JJ, Thibodeaux BA, Marquart ME, Girgis DO, Traidej M, O'Callaghan RJ. Effectiveness of ciprofloxacin, levofloxacin, or moxifloxacin for treatment of experimental Staphylococcus aureus keratitis. Antimicrob Agents Chemother. 2004;48(6):1948–1952.
[19] Furukawa M, Minekawa A, Haruyama T, et al. Clinical effectiveness of ototopical application of mupirocin ointment in methicillin-resistant Staphylococcus aureus otorrhea. Otol Neurotol. 2008;29(5):676–678.
[20] Cayé-Thomasen P, Stangerup S. Jørgensen G, Drozdziewic D, Bonding P, Tos M. Myringotomy versus ventilation tube in secretory otitis media: Eardrum pathology, hearing and Eustachian tube function 25 years after treatment. Otol Neurotol. 2008;29:649–657.
[21] Hall LJ. T-tube with tragus cartilage flange in long-term middle ear ventilation. Am J Otol. 1990;11(6):454–457.
[22] Duckert LG, Makielski KH, Helms J. Prolonged middle ear ventilation with the cartilage shield T-tube tympanoplasty. Otol Neurotol. 2003;24(2):153–157.
[23] Brackmann D, Shelton C, Arriaga M. Otologic Surgery 3rd edition: Cartilage Tympanoplasty. 3rd ed. Elsevier; 2010.

20 Canalplasty and Meatoplasty

Heng Wai Yuen

Abbreviations used in this chapter:

CSOE: chronic stenosing otitis externa
CT: computed tomography
EAC: external auditory canal
TMJ: temporomandibular joint

20.1 Introduction

Canalplasty refers to the surgical procedure that attempts to restore or create the natural contour and patency of the external auditory canal (EAC). Meatoplasty, on the other hand, describes the surgical creation of an enlarged external ear aperture. As the external ear aperture, or meatus, is in continuity with the bony and cartilaginous portions of the EAC, surgery on the EAC should almost always be accompanied by surgery on the external ear meatus. Thus, a canalplasty should be matched with an adequate meatoplasty. Canalplasty involves surgery on both the soft tissue as well as bony components of the EAC. Surgery on just one of these components is rarely adequate.

The indications for canalplasty include numerous pathologic conditions that may present as, or result in, canal stenosis or obliteration (▸ Table 20.1). These pathologies could be broadly categorized into bony or soft tissue in origin. Other conditions, such as keratosis obturans, although not causing canal stenosis, require canalplasty to prevent complications. For the purposes of this chapter, congenital aural atresia and congenital canal stenosis are not discussed (see Chapter 47 for a full discussion of these conditions).

Canalplasty is also performed during excision of benign soft tissue tumors of the EAC (e.g., squamous papilloma, seborrheic keratosis, or hemangioma). These tumors are fully excised with a small margin and full-thickness canal wall skin. A widened EAC facilitates postoperative surveillance. Split-thickness skin grafts may be necessary to cover any bare bone (see Chapter 48).

Canalplasty is an important part of other operations for chronic ear disease, especially tympanoplasty. In tympanoplasty, including underlay and overlay grafting techniques, canalplasty facilitates exposure and visualization of the entire tympanic membrane and annulus, especially the anterior portion. It provides access for canal skin elevation, evaluation of the ossicles, and secure placement of tympanic membrane grafts. Canalplasty also helps in postoperative care and follow-up examinations.

In keratosis obturans and EAC cholesteatoma, although there is no canal stenosis per se, there are crevices and bony overhangs in the EAC that cause accumulation of debris. Frequently, a significant area of bony canal is rendered bare and potentially devitalized. The bony EAC may also be expanded. At the same time, the meatus is too small, whether for proper inspection or for debridement. Therefore, canalplasty in combination with meatoplasty is necessary to smooth the canal contour and to enlarge the EAC opening. Any bare areas in the EAC are covered by a split-thickness skin graft. Removal of all disease must be achieved and the bony contours of the EAC smoothed out before covering bare areas in the EAC with a split-thickness skin graft. A meatoplasty matching the size of the canalplasty should be performed for ease of regular surveillance and debridement.

20.2 Patient Selection

Besides the inciting events (infection, trauma, etc.), early canal stenosis does not usually produce symptoms. Recurrent external otitis may occur later because the natural elimination of cerumen and desquamated epithelium from the EAC is impeded. Conductive hearing loss is a common symptom. This may result from occlusion of the EAC or when cerumen or debris tamponades against the tympanic membrane. Less

Table 20.1 Common indications for canalplasty

Bony stenosis	1. Exostosis 2. Osteoma 3. Fibrous dysplasia 4. Post-traumatic fracture
Soft tissue stenosis	1. Chronic stenosing otitis externa (CSOE) – secondary to recurrent or chronic inflammation. (Also known as post-inflammatory acquired atresia, obliterative otitis externa, or medial canal fibrosis.) 2. Trauma a) Fracture b) Burns c) Chemical injury 3. Iatrogenic causes a) Postoperative scarring b) Post-irradiation 4. Dermatological diseases (e.g., dermatitis, psoriasis, etc.) 5. Soft tissue neoplasms (benign, e.g., seborrheic keratosis, or malignant)
Others	1. Keratosis obturans 2. External canal cholesteatoma 3. As part of other operations (e.g., tympanoplasty, mastoidectomy)

commonly, cholesteatoma may develop medial to soft tissue stenosis.

In contrast to symptomatic bony stenosis, for which surgery is usually the only viable option, early soft tissue stenosis may be treated medically. This includes periodic dilation and stenting of the EAC with antibiotic- and steroid-impregnated expandable ear wicks. These wicks are replaced every 7 to 10 days for 6 to 8 weeks. Alternatively, the subcutaneous injection of steroid (triamcinolone) into the meatus may reverse or halt stenosis of the membranous EAC if applied early in the disease process. Patients who do not respond to these treatments are candidates for surgery.

All patients who undergo surgery require a preoperative audiogram to document the conductive hearing loss and any preexisting sensorineural hearing loss. A computed tomography (CT) scan of the temporal bone is performed to assess the location (lateral or medial), extent, and configuration of the stenosis. It is also useful in demonstrating possible cholesteatoma medial to the stenosis and evaluating any involvement of the middle ear and mastoid. In addition, the CT scan provides valuable preoperative information on the location of vital structures, such as the facial nerve.

20.3 Surgical Technique

20.3.1 Canalplasty

The goals of ear canal surgery are, first, to treat any concomitant infection (including associated cholesteatoma) and, second, to improve or reverse any conductive hearing loss. The principles of canalplasty for bony canal stenosis differ from those when soft tissue stenosis is the main indication. For example, in EAC stenosis due to exostosis, the canal skin is usually normal and should be preserved during canalplasty. This promotes the re-epithelization of the enlarged canal and may obviate the need for a split-thickness skin graft. In contrast, in soft tissue stenosis, especially in chronic stenosing otitis externa, the preservation of adjacent skin is not possible or desirable given that the canal skin is either contributing to the stenosis or is largely composed of fibrotic scar tissue; thus, full-thickness resection of canal wall skin is required.

The techniques of canalplasty and meatoplasty described herein are suitable for all indications, including tympanoplasty and tympanomastoidectomy.

Soft Tissue Exposure

An endaural-alone approach or a combination of endaural and postauricular approaches may be used for canalplasty. The endaural approach allows for canalplasty and meatoplasty simultaneously. The postauricular approach allows soft tissue flaps to be raised around the EAC; these flaps are useful when there is extensive exposure of mastoid cells.

After intubation and appropriate positioning, the patient's upper arm (hairless skin), hip, or thigh on the ipsilateral side is also prepared and draped accordingly to facilitate possible split-thickness skin graft harvesting (▶ Fig. 20.1).

The expected incisions and external ear canal are injected with 2% lidocaine with 1:80,000 epinephrine. The anterior canal wall, conchal bowl, and crus of the helix are also injected.

Pearls and Pitfalls

It is important to inject local anesthetic slowly with the needle in contact with bone. A too rapid or forceful injection would raise a wheal, further narrowing the already narrow canal lumen.

If an endaural incision is used, the surgery uses the same incision in the helicotragal groove and terminal incisure as for meatoplasty (see later discussion). This is then connected medially to a full-thickness radial EAC incision at 12 o'clock. The EAC is then held open with two self-retaining retractors placed perpendicularly to each other.

The postauricular incision is created approximately 1 cm posterior to the postauricular sulcus and carried down to the level of the temporalis fascia and periosteum in the standard manner. After incising the mastoid periosteum, the canal wall skin is then elevated off the underlying bone with a periosteal elevator. The EAC is entered posteriorly via an incision using a size 11 scalpel. The position of this incision is dictated by the location of the stenosis and should be placed just lateral to the stenosis. Otherwise, it is placed in a position beginning at about 5 mm medial to the suprameatal spine (▶ Fig. 20.2).

In many clinical situations (e.g., medial canal fibrosis) or if drilling of the anterior canal wall is anticipated, the canal incision is continued onto the anterior canal wall into a full circumferential incision (▶ Fig. 20.3). The skin of the EAC and soft tissue lateral to the incision are then elevated over the tympanic bone and retracted forward.

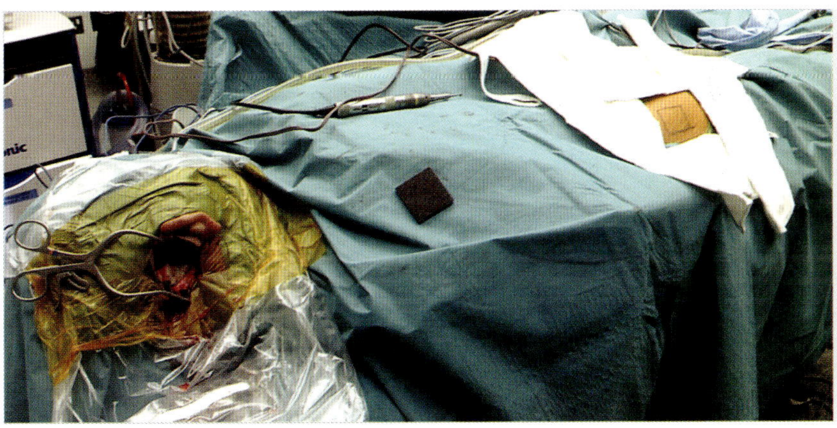

Fig. 20.1 While the patient is under general anesthesia, the right upper thigh is prepared for split-thickness skin graft harvest while surgery proceeds on the right ear.

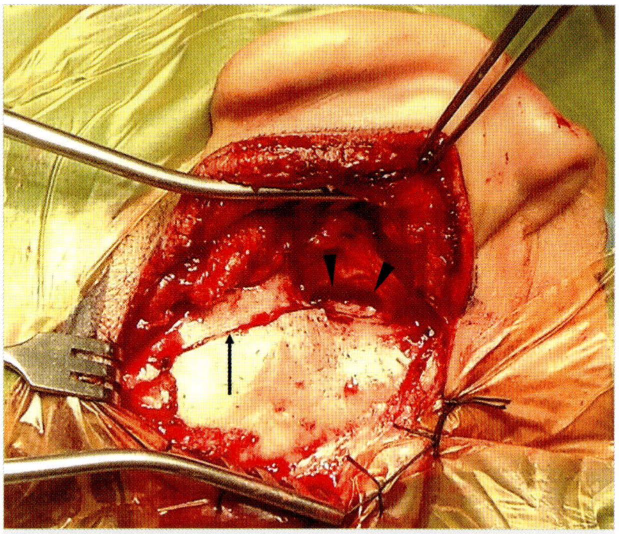

Fig. 20.2 Postauricular approach to canalplasty for EAC stenosis in a case caused by temporal bone fracture. The fracture line is seen (arrow). The EAC has been entered via a canal incision in the skin posteriorly (arrowheads). The ear and posterior canal flap are held forward with a self-retaining retractor.

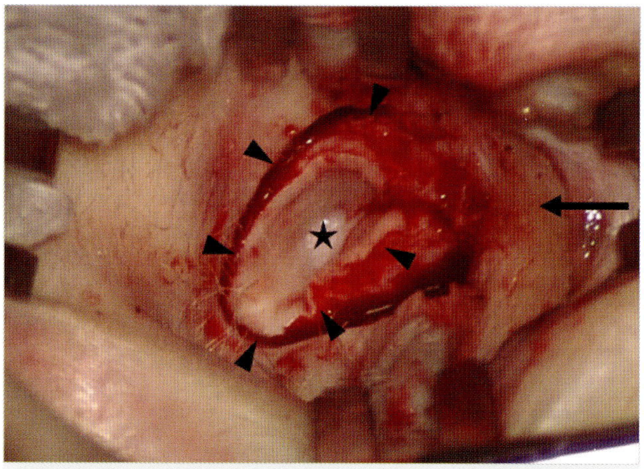

Fig. 20.3 An endaural approach to a case of medial canal fibrosis secondary to chronic inflammation. In this case, the endaural incision (arrow) is extended medially and is continuous with the circumferential canal incision (arrowheads) lateral to the area of fibrosis, which appears as a false fundus (asterisk).

Pearls and Pitfalls

It has been recommended that the anterior and posterior canal incisions be staggered to minimize the risk of circumferential stenosis. However, if the canal is further widened with drilling, the skin flaps are replaced properly, and there is meticulous postoperative care, there will be an extremely low risk of circumferential stenosis occurring.

Subsequently, the medial skin is carefully and circumferentially elevated off the underlying canal wall bone to the level of the tympanic annulus (▶ Fig. 20.4).[1] This exposes the whole EAC for canalplasty. In executing this step, some surgeons prefer to completely remove the anterior canal wall skin, to be later replaced as a skin graft, especially when canalplasty is performed as part of an overlay tympanoplasty (see Chapter 24).[2] If the canal wall skin is not removed, it is covered with a thick piece of Silastic sheeting or tin foil from a suture package to protect it from the rotating drill bur.

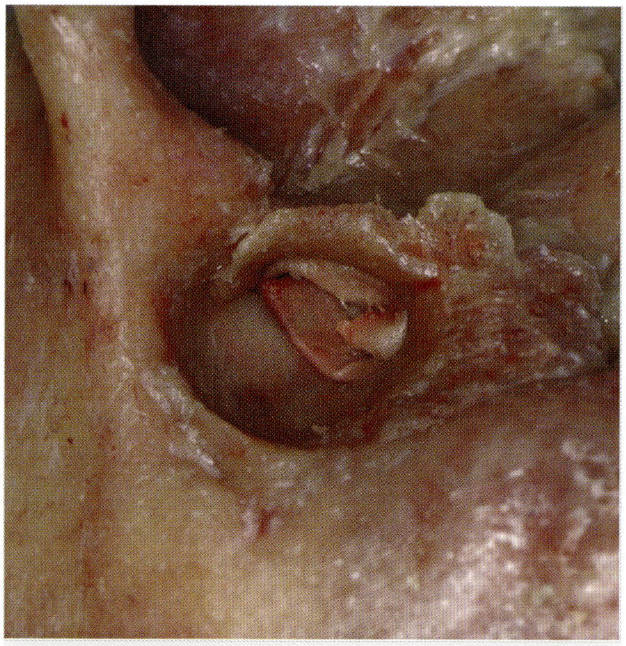

Fig. 20.4 Skin of the EAC is circumferentially elevated down to the level of the tympanic annulus. For underlay tympanoplasty, the anterior canal wall skin is left in place, protected by a Silastic disk during canal bone drilling, and redraped thereafter. For overlay tympanoplasty, the anterior canal wall skin is completely removed in continuum with the lateral epithelial layer of the tympanic membrane and later replaced as a free skin graft. (Used with permission from Atlas M, Eisenberg R. A Guide to Temporal Bone Dissection. 2nd Ed. Perth: Lions Ear 2004.)

Bone Drilling

The canalplasty begins by enlarging the canal laterally at the level of the suprameatal (Henle's) spine and the tympanosquamous suture, which can be quite prominent and obstructive in some cases. Once the major bone protuberances have been smoothed laterally, the surgeon will typically drill a deep superior trough into the zygomatic root through the tympanosquamous suture line and an inferior trough into the tympanic bone, both of which are immediately adjacent to the anterior canal wall bone. Drilling of these troughs creates an appearance that is sometimes referred to as "Mickey Mouse ears." Once these troughs are sufficiently deep to expose the annulus in the anterior-superior and inferior aspects, the anterior canal wall bone lying in between is then broadly removed to connect these troughs. In doing so, the penetration of the temporomandibular joint capsule is avoided while the entire anterior aspect of the annulus is exposed.

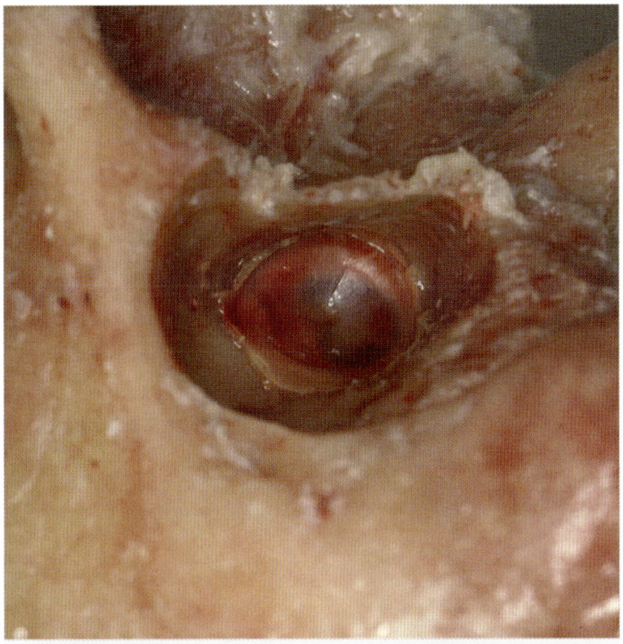

Fig. 20.5 Canalplasty is complete once the entire tympanic annulus can be viewed from a single vantage point without moving the microscope. (Used with permission from Atlas M, Eisenberg R. A Guide to Temporal Bone Dissection. 2nd Ed. Perth: Lions Ear 2004.)

Even after the cause of EAC stenosis has been addressed, the bony canal must be enlarged further to minimize the risk of recurrent stenosis. The canalplasty is complete when a funnel-shaped or truncated conical-shaped bony canal tapering medially is obtained and the complete tympanic annulus can be seen with one position of the microscope (▶ Fig. 20.5). In the event that exostoses of the external ear canal are present, it may be necessary to separately drill the posterior and superior aspect of the EAC more than is usually required (▶ Fig. 20.6).

Pearls and Pitfalls

While widening the posterior canal wall, it is best not to open the mastoid air cells to prevent canal retraction pockets or cholesteatomas. If mastoid air cells are opened and exposed, they should be covered by soft tissue flaps derived from around the EAC. The posterior-inferior mastoid periosteum may be elevated and transposed forward to overlie the exposed air cells.

After the surgical steps described above have been performed, the remnant medial canal skin is reset. Due to the newly enlarged bony canal wall, it may be necessary to create 12 o'clock and 6 o'clock radial incisions through the remnant canal wall skin in order for it to properly redrape after canalplasty. These incisions may also accommodate the subsequent creation of a tympanomeatal flap. Healing by secondary intention is usually adequate when more than half of the canal wall bone is covered by the skin flaps. Otherwise, the exposed surfaces are prone to secondary infection, granulation tissue, and recurrent stenosis from postoperative fibrosis. One method to prevent these occurrences is using split-thickness skin grafts to cover the exposed area.

Pearls and Pitfalls

In cases of very large exostoses, those involving the anterior wall are usually removed prior to the posterior ones. Care should be exercised when drilling in the region of the posterior bony annulus (to avoid injury to the chorda tympani and facial nerves), as well as in the anterior tympanomeatal angle close to the tympanic membrane (to avoid tympanic membrane perforation and contact with ossicles).

The techniques of canalplasty for other causes of bony stenosis (including osteoma and fibrous dysplasia) are similar to that for exostosis as described above.

Soft Tissue Stenosis

Chronic stenosing otitis externa (CSOE), also known as post-inflammatory acquired atresia or recurrent acquired atresia, may result from any injury or insult to the EAC skin, including chronic infection or previous ear surgery.[3] Stenosis or obliteration of the EAC may result. CSOE is prone to recurrence,[3,4] and an annual incidence of 0.6 per 100,000 has been reported in the literature.[5]

Stenosis of the canal may occur in the lateral portion of the EAC, in which case the medial part of the EAC may be filled with debris or even cholesteatoma; the tympanic membrane is usually intact. More commonly, the stenosis occurs in the medial portion of the EAC and involves the tympanic membrane. This form of CSOE is also known as post-inflammatory medial canal fibrosis or post-inflammatory medial meatal fibrosis.[6]

During surgery for both clinical situations, a circumferential canal incision is made lateral to the stenosis or false fundus through an endaural or postauricular incision as described previously. When the lateral EAC is stenosed, the fibrotic tissue is elevated off the bony EAC until normal skin is encountered lateral to the tympanic membrane. Any bare bone is grafted with a split-thickness skin graft. On the other hand, if the medial EAC is involved, dissection is performed circumferentially between the fibrous plug and the bony canal wall until the tympanic membrane annulus is reached. The correct plane of cleavage is identified, and a tube or column of fibrotic skin is removed together with the lateral squamous layer of the tympanic membrane, similar to what is undertaken in underlay tympanoplasty (▶ Fig. 20.7).[5]

Pearls and Pitfalls

Piecemeal removal of the fibrotic plug may be necessary for access and visualization medial to the stenosis. It is important to remove all abnormal fibrotic tissue to reduce the risk of recurrence.

The canalplasty is complete when the cause of stenosis is removed, the bony canal is enlarged, and the complete tympanic annulus can be seen with one position of the microscope.

Skin Grafting

The use of split-thickness skin grafts is discussed in detail elsewhere in this book. A brief outline is provided here. The

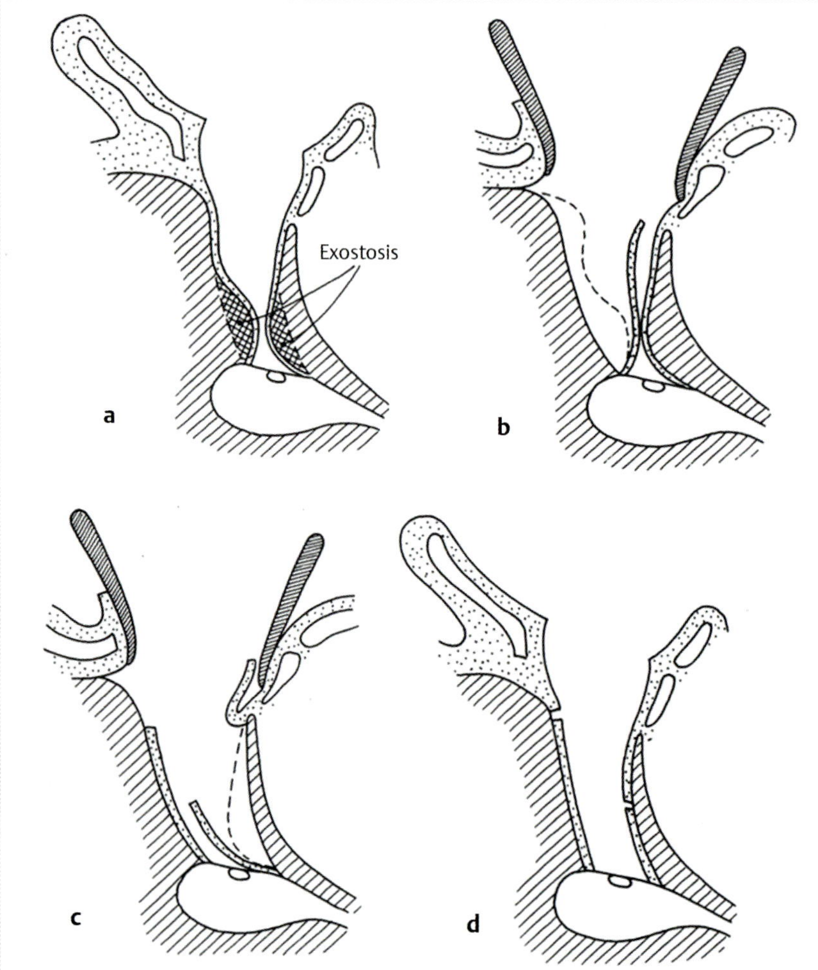

Fig. 20.6 Principles of canalplasty for exostoses. (a) Preoperative situation in which anterior and posterior exostoses cause canal stenosis. (b) The posterior, medially based skin flap is elevated, the exostosis removed, and the posterior canal wall widened. (c) Anterior skin flaps are similarly elevated and the anterior exostosis is removed and anterior canal wall drilled down. (d) After the canalplasty is completed, the skin flaps are replaced to line the enlarged ear canal. (Used with permission from Fisch U, May JS, Linder T, eds. Tympanoplasty, Mastoidectomy, and Stapes Surgery. New York, NY: Thieme, 2008.)

split-thickness skin graft is usually harvested from areas that are easily hidden under clothing (e.g., the medial upper arm, hip area, or upper thigh). The donor site is covered with an occlusive dressing and usually heals with little or no cosmetic defect. The harvested split-thickness skin graft is cut into tapering strips and used to line the exposed bone of the EAC, with the narrow end orientated medially. Strips of thin tapering silicone strips are placed over the split-thickness skin graft. This allows snug packing of the canal while maintaining the position of the split-thickness skin graft; it also helps to prevent blunting at the anterior angle.

Pearls and Pitfalls

When laying a split-thickness skin graft on the canal, it is important to place the keratinized epithelial surface upward, with the undersurface in contact with bone. The anterior tympanomeatal angle must be addressed with particular care to prevent blunting. Small pieces of absorbable gelatin packing are used to pack the skin graft firmly into the anterior and inferior sulcus.

20.3.2 Meatoplasty

Meatoplasty involves surgery on the skin and cartilage components of the external auditory meatus, especially in the region of the concha and crus of helix, to widen the lateral aperture of the EAC. The technique described here can be used with other procedures (e.g., canalplasty, tympanomastoidectomy).

Pearls and Pitfalls

The cartilaginous EAC is inclined posterior-superiorly while the bony part is inclined anterior-inferiorly; the axis of the EAC follows a lazy-S configuration, and the external auditory aperture is at a lower and more anterior position compared with the medial EAC. Hence, the most important part of the meatoplasty is the posterior-superior aspect.

First, an endaural incision is made at 12 o'clock, but unlike the usual endaural incision, it is directed posterior-superiorly towards and over the crus of helix without cutting it (▶ Fig. 20.8a). Skin is elevated off the underlying conchal cartilage and crus of helix with sharp-pointed scissors. A wedge of conchal cartilage and soft tissue incorporating the root of the crus of helix is resected to ensure sufficient posterior-superior exposure (▶ Fig. 20.8b). The conchal skin flaps are inverted and

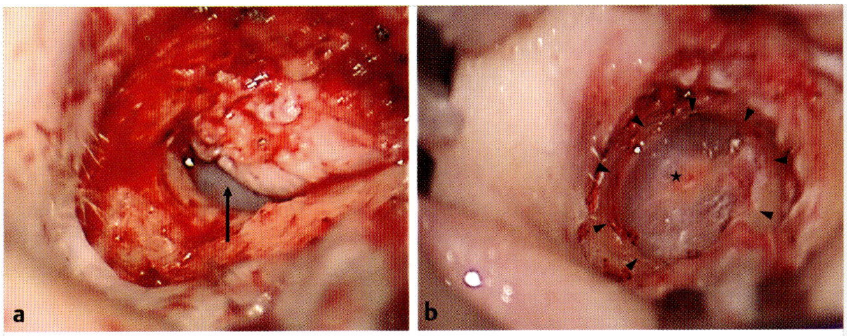

Fig. 20.7 Surgery for CSOE. (a) The fibrotic plug is elevated circumferentially to the level of the annulus. The squamous layer of the tympanic membrane is elevated laterally while preserving the fibrous layer (arrow) and the Shrapnell's membrane. (b) After the fibrous plug is completely removed, the bony EAC, including the anterior canal medial to the tragus, is exposed circumferentially (arrowheads) down to the tympanic annulus. The fibrous layer of tympanic membrane (asterisk) is preserved. These areas are covered with a split-thickness skin graft.

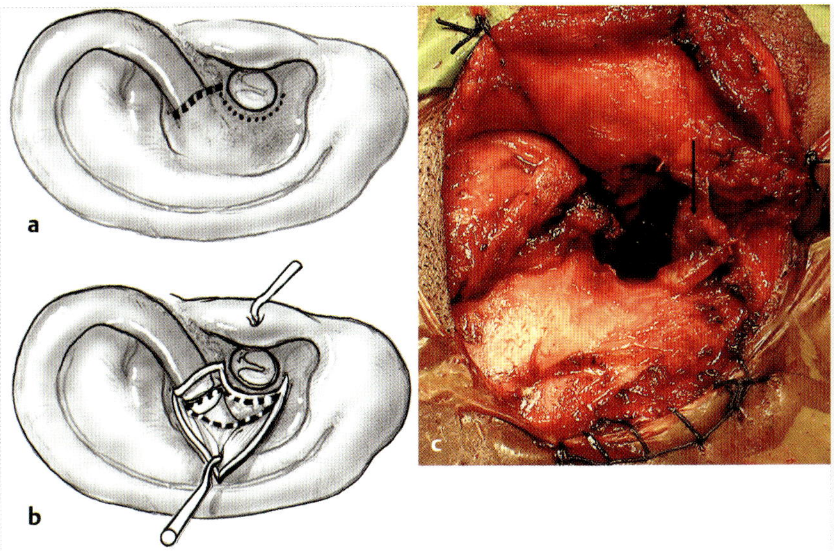

Fig. 20.8 Surgical steps for an endaural meatoplasty. (a) A meatoplasty begins with an endaural incision (dashed line). The medial part of this incision is full-thickness down to bone at 12 o'clock superiorly and connects with a canal incision or one made previously from the postauricular approach. Laterally, the incision extends into the soft tissue and is carried over the crus of helix without cutting it. (b) Skin is dissected off the underlying cartilage and soft tissue of the posterior canal skin and concha. The dissection is carried over the crus of the helix. The cartilage incorporating the crus of helix and soft tissue (dashed line) is excised. (c) When the meatoplasty is performed in combination with mastoidectomy, the skin flaps (arrow) are inverted and secured to the adjacent subcutaneous tissue with absorbable sutures, such that the external ear aperture is kept enlarged and the edges of the meatoplasty are skin-lined. The apex of the endaural incision is closed with nonabsorbable sutures.

anchored to the underlying soft tissue with absorbable sutures to create a rounded meatus (▸ Fig. 20.8c). The apex of the conchal incision may be closed with nonabsorbable suture to prevent any exposed cartilage. When combined with canalplasty alone, the skin flaps are not inverted and retaining sutures are not used. Instead, the skins flaps are laid onto the enlarged canal to promote re-epithelization. At the end of the surgery, the lateral part of the EAC and the meatoplasty are packed with a strip of ribbon gauze as a dressing and stent.

Pearls and Pitfalls

- To produce a lasting meatoplasty, adequate conchal cartilage must be resected. Simply incising through the cartilage alone, no matter how much or for how long packing is subsequently used, cannot produce and maintain an adequate meatal size because the cartilage would recoil and heal in proximity.
- During meatoplasty, it is important to ensure the elevated skin flaps are sutured back and inward, to create a rounded meatus, and that no cartilage is exposed (▸ Fig. 20.9). Exposed and protruding cartilage, especially inferiorly, can compromise the meatoplasty and may result in perichondritis.

A meatoplasty fails if an inadequate amount of cartilage is removed or if the site of fibrocartilaginous component removal is wrong. On the other hand, an excessively wide meatus should be avoided. Not only is this not aesthetically pleasing, some patients suffer vestibular symptoms caused by cold winds.

Variations in meatoplasty techniques revolve around similar principles to those described above. Some of these are suitable only for combination with canalplasty, whereas others could be combined with tympanomastoidectomy.

Fisch, May and Linder have described a popular technique for meatoplasty (▸ Fig. 20.10).[7] A linear incision is fashioned that extends posteriorly from the meatus in a slightly diagonal trajectory toward the sinodural angle. This incision penetrates both skin and cartilage of the concha. Sharp dissection is then undertaken superior and inferior to the incision to elevate the adjacent skin and perichondrium overlying the conchal cartilage. With the cartilage widely exposed, a large oval-shaped crescent is removed, minding the critical posterior-superior aspect. The margins of the previously elevated skin flaps are then rotated inward and sutured to the underlying surface of the concha such that all cartilage edges are covered.

Another popular technique is the so-called M-meatoplasty as described by Mirck.[8] This technique makes use of skin flaps around and within the EAC to enlarge the entrance of the EAC (▸ Fig. 20.11). Three conchal incisions and one radial membranous canal incision are made. The first incision is placed at the anterior edge of the cavum conchae at the entrance to the EAC. From the center of this first incision, two other incisions oriented as an inverted "V" are made. Skin is separated from the underlying cartilage to create three triangular conchal skin flaps. A crescent-shaped piece of conchal cartilage and subcutaneous tissue is resected. The upper and lower triangular conchal skin flaps are excised. Subsequently, a fourth connecting radial incision is made in the midline of the posterior aspect of the membranous canal wall, into which the remaining triangle of conchal skin is advanced to create an "M." The various connecting skin edges are sutured together with nonabsorbable sutures.

20.4 Postoperative Care

After canalplasty and meatoplasty, the patient may receive oral prophylactic antibiotics for 5 days. Strict water precautions are observed for a minimum of 2 weeks. The packing in the canal and meatus are removed together with the silicone strips at about 3 weeks, at which time the canal should be nearly re-epithelialized. After removal of packing, antibiotic-steroid otic drops should be applied twice daily for 10 days. The patient is seen every 2 weeks until the ear canal is healed. Granulation tissue in the canal should be cauterized with silver nitrate.

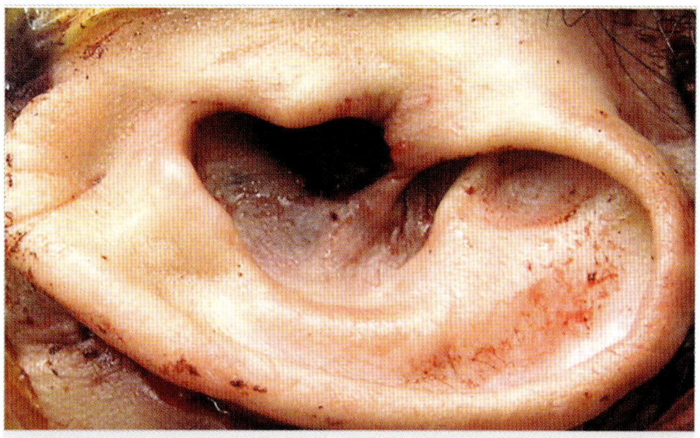

Fig. 20.9 The size of the meatus should match the size of the external ear canal or cavity that lies medial to it, with good posterior-superior exposure.

20.5 Complications

The main complications of canalplasty surgery include tympanic membrane perforation, sensorineural hearing loss, violation of the temporomandibular joint (TMJ), and facial palsy.

Iatrogenic perforation of the tympanic membrane can occur when the medial part of the fibrotic plug is elevated together with the squamous layer of the tympanic membrane. The perforation can be addressed with lateral placement of a split-thickness skin graft or grafted with fascia or perichondrium. Perforation of the tympanic membrane may also occur during drilling close to the tympanic membrane at the anterior tympanomeatal angle (e.g., during removal of anterior exostoses). Sensorineural hearing loss can develop when the drill or instrument inadvertently contacts the ossicular chain, especially the malleus. These complications may be prevented by using a silicone sheet or foil from a suture package to act as a barrier to protect the tympanic membrane.

Located immediately anterior to the EAC is the TMJ. While drilling in the anterior canal wall, exposure or violation of the TMJ can be avoided by removing more bone superiorly into the zygomatic root and inferiorly into the tympanic bone. Bone over the TMJ capsule is then carefully thinned with a diamond bur to leave an eggshell-thin layer of bone. A small area of exposed joint causes no problem aside from some minor temporary postoperative pain while chewing. Mild dehiscence of the TMJ may cause the herniation of fat and soft tissue into the EAC. The herniated tissue can be reduced with a bipolar cautery, and the defect is overlaid with a split-thickness skin graft. Tight canal packing is then applied. Larger dehiscence may cause the joint capsule to prolapse into the EAC during mandible movement. This can cause further stenosis. Such defects may be repaired with a piece of conchal cartilage, but this is challenging. Severe violation of the TMJ and capsule may result in joint dysfunction.

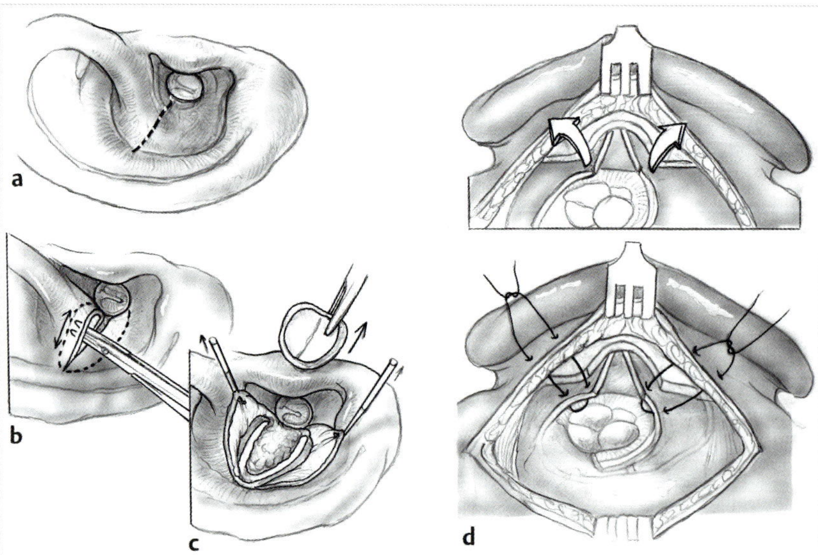

Fig. 20.10 The Fisch meatoplasty. (a) This technique is undertaken by making a radial diagonal incision that passes from the meatus toward the sinodural angle. This incision extends through skin and cartilage. (b) The adjacent skin and perichondrium are elevated to expose the conchal cartilage for resection. (c) A wedge of concha cartilage is resected. (d) After cartilage removal, the skin flaps are rotated inward and fixed with sutures to the underlying soft tissue, such that all cartilage edges are covered.

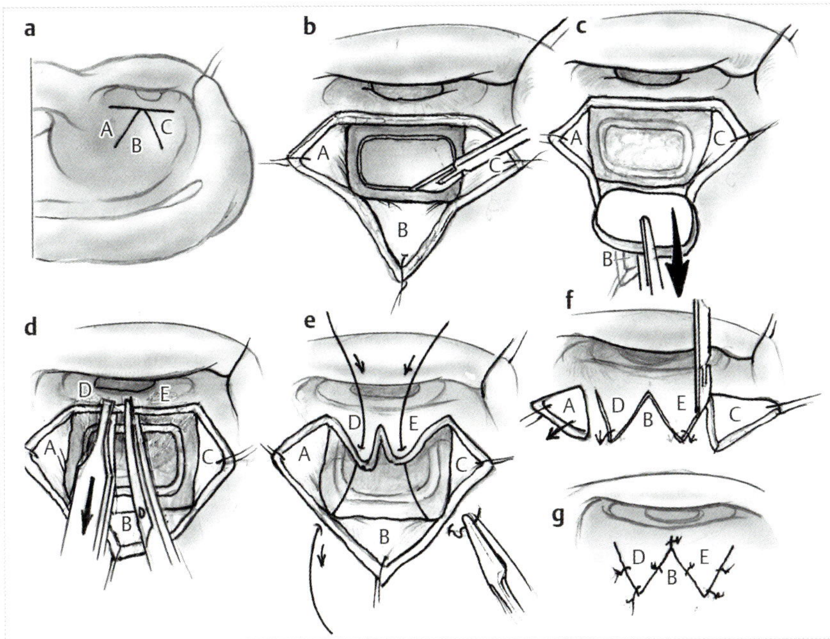

Fig. 20.11 The M-meatoplasty. (a) This is performed by creating an incision at the margin of the concha with two connecting incisions that form three adjacent triangles (marked A, B, & C). (b) Skin is elevated from the underlying concha such that (c) wide cartilage resection is afforded. (d) A radial incision is fashioned into the membranous EAC toward the bone-cartilaginous junction creating two additional triangles (marked D & E). (e) Triangle B is advanced in a V to Y fashion into the radial incision to expand the circumference of the meatus, while the apices of triangles D and E are sutured on either side of the base of triangle B. (f) Triangles A and C are excised. (g) The remaining skin edges are sutured in place with a resultant "M."

The facial nerve is at greatest risk during canalplasty at the posterior-inferior part of the tympanic annulus, where it is possible for the nerve to pass lateral to the tympanic ring.[9] Surgical experience and familiarity with surgical anatomy of the temporal bone, combined with the use of preoperative CT temporal bone scans and facial nerve monitoring, may reduce the likelihood of facial nerve injury. The proximity of the chorda tympani nerve to the posterior fibrous annulus causes taste disturbance to be a potential risk.

Skin grafting is often required during canalplasty surgery; however, these grafts may not always regain the normal migratory properties of natural EAC skin, especially if the tympanic membrane has been de-epithelialized. Patients who undergo extensive skin grafting in the ear canal with little to no residual native canal wall skin are predisposed to infection and accumulation of debris. These patients need surveillance every six months for the firstone to two years after the ear canal is healed and then annually thereafter.

20.6 Outcomes

Hearing results after surgical treatment of bony stenosis are often excellent. After repair of soft tissue stenosis, the air-bone gap closure is within 20 dB in 61% to 94% of cases.[5,6,10,11] The reported re-stenosis rates after corrective surgery for CSOE vary from 6.7% to 18.8%.[3,4,11] The absence of recurrence does not correlate with improved hearing thresholds.[4,6]

20.7 Conclusion

Understanding how to perform meatoplasty and canalplasty is critical to the management of the chronic ear. Key principles for canalplasty include preservation of as much native skin as possible, wide drilling of the bony canal such that the entire annulus is easily visualized from a single vantage point, and coverage of exposed bone with split-thickness skin grafts. For meatoplasty, it is essential to adequately widen the meatus in the posterior-superior aspect, with generous removal of concha cartilage, and to execute careful suture technique that affords a rounded and widened meatal opening without outwardly exposed cartilaginous edges.

References

[1] Atlas M, Eisenberg R. A Guide to Temporal Bone Dissection. 2nd Ed. Perth: Lions Ear & Hearing Institute; 2004.

[2] Rizer FM. Overlay versus underlay tympanoplasty. Part I: Historical review of the literature. Laryngoscope. 1997;107(12 Pt 2):1–25.

[3] Selesnick S, Nguyen TP, Eisenman DJ. Surgical treatment of acquired external auditory canal atresia. Am J Otol. 1998;19(2):123–130.

[4] Birman CS, Fagan PA. Medial canal stenosis—chronic stenosing external otitis. Am J Otol. 1996;17(1):2–6.

[5] Becker BC, Tos M. Postinflammatory acquired atresia of the external auditory canal: treatment and results of surgery over 27 years. Laryngoscope. 1998;108(6):903–907.

[6] Lin VY, Chee GH, David EA, Chen JM. Medial canal fibrosis: Surgical technique, results, and a proposed grading system. Otol Neurotol. 2005;26(5):825–829.

[7] Fisch U. Myringoplasty, meatoplasty and canalplasty. In: Fisch U, May JS, Linder T, eds. Tympanoplasty, mastoidectomy, and stapes surgery. New York, NY: Thieme, 2008:39–42.

[8] Mirck PGB. The M-meatoplasty of the external auditory canal. Laryngoscope. 1996;106(3 Pt 1):367–369.

[9] Adad B, Rasgon BM, Ackerson L. Relationship of the facial nerve to the tympanic annulus: A direct anatomic examination. Laryngoscope. 1999;109 (8):1189–1192.

[10] Slattery WH, III, Saadat P. Postinflammatory medial canal fibrosis. Am J Otol. 1997;18(3):294–297.

[11] Cremers WR, Smeets JH. Acquired atresia of the external auditory canal. Surgical treatment and results. Arch Otolaryngol Head Neck Surg. 1993;119 (2):162–164.

21 Cholesteatoma Dissection: Problems and Solutions

Bruce Black

Abbreviations used in the chapter:

CT: computed tomography
CWU: canal wall–up
EAC: external auditory canal

21.1 Introduction

Meticulous removal of disease is a requirement common to the various types of cholesteatoma surgery. Although this may be pursued via one of a variety of described techniques for surgical access, the choice of which remain controversial, the aims of cholesteatoma dissection remain constant: eradication of disease, restoration of function, and prevention of complications. Within limits, surgery should be simple, versatile, and reliable: simple, so that other otologists can master the technique; versatile, so the skills can be obtained from experience in the greatest number of cases; and reliable with regard to efficacy and durability. Removal of the squamous epithelial matrix is common to all methods. This requires particular aspects of preparation, instrumentation, exposure, and clearance techniques.

21.2 Preparation

Dissection of cholesteatoma matrix often requires full concentration that is demanding and intolerant of interruption. Thus, appropriate preparation and arrangement of the operating table and instrumentation (as described in Chapter 18), plus clear surgical planning, allow the surgeon to "settle into the saddle," avoid delays, and permit optimal dissection. For the novice cholesteatoma surgeon, it may be important to schedule more surgical time than what may be expected so as to avoid the need to perform the dissection hastily.

21.3 Instrumentation

Prompt access to the necessary instrumentation is essential for efficient cholesteatoma dissection. If working with a novice or in-training surgical assistant, it may be helpful to be involved in organizing a layout of instruments that places the frequently handled instruments (scalpel, suction, micro-picks) nearest the surgeon and the lesser handled at a greater distance (retractors, elevators, speculae, drill, diathermy). Also, numbering a few of the frequently used micro-picks (and maintaining a constant sequence) can help rapid identification and turnover.

Apart from surgeons' personal preferences and the usual instruments common to most otology sites, some instruments have particular application that readers may find useful during matrix dissection. These are listed in ▶ Table 21.1. All micro-picks should incorporate robust, stiff shafts if possible; flexible, "whippy" types are inadequate or dangerous in many circumstances. Some instruments with specific attributes deserve comment.

Dissection of matrix or mucosa is often difficult when advancing over the rim of the scutum, in confined cells, or

Table 21.1 Instrumentation

Specialized Instruments	Role
Hughes stapes mobilizer 223502 (KSG)	Matrix elevation over scutum and minor obstructions
Kley footplate knife 223400 (KSG)	Fine adhesion division; dissection on stapes superstructure, malleus, facial nerve
Large Plester sickle knife 223303 (KSG)	Extended reach; sharp dissection in anterior EAC angle, anterior attic (via attic defect)
3-mm 90-degree micro-pick (M)	Incudostapedial disarticulation; elevation of matrix off attic defect edges, stapes arch, malleus handle
Mini McGee fine alligator forceps 13–1040 (G)	Fine grasp of soft tissues
Up-biting alligator forceps (M)	Transcanal removal of attic ossicles
Holmgren self-retaining ear speculae 5 mm 123205 (KSG) 6 mm 123506 (KSG) 7 mm 123507 (KSG)	Transcanal exposure, dilatation of superficial soft tissues
Other commonly used micro-picks	Sheehy weapon 23–0339 (G) Rosen elevator (M) 260000 (G) Plester knife (M) 251–500 (G) House curette (M) 13–0568 (G) 45° .75 mm micro-pick (M) 13–0392 (G)
Suppliers: Karl Storz Gmb (KSG); Gyrus/Olympus (G); Multiple suppliers (M)	

around minor obstructions. A curved needle or fine sickle knife may be successful but may lacerate the more friable sacs. Alternatively, a Hughes stapes mobilizer (▶ Fig. 21.1) is advantageous. This resembles the Beales elevator but is narrower. Increasing its longitudinal curve beyond the supplied shape improves its use within the less accessible sites. When very fine needlepoint dissection is required in accessible sites, a Kley knife (▶ Fig. 21.1) is highly effective, especially when dissecting on or around ossicles. The razor-thin tip is especially effective for removing epithelium or drum remnants off the stapes and the handle of the malleus.

21.4 Case Evaluation

Cholesteatoma may be classified as congenital, acquired (attic, pars tensa, or combined), or atypical/unclassifiable (▶ Fig. 21.2). The presentation of the disease suggests its pattern, extent, and associated problems[1] and also the appropriate dissection steps. For example, a pars tensa pattern without attic extension may be best managed by transcanal removal via fine sharp dissection; limited attic disease may submit to an atticotomy approach and fine blunt elevation; extensive disease may require a mastoidectomy and more robust removal. Audiology and a computed tomography (CT) scan may provide further direction with respect to the ossicular chain status and mastoid aeration, respectively. Deciding the overall management strategy is best left until this evaluation is completed. This evaluation is essential to accurately counsel the patient preoperatively, but to do so effectively, the surgeon will need to forecast the situation that is present at the conclusion of disease clearance, that is, immediately before reconstruction, to be able to assess the effect of disease removal, the prognosis of the appropriate repairs, and, therefore, the final outlook.

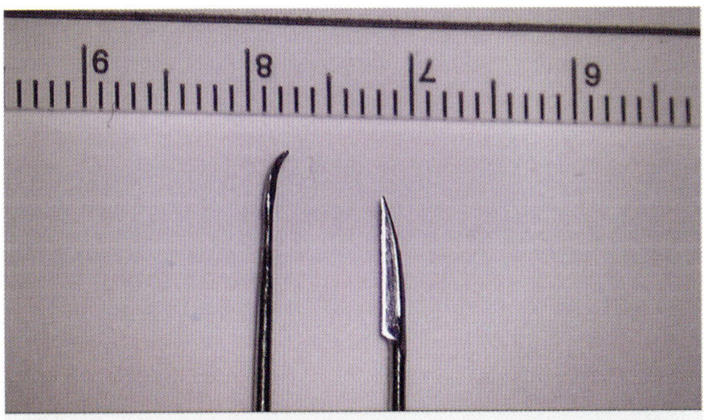

Fig. 21.1 Specialized dissection instrumentation. The Kley Knife (right) has a needle-sharp tip suited to fine dissection and a thin razor-sharp blade, useful in the confines of the oval window or similar sites. The Hughes elevator (left) allows matrix or mucosal elevation when progressing over the scutum or similar low-level obstacles or gentle, blunt dissection over vitals. Both are Karl Storz devices (Karl Storz GmbH and Co., Tuttlingen, Germany).

21.5 Cholesteatoma Surgical Scheme

Intraoperatively, a general stepwise flow to cholesteatoma surgery can be followed no matter which approach is favored. This involves the orderly sequence of (1) assessment of disease, (2) exposure of cholesteatoma, (3) removal of cholesteatoma, and (4) reconstruction of the defect.

Ideally, each step is completely finished before moving on to the next. Details of the first three of these are considered in the following discussion, with descriptions of the fourth covered in Part 4, Roundtable on Tympanic Membrane Reconstruction; Part 6, Roundtable on Tympanomastoidectomy; Part 7, Roundtable on Hybrid Tympanomastoid Surgical Techniques; and Chapter 41.

21.5.1 Assessment of Disease

Inspection of the tympanic membrane and exploration of the middle ear provide information about the nature, suspected origin, and extent of cholesteatoma that is helpful in anticipating the optimal surgical technique. Although preoperative imaging may provide useful information, at times it may be difficult to radiologically distinguish cholesteatoma from thickened mucosa, aural polyp, or middle ear secretions. Exploration also allows the surgeon to determine the status of the ossicular chain to avoid acoustic trauma during cholesteatoma exposure and dissection. Lastly, an initial assessment is made of the quality of hemostasis, which if greatly suboptimal, may impact intraoperative surgical decision-making.

21.5.2 Cholesteatoma Exposure

Several steps ensure adequate surgical access to the matrix for dissection that may be severely impeded or impossible should these be overlooked.

The essential first step in cholesteatoma removal surgery is adequate exposure of the stapes and its surrounds. Removal of matrix from this site is mandatory for a dry ear and functional hearing. In many cases this cannot be accomplished adequately

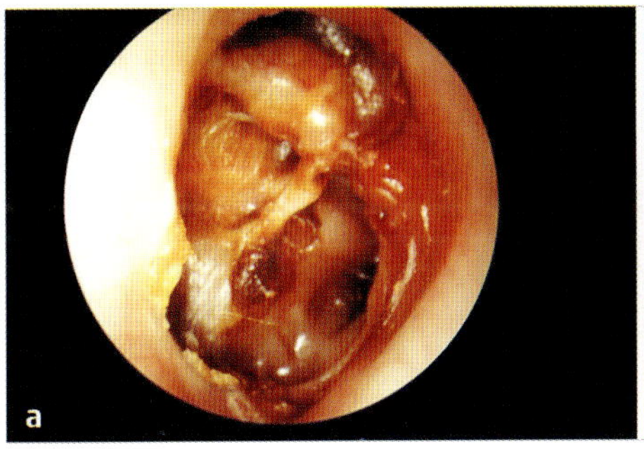

a

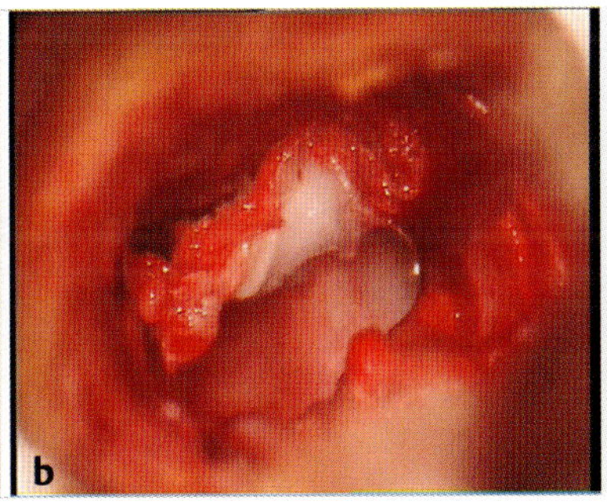

b

Fig. 21.2 (a) Advanced combined cholesteatoma due to long-standing tubal insufficiency. Gross tubal invagination is present, the ossicles are compromised, but mastoid extension may be limited into a poorly aerated cell system. (b) Atypical cholesteatoma pattern. Squamous epithelium covers the undersurface of the drum, possibly as a result of congenital origins, an adherent sac invagination, or epithelial migration via a drum perforation.

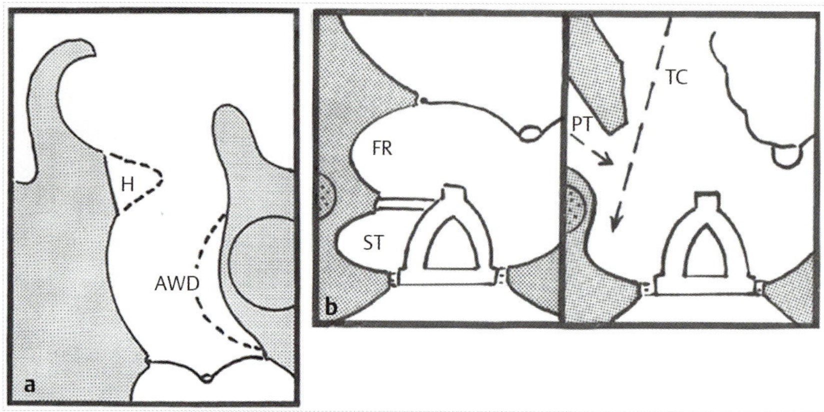

Fig. 21.3 (a) Transcanal access. A Hunsaker correction of superficial narrowing and an anterior EAC wall drill-back permit optimal long-term surveillance of the deep canal and facilitate management of external canal problems (debris, chronic myringitis). (b) Transcanal approach to the sinus tympani. The lateral approach offers the optimal approach to the sinus. Removing scutum back to the plane of the descending facial nerve can be supplemented by skeletonizing the nerve itself, for maximal access to the sinus itself.

via a posterior tympanotomy approach because the descending facial nerve often impedes optimal visualization to the posterior aspect of the oval window niche, the pyramidal process, and the ponticulus; mobilization of the facial nerve[2] is very rarely necessitated. The transcanal vantage point gives the best access for instrumentation of the posterior mesotympanum (including the sinus tympani), but this often requires careful modification of the ear canal and/or meatus to be ideal. Also, cholesteatoma surgery requires long-term postoperative observation. Therefore, where possible, an adequately wide and straight external auditory canal (EAC) lumen is advantageous, both during and after surgery.

The superficial narrowing of the EAC is common, especially in children, and may severely impede post-surgical observation of the pars tensa. Also, narrowing at this site may occur after canal wall–up (CWU) surgery, due to minor secondary ossification effects. Superficial meatoplasty may be necessary. Hunsaker's 1988 technique[3] is recommended: the relatively simple technique is transcanal, the final canal introitus size is predictable, and it is readily combined with deeper surgery.

A tortuous EAC is managed by a canalplasty that involves anterior wall drill-back. This facilitates access for initial stapes clearance and also permits postoperative access to the anterior sulcus in the event of myringitis, granulations, graft breakdown, or simple debris accumulation. The combination of superficial meatoplasty and anterior canalplasty exposure thus permits optimal operative and long-term management (▸ Fig. 21.3a).

If disease is noted in the posterior mesotympanum, a scutum drill-back is necessary. Anticipating this, the tympanomeatal flap is created more superficially (longer) than normal. Sufficiently wide scutum reduction, a step that is often inadequately performed by novice surgeons, affords visualization of the descending facial nerve, which may be skeletonized with a 2-mm diamond bur at its anterior aspect adjacent to the vestibule of the sinus tympani (▸ Fig. 21.3b). The resultant exposure, with proper patient rotation and positioning of the microscope, often permits inspection of the entire sinus tympani, requiring endoscopic assistance for dissection in a small minority. Drum composite grafting should follow scutum reduction to prevent pars tensa re-collapse.

Upon clearance of stapedial disease, management of attic disease may also be sought via the transcanal vantage point. However, the decision to use this method may be complicated by uncertainty as regards the extent of disease extension within the attic, into the mastoid, and/or into the supratubal recess[4]; endoscopy[5] may help in only a proportion of cases. Transcanal enlargement of the attic defect may permit the removal of smaller sacs, but open surgery or a CWU procedure is needed for deeper invaginations. An essential principle to consider is that, no matter which vantage point is chosen for cholesteatoma dissection in the attic, isolation of the cholesteatoma "neck" at its junction of the residual tympanic membrane and complete lateral exposure of the sac should be achieved prior to attempted disease removal. Adhering to this ideal will maximize the odds of definitively removing the sac as a single self-contained specimen. In contrast, blind piecemeal removal of matrix from "around the corner" of the scutum or from a limited and narrow posterior vantage point through the antrum are not recommended.

When postaural surgery is required, ample transmastoid attic exposure is needed (▸ Fig. 21.4). This approach is facilitated by the wide exposure of the root of the zygoma. The following steps as described provide sufficient access without trauma to either the temporalis fascia or the underlying squamous periosteum, both of which may be needed to provide vascular flaps for subsequent reconstructions.[6]

If CWU surgery is employed, it is important for the surgeon to widely remove all of the bone of the lateral attic wall, including drilling far into the anterior epitympanic wall for access to the perigeniculate region and supratubal recess. To be done properly, this requires the skeletonization of the middle fossa dura. In some cases, a low tegmen and/or an anteriorly displaced lateral sinus will impede CWU attic visualization. These problems may be countered by "egg-shelling" the bone overlying each with a large diamond bur, then displacing the semi-rigid result, or by similarly isolating an island of thin bone, which is then displaced. Bone wax is used to temporarily keep the structures out of the line of inspection. During the approach to the posterior attic, bleeding from a small branch of the middle meningeal artery in the dura above may be troublesome; this can also be managed with bone wax.

21.5.3 Matrix Removal

Sac Characteristics

The nature of the cholesteatoma sac itself will influence the dissection and removal methods employed. The matrix may be saccular, infiltrative, finely atrophic, friable, or a membranous

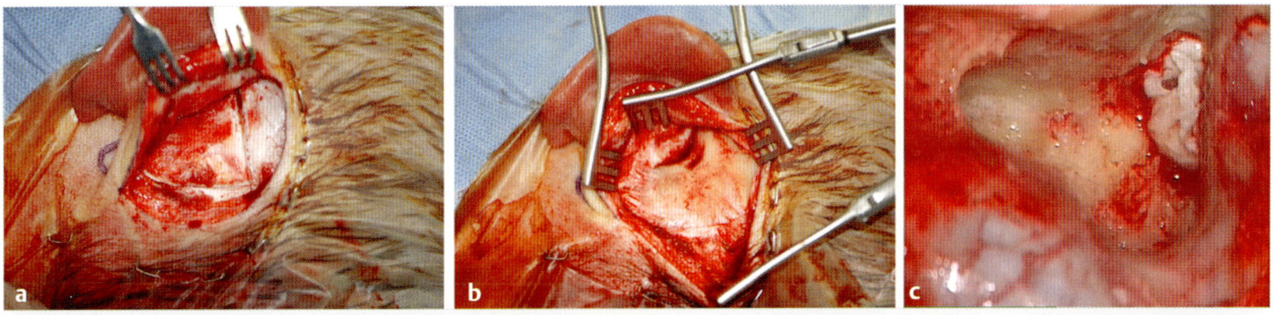

Fig. 21.4 (a) Postaural approach for CWU surgery, left ear. A hairline skin incision is followed by dissection in the avascular plane between skin and the underlying fascia-periosteal layer to expose the latter. A horizontal incision onto bone extends from the glenoid tubercle along the line of the avascular suprameatal crest, extending posteriorly 1–2 cm beyond the line of the skin incision. A second incision passes inferiorly from the crest along the posterior border of the mastoid to the tip. (b) Mastoid exposure. The mastoid periosteum is raised as an inverted-L flap. The temporalis fascia, muscle, and underlying pericranium are elevated intact, retaining vascular supply from the superficial and middle temporal arteries. These tissues can then be used for local vascular flaps if required. (c) Surgical approach to the attic. Vital structures to routinely identify include the lateral semicircular canal, then the posterior geniculate artery (central) that is a landmark identifying the site of the posterior genu. The descending facial nerve is seen immediately inferior.

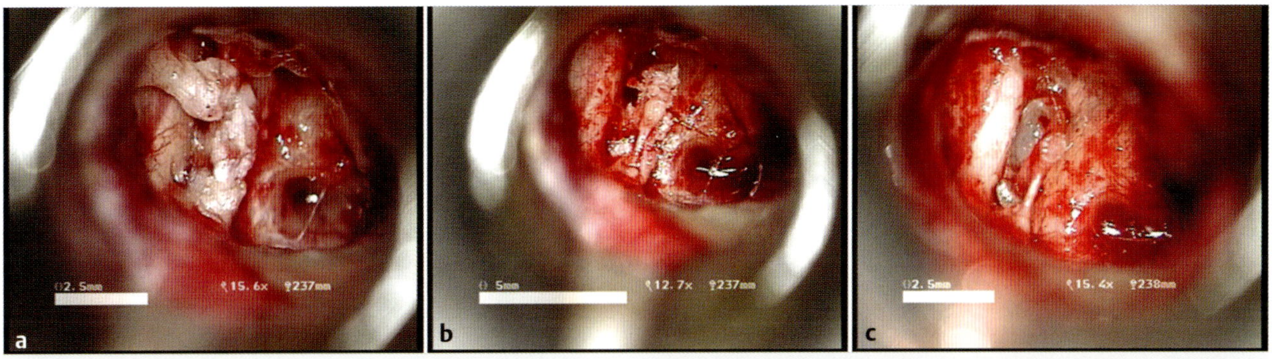

Fig. 21.5 Cholesteatoma matrix in the attic. (a) Friable-type matrix enveloping the incus and stapes superstructure, right ear. Previous congenital cholesteatoma removal. The lenticular process of the incus has necrosed. The facial nerve and its attendant vasculature are evident in the left field. (b) Removal of superstructure matrix via an incision from the pyramid to the stapes head. The stapedius tendon thus stabilizes the stapes. The two "wings" of matrix can be dissected off the superior and inferior aspects independently. (c) Final disease clearance. A fine Kley knife has been used to clear the matrix from the stapes itself and off the facial nerve above and the promontory below, working from posterior to anterior.

coating of the drum undersurface. Round/oval/globular sacs are common in attic and congenital cases. These have some tensile strength that permits gentle sac retraction with fine suction, plus sharp division of fine mucosal attachments that allows removal without rupture of the sac.

Infiltrative sac patterns are problematic in the anterior attic and in cellular mastoids, particularly around the semicircular canals. Fine, curved needle dissection may extract fine pockets but may carry some risk of local damage or residue. Likewise, infiltration around ossicles presents difficulties. Removal of the affected ossicle may be necessary, and when removed from the stapes or round window, chain repair is often best left until second-stage surgery.

Fine, atrophic squamous epithelium commonly results from drum collapse in pars tensa cases, secondary to chronic tubal insufficiency (▶ Fig. 21.2a). This is also a common problem in open cavity elimination surgery, where the tympanomastoid cavity lining is often particularly atrophic. The fine film may be fragile and adherent to the promontory, the remains of the ossicles, and the surrounding structures. Removal requires fine, sharp dissection to minimize trauma, but in the middle ear the mucosa should be spared if possible to limit subsequent adhesion formation. Absorbable gelatin film or Silastic may reduce postoperative adhesions although obliterative fibrosis often intervenes when mucosal loss is extensive and tubal failure persists. Suction will need to be delicate, using a fine lumen.

Friable sacs disintegrate with minor trauma. This less common fragile matrix variant is found in some congenital cholesteatoma cases and also when body tissues in general are of poor quality (▶ Fig. 21.5). Meticulous clearance is often necessary because the poor tensile strength impedes intact sac removal. Staged surgery to check for residual disease is mandatory in most of these cases.

Finally, squamous epithelium may line the medial aspect of the pars tensa (▶ Fig. 21.2b). The origins are uncertain; some seem originally congenital, others a result of invagination or epithelial migration though a perforation. The drum may exhibit the pearly sheen of cholesteatoma, but this may be obscured, the problem being detected only after failure of initial drum-grafting attempts. Limited access, excessive drum tissue mobility, or adherent disease may impede its fine, sharp dissection off the drum undersurface. Partial or total myringectomy may be required.

Choice of Technique

A range of instrumentation is available to remove the matrix itself: sharp points, blunt/rounded points, abrasives (cotton pledgets, ribbon gauze, diamond burs [rotating or stationary as a fine rasp]), suction, grasping forceps, micro-scissors, lasers, and drilling burs. Each has positives and negatives. Sharp knives/needles may be optimal for very fine dissection but less appropriate over some delicate, soft tissue vitals whereas blunt dissection is poorly adapted to difficult access sites or in fibrotic situations. Abrasives are effective over robust bony surfaces but less suitable upon vital or inaccessible sites. Suction is beneficial to retract matrix clear of dissection points but may shred less tensile disease, leaving residues, and should be used with great care near fistulae. Grasping forceps facilitate the removal of gross disease, particularly over non-vital areas such as the mastoid bowl, but are less appropriate in poorly accessible sites or if disease is adherent to vitals. Micro-scissors are used for sac incision, fine division of adhesions, or the development of soft tissue planes. All manipulative techniques should be used with care over vital structures, especially the stapes superstructure or footplate. Lasers are appropriate for the stapes superstructure or other fine removal sites but less appropriate over fistulae or some oval window situations, where perforations of the labyrinthine endosteum may result.

The choice of method ultimately used for a particular task may be determined by several additional factors: the pattern or nature of the matrix (as above), the underlying mucosa, access, local contours, the attached anatomy (e.g., ossicles), ease of dissection, or the availability of specific instrumentation (e.g., lasers, endoscopes).

Sac-type matrix frequently occludes access to the site involved, particularly in the mesotympanum and attic. Incising the sac and evacuating the contents collapses the sac, giving better access, which is further enhanced by progressive, grasping removal of elevated matrix as dissection proceeds. Conversely, fine or fragile disease dictates gentler dissection.

The status of the underlying mucosa is relevant. A plane between the sac and adjacent mucosa is frequently demonstrable and may permit removal without tearing either, but if not, dissection along the plane between the mucosa and the underlying bone offers the best chance of clearance without leaving residual foci, removing both mucosa and the sac by fine dissection, either sharp or blunt. Inflammation and mucosal edema thicken the mucosa, facilitating dissection.

Local contours frequently impede this dissection. These may be drilled off, but specific instrumentation, such as the Hughes or the large Plester knife, may be required to work around vital structures. Also, the structure to which the matrix is attached is relevant. For instance, drilling, grasping, or abrasive techniques may be optimal to clear extensive mastoid disease, but an attachment to a fistula or facial nerve requires a more delicate technique, avoiding tension on the site as much as possible.

The availability of specialized equipment may influence the method used. The necessity for laser equipment or facial nerve monitors remains controversial. The former is advantageous for adherent disease on the stapes superstructure; the latter should not replace optimal knowledge of anatomy. Monitors will not prevent nerve trauma in some cases and may prove distracting in many.

Special Sites

Several sites of particular interest are encountered during matrix clearance; these are identified below in bold text in the sequence in which they may be encountered.

Posterior Mesotympanum

The initial transcanal approach to the stapes is often complicated by drum retraction into the facial recess and sinus tympani, which hinders elevation without tearing the epithelium. Reducing the rim of the overhanging scutum with a diamond bur, then displacing the thinned bone and underlying mucosa-matrix medially with a fine, rounded (Hughes) elevator, displaces the overlying matrix out of the facial recess and sinus tympani in continuity. Such elevation, working from the lower end of the retraction/sac superiorly toward the oval window, provides progressive visualization of the round window, then the stapes and its surrounds, with the least risk of tearing the matrix, leaving residual foci. The round window site requires caution, to avoid penetration of the membrane, given that the position and orientation of this is variable and may be relatively superficial. If the matrix is adherent, the surrounds should be cleared, then the overlying patch should be removed with fine, sharp or blunt dissection. Upon approach to the oval window, the pyramid and the stapedius tendon are useful landmarks that help locate the head of the stapes, which may be obscured by edema or enveloping matrix (▶ Fig. 21.5b).

Following the bony contours superior to the pyramid leads to the horizontal facial nerve, which should be clearly identified prior to working deeper in the oval window site. Dissection along the sheath of the facial nerve with a fine, rounded elevator carries little risk, even when the nerve is dehiscent, as frequently occurs.[7,8] If the incus is fixed, diseased, or necrotic (▶ Fig. 21.5a), it is best removed at this stage. Removal aids identification of the stapes head and facilitates deeper peristapedial dissection. Elective removal of an intact incus is desirable if extensive attic disease is present and also to isolate the stapes from potential drill trauma if the attic is to be cleared via a postaural approach.

The ultra-fine tip of the Kley knife is advantageous to clear the disease off the stapes superstructure, working posterior forward (▶ Fig. 21.5b) along the planes between the stapes and promontory or facial nerve, using the stapedius tendon to stabilize the superstructure during dissection and fine suction to retract the matrix. Clearance of matrix off the stapes superstructure or footplate may demand the highest skills; manipulation, subluxation, footplate fracture, or residual foci are significant dangers of this situation (▶ Fig. 21.5c). A laser may facilitate the clearance by detachment of the stapes arch, especially when disease has invaginated through the arch itself, but if this equipment is not available, manual clearance using straight, angled, or 90-degree micro-picks requires considerable delicacy to avoid cochlear trauma from stapes manipulations.

Irremovable matrix on the stapes arch presents formidable problems and is often best left until a sterile second-stage situation, when a more easily defined pearl may be present, or at which time the arch may have necrosed away. Without an available laser, the manual removal of an intact stapes arch is particularly difficult and risks a footplate fracture or avulsion. Usually, this should be attempted only when disease cannot be removed by other methods, when it is imperative to do so, and is best left to the end of the procedure, with a fine soft tissue graft at the ready in case footplate removal inadvertently occurs. Avoiding the latter requires a balance between removal technique, footplate stabilization, and cochlear protection, which a laser achieves comfortably. Alternatively, a gentle grasp (mini-McGee forceps) on the posterior crus and slow drilling with a 0.5-mm diamond bur suffice to divide the posterior arch. The anterior crus can then be crushed and removed. Adequate exposure is essential, as per ▶ Fig. 21.5c.

Covert crural necrosis may be noted during sac removal; delicate palpation of the stapes head may reveal hypermobility in this instance. Alternatively, a slightly stiff superstructure commonly warns of subtle fixation that may defy mobilization efforts and thus frustrate ossiculoplasty outcomes. Fibrous attachments can be divided piecemeal or removed by using a laser, but these tend to recur due to loss of mucosa and the narrow confines of the stapes site. Tympanosclerosis, although commonly "cheesy" in consistency and often not difficult to remove, may still be accompanied by secondary ossification, requiring removal with a micro-drill. Both may cause subsequent stapes re-fixation.

In the absence of superstructure, the sac may be adherent to the footplate. Particularly fine, sharp dissection along the plane of the footplate without pressure and with minimal traction from suction avoids footplate mishaps. The footplate is frequently fragile and easily broken. Oval window fistulae are another uncommon difficulty to be avoided at this time. Footplate mishaps require soft tissue coverage and immediate parenteral antibiotic (gentamicin or ciprofloxacin) cover; ossiculoplasty should be left to second-stage surgery rather than risk cochlear penetration from a prosthesis placed on an unstable site. Overall, the stapes that is compromised by disease or surgery represents a severe outcomes threat.

Uncommonly, severe drum retraction may develop hypotympanic cell invagination. Considerable scutum reduction plus a postaural approach may be necessary for access. As above, the optimal clearance involves elevation of the underlying mucosa in toto. Cautious diamond drilling of the inferior otic capsule and endoscopic inspection may facilitate exposure and removal, but involvement of this site usually dictates second-stage reinspection. Rarely, skull base expertise may be required.

Attic Invagination

Attic cholesteatoma may occur from traction via the notch of Rivinus or from attic extension via a pars tensa collapse. Both may be managed from the transcanal vantage point; however, the decision on whether or not to combine this exposure with a postaural approach will depend on the background, bias, and experience of the surgeon. Assessment of the extent or pattern of the pocket may be difficult before surgery. Computed tomography scans may not help if infection, effusion, or attic fibrosis hinders the image interpretation.[4] Keratin accumulation may preclude endoscopic inspection to assess the depth of the pocket although this technique may help plan care of less occluded cases. If the sac is small, transcanal removal via only limited scutum removal may suffice.

Deeper sacs may cause difficulty: the surgeon reaches a point where a decision on open or closed surgery is necessary. Limited, blind elevation of the sac is possible using the Hughes device, a 3-mm 90-degree right angle pick, or similar curved instrumentation. This can be undertaken, drawing the sac away from the edges of the defect with a fine sucker, while gently clearing the underlying fine soft tissue attachments until the apex of the sac is delivered. However, this technique is viable only if the sac is maintained in continuity; once ruptured, direct observation of further clearance is necessary to avoid the problem of residual disease. Retention of the head of the malleus and incus may be achieved in simpler and limited cases, but if the sac has invaginated around these structures, it is generally safer to remove these to permit better inspection, particularly of the anterior attic area, normally as a part of more advanced surgery.

Mastoid Disease

When disease has extended into the antrum or mastoid, a decision for open or closed management is required to clear the diseased cell system. During mastoid surgery the dissection methods change to more robust techniques. Large sacs may be incised and keratin evacuated to enhance exposure. In the mastoid itself, removal of matrix using suction and blunt dissection, followed by drilling and polishing the underlying cells or bone, is generally highly successful: residual disease in this area is relatively uncommon.

Retro-labyrinthine extension is an unusual problem encountered at this time. Access being impeded, CWU surgery is invalid unless the remaining disease can be removed with certainty. The choice is thus open-cavity surgery or labyrinthectomy, the latter if intracranial problems threaten or if severe sensorineural deafness precludes restoration of useful hearing.

As the dissection approaches the antrum ad aditus, identification of the lateral semicircular canal, the posterior geniculate artery,[9] then the descending facial nerve should be routine steps to avoid trauma to the nerve. Dissection becomes more cautious at this stage. Fine, sharp dissection, abrasive methods, and gentle suction, followed by fine diamond-drill polishing, are the preferred methods. Over non-vital structures, dissection using the tip of the sucker itself or rasping with a stationary diamond bur is effective. During this phase in CWU cases, care should be observed not to perforate or excessively thin the posterior-superior canal wall; perforation or resorption of this section is a common problem,[10,11] especially in tortuous canals when attic access is difficult.

Advancing into the antrum, the approach to the lateral semicircular canal also requires some care. Fistulae are a common occurrence in cholesteatomas, particularly those with larger sacs that involve the mastoid. [12,13] The defects are present usually on the lateral or superior aspect of the lateral canal.[14,15] Clinical assessment and CT scans, if employed, may not detect these. Therefore, elevating matrix over the bulge of the lateral canal should be performed with vigilance to avoid traumatizing

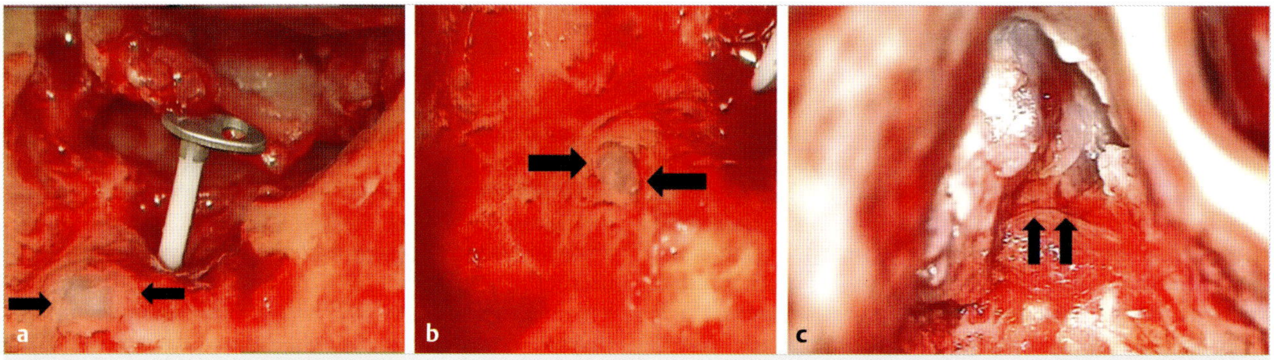

Fig. 21.6 (a) Lateral semicircular canal fistula, right ear, mastoidectomy reconstruction case. Matrix has been left on the fistula (lower left field), pending completion of other procedures. A total ossicular replacement prosthesis is in situ. The vessels of the horizontal facial nerve are visible superior to the prosthesis. (b) Fistula site after removal of the matrix patch. (c) Giant lateral canal fistula (central), right attic. Concurrent, extensive dural exposure covered by cholesteatoma. Extensive attic granulations precluded dural clearance prior to removal of disease from the fistula.

a fistula site. The latter may be suspected by direct inspection through the matrix (▶ Fig. 21.6a) once the keratin contents of the sac have been removed, by altered canal contours, by a larger-than-expected aditus, or from the "blue-lined" thinning of the canal bony casing, observed when the overlying matrix is elevated as the fistula site is approached.

If a fistula is strongly suspected, an "island" of matrix over the site should be left (▶ Fig. 21.6) until all other clearance and reconstruction nears completion.[12,13,14,15] Definitive management is controversial. In most cases, developing a plane between the otic capsule endosteum and the matrix by using gentle blunt dissection and fine suction can clear the matrix patch, which is then covered with soft tissue or bone paté. If the matrix is adherent during CWU surgery, a scrap may be left over the fistula site. At second-stage surgery, this epithelial patch has often vanished or has formed a small pearl that is easily cleared. The fistula is often found to have ossified over or is covered with robust soft tissues. Rarely, matrix invagination into the labyrinth may be found at primary surgery. This may dictate either labyrinthectomy, especially if substantial sensorineural losses have occurred, or a conversion to open surgery although the latter risks substantial vertigo if cavity suction toilet aftercare is necessary.

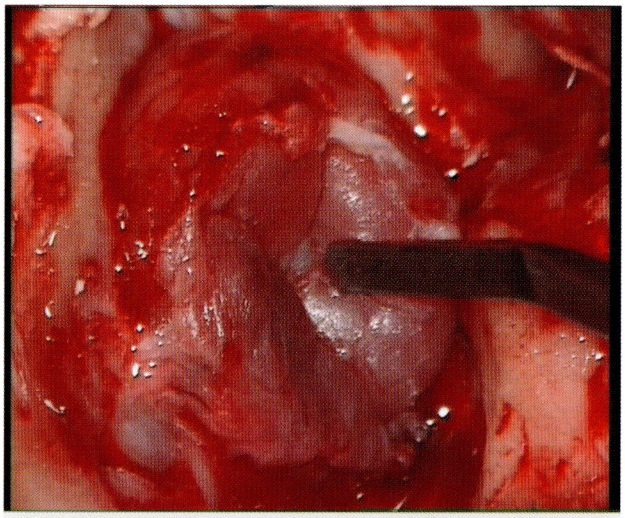

Fig. 21.7 Extensive middle fossa dural exposure by cholesteatoma, right ear. The Rosen elevator indicates a central defect extending into the middle cranial fossa with demonstration of the depth of the intracranial extension by gentle probing. The dura could be cleared by alligator micro-scissor dissection, but the extension requires neurosurgical expertise.

Attic Disease

Advancing beyond the lateral canal into the attic, the horizontal facial nerve is the next critical landmark and is often identified by the vessels within (▶ Fig. 21.5a; ▶ Fig. 21.6a). If matrix has not been cleared via the initial transcanal approach, the frequent dehiscence of this structure[7,8] dictates care, using clearance methods similar to those used to remove fistula matrix. Elsewhere, the attic can be cleared by fine, sharp dissection or gentle abrasion, followed by diamond-drill polishing. Particular care to avoid residual foci should be taken around the processus cochleariformis and the tensor tendon.

Anterior attic clearance may require limited scutum reduction and also removal of "Sheehy's cog." If there is doubt regarding removal of matrix off the edges of the attic defect or scutum, these can be polished with the shoulder of a 3-mm diamond bur or scoured with a thin gauze strip passed through the attic defect.

Dural exposure by cholesteatoma is not infrequent (▶ Fig. 21.6c; ▶ Fig. 21.7). Removal with finely tipped, sharp dissection (e.g., the Kley knife) usually suffices to clear the site, but adherent disease may require alligator micro-scissor dissection or even limited resection and repair with soft tissue or cartilage grafts. Penetration of matrix into the middle fossa mandates neurosurgical expertise (▶ Fig. 21.7). Further anteriorly, the middle fossa dura dips inferiorly immediately anterior to the "cog" and should be avoided during final diamond-bur bone polishing in the anterior attic. If the attic roof bone is thinned extensively, a brain hernia may result (▶ Fig. 21.8). These should be retracted at second-stage surgery to ensure the absence of residual disease.

Other Postaural Approach Sites

Clearance of other sites may require a postaural approach. Invagination into the Eustachian orifice (▶ Fig. 21.2a) may form

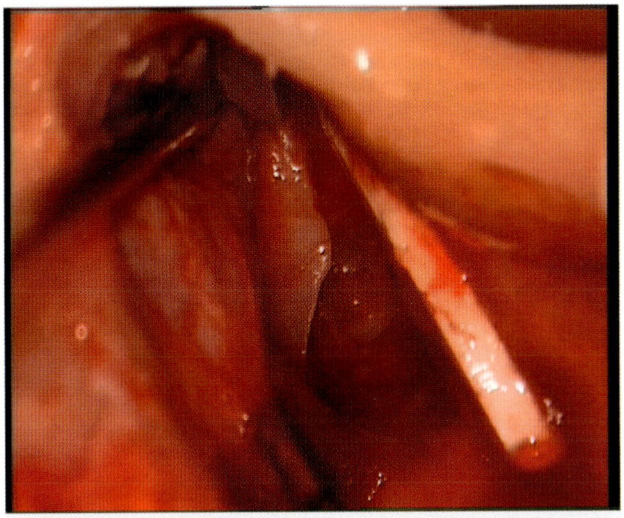

Fig. 21.8 Brain hernia, right attic, seen filling the attic at second-stage CWU surgery, subsequent to dural exposure at previous CWU surgery. A hydroxyapatite attic repair plate is present. Attic visualization is totally obscured.

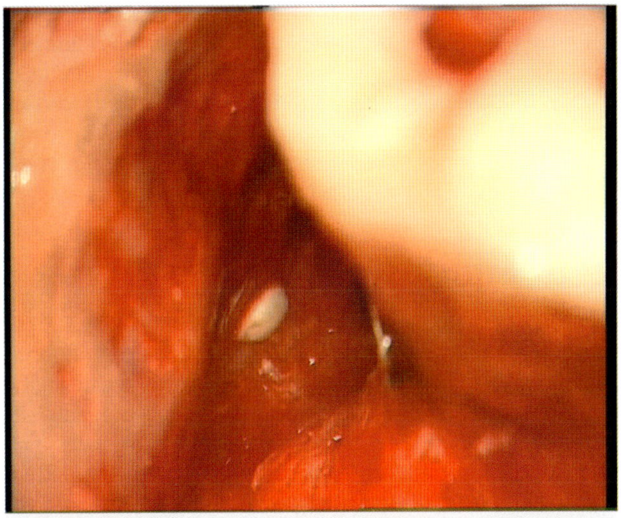

Fig. 21.9 Residual cholesteatoma, right aditus, easily removed intact by clearing the underlying mucosa. Small lesions may be missed by MRI scans.

a saccular retraction that is relatively easily removed, but, alternatively, matrix may be adherent to the lateral wall of the orifice. Reduction of the anterior scutum may not give adequate visualization in such cases; endoscopic monitoring may help. Using a long, curved needle or Plester sickle knife for limited, blind meticulous elevation of the lateral tubal mucosa usually achieves clearance of the overlying matrix. When deeply penetrating disease coats the medial wall, the carotid artery will lie medially.

Retention of the malleus handle may be desirable if an assembly-type ossiculoplasty is preferable. This may be enveloped by disease (▶ Fig. 21.2a) that may be difficult to remove during the transcanal stapes clearance phase, and a postaural approach may be necessary. The collapsed posterior drum is elevated and reflected forwards to expose the periosteum of the posterior surface of the handle. This is then incised from the lateral process to the umbo using a sharp-tipped knife/needle (the Kley knife is ideal), then gently elevated off the handle using either a curved, blunt elevator (e.g., the extra-curved Hughes) or the 3-mm 90-degree pick to complete elevation of the drum off the anterior surface. Robust fibrous attachment at the umbo may cause difficulty. This technique is also applicable to congenital cases where the sac may be adherent to the handle. If removal cannot be accomplished without substantial risk of residual disease, removal of the handle and subsequent composite grafting of the drum is a safer route.

21.6 Subsequent Surgery

Residual cholesteatoma commonly presents as a rounded "pearl," typically in either the attic or the middle ear (▶ Fig. 21.9). Usually, the lesion can be removed intact by sharp dissection elevation of a patch of the underlying mucosa, then optionally diamond-drilling the site for further certainty. If the matrix is more difficult to access, clearance of the attached structures may be necessary, requiring further repairs; some cases will need third-stage reinspection.

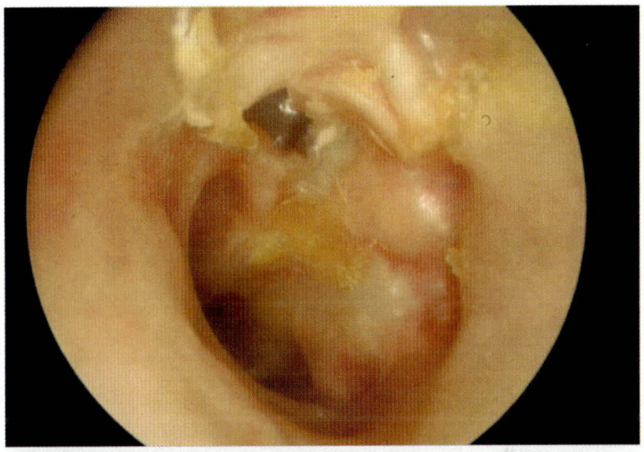

Fig. 21.10 Recurrent cholesteatoma, left attic, subsequent to CWU surgery. Chronic tubal insufficiency has caused gross drum collapse and invagination into the attic after necrosis of cartilage attic wall repairs. The sac remains free of keratin, and postaural removal may not be difficult although the depth may be extensive.

Recurrent disease may penetrate the tiniest tissue defects, probably as a result of ongoing tubal insufficiency, which is noted regularly in the postoperative[1] period. Significantly different middle ear or attic-mastoid patterns are seen. The former is common to both open and closed techniques and tends to self-marsupialize without major complications or surgery. If necessary, the sac is excised via a tympanomeatal flap approach, clearing the sac with delicate sharp dissection from the stapes, if necessary, as in primary disease, and perhaps removing an ossicular prosthesis. Excision of the affected drum origin may require further composite grafting to prevent recurrence.

Conversely, the potentially dangerous (and controversial) attic-mastoid penetration is mainly a problem of closed techniques; most of these recurrences require revision surgery. Four patterns of penetration occur: an extension of pars tensa collapse, recurrence through a patent attic defect, canal wall absorption, and sacs that penetrate around, under, or through EAC repairs (▶ Fig. 21.10).[1,16] The recurrent sac, although often extensive, may not contain keratin and may adhere only tenuously to the adjacent structures, which permits fine, blunt elevation in most cases. Fortunately, in many cases the contours of the site have been smoothed at the prior surgery, and infection may be absent, resulting in minimal bleeding and an easily observed site that is relatively easily cleared. The site of origin requires precise repairs to avoid repetition.

21.7 Conclusion

Removal of matrix is a demanding and often difficult task. Optimal surgery results from logical planning, practiced performance, and constant refinement of technique as technological advances emerge. Familiarity with the anatomy, adequate site exposure, and some specialized instrumentation are necessities. The surgery must address each case individually: the pattern and nature of the disease, the specific site problems, and the associated pathology. The particular removal technique is tailored to the micro-situation addressed.

References

[1] Black B, Gutteridge I. Acquired cholesteatoma: Classification and outcomes. Otol Neurotol. 2011;32(6):992–995.

[2] Pensak ML, Friedman RA. Fallopian bridge technique in surgery for chronic ear disease. Laryngoscope. 1997;107(11 Pt 1):1451–1456.

[3] Hunsaker DH. Conchomeatoplasty for chronic otitis externa. Arch Otolaryngol Head Neck Surg. 1988;114(4):395–398.

[4] Lee DH, Kim CS, Park CW, Chung DY. Is preoperative computed tomographic density measurement of soft tissues helpful in the diagnosis of cholesteatoma? Ann Otol Rhinol Laryngol. 2012;121(12):792–797.

[5] Tarabichi M, Nogueira JF, Marchioni D, Presutti L, Pothier DD, Ayache S. Transcanal endoscopic management of cholesteatoma. Otolaryngol Clin North Am. 2013;46(2):107–130.

[6] Black B. Mastoidectomy Reconstruction: Problems and Solutions. In: Magnan J., Chays A. Proceedings of the Sixth International Conference on Cholesteatoma and Ear Surgery, Cannes 2000. Marseille, Label Production. 2001;813–829.

[7] Magliulo G, Colicchio MG, Appiani MC. Facial nerve dehiscence and cholesteatoma. Ann Otol Rhinol Laryngol. 2011;120(4):261–267.

[8] Moody MW, Lambert PR. Incidence of dehiscence of the facial nerve in 416 cases of cholesteatoma. Otol Neurotol. 2007;28(3):400–404.

[9] Black B. Posterior geniculate artery: a surgeon's guide to the facial nerve. Am J Otol. 1992;13(1):78–79.

[10] Weinberg J, Sadé J. Posterior wall atrophy. A late silent complication of the combined approach tympanoplasty operation. Am J Otol. 1982;3(4):315–317.

[11] Sanna M, Gamoletti R, Bortesi G, Jemmi G, Zini C. Posterior canal wall atrophy after intact canal wall tympanoplasty. Am J Otol. 1986;7(1):74–75.

[12] Falcioni M, Frisina A. Taibah a., et al. Surgical Treatment of Labyrinthine Fistula in Chronic Ear surgery. In: Magnan J, Chays A. Proceedings of the Sixth International Conference on Cholesteatoma and Ear Surgery, Cannes 2000. Marseille, Label Production. 2001:859–862.

[13] Trabalzini F, Albu S, Cristalli G, et al. Management of Labyrinthine Fistula in Cholesteatoma. In: Magnan J, Chays A. Proceedings of the Sixth International Conference on Cholesteatoma and Ear Surgery, Cannes 2000. Marseille, Label Production; 2001:863–865.

[14] Portier F, Lescanne E, Racy E, Nowak C, Lamblin B, Bobin S. [Studies of labyrinthine cholesteatoma-related fistulas: report of 22 cases] J Otolaryngol. 2005;34(1):1–6.

[15] Gocea A, Martinez-Vidal B, Panuschka C, Epprecht P, Caballero M, Bernal-Sprekelsen M. Preserving bone conduction in patients with labyrinthine fistula. Eur Arch Otorhinolaryngol. 2012;269(4):1085–1090.

[16] Black B. Prevention of recurrent cholesteatoma: use of hydroxyapatite plates and composite grafts. Am J Otol. 1992;13(3):273–278.

Part 4

Roundtable on Tympanic Membrane Reconstruction

22 Overview and Introduction

John L. Dornhoffer and Michael B. Gluth

22.1 Introduction

The following three chapters of this surgical roundtable discuss important techniques for the reconstruction of the tympanic membrane. This type of surgical intervention is generally called a Type I tympanoplasty, according to the classification of Wullstein, but it can also be referred to as a myringoplasty when the surgery is isolated to the drumhead and no attempt is made to open or manipulate the middle ear space through the development of a tympanomeatal flap. The nomenclature used for the different surgical techniques generally is based on one of several factors: the graft material used (e.g., cartilage tympanoplasty, fat graft myringopasty), the position of the graft relative to the remnant drum (e.g., underlay or overlay tympanoplasty), and/or the surgical approach utilized (e.g., postauricular, endaural, trans-speculum). Whereas each has its advantages and disadvantages, modern tympanoplasty techniques all have common ground in that they endeavor to reconstruct the deficient middle fibrous layer of a tympanic membrane perforation or retraction pocket with graft materials that then act as a scaffold for lateral epithelial growth. Although simplified myringoplasty techniques that utilize non-grafted temporary scaffold materials, such as a thin paper patch, can be used for small perforations, they are relatively limited in application and simple to learn. Thus, patch myringoplasty techniques are not a focus of Part 4.

22.2 Surgical Approach

The importance of assuring proper visualization and exposure to surgically manipulate the tympanic membrane and middle ear may seem obvious, but if taken for granted, surgical results can be compromised. Line-of-sight visualization in itself does not always signify adequate exposure. The surgeon must ensure that instruments are allowed to enter the microscopic field at a sufficiently open lateral angle so as not to impede binocular vision or require awkward manipulation. Although minimally invasive approaches can be desirable, these should only be utilized if they provide equally sufficient access and exposure to the surgical target. The morbidity associated with even the widest tympanoplasty access route (postauricular with canalplasty) is generally not high.

Although each chapter in this part includes some discussion of approach, a few general comments are in order. The surgical approach for tympanoplasty is dictated by the degree of pathology in combination with the anatomical makeup of the ear canal and eardrum of the individual. These are usually described as the postauricular approach, which involves a skin incision behind the ear, and the transcanal approach, which involves various types of techniques with minimal external incisions. The latter can be further divided into trans-speculum and endaural, which are similar in concept but with each having its advantages and disadvantages.

The trans-speculum approach is the least invasive in the sense that the only external incision required is that used to harvest the graft material, but it requires a fair degree of technical skill. First of all, it is necessary to learn to support the speculum with the nondominant hand that is usually also used to manipulate the middle ear suction. Some surgeons utilize a speculum holder that connects to the surgical table, but this is time-consuming to set up and cumbersome under local anesthesia cases where the patient may move slightly and take it out of adjustment. Likewise, the added length of the speculum above the concha makes it difficult for the surgeon to stabilize his/her hands against the patient's head. Thus, trans-speculum tympanoplasty is typically reserved for very simple posterior perforations.

The endaural approach adds a lateral 12 o'clock radial incision to the tympanomeatal flap that extends into the terminal incisure area and allows placement of self-retaining retractors, which reduces the depth of the surgical field, affording more hand stability. A limited endaural incision, as would be utilized for tympanoplasty, only generates a small externally visible scar that is hidden in the natural skin crease of the helicotragal groove. Thus, if properly executed, cosmesis should not be an issue with endaural surgery unless the incision is extended superiorly around the pinna, as has been described for mastoidectomy. Endaural access can be used for most perforations, especially if combined with a canalplasty procedure. The disadvantages of endaural exposure center around the 12 o'clock incision because if this made too deeply, the temporalis muscle can be injured, leading to increased postoperative pain. An endaural incision also requires additional time for suturing during wound closure as well as postoperative packing to prevent webbing of the superior external auditory meatus.

The postauricular approach involves a C-shaped incision that is placed behind the pinna. It is cosmetically preferable to place this incision at least 1 cm behind the postauricular sulcus to prevent disruption of the natural concha-mastoid angle, which may result from subsequent scar contracture if it is too close to the pinna. At times, it is favorable to extend the incision further posterior to hide it in the hairline. Commonly, the ear canal is approached within a surgical plane that is immediately deep to the postauricular muscle fibers, and often this is combined with a layered T-shaped periosteal flap over the mastoid cortex. Various canal incisions have been described to allow concomitant anterior reflection of the pinna and creation of a tympanomeatal flap. The choice of a canal incision scheme is probably less important than the degree of care applied when elevating a tympanomeatal flap to prevent undue soft tissue trauma. Postauricular surgery affords wide circumferential exposure to the entire external auditory canal, as needed for canalplasty, tympanoplasty, mastoidectomy, and the harvest of temporalis fascia, all through a single incision.

All of the approaches for tympanoplasty can be performed under local anesthesia, and the decision for anesthesia type should not be a determinant of surgical approach in most cases. It should be noted that the surgical approach is not to be dictated by the pathology alone, nor by anatomical considerations in isolation, but, rather, by a combination of both. A subtotal perforation that is easily visualized in a large, straight canal can be repaired through a transcanal approach as long as the entire annulus and eardrum remnant can be easily seen from a single vantage point without moving the microscope. On the other hand, a small anterior perforation with an obstructing anterior canal bulge is best repaired through postauricular access, often with the addition of a canalplasty. A reasonable pearl of wisdom would be that "when in doubt, go postauricular." The morbidity is minimal, it adds very little surgical time, and it is the most versatile of all the approaches.

22.3 Graft Material

The tympanic membrane is the major element of the middle ear transformer mechanism, acting as a barrier between the sound pressure of the ear canal and the middle ear. Its motion, which has been studied with laser vibrometry and stroboscopic holography, is both complex and variable depending on the frequency of stimulation.[1,2] At frequencies up to 1000 Hz, the tympanic membrane tends to vibrate in one consolidated phase, but as frequency rises further, its vibration splits into a state of phase subdivision, with overall diminished efficiency.

Although it is intellectually satisfying to assert that reconstruction of the tympanic membrane must endeavor to exactly re-create these native vibratory patterns, in truth it is unknown if this is possible or even necessary. Numerous tympanic membrane graft materials have been used that are quite dissimilar to the native drumhead in rigidity and thickness, yet excellent acoustic outcomes have been attained. For example, reconstruction with large cartilage grafts has been reported to result in hearing outcomes equal to those with more pliable temporalis fascia,[3,4,5,6] including occurrences of complete air-bone gap closure in the speech frequencies. Further complicating the situation is uncertainty regarding the interplay between an aphysiologic reconstructed tympanic membrane and the underlying aphysiologic reconstructed ossicular chain in collectively providing acoustic gain.[7] Inconsistencies between observed clinical outcomes and predicted tympanoplasty outcomes based on tympanic membrane acoustic models highlight the fact that there is still much to be learned.

Although nearly any mesenchymal tissue can and has been used for tympanoplasty, the most commonly used grafting material is temporalis fascia, which is desired for its pliability. This is harvested, via either an endaural or postauricular incision, as the glistening whitish layer of fascia immediately overlying the temporalis muscle fibers. After harvest, it is generally pressed thin and set aside for drying, which may promote ease of trimming and placement. Readily available alternatives to temporalis fascia that are also thin and pliable include pressed perichondrium, periosteum, and muscle. Cadaveric acellular dermal matrix (AlloDerm, LifeCell Corp, Branchburg, New Jersey)[8] has also been used with success and may be particularly useful in situations where harvest of a tissue graft is not desired.

Auricular cartilage grafts are very useful in tympanoplasty[9,10] and may be harvested from various sites but are typically taken from the tragus and the concha. These can be applied as composite grafts with overlying perichondrium intact or having the perichondrium removed in combination with concurrent application of fascia; however, the editors' bias is to apply composite cartilage and perichondrial grafts that have been stripped of perichondrium on the medial surface but have adherent perichondrium or overlying fascia on the lateral surface.[11] In the editors' experience, the medial surface of such grafts tends to be more resistant to involvement with postoperative middle ear adhesions than either fascia or perichondrium.

The choice of graft material is impacted by the complexity of the reconstruction and the activity of any underlying chronic ear disease. When planning a tympanoplasty procedure, it is important for the surgeon to consider not only the graft characteristics that directly impact hearing via the acoustic properties of the resultant reconstructed drumhead, but also the characteristics that impact its ability to resist future disease, such as retraction, adhesions, or repeat perforation given that these will also affect the ultimate hearing result. In higher-risk situations, cartilage tympanoplasty techniques may provide more durable results.[12,13] A high-risk perforation might be considered one that is larger than 50%, an anterior perforation, a perforation draining at the time of surgery, a recurrent perforation,[14,15] or a perforation in the setting of permanent absent Eustachian tube function. Other situations in which cartilage is useful are the atelectatic ear, retraction pockets, a lateralized tympanic membrane, and cholesteatoma, as re-atrophy and perforation are common over the long term when fascia is used solely in the reconstruction.[16]

22.4 Graft Placement

22.4.1 Underlay or Medial Graft Placement

Underlay tympanoplasty is the most widely used tympanic membrane repair technique and is suitable for perforations of all sizes and locations. The concept of underlay grafting involves placement of graft material immediately underneath the residual native drumhead in a manner that accounts for the entire defect and all perforation margins. Three forces typically support this graft: (1) medial support is obtained via absorbable middle ear packing material; (2) adhesion occurs between the graft and the undersurface of the adjacent native drumhead and between the graft and lateral packing material through the perforation; and (3) the peripheral aspect of the graft is anchored in place between the tympanic annulus/canal skin and the underlying bone of the external auditory canal. Anchoring almost always involves the posterior canal wall and tympanomeatal flap but has also been described at various anterior points.[17,18]

The advantages of underlay grafting include simplicity, rapid execution, and a high rate of reported success. However, failures do occur, and these are most often related to overreliance on middle ear packing materials. If peripheral annulus anchoring is insufficient, packing may fail to prevent medial graft displacement and point separation of the graft from the perforation edge. This seems to be a particular risk when repairing an anterior or subtotal perforation. In the editors' experience, large rigid cartilage grafts are less likely than fascia or perichondrium to displace medially when placed anteriorly. Furthermore, canalplasty is an underutilized technique that allows precise graft placement and access for anterior-superior annulus elevation that will facilitate underlay anchoring and prevention of graft collapse, which is a common cause of tympanoplasty failure in this area.

22.4.2 Overlay or Lateral Graft Placement

The basic concept of overlay or "lateral grafting" involves de-epithelialization of the tympanic membrane remnant while preserving what exists of the native middle fibrous layer. This preserved middle layer remnant is then used as partial medial support upon which grafting materials are set. Most common overlay graft techniques are combined with canalplasty to remove the bulge of the anterior canal wall. Usually, this canal wall skin is removed and reset near the end of the surgery as a free graft. Overlay techniques are robust and can be applied to all perforations, but they are especially useful in dealing with anterior and subtotal defects.[19] They have the advantage of being relatively resistant to graft failure due to inadequate medial support and inward graft migration during the healing phase that is sometimes seen with underlay techniques.

The disadvantages of the overlay technique include anterior canal blunting, graft lateralization, and intratympanic keratin inclusion cysts. Blunting can be functionally understood as dense scarring of the anterior tympanic membrane that results in reduction of the functional surface area of the drumhead and "pseudo-malleus fixation" caused by adhesion between the manubrium and the anterior canal wall. This risk can be minimized by proper canalplasty to widen the anterior tympanomeatal angle, coverage of all exposed bone with canal skin or skin grafts, and careful placement of packing in this area after graft placement. Graft lateralization refers to the lateral movement of the graft during the healing process away from the level of the native eardrum and ossicular chain, resulting in recurrent conductive hearing loss, which is often maximal. This is a particular risk when overlay grafting is undertaken in an ear that lacks a malleus manubrium to anchor the graft. Finally, epithelial retention cysts can occur if insufficient care is taken to remove all the epithelium from the remnant fibrous layer of the tympanic membrane.

22.5 Revision Tympanoplasty

When performing revision tympanoplasty, there are several useful pearls to be considered to maximize the chance of ultimately achieving a successful reconstruction. First, it is advisable during a revision surgery to seek maximum exposure by means of a postauricular approach. If the perforation involves the anterior aspect of the drumhead, which is common in a previously failed repair, a canalplasty is strongly recommended.

Second, undesirable elements of the remnant tympanic membrane should be aggressively removed. As a general rule it is preferable to resect and create a large perforation or to replace the entire tympanic membrane as opposed to attempting the repair of a small perforation that is part of a severely diseased drumhead. This includes the removal of all myringitis, thickened prior graft material, devascularized myringosclerotic perforation margins, and scar tissue. It is also preferable to remove any elements of a previous tympanoplasty that impart an irregular contour and are apt to accumulate debris and infection, especially raised edges of cartilage.

Another common consideration in revision tympanoplasty is the correction of the lateralized tympanic membrane. This typically involves the complete removal of the lateralized drumhead and reestablishment of a new graft using underlay techniques, with anchoring under the majority of the annulus and under the malleus. Cartilage tympanoplasty techniques have proven particularly useful in this situation as the rigid material allows precise fixation medial to the bony annulus, and the graft can often be securely set under the anterior tympanic spine.[20] Small split-thickness skin grafts are used to cover exposed external canal bone and the drumhead to promote rapid healing and minimize the scar formation that leads to lateralization, which is particularly critical at the anterior tympanomeatal angle.

Tympanoplasty may be particularly difficult in the setting of long-standing severe tympanic membrane atelectasis, wherein the malleus may be severely rotated onto and even partially fixed to the promontory. It is possible in this situation for the malleus to have undergone a degree of remodeling, such that attempts at manual lateralization of the manubrium are in vain, with resultant restricting contact of the malleus head against the medial epitympanic wall. Thus, it may be useful to remove the incus and amputate the malleus head to restore the manubrium to a height favorable for tympanoplasty, even if the ossicular chain is still intact and disarticulation is required. The expected hearing result from the resultant tympanoplasty with ossicular reconstruction should be at least as favorable as a Type I tympanoplasty that involves a severely diseased malleus.[21]

A final situation to consider is the challenge of performing tympanoplasty when microvascular nutrient blood supply is poor, such as with a radiated surgical field or in the setting of a past welding slag injury. These situations are further worsened if the malleus and its tympanic blood supply have been taken, if the patient has poorly controlled diabetes, or if the patient is a smoker. In such instances, it may be useful to introduce a new source of blood supply by performing tympanoplasty with partial inlay of a thin vascularized soft tissue flap, such as the middle temporal artery flap[22] (discussed in Chapter 41). Although the thickness of this flap is somewhat less than ideal from an acoustic standpoint, it is nonetheless sufficiently thin to afford a reasonable healing result while optimizing the chance of tympanic membrane healing and achievement of a dry ear.

22.6 Which Technique to Use?

The decision regarding which technique to use for tympanoplasty is influenced by several factors, not the least of which is the experience of the surgeon and the philosophy of the parent training institution. There is no question that good results can be obtained with each of the techniques discussed in the following chapters if surgery is meticulously executed. However, there are in fact relative advantages to one technique over another and situations where the choice of a particular approach will impact the chance of a favorable long-term outcome. Thus, it behooves otologic surgeons to become familiar and proficient with as many of these techniques as possible to expand one's ability to deal with complications and revision surgery, which are inevitable when managing a high-volume chronic ear surgical practice.

References

[1] Aarnisalo AA, Cheng JT, Ravicz ME, Furlong C, Merchant SN, Rosowski JJ. Motion of the tympanic membrane after cartilage tympanoplasty determined by stroboscopic holography. Hear Res. 2010;263(1–2):78–84.

[2] Aarnisalo AA, Cheng JT, Ravicz ME, et al. Middle ear mechanics of cartilage tympanoplasty evaluated by laser holography and vibrometry. Otol Neurotol. 2009;30(8):1209–1214.

[3] Dornhoffer JL. Hearing results with cartilage tympanoplasty. Laryngoscope. 1997;107(8):1094–1099.

[4] Gerber MJ, Mason JC, Lambert PR. Hearing results after primary cartilage tympanoplasty. Laryngoscope. 2000;110(12):1994–1999.

[5] Kyrodimos E, Sismanis A, Santos D. Type III cartilage "shield" tympanoplasty: an effective procedure for hearing improvement. Otolaryngol Head Neck Surg. 2007;136(6):982–985.

[6] Ozbek C, Ciftçi O, Tuna EE, Yazkan O, Ozdem C. A comparison of cartilage palisades and fascia in type 1 tympanoplasty in children: anatomic and functional results. Otol Neurotol. 2008;29(5):679–683.

[7] Morris DP, Bance M, Van Wijhe RG. How do cartilage and other material overlay over a prosthesis affect its vibration transmission properties in ossiculoplasty? Otolaryngol Head Neck Surg. 2004;131(4):423–428.

[8] Downey TJ, Champeaux AL, Silva AB. AlloDerm tympanoplasty of tympanic membrane perforations. Am J Otolaryngol. 2003;24(1):6–13.

[9] Dornhoffer J. Cartilage tympanoplasty: Indications, techniques, and outcomes in a 1,000-patient series. Laryngoscope. 2003;113(11):1844–1856.

[10] Tos M. Cartilage tympanoplasty methods: Proposal of a classification. Otolaryngol Head Neck Surg. 2008;139(6):747–758.

[11] Dornhoffer JL. Cartilage tympanoplasty. Otolaryngol Clin North Am. 2006;39 (6):1161–1176.

[12] Beutner D, Huttenbrink KB, Stumpf R, et al. Cartilage plate tympanoplasty. Otol Neurotol. 2010;31(1):105–110.

[13] Cabra J, Moñux A. Efficacy of cartilage palisade tympanoplasty: Randomized controlled trial. Otol Neurotol. 2010;31(4):589–595.

[14] Boone RT, Gardner EK, Dornhoffer JL. Success of cartilage grafting in revision tympanoplasty without mastoidectomy. Otol Neurotol. 2004;25(5):678–681.

[15] Moore GF. Candidate's thesis: Revision tympanoplasty utilizing fossa triangularis cartilage. The Laryngoscope. 2002;112(9):p. 1543–54.

[16] Jesic SD, Dimitrijevic MV, Nesic VS, Jotic AD, Slijepcevic NA. Temporalis fascia graft perforation and retraction after tympanoplasty for chronic tubotympanic otitis and attic retraction pockets: factors associated with recurrence. Arch Otolaryngol Head Neck Surg. 2011;137(2):139–143.

[17] Jung TT, Park SK. Mediolateral graft tympanoplasty for anterior or subtotal tympanic membrane perforation. Otolaryngol Head Neck Surg. 2005;132 (4):532–536.

[18] Kartush JM, Michaelides EM, Becvarovski Z, LaRouere MJ. Over-under tympanoplasty. Laryngoscope. 2002;112(5):802–807.

[19] Angeli SI, Kulak JL, Guzmán J. Lateral tympanoplasty for total or near-total perforation: Prognostic factors. Laryngoscope. 2006;116(9):1594–1599.

[20] Boone R, Dornhoffer J. Surgical correction of the lateralized tympanic membrane. Laryngoscope. 2002;112(8 Pt 1):1509–1511.

[21] Hol MKS, Nguyen DQ, Schlegel-Wagner C, Pabst G, Linder TE. Tympanoplasty in chronic otitis media patients with an intact, but severely retracted malleus: A treatment challenge. Otol Neurotol. 2010;31(9):1412–1416.

[22] Gluth MB, Sunde J. Vascularized reconstruction of partial external auditory canal wall defects using the middle temporal artery flap. Otol Neurotol. 2014;35(1):e31–e35.

23 Underlay and Related Techniques

Seilesh C. Babu and Brent J. Benscoter

Abbreviations used in this chapter:

ABG: air-bone gap

23.1 Introduction

This chapter will cover the underlay tympanoplasty, defined as the reconstruction of the tympanic membrane via placement of graft material medial to the tympanic membrane defect, with the graft positioned medial to any remnant middle fibrous layer and the annulus. This is the most commonly utilized tympanoplasty technique and is in contrast to the lateral graft (overlay) technique, which places the graft lateral to any remnant middle fibrous layer and the annulus. The over-under technique, also addressed in this chapter, is a variation of the underlay approach that allows management of anterior or large central perforations involving the malleus. With this technique, the periosteum and epithelium are taken off the malleus, thereby improving exposure of the anterior mesotympanum. The graft is then placed lateral to the malleus but still medial to the annulus. A summary of the advantages and disadvantages of the various techniques for tympanoplasty is shown in ▶ Table 23.1.

23.2 Patient Selection

The key to a successful underlay technique is secure anchoring of the graft, either under the annulus and/or with support of middle ear packing material. The two most important factors in determining the likely outcome are the etiology of the perforation and the status of the middle ear once all disease has been eradicated. Traumatic tympanic membrane perforations demonstrate a spontaneous healing rate of 78%–95% at 12 months, with an increase in healing with paper patch myringoplasty.[1,2,3] Some perforations may be managed in the office setting with a fat myringoplasty. These would be small, posterior perforations (5%–10% in size) in patients who may not wish to undergo surgical repair. The success rate, especially with chronic perforations, is improved with surgical repair using a formal tympanoplasty technique.

It is important to distinguish dry central perforations with a good middle ear space and aeration from other complicating factors, such as cholesteatoma, severe mucosal disease, Eustachian tube dysfunction, tobacco usage, and ossicular chain abnormalities. These other factors may decrease the likelihood of success with tympanic membrane reconstruction. Absolute contraindications for tympanoplasty include poor health, uncontrolled severe middle ear or mastoid infection, and uncontrolled cholesteatoma necessitating mastoidectomy as well. The status of the contralateral ear should always be considered because operating on an only-hearing or better-hearing ear should be avoided except in rare cases due to the risk of irreversible hearing loss with surgery. Relative contraindications included Eustachian tube dysfunction and smoking, where long-term failure approaches 60%.[4]

The traditional underlay grafting technique can be used in most perforations, especially those posteriorly located (▶ Fig. 23.1). Difficulty arises when working with perforations that are anterior or adjacent to the malleus (▶ Fig. 23.2). The improved exposure with the over-under variation is ideal in total perforations, large anterior perforations, perforations involving the malleus or umbo, or where better visualization of the anterior mesotympanum is necessary. Placement of the graft and packing material is easier with the over-under variation, compared with the traditional underlay technique given that one can anchor the graft under the annulus and "lock" it into position over the malleus, preventing medialization of the graft.

The lateral grafting technique has similar benefits but requires more work on the canal for wider exposure and is technically more difficult to teach.

Table 23.1 Advantages and disadvantages of underlay, overlay, and over-under techniques for tympanoplasty

Technique	Advantages	Disadvantages
Underlay	• No risk of blunting of the anterior sulcus • No lateralization • Simple technique • High success rate	• Inadequate visualization of anterior middle ear • Less suitable for large anterior perforations
Overlay	• Suitable for perforations of all sizes and locations • No reduction of middle ear space • Very high success rate	• Risk of blunting • Risk of graft lateralization • Risk of epithelial pearls • Healing time is longer • Technically challenging
Over-Under	• Suitable for perforations of all sizes and locations • Superior exposure of entire middle ear • No blunting • Minimal risk of lateralization • No reduction of middle ear space • Very high success rate	• Need for malleus manipulation • Risk of vibrational trauma to ossicular chain • Risk of lateralization

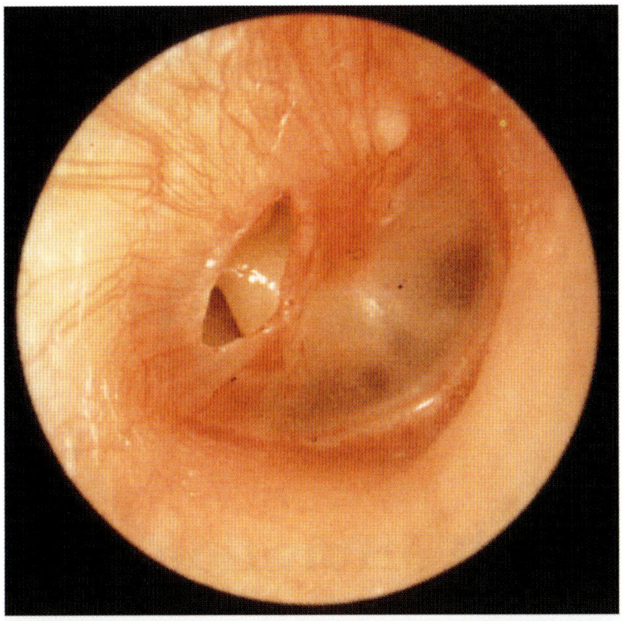

Fig. 23.1 Clinical example of a small right posterior tympanic membrane perforation suitable for underlay tympanoplasty technique.

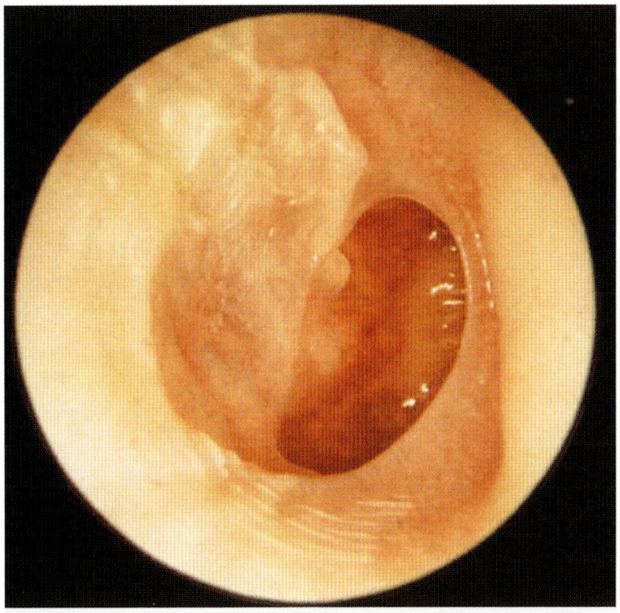

Fig. 23.2 Clinical example of a large right anterior tympanic membrane perforation suitable for the over-under tympanoplasty technique.

23.3 Surgical Technique

23.3.1 Underlay Technique

The first decision the surgeon must make is whether the tympanoplasty can be performed purely transcanal or if a wider approach, such as postauricular, should be used. A transcanal approach may be an option if the canal is of adequate size, usually accommodating at least a 5 mm or larger speculum. The anterior overhang must also be considered in relation to the location of the perforation given that it can obstruct the view substantially. Finally, an incision must be made to harvest temporalis fascia, and enlarging the incision to perform a complete postauricular approach can often ensure a significantly better view and, hence, a better outcome.

Approximately 1 mL of 1% lidocaine with 1:100,000 epinephrine is injected into the posterior/superior ear canal in the area of the vascular strip. Inserting the needle laterally into the thicker soft tissue of the canal and infiltrating the solution slowly will help to prevent formation of blebs in the ear canal. Most surgeons make canal incisions, whereas some will raise the canal skin from behind prior to making any canal incisions. If canal incisions are made first, the vascular strip medial incision is made approximately 4 mm lateral to the tympanic annulus. Incisions are then made superiorly along the tympanosquamous suture line at approximately 12 o'clock and posterior-inferiorly along the tympanomastoid suture line at approximately 4 o'clock in a left ear (▶ Fig. 23.3). An epinephrine-soaked piece of absorbable packing is placed into the canal for hemostasis.

A postauricular incision is made 5 mm behind the postauricular sulcus. It is often easiest to find the correct surgical plane superiorly by identifying the loose areolar tissue and following the plane inferiorly. A retractor holds the ear forward to expose the temporalis fascia. A graft may be taken at this time to allow it to dry, or it may be delayed until the exact size of the perforation is established. Either temporalis fascia or loose areolar tissue may be obtained as graft material. The amount to harvest depends on the size of the perforation. If too much is taken, revision surgery will be difficult without any remaining tissue to harvest. Once harvested, the graft should be thinned and cleaned. Placement in a press can be used to thin the graft. Usually the graft can be dried under a heat lamp for 10–12 minutes, after which it is cut to size. Other graft materials may be utilized, such as loose areolar tissue, periosteum, cartilage, and processed dermal/epidermal tissue, such as Alloderm (LifeCell Corp, Branchburg, New Jersey). Graft material is surgeon-dependent, and in revision cases is dependent on the quality of remaining tissue.

A T-shaped incision is made through the temporalis fascia along the linea temporalis and inferiorly down to the mastoid tip with a monopolar cautery, ensuring correct orientation so as not to enter the ear canal with the instrument or injure the facial nerve as it exits the stylomastoid foramen. An elevator is used to elevate the fascia and push the vascular strip forward. Once the notch of Rivinus is identified, the microscope is brought in and an elevator and suction are used to further elevate the vascular strip and identify any incisions that were made. These incisions can then be completed, and the vascular strip is everted laterally.

Prior to any skin elevation, to maintain a taut tympanic membrane remnant, the size of the perforation is assessed and the edges of the perforation are denuded of squamous epithelium (▶ Fig. 23.3). Migrating epithelium often requires enlarging the perforation to ensure that there is healthy tissue at the periphery to improve graft take and reduce the chance of cholesteatoma formation. The tympanomeatal flap is further elevated down to the fibrous annulus. If significant anterior bony overhang exists, a canalplasty (see Chapter 20) can be performed to

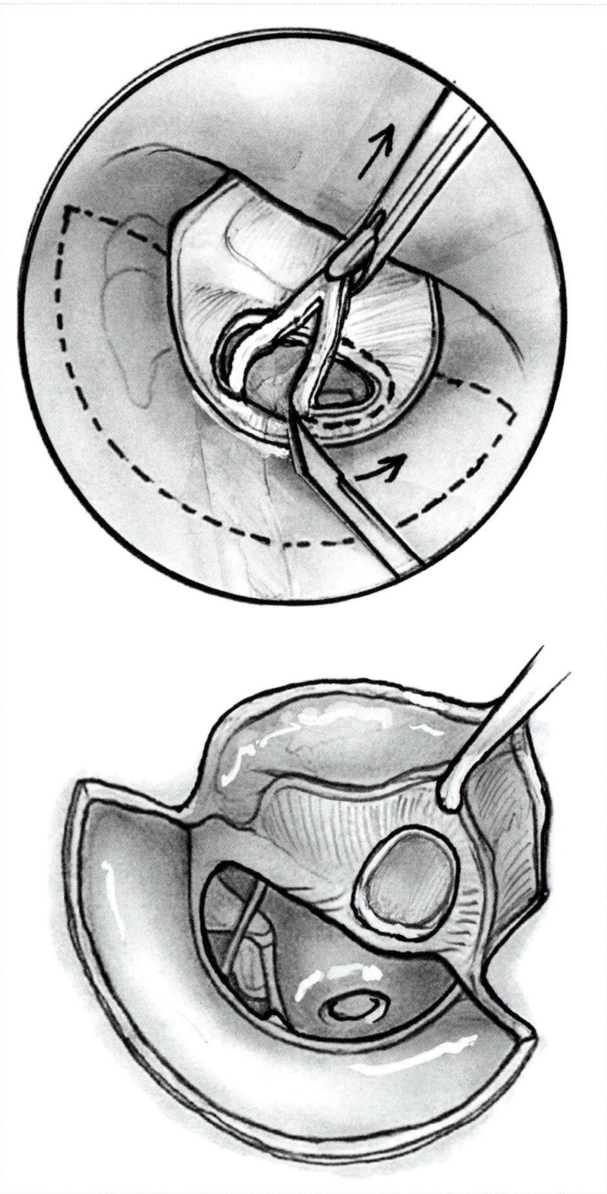

Fig. 23.3 Underlay tympanoplasty technique with the edges of the tympanic membrane perforation being denuded followed by elevation in preparation for graft placement. Care must be taken to ensure that no epithelium has migrated onto the undersurface of the tympanic membrane remnant. Canal incisions are marked with dashed line.

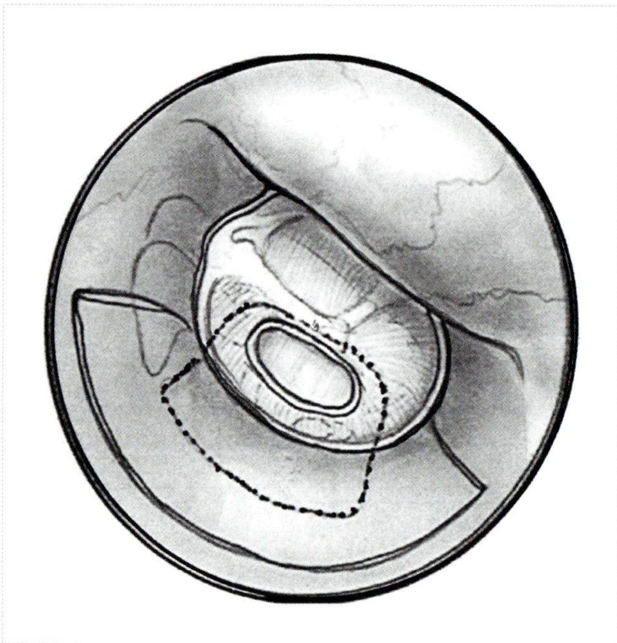

Fig. 23.4 Underlay tympanoplasty technique showing graft in place with tympanomeatal flap placed back into position.

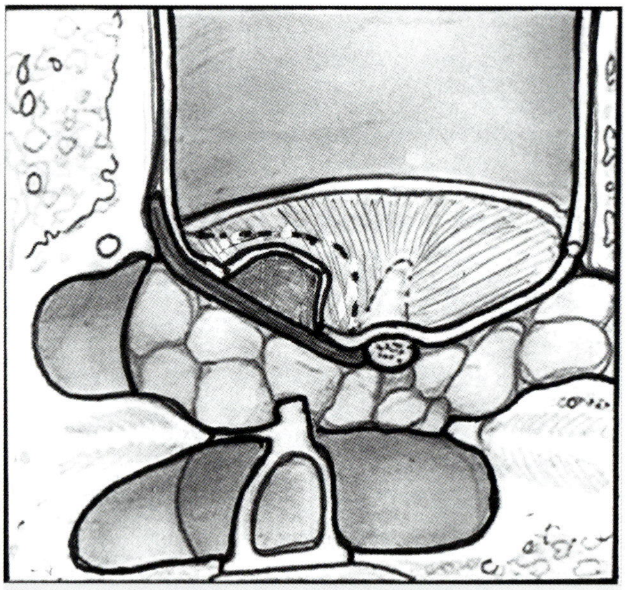

Fig. 23.5 Underlay tympanoplasty technique, lateral view with middle ear packing showing graft abutting malleus and continuing laterally under annulus.

improve anterior canal and tympanic membrane visualization. The middle ear is entered and the tympanic membrane remnant is elevated, taking care to protect the chorda tympani nerve.

Packing the middle ear with absorbable packing will support the graft. The dried graft material of choice is then placed medial to the tympanic membrane, and residual edges are placed back in position. Care must be taken to ensure the graft is in contact with the edges of the perforation, especially anterior-inferiorly, where visualization may be difficult but is paramount for success (▶ Fig. 23.4; ▶ Fig. 23.5). Anchoring the graft material with small pieces of absorbable packing laterally will hold it in place.

23.3.2 Over-Under Variation

Perforations anterior-superiorly or those involving the manubrium of the malleus can be quite challenging to repair. A slit in the graft material can accommodate the malleus but can leave redundant graft material or have problems healing around the bone when performing a medial technique. In these instances, a variation can be performed termed an "over-under tympanoplasty." This approach allows wide exposure to the anterior

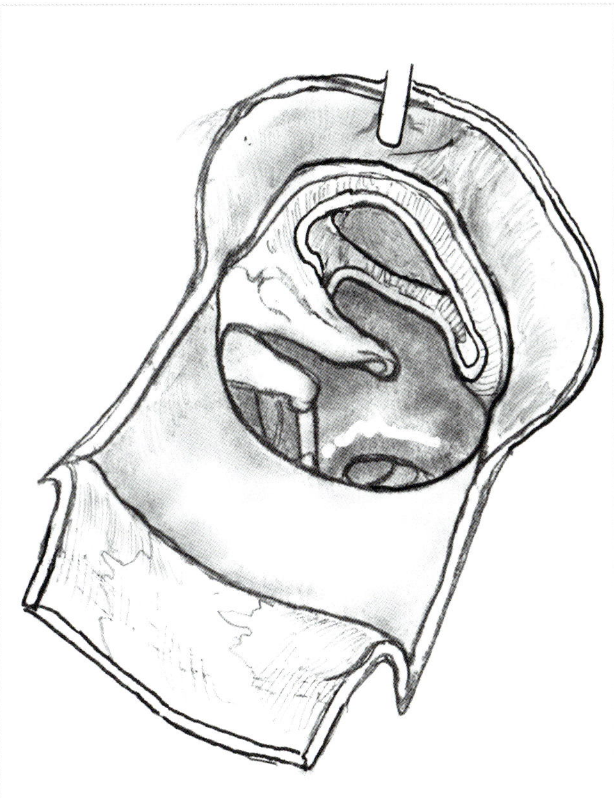

Fig. 23.6 Over-under tympanoplasty technique showing tympanic membrane remnant elevated anteriorly off the malleus.

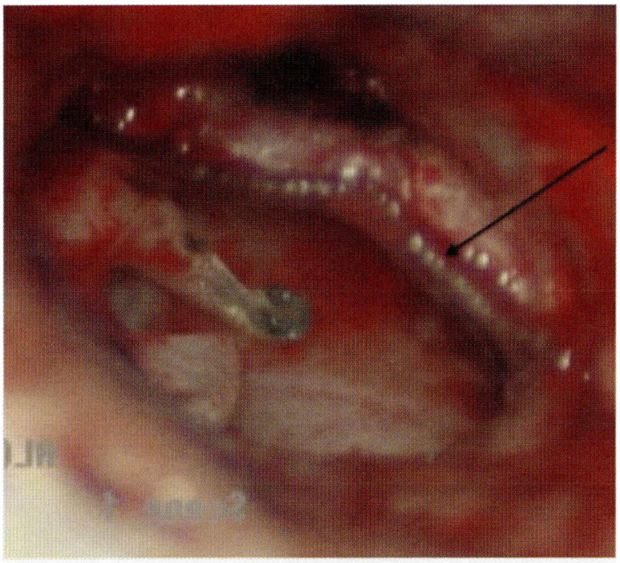

Fig. 23.7 Intraoperative view of over-under tympanoplasty technique showing tympanic membrane remnant elevated anteriorly off the malleus. Arrow indicates the graft in place medial totympanomeatal flap.

aspect of the middle ear, tympanic membrane, and even the Eustachian tube. The over-under variation improves visualization and reduces the risk of blunting that may be seen from the lateral tympanoplasty technique.

In the over-under tympanoplasty, the tympanic membrane or remnant is taken off the malleus completely (▶ Fig. 23.6; ▶ Fig. 23.7). This is performed by creating a subperiosteal plane along the neck of the malleus and elevating this periosteum with the tympanic membrane in an inferior direction toward the umbo. This meticulous process can be aided with the use of a sharp needle and gentle counter traction with suction in the opposite hand. The fibrous tissue attached at the umbo can be separated sharply with scissors or with a laser. A CO_2 laser, with either the micromanipulator on the microscope or the handheld handpiece (Omniguide, Cambridge, Massachusetts), can assist in less traumatic dissection along an intact ossicular chain. Care must be taken with this approach so that vibratory trauma is not transmitted along an intact chain. Once dissection is complete and the tympanic membrane is separated from the malleus, disease anterior to the malleus is removed. Absorbable packing material is placed in the middle ear space and the graft is placed "over," or lateral to the malleus, and "under," or medial to the anterior fibrous annulus (▶ Fig. 23.8; ▶ Fig. 23.9). With very anterior or marginal perforations, anterior canal skin must be elevated laterally. The graft must then be tucked under the anterior ear canal skin before it is laid back into place.

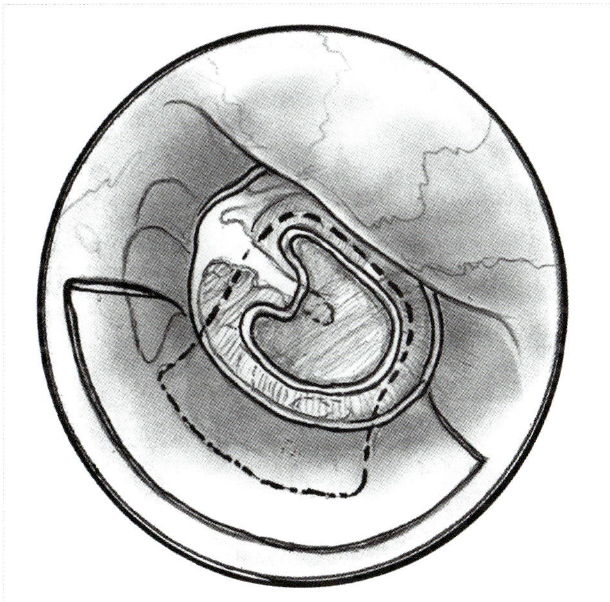

Fig. 23.8 Over-under tympanoplasty technique showing graft placement with the tympanomeatal flap placed back into position.

After the graft is initially placed, it is then typically easiest to lift up the entire graft posteriorly to anteriorly to allow any additional packing of the middle ear with saline-soaked absorbable packing to support the graft medially. The graft is then placed back down and antibiotic-soaked absorbable packing is placed lateral to the graft as well. The retractor is removed, and the vascular strip is unfurled and placed against the posterior bony canal wall. Using an ear speculum, the ear is inspected to ensure that the vascular strip is in the proper place, not lying over other epithelium, and not curled posteriorly.

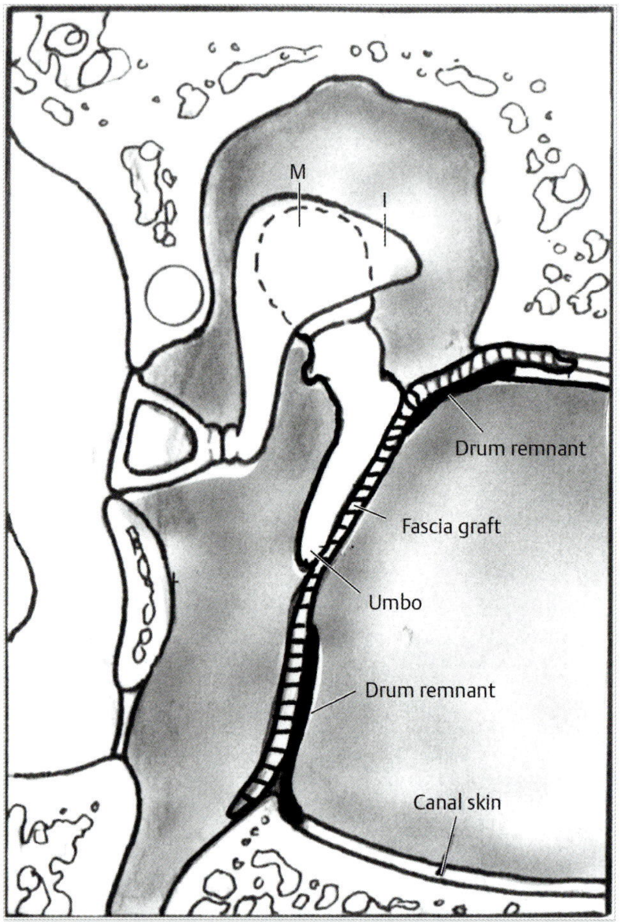

Fig. 23.9 Over-under tympanoplasty technique, lateral view, showing graft lateral to the malleus but under the tympanic membrane remnant and annulus.

23.4 Postoperative Care

Patients are typically discharged the same day as the surgery, barring unexpected nausea or vomiting. The mastoid or cup dressing is removed on the first postoperative day. The patient is allowed to get the incision wet approximately 4 days after surgery, but strict dry ear precautions must be kept for the first month. The patient is prescribed antibiotic drops and is instructed to apply 4–6 drops of the medication to the ear packing twice a day until the first follow-up visit. Patients are typically seen 1 week after surgery, at which time the majority of absorbable packing is removed. Absorbable packing is left in place over the canal incisions and over the site of the perforation. Patients are usually seen again 2–3 weeks later. An audiogram is not obtained until 4–6 months postoperatively.

Occasionally some graft separation can be noted in the early postoperative period and may be treated in the office by the meticulous dissection of epithelial remnants to flatten them back down medially. Absorbable packing may also be placed over the area of concern to keep the area moist and secure. A wet or infected graft or ear canal can be treated more aggressively with antibiotic solution or powdered material.

23.5 Complications

Tympanoplasty has relatively few complications, and most are preventable by a well-thought out surgical plan, meticulous intraoperative dissection, and frequent postoperative follow-up care. Complications related specifically to the underlay technique include medial graft displacement, acoustic trauma, persistent perforation, or cholesteatoma. Medial graft displacement is most likely due to lack of anchoring along the tympanic membrane edges/remnant or lack of enough middle ear packing support. Acoustic trauma from manipulation of the tympanic membrane and malleus is a concern that requires meticulous dissection. The risk is slightly higher in the over-under variation, with dissection off of the malleus, but can be lessened by supporting the malleus with the suction and with the use of the laser.

Anterior perforation failure rate can be higher with an underlay technique due to decreased visualization and possible lack of a tympanic membrane remnant. This is especially true with anterior marginal perforations, and often the best technique to prevent a gap between the graft and the anterior canal wall skin is to back elevate the skin of the canal to enable it to rest over the graft. This problem can also cause anterior tympanic membrane blunting. The over-under technique reduces the risk for this in that it improves visualization, allows easier middle ear packing, and allows the large graft to be placed in entirety without requiring an incision for the malleus.

Cholesteatoma or intratympanic cyst formation may occur and is likely related to inadequate rimming of the margin of the perforation or inadequate resection of an ingrowth cholesteatoma around the perforation edges on the medial side of the tympanic membrane remnant. Ridges or imperfections in the graft may also allow for small epithelial keratin pearls.

A specific risk with the over-under technique is lateralization of the graft material, hence, lack of connection between the healed tympanic membrane and the malleus. Although occurring most commonly at the annulus, the amount can be varied, thus causing varying degrees of conductive hearing loss. The key to preventing this complication is adequate packing, both medially and laterally. Often more pressed out, dried pieces of absorbable packing are used, which are tucked under the umbo. Firm packing is also placed lateral to the graft to apply medial pressure as well.

23.6 Outcomes

Outcome results may be categorized in multiple ways. In general, surgery should produce a dry ear with normal hearing in 93% to 97% of cases.[5] Although the initial goal of all ear surgery is to produce a safe, dry ear, other outcomes include graft take. For an underlay technique, the graft take is reported to be between 93% to 97.6% for primary surgeries, especially in experienced surgical hands.[5,6,7] Using the over-under tympanoplasty technique, Kartush, Michaelides, Becvarovski, and LaRouere reported a success rate of 100% initial graft take in 120 patients, with delayed failure in 12 patients (10%) secondary to continued Eustachian tube dysfunction.[8] The mean postoperative air-bone gap (ABG) was 5.3 dB. Another study compared over-under tympanoplasty to the standard underlay technique and found superior graft take with the over-under method (94.9% versus 91.5%) at 11 months.[9] Both groups had similar hearing results. It should be noted that success with these techniques is reported by experienced surgeons who have performed these procedures numerous times. Specifically with the over-under technique, dissection off of the malleus can be quite challenging, and surgeons may show improved results with decreased risks over time.

In general, all study results should be interpreted with caution because there are many causes of "failure." This is particularly true of revision surgery. Causes can include surgical technique, chronic Eustachian tube dysfunction, cholesteatoma, postoperative healing issues (including infection), and other patient factors such as smoking. Many of the studies group different diagnoses into the reported group, so numbers may not be comparable to a specific patient depending upon the disease process. Many reports also use a variety of graft types and techniques, making direct comparisons difficult.

References

[1] Park MK, Kim KH, Lee JD, Lee BD. Repair of large traumatic tympanic membrane perforation with a Steri-Strips patch. Otolaryngol Head Neck Surg. 2011;145(4):581–585.

[2] Lou ZC, Lou ZH, Zhang QP. Traumatic tympanic membrane perforations: a study of etiology and factors affecting outcome. Am J Otolaryngol. 2012;33(5):549–555.

[3] Lou ZC, Tang YM, Yang J. A prospective study evaluating spontaneous healing of aetiology, size and type-different groups of traumatic tympanic membrane perforation. Clin Otolaryngol. 2011;36(5):450–460.

[4] Becvarovski Z, Kartush JM. Smoking and tympanoplasty: Implications for prognosis and the Middle Ear Risk Index (MERI). Laryngoscope. 2001;111(10):1806–1811.

[5] Glasscock ME, III, Jackson CG, Nissen AJ, Schwaber MK. Postauricular undersurface tympanic membrane grafting: a follow-up report. Laryngoscope. 1982;92(7 Pt 1):718–727.

[6] Cueva RA. Areolar temporalis fascia: A reliable graft for tympanoplasty. Am J Otol. 1999;20(6):709–711.

[7] Dornhoffer J. Cartilage tympanoplasty: indications, techniques, and outcomes in a 1,000-patient series. Laryngoscope. 2003;113(11):1844–1856.

[8] Kartush JM, Michaelides EM, Becvarovski Z, LaRouere MJ. Over-under tympanoplasty. Laryngoscope. 2002;112(5):802–807.

[9] Yigit O, Alkan S, Topuz E, Uslu B, Unsal O, Dadas B. Short-term evaluation of over-under myringoplasty technique. Eur Arch Otorhinolaryngol. 2005;262(5):400–403.

24 Overlay Tympanoplasty Technique

Audrey P. Calzada and Eric P. Wilkinson

Abbreviations used in the chapter:

TMJ: temporomandibular joint

24.1 Introduction

The overlay, or lateral graft, tympanoplasty technique was established as a reliable method to reconstruct the tympanic membrane in 1961 when Storrs published the first series using temporalis fascia for the graft.[1] This technique was then adopted by others, with a > 90% graft take reported in subsequent years.[2]

24.2 Patient Selection

The main advantage of the overlay tympanoplasty technique is full visualization of the anterior tympanic sulcus in patients with total, subtotal, or anterior tympanic membrane perforations. The technique is advantageous in cholesteatoma surgery and in cases of severe tympanosclerosis when the tympanic membrane remnant is diseased, warranting complete resurfacing with fascia. The lateral graft tympanoplasty technique has a high graft success rate and can be utilized in every chronic ear scenario.

24.3 Surgical Technique

Although lateral graft tympanoplasty is feasible using local anesthesia, the majority of cases are done under general anesthesia to maximize patient comfort. The table is placed in a slight Trendelenburg position and rolled toward the surgeon to increase visualization of the posterior-superior quadrant of the tympanic membrane and ear canal where the vascular strip and ossicles are located. Under microscopic vision, the bony cartilaginous junction of the ear canal skin is injected in 4 quadrants with local anesthetic using 1% lidocaine with 1:100,000 epinephrine. The postauricular sulcus is also infiltrated with local anesthetic. The following eight steps provide the framework of the overlay tympanoplasty technique.[3]

24.3.1 Step 1: Transmeatal Incisions

After local anesthetic injection, transcanal incisions are made along the tympanosquamous suture line (anterior-superiorly) and the tympanomastoid suture line (posteriorly) using either a No. 1 knife (sickle) or a No. 64 Beaver knife (▶ Fig. 24.1a). A line extended from the short process of the malleus superiorly is a good approximation of the tympanosquamous suture line. These two suture lines demarcate the vascular strip portion of the ear canal skin, which is thicker and tends to swell to a greater degree after infiltration with local anesthetic (▶ Fig. 24.1b). A medial incision connecting the vascular strip using a No. 72 Beaver knife can be made but is not necessary.

24.3.2 Step 2: Postauricular Exposure and Removal of Fascia

A standard incision is made in the postauricular sulcus and extended superiorly 1 cm above the level of the postauricular fold. The incision is carried inferiorly toward the mastoid tip at the level of the ear lobule. Skin flaps are raised anteriorly and posteriorly at the level of the temporalis fascia once the areolar tissue is dissected off the underlying true temporalis fascia. A No. 15 blade is used to incise the temporalis fascia 1 cm above the linea temporalis, and Metzenbaum scissors are used to harvest a 2 cm x 2 cm piece of fascia, which is then pressed and spread out. It is important to remove any adherent muscle or areolar tissue from the harvested graft, which is then set aside under a heat lamp to dehydrate.

Incisions are made through the soft tissue overlying the mastoid bone at the linea temporalis and extended inferiorly toward the mastoid tip just below the level of the ear canal. It is good practice to manually palpate the mastoid tip while making this incision to ensure the stylomastoid foramen is not in close proximity. The periosteum is elevated anteriorly using a Lempert elevator to expose the ear canal skin. A self-retaining retractor is placed to retract the auricle forward.

The canal skin is elevated using a narrow elevator until the transcanal incisions demarcating the vascular strip are encountered. The vascular strip is gently elevated off the canal bone and tympanic membrane and placed in the retractor (▶ Fig. 24.1c). A Perkins retractor can be useful to retract the auricle and the vascular strip anteriorly without traumatizing the ear canal skin.

24.3.3 Step 3: Removal of Canal Skin

With the retractor in place, a semilunar incision is made in the remaining ear canal skin using the No. 64 Beaver knife just lateral to the bony cartilaginous junction. Hair-bearing canal skin measuring 1–2 mm and lateral canal cartilage are included to ensure complete skin removal from the lateral bony ear canal. To accomplish this, the blade is beveled toward the bony portion of the ear canal to develop the correct plane of dissection (▶ Fig. 24.2a). Using a round knife, the periosteum and canal skin are elevated from the canal bone down to the annular ligament (▶ Fig. 24.2b). The tympanic annulus should be left in place anteriorly given that this structure will support the graft. Posteriorly, removal of the annulus has no consequence. Of special note in children, it is best to begin the lateral anterior canal skin incision posterior-inferiorly to avoid injury to their developing cartilaginous ear canal.

Once the ear canal skin is elevated down to the annulus, the tympanic membrane remnant is de-epithelialized in continuity with the canal skin. Only the outer epithelial layer of the tympanic membrane must be removed; the middle and inner fibrous layers are left in place. Using small cup forceps, the outer layer of the remnant tympanic membrane anterior-superiorly is grasped and gently peeled off the short process of the

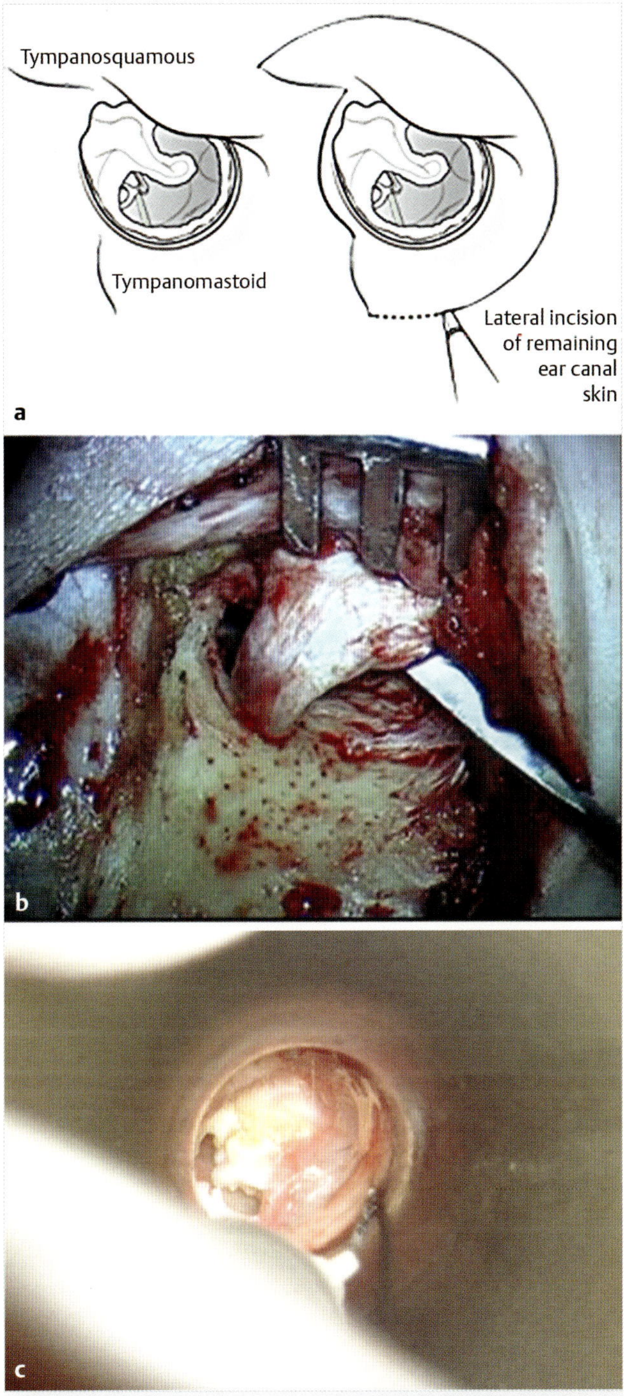

Fig. 24.1 Vascular strip. (a) Incisions along the tympanosquamous (TS) and tympanomastoid (TM) suture lines, which define the vascular strip, are depicted for a right ear. (b) Injection of local anesthetic into the vascular strip of a left ear. Characteristic ballooning of the thick vascular strip skin is observed. (c) Intraoperative photograph in a right ear, showing elevation of the vascular strip after postauricular exposure is obtained.

malleus. It is imperative that the vector of force is parallel to the short process of the malleus (▶ Fig. 24.2c). Once the plane between the outer epithelial layer of the tympanic membrane and the middle fibrous layer is developed, a round knife is positioned perpendicularly along the annulus and medial bony canal to continue the de-epithelialization anteriorly and inferiorly until the entire skin specimen is freed and can be removed (▶ Fig. 24.2d). The round knife should be kept in contact with the medial ear canal bone at all times to ensure complete skin removal. The periosteum and canal skin are set aside and kept moist in saline-soaked gauze.

24.3.4 Step 4: Enlargement of the Ear Canal; Canalplasty

Using a combination of four cutting and three diamond drill bits with continuous suction irrigation, the ear canal is enlarged by removing the anterior and inferior canal bulges. Removing the anterior and inferior bony overhangs is imperative to allow for complete 360-degree visualization of the tympanic annulus to ensure both complete de-epithelialization and optimal graft placement. Equally important is drilling medially to enlarge the acute angle, which exists anteriorly (▶ Fig. 24.3). Creating a more obtuse anterior sulcus will prevent postoperative blunting. This is best accomplished with a small diamond drill bit (2 diamond). Other than removing the spine of Henle posterior-laterally, there is usually no benefit to removing any canal bone posteriorly. Occasionally, posterior canalplasty is necessary to visualize the posterior annulus, but care must be taken to avoid injury to the vertical segment of the facial nerve.

When performing canalplasty, the anatomic structures surrounding the external auditory canal should not be violated. The periosteum of the temporomandibular joint (TMJ) abuts the external auditory canal anteriorly; the jugular bulb is located inferiorly to the canal; the vertical segment of the facial nerve is posterior-inferiorly in the canal and can run lateral to the annulus in this area; lastly, the tegmen tympani can be low-lying and encountered when drilling the superior portion of the canal.

24.3.5 Step 5: De-epithelialization of the Remnant Tympanic Membrane

Once 360-degree visualization of the annulus is obtained, complete de-epithelialization of the remnant tympanic membrane must be accomplished by carefully examining the ear canal bone adjacent to the bony annulus. Anterior-inferiorly, the skin is tightly adherent to the bone just lateral to the annulus, where a small neurovascular bundle penetrates the bone. Once the medial bony canal is cleared of any skin remnants, the tympanic membrane is checked for skin (▶ Fig. 24.4). When there is a question of complete de-epithelialization, a portion of the remnant tympanic membrane is removed. In cases with severe tympanic membrane retraction, it may be prudent to also remove the chorda tympani to prevent leaving a remnant of skin in the middle ear.

24.3.6 Step 6: Placement of the Fascia

Prior to placing the previously harvested temporalis fascia, the middle ear is packed with small pieces of absorbable packing soaked in fluoroquinolone-containing otic drops. The absorbable packing should be placed in the middle ear to the level of the annulus and not over-packed. The dehydrated fascia is

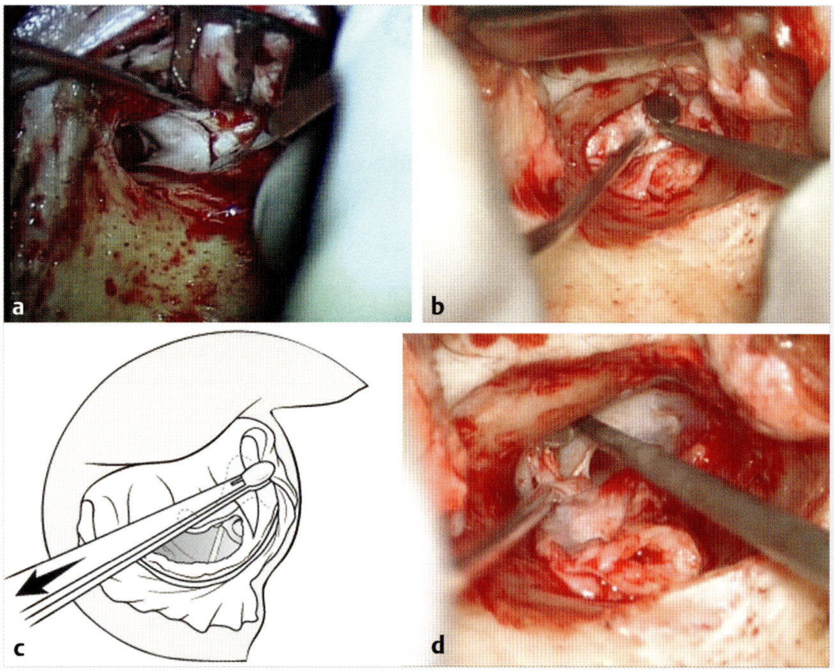

Fig. 24.2 Removal of canal skin. (a) The No. 64 Beaver knife is used to incise the remaining ear canal skin 1 to 2 mm lateral to the bony cartilaginous junction of the ear canal. Notice the blade is beveled toward the bony portion of the ear canal. (b) A round knife is used to elevate the ear canal skin medially toward the annulus. (c) Left ear; cup forceps are used to grasp the outer epithelial layer of the tympanic membrane just anterior to the short process of the malleus. Note the vector of force is directed parallel to the short process of the malleus. (d) Left ear; the round knife is positioned perpendicularly along both the annulus and the medial bony ear canal to peel the epithelial layer of the tympanic membrane off in continuity with the canal skin.

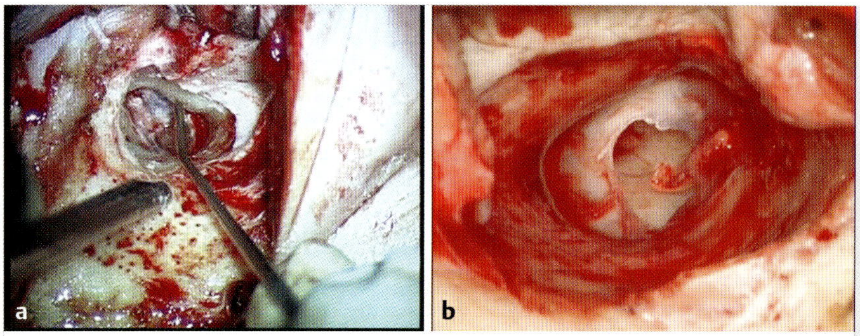

Fig. 24.3 Canalplasty. (a) Anteriorly, the superior and inferior aspects of the bony ear canal have been drilled away in a right ear, creating the classic "Mickey Mouse" ears. The Gimmick is pointing to the area of the temporomandibular joint that lies halfway between the superior and inferior troughs and halfway from medial to lateral (annulus to bony cartilaginous junction). (b) In a left ear, this is how the ear canal should appear after adequate canalplasty, removing the anterior overhang as much as possible without violating the temporomandibular joint. In this case, the temporomandibular joint slightly obscures visualization of the entire anterior annulus, but we have created an obtuse angle anterosuperiorly adjacent to the head of the malleus.

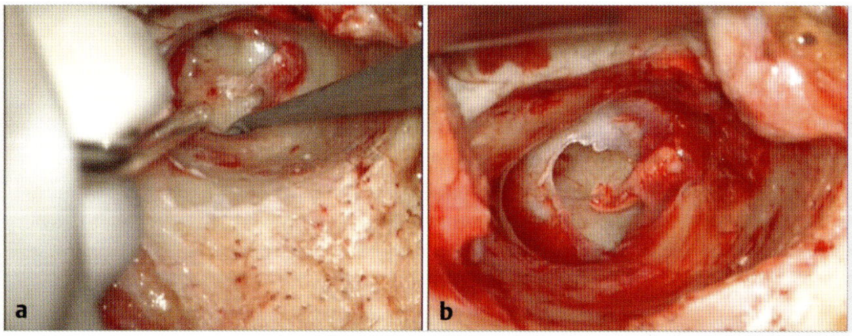

Fig. 24.4 De-epithelialization. (a) A stapes curette can be used to remove remaining epithelial elements from the underside of the annulus. (b) Left ear; this is how a completely de-epithelialized tympanic membrane should appear. One can also choose to remove the remnant fibrous layers of the tympanic membrane, leaving only the annulus.

trimmed to approximately 1.3 cm x 1.5 cm, which is about the size and shape of the thumb nail bed. A slit is then cut in the fascia to allow for placement medial to the malleus handle (▶ Fig. 24.5a). The fascia is then grasped with fine alligator forceps in the center of the slit and transiently immersed in saline solution. The graft is then placed over the perforation and medial to the malleus handle.

A Rosen needle is useful for slipping the slit edge of the fascia medial to the short process of the malleus. The fascia is then carefully arranged along the annulus anteriorly and inferiorly. It should extend no further than 1 mm beyond the bony wall anteriorly. The anterior flap is then turned back over the exposed manubrium (▶ Fig. 24.5a; ▶ Fig. 24.5b; ▶ Fig. 24.5c).

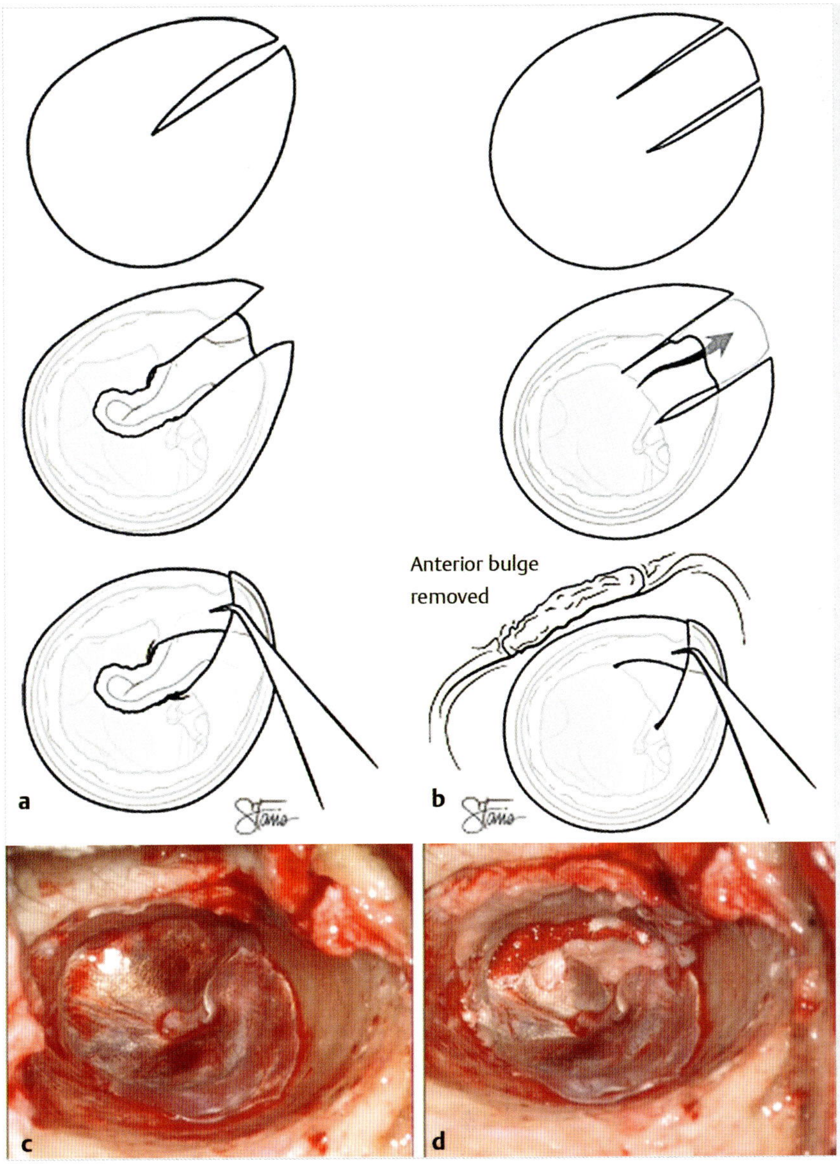

Fig. 24.5 Placement of fascia and skin. (a) A slit in the fascia is cut and then slipped medially to the short process of the malleus using a Rosen needle. The tympanic membrane flaps are then folded over each other. (b) In a patient without a malleus short process, a rectangular piece of the fascia is cut as shown to slip medially into the epitympanum. The fascia flaps are then folded over one another. (c) Intraoperative photograph of a left ear after placement and positioning of the graft. (d) The ear canal skin is then replaced anteriorly and inferiorly. The skin is positioned slightly more medially so that it overlaps the fascia by 1 to 2 mm. Small pieces of Gelfoam are placed along the skin to hold it in place.

24.3.7 Step 7: Replacement of Canal Skin

The canal skin removed earlier in the case is trimmed of any frayed edges and replaced in the bony ear canal. The skin is placed slightly more medially than its native position so that it overlaps the fascia by approximately 1 mm to promote epithelialization (▶ Fig. 24.5d). The skin should be completely unfurled to avoid the development of small epithelial cysts postoperatively. A small, dry, rolled-up piece of absorbable packing is then placed into the anterior sulcus. The rest of the canal is then packed with pledgets of slightly moist absorbable packing. The posterior-superior quadrant of bone is left unpacked for replacement of the vascular strip.

24.3.8 Step 8: Replacement of the Vascular Strip

The vascular strip is released from the retractor and tucked anteriorly in the canal over the absorbable packing. Several sutures are placed to reapproximate the mastoid soft tissue and periosteum to reposition the auricle. A nasal speculum is then used in the meatus to visualize and replace the vascular strip to its native position with cup forceps. Absorbable packing is then used to fill the rest of the canal, with a piece of cotton placed laterally. The postauricular incision is closed, and a mastoid pressure dressing is applied.

24.4 Postoperative Care

Patients are routinely discharged 2 to 3 hours after surgery once they have adequately recovered from general anesthesia. They are instructed to remove the mastoid pressure dressing 24 hours after surgery and to change the cotton ball in the ear canal as needed. Patients are also counseled to refrain from blowing their nose and to keep the operated ear and incision site dry. Air travel is permissible 2 days after surgery, but patients are counseled to remain awake and chew gum during altitude changes.

Postoperative visits occur 7 days after surgery. During this visit, the cotton ball is removed, and the incision is examined. Patients are instructed to start using fluoroquinolone-containing otic drops 3 weeks after the surgery to liquefy the packing. A second postoperative visit is scheduled 6–8 weeks after the surgery date, when the remnants of the packing are cleaned and the ear canal and graft are examined.

24.5 Complications

Although the overlay tympanoplasty technique provides excellent exposure, versatility, and an excellent graft take, there are several disadvantages to this technique. Compared with other approaches, drawbacks include the requirement of increased technical skill with precise microsurgical dissection, a longer healing time, and the potential for compromised hearing outcomes from graft blunting and/or lateralization.

Technical skill and knowledge of the anatomy is imperative to avoid postoperative complications, such as TMJ pain and sensorineural hearing loss. One of the more common complications is exposure of the TMJ periosteum and/or fat while removing the anterior bony canal overhang during canalplasty. As long as the periosteum of the joint capsule remains intact, few patients have postoperative problems; however, violation of the capsule, with fat exposure, can result in prolonged postoperative TMJ pain and aggravating clicking sensations with talking or chewing. The best treatment is avoidance in this case given that outcomes of repair of the anterior bony canal wall are mediocre at best.

The most serious complication that can occur with the overlay tympanoplasty technique is complete sensorineural hearing loss, which occurs rarely. More common is high-frequency sensorineural hearing loss, which can occur up to 3% of the time.[4] Direct ossicular damage and subsequent sensorineural hearing loss with disruption of the oval window can theoretically occur with the drill bit while completing the canalplasty in the anterior and superior sulci near the short process of the malleus. This can be avoided with meticulous attention to surgical technique and the use of appropriate-size drill bits when drilling medially in the canal.

Complications related to healing include graft lateralization, anterior sulcus blunting, epithelial cysts, and granular myringitis.

Graft lateralization usually is not apparent until 6–12 months after surgery and most commonly results from the fascia not being tucked adequately medial to the malleus handle. A lateralized graft looks like a smaller eardrum, which is mobile and lies at a direct angle to transcanal visualization. Treatment involves revision overlay tympanoplasty, with placement of the graft under the malleus handle in the setting of persistent postoperative conductive hearing loss.

Anterior sulcus blunting after overlay tympanoplasty occurs from excess fibrous scarring, which causes a rounding of the angle between the anterior external auditory canal wall and the lateral aspect of the anterior tympanic membrane. This occurs to a minor degree after every lateral graft tympanoplasty without any problem; however, when anterior sulcus blunting is prominent, the sound transfer function of the vibrating tympanic membrane is decreased, resulting in a conductive hearing loss.[5] In certain cases, blunting of the edge of the graft can even involve the malleus handle and limit ossicular mobility. Anterior sulcus blunting has been correlated to conductive hearing losses ranging from 20 dB to 60 dB.

Prevention of blunting requires meticulous drilling during the canalplasty to open the anterior canal wall angle. The anterior canal wall must be drilled up to the short process of the malleus anteriorly and superiorly to create a platform for the graft. Additional maneuvers to prevent blunting include replacing the canal skin to overlap the graft, as previously described, and placing a rolled-up piece of dried absorbable packing on the anterior sulcus once the graft and skin are placed.

Severe anterior sulcus blunting appears as an immobile anterior tympanic membrane without delineation between the canal wall and the edge of the eardrum. It has a concave configuration and occurs anterior-superiorly. This finding in association with a conductive hearing loss persisting more than 6 months requires reoperation.

Epithelial cysts can form on the tympanic membrane or ear canal postoperatively if the replaced ear canal skin is not completely unfurled intraoperatively. These either spontaneously rupture or can be treated easily with marsupialization in the clinic setting using a Rosen needle. Annular cholesteatomas, epithelial cysts that occur between the remnant tympanic membrane and the fascia after inadequate de-epithelialization of the remnant eardrum, can also occur postoperatively. These tend to grow over several years and occur most commonly anterior-inferiorly as a concave mass where the skin is more tightly adherent to the bone. Complete skin removal in this area is more difficult because of the small neurovascular bundle that enters the ear canal at this location. Annular cholesteatomas are treated with incision and cyst evacuation.

Postoperative graft mucosalization, or granular myringitis, appears as a moist, weeping tympanic membrane graft, which persists for months post-surgery. In these cases, patients can have otorrhea and various degrees of conductive hearing loss if the tympanic membrane is thickened and has decreased compliance. This can be prevented by using true temporalis fascia and debriding the graft of adherent muscle and temporoparietal fascia prior to dehydration. Mucosalization of the graft is treated with combinations of antibiotic drops and powders, and strict dry ear precautions should be followed. In recalcitrant cases, reoperation is performed.

As emphasized previously, most, if not all, complications of the overlay tympanoplasty technique can be avoided using precise surgical skills coupled with complete anatomical knowledge. Technical pearls and some of the more common pitfalls are summarized in Table 24.1.

24.6 Outcomes

The overlay tympanoplasty technique has been established in both our experience and in the literature as a reliable and versatile technique to accomplish disease eradication and a successful graft take rate. Successful graft take rates, defined as no recurrent perforation, range from 91% to 97% in the literature.[4,6,7,8,9] The two largest series evaluating the overlay technique both had successful graft take rates of 97%.[4,8]

In the more recent review of lateral graft outcomes, 147 overlay grafts were performed in cases of subtotal perforation, mesotympanic cholesteatoma, extensive tympanosclerosis, and

Table 24.1 Pearls and pitfalls of overlay tympanoplasty

Pearls	Pitfalls
• Use true temporalis fascia for the graft and remove all muscle and temporoparietal fascia.	• Granular myringitis
• The TMJ "bulge" is halfway between the superior and inferior limits of the tympanic membrane and halfway from the lateral canal to the medial annulus.	• Violating the TMJ periosteum causes postoperative pain and clicking
• Drill the medial anterior sulcus to create an obtuse angle up to the short process of the malleus.	• An acute anterior sulcus angle causes blunting
• Stapes curette to the underside of the remnant tympanic membrane and annulus to remove all epithelium, especially anterior-inferiorly.	• Epithelial cysts, annular cholesteatomas
• Ensure the graft is tucked medially to the short process of the malleus (or slipped medial into the epitympanum if the malleus is absent).	• Graft lateralization
• Overlap replaced canal skin with the graft medially by 1 mm.	• Anterior sulcus blunting

revision surgery after previous graft failure. The graft success rate was 96.6% in this patient population, representing a subset of more complicated chronic ear disease.[8] Of the 5 cases with re-perforation, 3 were successfully revised with overlay grafts.

The main critique of the overlay tympanoplasty technique is delayed wound healing in the form of epithelial pearls, graft lateralization, blunting, and myringitis, which can occur in up to 26% of patients.[8] However, the incidence of reoperation due to wound healing issues is exceedingly low as most are either asymptomatic or resolve with conservative management.[4,6,8,9]

The association of worse graft outcomes with preoperative factors is variably reported. Inferior graft outcomes have been reported to be associated with children, wet ears, cholesteatoma, and ossicular involvement with disease. However, in a more recent controlled study, the success of graft incorporation was independent of demographic and disease variables,[6] and a higher take rate with lateral graft tympanoplasty in children has even been noted.[7]

When comparing the results of the overlay tympanoplasty technique to the underlay technique, several randomized comparative studies have attempted to show the superiority of one over the other, with differing results.[7,9] Although there are many methods by which tympanoplasty can be performed, in our experience, the overlay tympanoplasty is an essential technique whereby complete visualization of the anterior sulcus and reliable postoperative graft take rates ensure a high degree of success in managing the chronic ear.

References

[1] Storrs LA. Temporalis muscle fascia and denatured fat grafts in middle-ear surgery. Laryngoscope. 1963;73:699–701.

[2] Sheehy JL, Glasscock ME, III. Tympanic membrane grafting with temporalis fascia. Arch Otolaryngol. 1967;86(4):391–402.

[3] Fayad JN, Sheehy JL. Tympanoplasty – Outer Surface Grafting Technique. In: Otologic Surgery 3rd Edition. Philadelphia, PA: Saunders; 2010:119–129.

[4] Sheehy JL, Anderson RG. Myringoplasty. A review of 472 cases. Ann Otol Rhinol Laryngol. 1980;89(4 Pt 1):331–334.

[5] Mullin DP, Ge X, Jackson RL, Liu J, Pfannenstiel TJ, Balough BJ. Effects of tympanomeatal blunting on sound transfer function. Otolaryngol Head Neck Surg. 2011;144(6):940–944.

[6] Angeli SI, Kulak JL, Guzmán J. Lateral tympanoplasty for total or near-total perforation: prognostic factors. Laryngoscope. 2006;116(9):1594–1599.

[7] Rizer FM. Overlay versus underlay tympanoplasty. Part II: The study. Laryngoscope. 1997;107(12 Pt 2):26–36.

[8] Ryan JE, Briggs RJ. Outcomes of the overlay graft technique in tympanoplasty. ANZ J Surg. 2010;80(9):624–629.

[9] Singh M, Rai A, Bandyopadhyay S, Gupta SC. Comparative study of the underlay and overlay techniques of myringoplasty in large and subtotal perforations of the tympanic membrane. J Laryngol Otol. 2003;117(6):444–448.

25 Cartilage Tympanoplasty

John L. Dornhoffer

Abbreviations used in this chapter:

CT: computed tomography
TM: tympanic membrane
TORP: total ossicular replacement prosthesis

25.1 Introduction

The use of cartilage in middle ear surgery is not a new concept and has been recommended on a limited basis to manage retraction pockets for many years.[1,2] More recently, however, it has been increasingly described for the reconstruction of large portions of the pars tensa of the tympanic membrane (TM) in cases of recurrent perforation, atelectasis, and cholesteatoma.[3,4] Although one might anticipate a significant conductive hearing loss with cartilage due to its thickness and rigidity, several studies have reported results to the contrary, suggesting hearing results with cartilage to be no different than those with fascia.[3,4] The cartilage graft retains its rigid quality and resists resorption and retraction, even in the milieu of continuous Eustachian tube dysfunction.

Two distinct techniques are commonly employed for cartilage reconstruction of the TM: the perichondrium/cartilage island flap, which uses tragal cartilage; and the mosaic technique, which uses cartilage from the tragus or cymba. The choice of technique is typically dictated by the specific middle ear pathology or, in cases where the TM reconstruction is in conjunction with ossiculoplasty, the status of the ossicular chain. The mosaic technique is preferred in cases of cholesteatoma and when ossicular reconstruction is needed in the malleus-present situation. In this situation an exact fit is necessary to prevent cholesteatoma recurrence. The perichondrium/cartilage island flap is preferred for management of the atelectatic ear and the high-risk perforation. This chapter describes the two techniques in detail, followed by descriptions of the modifications that should be taken in response to specific surgical indications.

25.2 Patient Selection

Generally speaking, cartilage is used as a graft material in any ear considered to be at high risk for failure with traditional techniques utilizing temporalis fascia or perichondrium. Included in this would be the high-risk perforation, the atelectatic ear, and cholesteatoma. The high-risk perforation comprises a revision surgery, a perforation anterior to the annulus, a perforation draining at the time of surgery, a perforation > 50%, or a bilateral perforation, all of which have been shown to be associated with increased failure rates using traditional techniques.[5,6] The atelectatic ear is one of the most important indications for cartilage tympanoplasty, and numerous reports have established its efficacy over fascia in this situation.[1,2] For similar reasons, the use of cartilage to reconstruct and reinforce the scutum and posterior half of the eardrum in cholesteatoma surgery has reduced the incidence of recurrent atrophy and retraction pockets in these difficult cases.

Cartilage tympanoplasty has proven to be efficacious in both pediatric and adult patients, with special precautions used in the former group. The general approach to pediatric patients is to avoid repairing the TM during the otitis-prone years (< 3 years of age). If the contralateral ear is normal, routine tympanoplasty is performed at age 4 years.[7] If the contralateral ear is abnormal at this time, adenoidectomy is considered, and tympanoplasty is generally deferred until age 7 years.[8] If contralateral disease is still present at this time, cartilage tympanoplasty is performed on the worse-hearing ear because a perforation in the contralateral ear has been shown to be associated with a high risk for failure.[9]

As part of the preoperative preparation, all patients are encouraged to perform the Valsalva maneuver (or use the Otovent [Invotec International, Jacksonville, Florida] in younger children). Those unable to insufflate the ear are placed on nasal steroids 6 weeks prior to surgery, and these are continued in the postoperative period until an aerated middle ear cleft is documented. Although we have found no difference in graft take between those who can and cannot perform the Valsalva maneuver, we have found a slightly increased need (7%) for postoperative tube insertion in the Valsalva-negative group. Likewise, an attempt is made to optimize concomitant sinonasal disease (allergy, chronic sinusitis) prior to ear surgery, and smoking cessation is encouraged where applicable. The draining ear is treated with antibiotic/steroid-containing topical solutions and aural toilet for 6–8 weeks prior to surgery. While every attempt is made to dry an ear prior to surgical intervention, it is not considered a prerequisite for tympanoplasty.

25.3 Surgical Technique

25.3.1 General Considerations

The surgical approach for cartilage tympanoplasty does not differ from that for traditional otologic surgery and is dictated by the extent and location of the disease. The postauricular approach is utilized in most patients as these cases, by definition, tend to have more extensive middle ear pathology. A small, localized, posterior retraction or perforation can be performed through a transcanal or endaural incision, but great care must be taken to assure that the depths of the retraction can be reached. Likewise, the placement of the cartilage graft utilizes the underlay technique, so that no special tympanomeatal flaps or skin incisions are required.

Some general observations should be made regarding the differences in cartilage that occur with aging. The cartilage thickness of the tragus and cymba are not appreciably different between children and adult patients, but the perichondrium seems to be more adherent in children. For this reason, when the perichondrium is removed from one side when fashioning the graft (described below), care must be taken to ensure the correct plain is dissected, especially in the pediatric patient. Likewise, cartilage is more pliable in children, making it slightly easier to work with than adult cartilage, which can become

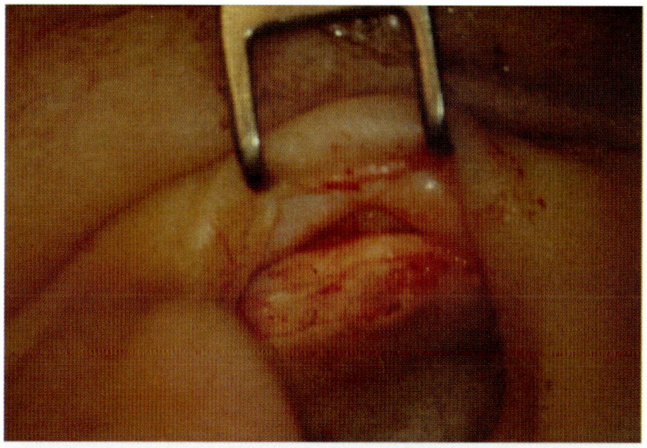

Fig. 25.1 Harvest of cartilage, leaving small rim of cartilage in dome for cosmesis (right ear).
Used with permission from Dornhoffer JL. Cartilage tympanoplasty: indications, techniques, and outcomes in a 1000-patient series. Laryngoscope 2003;113:1844–1856.

somewhat brittle in patients over 65 years of age. For this reason, during the fashioning of the graft, it is generally a good practice to manipulate and hold the cartilage with fingers instead of forceps, and toothed-forceps should not be used at any time to grasp the cartilage to avoid fracture.

As a general rule, the perichondrium is left attached to the side of the cartilage that faces the ear canal, regardless of which technique is used. It is believed that the perichondrium improves graft stability and facilitates the ingrowth of fibrous tissue and epithelialization. It should be noted, however, that with the mosaic technique, perichondrium has been removed from both sides of the cartilage on occasion due to untoward curling of the graft, which will typically curve toward the side with the perichondrium. No ill effect has been noted, other than increased fragility of the graft during formation and placement.

25.3.2 The Perichondrium/Cartilage Island Flap

The general technique of reconstruction using the perichondrium/cartilage island flap begins with harvest of the cartilage from the tragal area.[10] This cartilage is ideal because it is thin, flat, and in sufficient quantities to permit reconstruction of the entire TM. The cartilage is used as a full-thickness graft and is typically slightly less than 1 mm thick in most cases. Although it has been suggested that a slight acoustical benefit could be obtained by thinning the cartilage to 0.5 mm,[11] this advantage is offset by the unacceptable curling of the graft, which occurs when the cartilage is thinned and perichondrium is left attached to one side.

An initial cut through skin and cartilage is made on the medial side of the tragus, leaving a 2-mm strip of cartilage in the dome of the tragus for cosmesis (▶ Fig. 25.1). The cartilage, with attached perichondrium, is dissected medially from the overlying skin and soft tissue by spreading a pair of sharp scissors in a plane that is easily developed superficial to the perichondrium on both sides. It is necessary to make an inferior cut as low as possible to maximize the length of harvested cartilage. The cartilage is then grasped and retracted inferiorly, which delivers the superior portion from the incisura area. The superior portion is then dissected out while retracting, which produces a piece of cartilage typically measuring 15 mm x 10 mm in children and somewhat larger in adults.

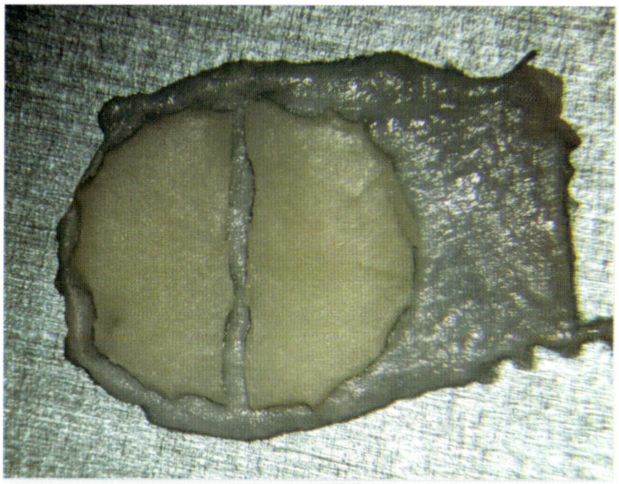

Fig. 25.2 Prepared perichondrium/cartilage island graft, showing strip of cartilage removed to facilitate malleus.
Used with permission from Dornhoffer JL. Cartilage tympanoplasty: indications, techniques, and outcomes in a 1000-patient series. Laryngoscope 2003;113:1844–1856.)

The perichondrium from the side of the cartilage furthest from the ear canal is dissected off, leaving the thinner perichondrium on the reverse side. A perichondrium/cartilage island flap is then constructed in the following manner.[10] Using a round knife, cartilage is dissected from the graft to produce an eccentrically located disc, approximately 7–9 mm in diameter, that will be used for total TM reconstruction. A flap of perichondrium is produced posteriorly that will eventually drape over the posterior canal wall. A complete strip of cartilage 2 mm in width is then removed vertically from the center of the graft to accommodate the entire malleus handle (▶ Fig. 25.2). The creation of two cartilage islands in this manner is essential to enable the reconstructed TM to bend and conform to the normal conical shape of the TM. When the ossicular chain is intact, an additional triangular piece of cartilage is removed from the posterior-superior quadrant to accommodate the incus. This excision prevents the lateral displacement of the posterior portion of the cartilage graft that sometimes occurs because of insufficient space between the malleus and incus.

The entire graft is placed in an underlay fashion, with the malleus fitting in the groove and actually pressing down into and conforming to the perichondrium, as shown in ▶ Fig. 25.3. The cartilage is placed toward the promontory, with the perichondrium immediately adjacent to the TM remnant, both of which are medial to the malleus. Failure to remove enough cartilage from the center strip will cause the graft to fold up at the center instead of lying flat in the desired position. Likewise, if the strip is insufficient, the cartilage may be displaced medially instead of assuming a more lateral position in the same plane as the malleus.

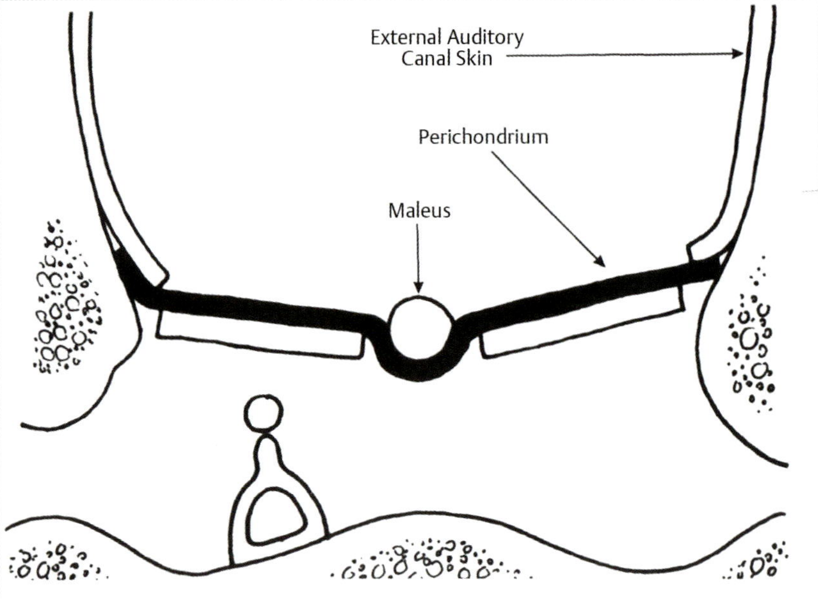

Fig. 25.3 Lateral line drawing demonstrating proper placement of graft.
Used with permission from Dornhoffer JL. Cartilage tympanoplasty: indications, techniques, and outcomes in a 1000-patient series. Laryngoscope 2003;113:1844–1856.

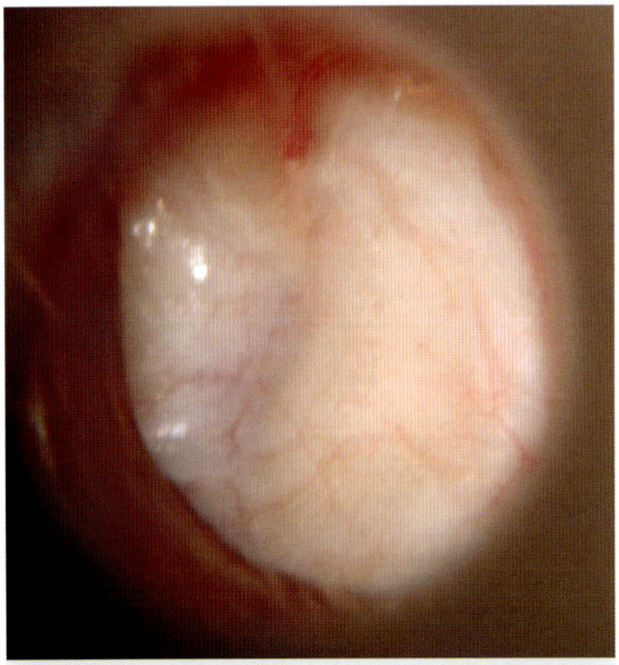

Fig. 25.4 Postoperative ear with perichondrium/cartilage island graft (left ear).
Used with permission from Dornhoffer JL. Cartilage tympanoplasty: indications, techniques, and outcomes in a 1000-patient series. Laryngoscope 2003;113:1844–1856.

Gelfoam (Upjohn Laboratories, Kalamazoo, Michigan) is packed in the middle ear space underneath the anterior annulus to support the graft in this area, and the posterior flap of perichondrium is draped over the posterior canal wall. Middle ear packing is avoided on the promontory and in the vicinity of the ossicular chain. One piece of Gelfoam is placed lateral to the reconstructed TM, and antibiotic ointment is placed in the ear canal (▸ Fig. 25.4).

25.3.3 The Mosaic Technique

When the mosaic technique is used for reconstruction of the TM, cartilage can be harvested from either the tragus or the cymba. Cartilage from the cymba area of the conchal bowl is used if the surgical approach involves a postauricular incision. Tragal cartilage is used if the approach is transcanal or endaural. The cartilage of the cymba is similar to the tragus in that it has an acceptable thickness of about 1 mm, in contrast to other areas of the concha, which are thicker and irregular. Cymba cartilage is more curved, however, which makes it particularly suitable for this technique, which, unlike the perichondrium/cartilage island flap technique, does not require one large, flat piece of cartilage.

The cartilage is cut into several slices that are subsequently pieced together, like a jigsaw puzzle, to reconstruct the TM (▸ Fig. 25.5; ▸ Fig. 25.6). A large area of conchal eminence can be exposed by elevating the subcutaneous tissue and postauricular muscle from the conchal perichondrium. The cymba cartilage is the prominent bulge at the superior aspect of the concha (▸ Fig. 25.7). A circumferential cut the size of the anticipated graft is made through the perichondrium and cartilage, but not through the anterior skin. The perichondrium is removed from the postauricular side, and the cartilage, with the perichondrium on the anterior aspect, is dissected from the skin. This technique is also used for harvesting cartilage for canal wall reconstruction when the retrograde mastoidectomy technique is used for cholesteatoma surgery.

The mosaic technique described here differs somewhat from the palisade tympanoplasty of Heermann, Heermann, and Kopstein.[12] Instead of placing rectangular strips of cartilage side to side, an attempt is made to cut one major piece of cartilage in a semi-lunar fashion, which is placed directly against the malleus on top of the prosthesis (▸ Fig. 25.8a; ▸ Fig. 25.8b). This acts to reconstruct a major portion of the posterior half of the TM and serves as a foundation for the rest of the cartilage pieces. A second semi-lunar piece is placed between this first piece and the canal wall to reconstruct the scutum precisely (▸ Fig. 25.8c).

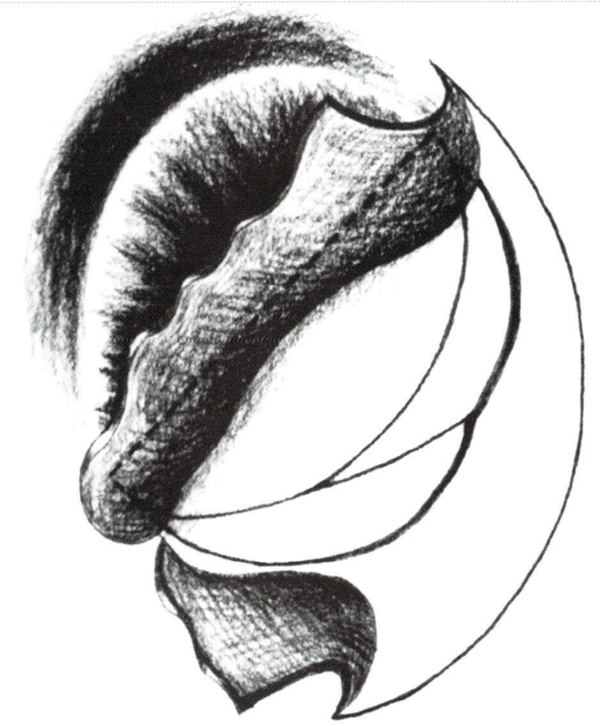

Fig. 25.5 Schematic of mosaic technique (right ear).
Used with permission from Dornhoffer JL. Cartilage tympanoplasty: indications, techniques, and outcomes in a 1000-patient series. Laryngoscope 2003;113:1844–1856.

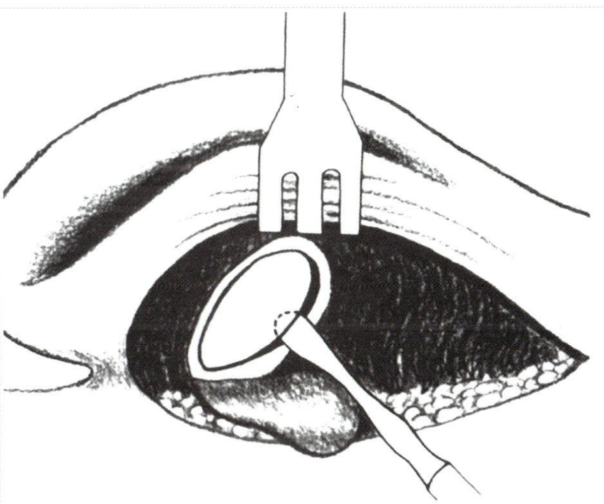

Fig. 25.7 Harvesting of cymba cartilage with postauricular incision (right ear).
Used with permission from Dornhoffer JL. Cartilage tympanoplasty: indications, techniques, and outcomes in a 1000-patient series. Laryngoscope 2003;113:1844–1856.

Any spaces that result between this cartilage and the canal wall or scutum are filled in with small slivers of cartilage to prevent prosthesis extrusion and recurrent retraction (▸ Fig. 25.8d). The reconstruction is then covered with the previously harvested perichondrium draped over the posterior canal wall (▸ Fig. 25.9).

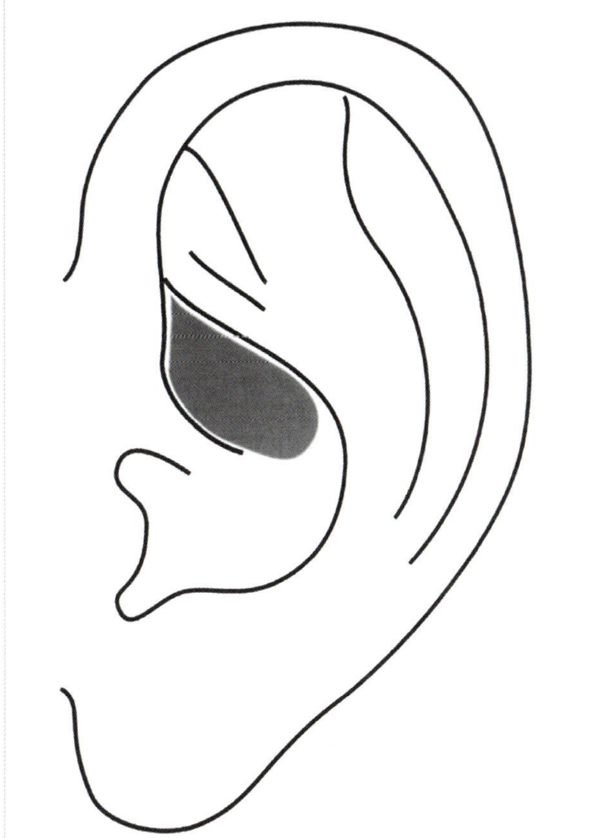

Fig. 25.6 Schematic illustrating location of cymba cartilage (left ear).
Used with permission from Dornhoffer JL. Cartilage tympanoplasty: indications, techniques, and outcomes in a 1000-patient series. Laryngoscope 2003;113:1844–1856.

Although this technique can be used for TM reconstruction without ossicular reconstruction, it is favored when ossiculoplasty is performed in a malleus-present situation and is especially suitable for cholesteatoma surgery. Because the prosthesis is placed prior to the cartilage reconstruction, the mosaic technique allows direct visualization and contact of the notched prosthesis to the manubrium handle, which has been shown to provide superior hearing results.[13] The prosthesis acts as a scaffolding on which the cartilage is placed, which serves to reconstruct the TM as well as prevent prosthesis extrusion. It likewise allows a precise and water-tight fit between the reconstructed TM and the canal wall in the posterior area, where recurrent cholesteatoma most frequently occurs. Typically, in these situations, the anterior half of the TM is not altered or is grafted with conventional materials to allow cholesteatoma surveillance and possible intubation in the postoperative period if necessary.

25.4 Postoperative Care

At 1–2 weeks post-surgery, the packing material of Gelfoam and antibiotic ointment is completely suctioned from the external canal. Antibiotic/steroid-containing drops are used for an additional 2 weeks to clear the ear of residual ointment and

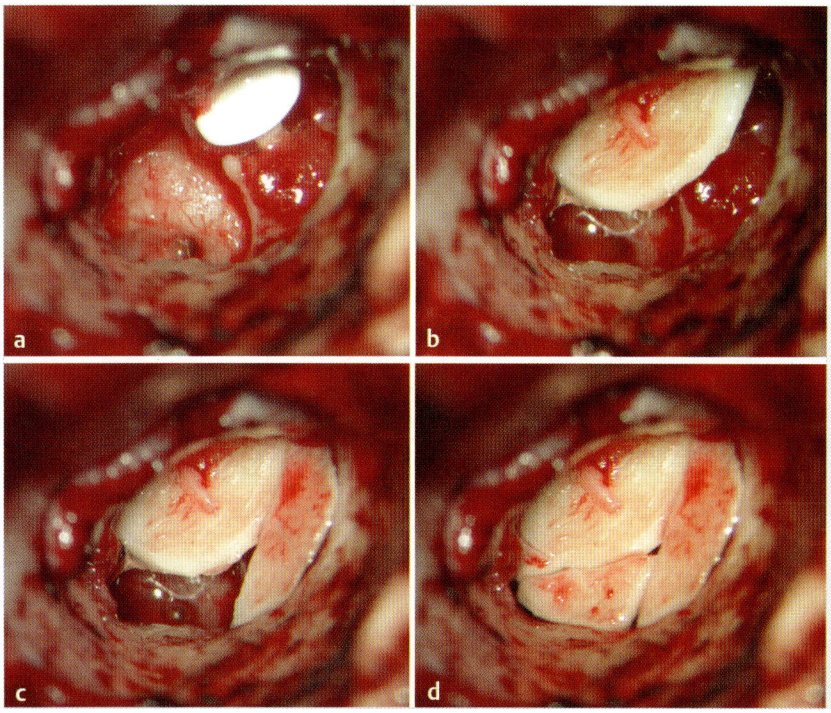

Fig. 25.8 Series demonstrating sequence of mosaic reconstruction (left ear). (a) Total ossicular replacement prosthesis (TORP) in place. (b) Initial cartilage placement. (c) Reconstruction of the scutum. (d) Reconstruction of remainder of posterior TM.
Used with permission from Dornhoffer JL. Cartilage tympanoplasty: indications, techniques, and outcomes in a 1000-patient series. Laryngoscope 2003;113:1844–1856.

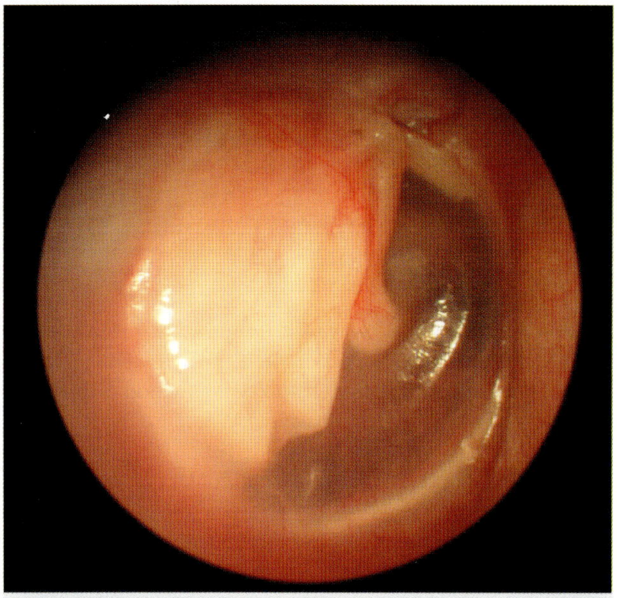

Fig. 25.9 Postoperative appearance of TM after mosaic reconstruction (right ear).
Used with permission from Dornhoffer JL. Cartilage tympanoplasty: indications, techniques, and outcomes in a 1000-patient series. Laryngoscope 2003;113:1844–1856.

Gelfoam, the latter of which can lead to granulation and fibrous tissue formation if inadequately removed from the TM. The adult patient is instructed to begin the Valsalva maneuver, and children are instructed to use the Otovent, 3 times a day beginning 2–3 weeks after the surgery.

A postoperative audiogram is obtained 6–8 weeks post-surgery, at which time the TM is examined. It should be mentioned that impedance tympanometry is unreliable after cartilage tympanoplasty and will generally yield a low-volume type B tympanogram, despite normal hearing, due to the noncompliant nature of the graft. It is therefore necessary to check air and bone conduction after the surgery and use hearing levels to determine whether an effusion is present. If the hearing result is good and the TM is clear, the ear is examined at 6 months and again at 1 year from the date of surgery. If an effusion is present based on observation or conductive hearing loss, nasal steroids are added, the Valsalva (Otovent) encouraged, and the ear examined at 3 months. If, in a case of postoperative conductive hearing loss, it is unclear whether an effusion is present due to the opacity of the TM, a computed tomography (CT) scan is sometimes necessary to assess the status of the middle ear. If an effusion is present at that time, the ear is intubated.

25.5 Complications

25.5.1 Intraoperative Complications

Intraoperative difficulties center around poor graft fit or difficult graft placement. If the perichondrium/cartilage island graft is inadvertently made too small, the problem can be rectified in one of two ways. The most effective is to piece leftover cartilage slivers between the cartilage island and annulus using the mosaic technique in connection with the island technique. This works particularly well when the posterior island is too small. The second way to rectify a too-small graft is to cover the entire graft with the perichondrium that was previously harvested from one side and tuck it under the annulus as an underlay graft. Although this results in two layers of perichondrium over the cartilage, no detrimental effect on hearing has been noticed with this slightly thicker graft, and it is used on occasion.

Poor fit more commonly results when the island flap is made too large, especially the anterior island. Because the bony annulus is blunt and thicker anterior-superiorly, if the anterior island is too large, it will be pushed medially by the ridge of bone, making a step-off just anterior to the malleus neck. Although at first it may appear that this problem could be rectified by additional Gelfoam packing anteriorly, grasping the graft with cup-forceps and pulling it laterally through and into the defect will reveal that it is actually being held medially by the anterior bony annulus. Once this is identified, it is easily corrected by making the graft smaller and ensuring a precise fit to the bony annulus.

A problem with placement can occur with an intact chain exhibiting a medially rotated malleus, which is usually encountered with the atelectatic ear. This can be overcome in one of two ways. The first is to remove 1 mm of the manubrium at the umbo with the malleus head amputator (malleus "nippers"). This does not affect hearing and allows medial placement of the graft. Attempting to lateralize the malleus with an intact chain should be discouraged due to the possibility of acoustic trauma. The second way to resolve this problem is to remove a slightly wider strip of cartilage (2 mm) to facilitate the malleus handle. This allows the more medial malleus to indent further into the perichondrium, permitting the cartilage plates to move more laterally in the reconstruction and avoiding contact with the promontory. This also allows the anterior island of cartilage more flexibility in positioning, which is necessary to make good contact with the anterior annulus. It has been the author's experience that the reconstructed TM frequently pulls the malleus laterally during healing, even when the graft is making contact with the promontory at the level of the malleus manubrium after graft placement.

The other pitfall specific to the atelectatic ear concerns management of the atrophic TM. After elevating the atrophic TM off the promontory, it is tempting to insert the cartilage medial to the intact TM. It is important, however, to remove at least a portion of the atrophic TM anterior and posterior to the malleus to ensure that the cartilage flap is incorporated into the reconstructed TM.

25.5.2 Postoperative Complications

The most significant pitfall seen in the postoperative period is persistent effusion with conductive hearing loss, requiring intubation of the reconstructed eardrum. This is seen in about 7–10% of cases and can be problematic in cases where the entire TM is reconstructed with the cartilage/perichondrium island flap. (As mentioned earlier, the tympanogram, generally low-volume type B, will often be unreliable in the postoperative situation due to the noncompliant graft. Therefore, the hearing result is the best indicator of middle ear function, and, in some cases, especially when the conductive loss is intermediate or difficult to ascertain, a CT scan may be needed to assess the middle ear.) Although the TM remains relatively insensate after cartilage reconstruction, it is often necessary to take the patient to the operating room for eardrum intubation because tube placement can be difficult. If enough room exists between the anterior annulus and the cartilage graft, a traditional myringotomy can be made, with more depth frequently found in the anterior-superior quadrant. It is more often necessary, however, to remove an ellipse of cartilage with a sickle knife or laser for adequate tube fit. It should be noted that due to the thickness of the cartilage graft, grommet tubes are not applicable to this situation, and Silastic T-tubes are more frequently used. More recently, a titanium tube (Razrbac Tube, Grace Medical Inc., Memphis, Tennessee) has been designed specifically for use in ears reconstructed with cartilage tympanoplasty. The tube extends through the cartilage but has more rigidity than a Silastic tube to prevent compression by the rigid graft.

In cases of more pervasive Eustachian tube dysfunction, such as in patients with craniofacial abnormalities (including Down syndrome), previous head and neck cancer involving the nasopharynx, or a history of multiple ear surgeries, a T-tube is inserted in the cartilage graft during the initial surgery. The perichondrium/cartilage island graft is harvested and prepared as previously described. Using a round knife, a window that is large enough to allow placement of a Xomed Modified Goode T-tube (Xomed Surgical Products, Jacksonville, Florida) is cut into the anterior cartilage island. A straight pick is then placed into the cartilage window to dilate the perichondrium to allow tube placement. Prior to inserting the graft, the tube is placed into the cartilage window and brought out through the perichondrial surface. If the malleus is present, the end of the tube is first angled under the manubrium with small alligator forceps. After hooking the tube under the malleus, the graft is slid forward into place. If the malleus is absent, the graft/tube complex is slid directly into its final position (▶ Fig. 25.10).

Should a T-tube be removed either accidentally or purposely from the ear reconstructed with cartilage, the TM heals with a monomeric membrane; however, the cartilage defect remains. If tube reinsertion is needed, a myringotomy is first performed through the monomeric membrane. The tube is then reinserted at the original site by grasping the end of the T-tube with alligator forceps and pushing the flanges through the cartilage defect. Since the TM is relatively rigid from the cartilage reconstruction, it does not medialize when pressure is placed laterally. This increased rigidity greatly facilitates secondary tube insertion.

Another problem that may occur postoperatively concerns the patient undergoing reconstruction after cholesteatoma removal. One serious disadvantage of using cartilage for reconstruction in

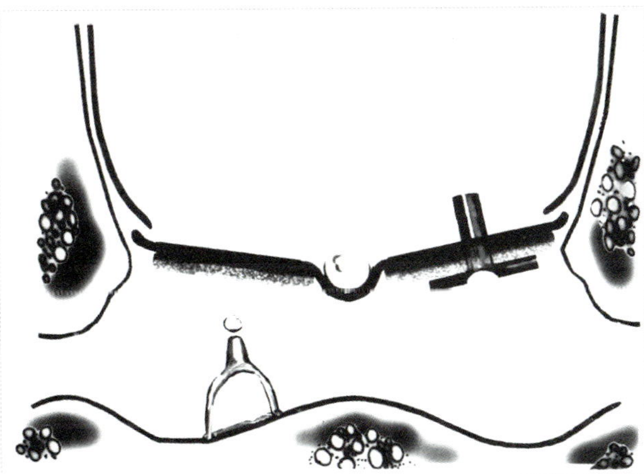

Fig. 25.10 Schematic showing technique of cartilage tympanoplasty with intraoperative placement of T-tube.
Used with permission from Dornhoffer JL. Cartilage tympanoplasty: indications, techniques, and outcomes in a 1000-patient series. Laryngoscope 2003;113:1844–1856.

cholesteatoma surgery is that it creates an opaque TM posteriorly, which could potentially hide residual disease. This is a problem that should be recognized, and surgical discretion should be used. If major disruption of the cholesteatoma sac occurs at extirpation, one must consider the advisability of performing a second-look surgery at a later date. However, this also applies to cholesteatoma surgery in general, not just in cases where cartilage is used in the reconstruction. One must also recognize the fact that most residual disease occurs in the epitympanum, an area that is hidden by the bony canal wall and scutum when canal wall-up surgery of any type is performed.[14] Although posterior cartilage TM reconstruction can delay the diagnosis of residual cholesteatoma, the disease will become manifest either anteriorly or as a recurrence of a conductive hearing loss, and there should be no major complications as a result of this delay in diagnosis.[15,16]

Revision surgery following cartilage tympanoplasty is generally straightforward. The tympanomeatal flap is elevated in the usual fashion, and the fibrous annulus is identified. The mucosa is incised, the middle ear entered, and the posterior portion of the eardrum is lifted up. This technique is similar to elevating a TM with posterior myringosclerosis, as long as an adequate strip of cartilage was removed to facilitate the malleus in the initial surgery. This allows the graft to hinge at the malleus during revision surgery. Removing the perichondrium from the medial surface of the graft prior to placement allows the smooth surface of the cartilage to become mucosalized and actually prevents adhesions, similar to the action of Silastic sheeting, so scarring is generally less than what is seen with other graft materials, especially in cases with mucosal disruption on the promontory.

25.6 Outcomes

Successful graft take can be anticipated in well over 95% of patients undergoing cartilage tympanoplasty. Short-term (< 3 months) graft failures are exceedingly rare, even in an infected environment, where the increased durability of the cartilage is a distinct advantage. If long-term failures occur, they are usually seen in the non-grafted portion of the TM, between the cartilage graft and the normal TM or between the cartilage graft and the bony annulus. If revision is necessary, a small piece of cartilage can be placed using the mosaic technique, after freshening the edges of the perforation.

Although the ossification of the cartilage graft has not proven to be a problem, the graft does soften somewhat over time. Usually, this softening is inconsequential, and the graft maintains its shape and integrity with little remodeling. However, when the ossiculoplasty is performed with cartilage pieces, problems can occur with a poorly fitted prosthesis. If significant pressure is exerted on a focal area, as with a sharp edge of a prosthesis that is tilted or too long, the cartilage can focally absorb at the pressure point, leading to prosthesis exposure. Although its rigidity would seem to afford a degree of protection, cartilage should not be considered to be a safety net for an ill-fitting prosthesis.

Given the good anatomical results, more attention has recently been given to the acoustic properties of cartilage compared with more traditional grafting materials. In a retrospective comparison between perichondrium and cartilage in type I tympanoplasties, we reported no significant difference in hearing between groups.[10] Our larger series of over 1000 cases continued to demonstrate encouraging results,[17] which have been supported by others who have shown excellent closure of the air-bone gap with cartilage tympanoplasty techniques.[9,10] Given the postoperative appearance of the TM after cartilage tympanoplasty, it is admittedly surprising that no hearing loss is incurred. There is no satisfactory explanation for this phenomenon, other than that the dictum of "form follows function" appears not to apply to cartilage tympanoplasty.

References

[1] Glasscock ME III, Hart MJ. Surgical treatment of the atelectatic ear. In: Friedman M, ed. Operative Techniques in Otolaryngology–Head and Neck Surgery. Philadelphia: WB Saunders, 1992:15–20.

[2] Levinson RM. Cartilage-perichondrial composite graft tympanoplasty in the treatment of posterior marginal and attic retraction pockets. Laryngoscope. 1987;97(9):1069–1074.

[3] Milewski C. Composite graft tympanoplasty in the treatment of ears with advanced middle ear pathology. Laryngoscope. 1993;103(12):1352–1356.

[4] Duckert LG, Müller J, Makielski KH, Helms J. Composite autograft "shield" reconstruction of remnant tympanic membranes. Am J Otol. 1995;16(1):21–26.

[5] Black B. Ossiculoplasty prognosis: the spite method of assessment. Am J Otol. 1992;13(6):544–551.

[6] Goldenberg RA. Hydroxylapatite ossicular replacement prostheses: preliminary results. Laryngoscope. 1990;100(7):693–700.

[7] Buchwach KA, Birck HG. Serous otitis media and type 1 tympanoplasties in children. A retrospective study. Ann Otol Rhinol Laryngol Suppl. 1980;89(3 Pt 2):324–325.

[8] Bailey HA, Jr. Symposium: Contraindications to tympanoplasty. I. Absolute and relative contraindications. Laryngoscope. 1976;86(1):67–69.

[9] Raine CH, Singh SD. Tympanoplasty in children. A review of 114 cases. J Laryngol Otol. 1983;97(3):217–221.

[10] Dornhoffer JL. Hearing results with cartilage tympanoplasty. Laryngoscope. 1997;107(8):1094–1099.

[11] Zahnert T, Hüttenbrink KB, Mürbe D, Bornitz M. Experimental investigations of the use of cartilage in tympanic membrane reconstruction. Am J Otol. 2000;21(3):322–328.

[12] Heermann J Jr Heermann H, Kopstein E. Fascia and cartilage palisade tympanoplasty. Nine years' experience. Arch Otolaryngol. 1970;91(3):228–241.

[13] Dornhoffer JL, Gardner E. Prognostic factors in ossiculoplasty: A statistical staging system. Otol Neurotol. 2001;22(3):299–304.

[14] Smyth GD. Cholesteatoma surgery: the influence of the canal wall. Laryngoscope. 1985;95(1):92–96.

[15] Parisier S, Hanson M. Pediatric cholesteatoma: Results of individualized single surgery management. In: Sanna M, ed. Fifth International Conference on Cholesteatoma and Mastoid Surgery. Alghero-Sardinia, Italy: CIC Edizioni Internazionali, 1997:375–385.

[16] Hirsch BE, Kamerer DB, Doshi S. Single-stage management of cholesteatoma. Otolaryngol Head Neck Surg. 1992;106(4):351–354.

[17] Dornhoffer J. Cartilage tympanoplasty: indications, techniques, and outcomes in a 1,000-patient series. Laryngoscope. 2003;113(11):1844–1856.

Part 5

Roundtable on Ossiculoplasty

26 Overview and Introduction

John L. Dornhoffer and Michael B. Gluth

26.1 Introduction

Ossiculoplasty, also known as ossicular chain reconstruction, requires dexterity, precision, and a working knowledge of tympano-ossicular anatomy and physiology. In the following chapters of this surgical roundtable discussion, experts in the craft of ossiculoplasty will outline various techniques to manage the full spectrum of ossicular dysfunction found in the chronic ear. To properly grasp and apply the techniques described, it is critical that the reader understands a few essential concepts that dictate how ossiculoplasty is applied and how hearing outcomes should be judged. Furthermore, the material in Chapter 8 (Biomaterials in Tympanomastoid Surgery) and Chapter 9 (Middle Ear Mechanics in Hearing Reconstruction) will further augment the information presented here on ossiculoplasty.

26.2 Middle Ear Environment

Although several factors, such as surgical technique and the qualities of the prosthesis, can affect ossiculoplasty hearing outcomes, there is no question that the condition of the middle ear is the most important determinant of long-term results.[1,2,3] Unfortunately, this is also the most difficult concept for both novice and experienced ear surgeons to understand. For example, even the most elegant and meticulously executed ossiculoplasty will be relegated to a poor hearing result if the middle ear space is not aerated postoperatively. By considering these factors during the preoperative assessment, patient stratification, realistic expectations, and informed consent are facilitated.

Although there is no universal agreement as to which factors are most important for success in ossiculoplasty, a review of the available classification schemes on middle ear risk and other reports on long-term ossiculoplasty outcomes will reveal certain trends.[1,2,4,5] Specifically, revision surgery, middle ear fibrosis, active middle ear drainage, and underlying untreated Eustachian tube dysfunction appear to impart a worse prognosis. As such, control of some of these factors should be pursued in the preoperative period if possible.

The extent of damage to the ossicular chain will also impact outcomes in that there is an apparent trend toward worse outcomes if the malleus manubrium is absent, even when statistically corrected for underlying disease severity.[1,2,5] Benefits of the intact malleus manubrium may include preserved tympanic blood supply, more rapid tympanic membrane healing, a lower rate of eardrum lateralization, and possibly improved acoustic gain if the malleus is incorporated into the ossiculoplasty scheme. Although the status of the stapes superstructure is frequently mentioned as being an important factor due to the stability that it can afford, this is controversial and the role of the superstructure in determining hearing outcomes is not nearly as well established in the literature as that of the malleus manubrium.[2,6]

26.3 Judging Ossiculoplasty Outcomes

Is a 17-dB air-bone gap a good result after ossiculoplasty? Conventional teaching might say "yes" since many reports in the literature traditionally present hearing outcomes within the premise that success is judged by the percentage of subjects having a postoperative air-bone gap < 20 dB. Although the traditional application of bracketed air-bone gap subgroups (≤ 10 dB, 11–20 dB, 21–30 dB, > 30 dB) may be useful in reporting results of stapes surgery where the middle ear environment is consistently favorable, it is not an ideal way to assess ossiculoplasty outcomes in chronic ear disease due to middle ear variability. Reality is that judgment of a 17-dB air-bone gap can only be made within the context of the underlying ear. In a severely affected chronic ear with fibrocystic sclerosis of the mucosa, tympanosclerotic fixation of the ossicular chain, and a previous canal wall-down mastoidectomy, such a result would be quite good. On the other hand, a 17-dB air-bone gap after simple ossiculoplasty in an aerated and stable middle ear cleft should not be considered a particular success.

One major problem that impedes interpretation of the ossiculoplasty literature is the issue that hearing outcomes are commonly presented without an accompanying analysis of the middle ear environment. Without using one of the various published middle ear risk indices to frame the quality of results, meaningful interpretation is not possible. In 2012, the editors of this textbook published an example of how "contextual" ossiculoplasty analysis can be undertaken.[7] In this report, we applied Dornhoffer's Ossiculoplasty Outcomes Parameter Staging (OOPS) Index[5] to calculate the predicted hearing outcome for a cohort of patients based on underlying middle ear risk factors. A surgeon's actual ossiculoplasty hearing outcomes were then compared with these predicted results to judge the quality and reproducibility of a standardized ossiculoplasty technique. It would be possible to perform a similar analysis using other published grading scales, such as Black's SPITE method.[2]

26.4 Primary versus Staged Ossiculoplasty

Controversy exists as to whether reconstruction of the ossicular chain should be performed as a primary technique during the same setting as tympanic membrane repair or if it should be staged as part of a separate procedure. Compelling data does not exist to support one over the other. Proponents of primary ossiculoplasty, including the editors of this textbook, assert that the presence of a middle ear prosthesis can impart advantages during the healing phase by supporting the overlying tympanic membrane graft (especially cartilage) and by acting as a strut to preserve middle ear volume. In the uncommon scenario where an unfavorable hearing result is encountered after primary ossiculoplasty, it is then possible to remove and reposition the prosthesis during a second-look procedure.

Staged reconstruction, on the other hand, offers the surgeon the advantage of assuring stability of the middle ear envelope prior to proceeding with ossiculoplasty. When the middle ear environment is deemed particularly poor during primary surgery or when a second-look procedure is already indicated for cholesteatoma, a staged approach may be particularly sensible. Advocates of staged reconstruction will typically place Silastic sheeting within the middle ear cleft to prevent formation of adhesions. This sheeting is later removed during a second stage when ossiculoplasty is performed.

26.5 Classification of Tympanoplasty

Wullstein introduced the classic scheme used to classify the various subtypes of tympano-ossicular reconstruction; Merchant later modified this classification to comply with modern surgical techniques.[8] To understand the literature pertaining to tympano-ossicular reconstruction, it is helpful for a surgeon to possess at least a basic understanding of Merchant's Modified Wullstein Classification, as follows.

26.5.1 Type I Tympanoplasty

Repair of the tympanic membrane in the setting of an intact native ossicular chain.

26.5.2 Type II Tympanoplasty

Repair of the tympanic membrane in combination with any type of ossiculoplasty procedure that preserves the integrity of the malleoincudal lever mechanism. The most common example of this is repair of a dysfunctional (eroded) incudostapedial articulation. This modified classification of type II tympanoplasty differs from the classic description that depicted the uncommon scenario of tympanic membrane grafting applied directly upon the intact long process of the incus.

26.5.3 Type III Tympanoplasty

Repair of the tympano-ossicular mechanism by a means that does not preserve the integrity of the malleo-incudal lever mechanism. Type III tympanoplasty includes the vast majority of techniques described for routine ossicular chain reconstruction and it has thus been further subdivided according to ossiculoplasty technique, as described below.

Stapes Columella Subtype

This refers to any reconstruction scheme that places the superstructure of the stapes in direct contact with the tympanic membrane.

Minor Columella Subtype

This involves placement of an inter-positional graft or prosthesis to establish continuity between the tympanic membrane/ malleus manubrium and the superstructure of the stapes. Examples of this include the use of a synthetic partial ossicular replacement prosthesis (PORP) or sculpted ossicular (incus or malleus head) autograft.

Major Columella Subtype

This procedure is exactly the same as the minor columella subtype except that the stapes superstructure is absent; thus, with a major columella subtype the inter-positional graft or prosthesis is set upon the stapes footplate. An example of this is the use of a synthetic total ossicular replacement prosthesis (TORP).

26.5.4 Type IV and Type V Tympanoplasty

Type IV tympanoplasty involves the repair of the tympanic membrane without ossicular chain reconstruction in a manner where the stapes footplate is exteriorized into the external auditory canal, while simultaneously the round window is shielded within a small middle ear cleft termed the *cavum minor*. The modern Type V tympanoplasty is identical to Type IV aside from the fact that it involves the staged removal of a fixed stapes and soft tissue grafting of the oval window. This is in contrast to a traditional Type V, which involves fenestration of the lateral semicircular canal.

References

[1] Yung M, Vowler SL. Long-term results in ossiculoplasty: An analysis of prognostic factors. Otol Neurotol. 2006;27(6):874–881.

[2] Black B. Ossiculoplasty prognosis: the spite method of assessment. Am J Otol. 1992;13(6):544–551.

[3] Demir UL, Karaca S, Ozmen OA, Kasapoglu F, Coskun HH, Basut O. Is it the middle ear disease or the reconstruction material that determines the functional outcome in ossicular chain reconstruction? Otol Neurotol. 2012;33 (4):580–585.

[4] Albu S, Babighian G, Trabalzini F. Prognostic factors in tympanoplasty. Am J Otol. 1998;19(2):136–140.

[5] Dornhoffer JL, Gardner E. Prognostic factors in ossiculoplasty: A statistical staging system. Otol Neurotol. 2001;22(3):299–304.

[6] Vincent R, Rovers M, Mistry N, Oates J, Sperling N, Grolman W. Ossiculoplasty in intact stapes and malleus patients: a comparison of PORPs versus TORPs with malleus relocation and Silastic banding techniques. Otol Neurotol. 2011;32(4):616–625.

[7] Gluth MB, Moore PC, Dornhoffer JL. Method and reproducibility of a standardized ossiculoplasty technique. Otol Neurotol. 2012;33(7):1207–1212.

[8] Merchant SN. Ossiculoplasty and Tympanoplasty in Chronic Otitis Media. In: Nadol J.B., McKenna M.J. Surgery of the Ear and Temporal Bone. Philadelphia, PA: Lippincott, Williams, & Wilkins; 2004:305–324.

27 Reconstruction of the Incudostapedial Articulation

Jan-Christoffer Lüers and Karl-Bernd Hüttenbrink

Abbreviations used in this chapter:

ABG: air-bone gap

27.1 Introduction

27.1.1 Anatomy

The incudostapedial joint connects the incus and stapes and represents the smallest interosseous joint in the human body. Like any other joint, it comprises hyaline cartilage, a synovial membrane, and an articular capsule. The diarthrodial joint is formed by the convex lenticular process of the incus on the one side and by the concave stapes head on the other side, thus forming a ball and socket joint. The lenticular process connects to the long process of the incus in a 90-degree angle (range, 75–105 degrees) and is composed of a thin stem deriving from the long process of the incus and a cap that forms the functional articular surface towards the stapes.[1] In fact, the incudostapedial joint capsule not only envelops the lenticular process, but it also incorporates part of the long process into the joint complex (▶ Fig. 27.1; ▶ Fig. 27.2).[2]

27.1.2 Physiology

Like any other joint of the ossicular chain, the incudostapedial joint has two main functions. First, the joint facilitates sound conduction from the incus to the stapes, for which a stiff and soundproof connection between the lenticular process and the stapes head is necessary. Second, the joint allows gliding movements between the articular surfaces. It is through this gliding movement that the stapes is decoupled from the rest of the ossicular chain, and, hence, the inner ear is decoupled from the large movements of the tympanic membrane, which are caused by changes of ambient atmospheric pressure.[3]

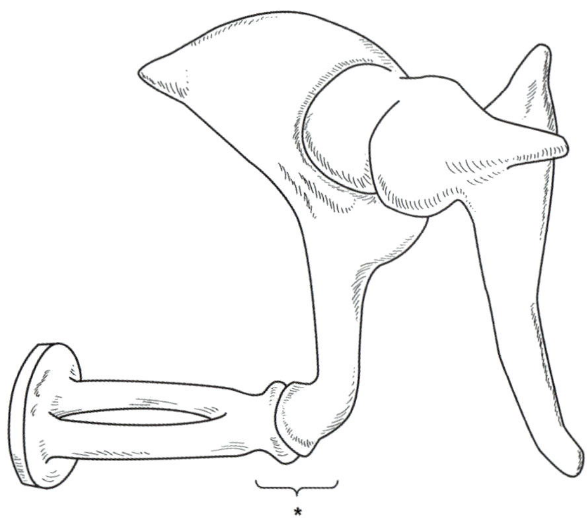

Fig. 27.1 The incudostapedial joint complex. This is a key factor in controlling ambient atmospheric pressure variations in the middle ear as it can decouple the stapes from the rest of the ossicular chain.

Among all the delicate structures of the ossicular chain, the long process of the incus is the most vulnerable for developing chronic otitis media with or without cholesteatoma.[4] As the ossicles have, unlike other bones, no capacity for self-regeneration, any discontinuity of the ossicular chain can only be repaired by surgical intervention,[2] and any attempt to repair the incudostapedial joint must take into account the specific characteristics of this area of the ossicular chain. However, the micro-mechanism of the incudostapedial joint, with its gliding joint movement and possible decoupling of the stapes and inner ear, is currently not replicated by any reconstruction technique.

27.2 Surgical Technique

The choice of the reconstructive technique depends on the extent of the defect, which can be just a slightly eroded joint (with a preserved soft tissue bridge between the incus and stapes), or a missing lenticular process, or an increased erosion of the long process of the incus. In principle, the surgeon has two possibilities for treating a damaged incudostapedial articulation.

With smaller defects, the original ossicular chain can be rebuilt by the reconstruction of the defective part of the long process of the incus (bridging technique). With larger defects, the sound conducting apparatus must be restructured by bypassing the incus and insertion of a prosthesis (interposition technique). The bridging technique derives from the former type II tympanoplasty according to the Wullstein classification. Although the original type II describes a direct contact between the tympanic membrane and the incus rudiment, this modification restores the continuity of the ossicular chain. The interposition technique, on the other hand, corresponds to the tympanoplasty type III Wullstein classification.[5] To date, none of the various surgical techniques to treat a damaged incudostapedial articulation have received universal acceptance.

With the bridging technique, the small defect of the long incus process is reconstructed so that the malleus-incus complex with its joint is still operational for sound conduction. The main advantages of the bridging technique are the preservation of the normal tri-ossicular configuration, allowing the full sound energy to be collected from the complete tympanic membrane via the malleus's handle. Thus, the bridging technique preserves a rather physiological constitution of the ossicular chain and represents the most straightforward way for handling a damaged incudostapedial joint. Most often, autologous materials, synthetic prostheses, and bone cement are used for this technique.

With the interposition technique, the sound is transmitted from parts of the eardrum via an interposition graft directly to the head of the stapes. Hence, interposition techniques are independent of a functional malleoincudial joint, which is

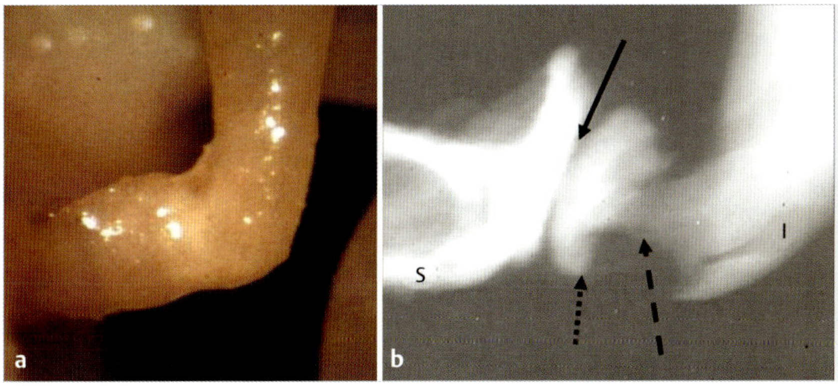

Fig. 27.2 Anatomy of the incudostapedial joint. The 90° angle is shown in a temporal bone specimen (left). On X-rays (right), the stem (dashed arrow) and the cap (dotted arrow) of the lenticular process next to the joint space (solid arrow) become visible. The articular surfaces of stapes (S) and incus (I) form the functional zone of the incudostapedial joint.

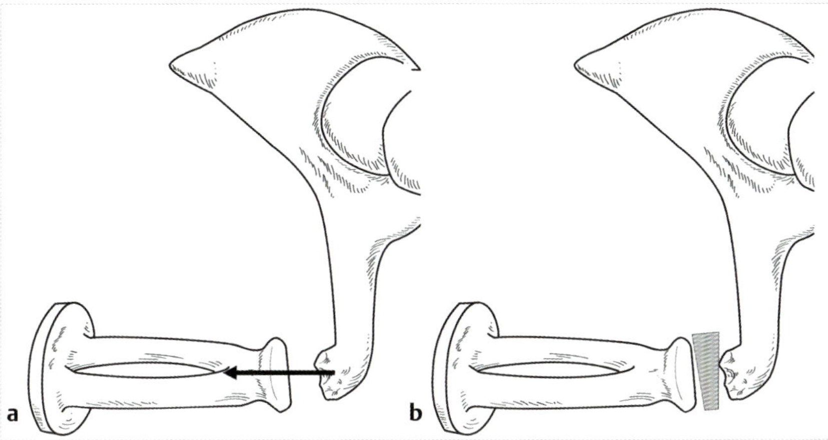

Fig. 27.3 Ideal situation for a bridging technique: Only the lenticular process is missing, but the long incus process is fully preserved. Hence, the action of the force runs through the stapes axis (left image) and the gap can be bridged with an interposition graft, preferably a piece of bone (right image).

bypassed. Prostheses made of autologous bone and synthetic materials are the constitutive materials.

27.2.1 Autologous Materials

The significant advantages of using autologous materials for reconstruction are the ease of availability, the absent risk of transmitting disease, their biocompatibility, and their cost-effectiveness. Potential disadvantages include displacement, absorption, and time required to sculpt the prosthesis.[6]

Bridging Technique

When the incudostapedial joint is only dislocated, a joint stabilization with perichondrium or temporalis fascia has been described,[7] but no long-term results are available. If only the lenticular process is missing, with the majority of the long process of the incus hovering on top of the stapes head, the gap can be bridged with an interposition graft. Here, a piece of (cortical) bone pushed into the gap between the incus and stapes represents the most effective option as it leads to a very firm sound connection. Alternatively, a piece of tragal or conchal cartilage, (depending on the approach), can be used as an interposition graft. In the course of time, however, cartilage might show inferior acoustic results due to softening (▶ Fig. 27.3).[8]

If the erosion of the long process of the incus has increased to a degree, where its edge is no longer on top of the stapes head circumference, then a simple bony interposition graft poses the risk of tilting and, subsequently, ineffective transmission with a piston-like movement between the incus and stapes (▶ Fig. 27.4). As a solution, a 1-mm thick piece of cartilage can be cut in a U-shape and a small 1-mm diameter groove drilled centrally into the undersurface of its apex. Although the small groove encompasses the stapes head, the two cartilage legs clasp the remaining part of the long process of the incus, thus preventing dislocation. The lateral surface of the cartilage has direct contact to the tympanic membrane on top and, hence, allows for additional direct sound transmission (the original Wullstein type II tympanoplasty).[9]

Interposition Technique

If the long process of the incus is too short for bridging, then autologous materials can be positioned between the stapes and tympanic membrane for a direct sound transmission. The correct size of this prosthesis is crucial. If the graft is too short, a loose contact with loss of acoustic energy will result. If the graft is too long, the stapes will be pushed inward, leading to a stiffening of the annular ligament, with a reduction of sound transmission, mostly in the lower frequencies.

When available, the autologous incus body, unless extensively involved or eroded by cholesteatoma, represents the gold standard as material for partial ossicular reconstruction as it combines optimal biostability with good acoustic transfer function (see Chapter 28). The incus body must be transformed into a prosthesis with a 1-mm groove in its lower end for placing it on top of the stapes head. The short process is shortened and can be provided with a small oblique groove to engage the

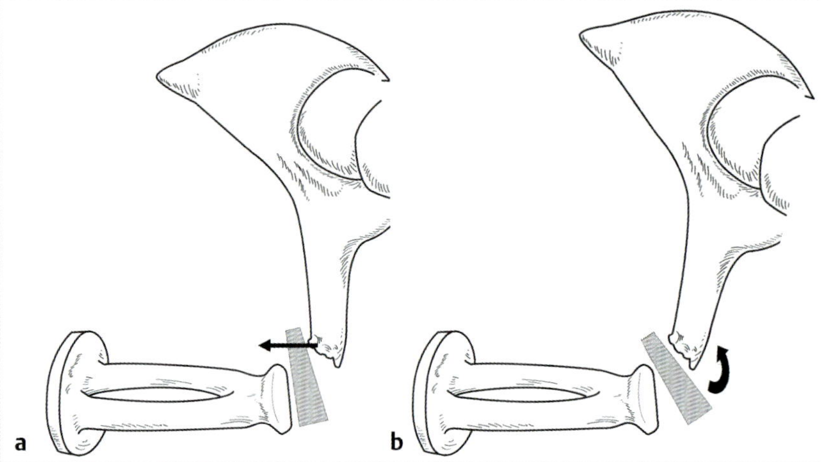

Fig. 27.4 If the edge of the eroded long incus process is out of the stapes head circumference, then the action of the force runs parallel to the stapes action (arrow on left image). Hence, a bony interposition graft poses the risk of tilting and thus ineffective sound transmission (arrow on right image indicates the movement of the graft).

malleus's handle. However, although an autograft of the repositioned incus might provide continuity of the ossicular chain, the fixation to the remnants of the ossicular chain remains a critical issue.[2] In addition, the sculpted auto-incus can partially erode or fuse to one of the bony walls around the oval window niche.[10]

27.2.2 Synthetic Prostheses

Synthetic alloplastic prostheses have been inserted into the middle ear since the origin of ossiculoplasty in the 1950s, and numerous materials (e.g., plastics, ceramics, various types of metals, etc.) and innovative forms have been proposed. Any middle ear prosthesis must fulfill high demands in terms of biocompatibility and acoustic-mechanic properties to enable optimal sound transmission (see Chapter 29). Following these demands, middle ear prostheses made of titanium or hydroxyapatite appear most suitable and are commonly used by otologic surgeons worldwide.[11]

Bridging Technique

A small defect might be filled with medical glue (e.g., fibrin tissue adhesive)[12] or cement (e.g., hydroxyapatite, glass ionomeric).[13] Prior to using the cement, any soft tissue or unstable bony debris has to be removed from the ossicles to obtain a smooth, dry, and solid bony surface. After the components are mixed, the cement keeps an ideal pasty consistency for a couple of minutes (working time) before it completely hardens. Notably, the various commercially available cements are distinguished from one another based on their handling characteristics and setting times.[13] Bone cement and other alloplastic materials may also be combined in such a way that a wire prosthesis or an absorbable suture is initially positioned between the stapes head and the long incus process; the bone cement is then modeled around the assembly with the wire or suture acting as a guide (▶ Fig. 27.5).

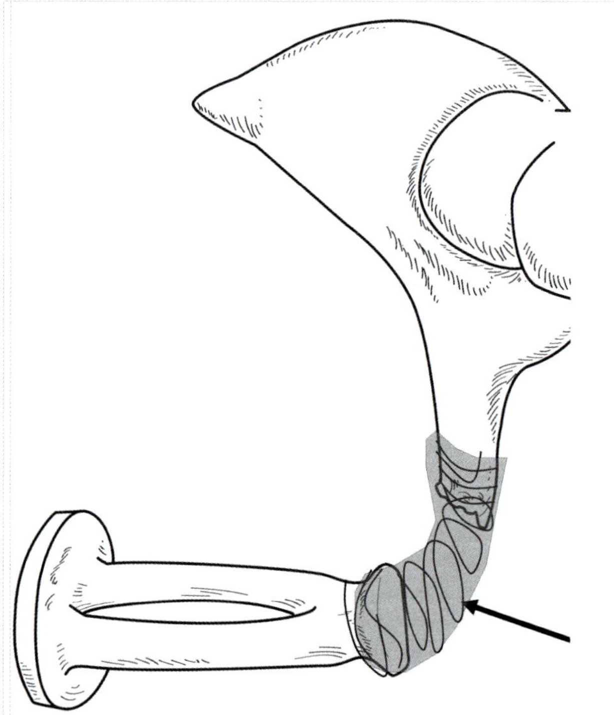

Fig. 27.5 If bone cement is to be used as bridging material, a wire or a suture (arrow) positioned between stapes and long incus process may give extra support for the cement during the modelling process.

The next option to bridge a gap between the stapes and incus are titanium-angled prostheses, with or without a clip mechanism for contact to the stapes's head (▶ Fig. 27.6). The clip was developed from the earlier bell-shaped angular prosthesis to simplify the handling of the prosthesis application, as it automatically adjusts to a stable final position on the stapes. Hence, most of the surgical challenge is limited to the crimping of the small titanium bands around the incus long process, a procedure known to the otologic surgeon due to its similarity to the fixation of a stapes piston. Afterward, the whole assembly is covered with a thick piece of cartilage to bridge the distance toward the tympanic membrane[14] (additional Type II tympanoplasty).

Interposition Technique

A stable coupling of the alloplastic prosthesis on the stapes head is of utmost importance for effective sound transport. Bell-shaped prostheses are more prone to a loose contact, even after stabilization by the application of absorbable gelatin

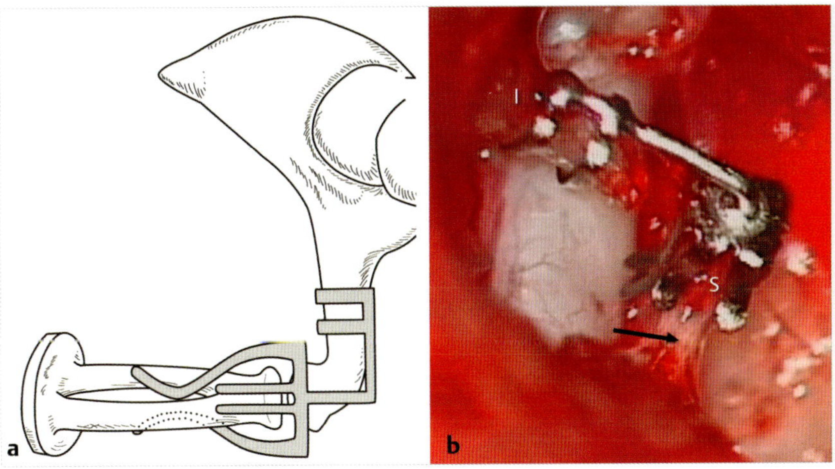

Fig. 27.6 Schematic display and intraoperative view of an angular clip prosthesis. Two titanium bands are crimped around the rest of the eroded long process of the incus (I) while the clip sits on the stapes (S). The stapedial tendon (arrow) is encompassed by two short legs of the clip, leading to further stabilization.

sponge.[15] A crimping of the bell around the stapes head is risky and can result in crushing the delicate bone. The clip mechanism allows a standardized, stable, and atraumatic coupling to the stapes head. The easy removal of the prosthesis in case of revision surgery is a further advantage.[16]

Any prosthesis should be positioned and, hence, operate in line with the stapes vertical axis. If not, the prosthesis and the stapes might tilt sideways, and ineffective rocking movements can result. The desired piston-like excitation is most likely to be obtained with a prosthesis that couples vertically up from the stapes head toward the overlying tympanic membrane, which should be stabilized with cartilage on top of the prosthesis's plate. If the malleus is not positioned too far anteriorly or retracted, an additional contact with a notch at the plate can be advantageous.

27.3 Postoperative Care

Pure tone audiometry with testing of the bone conduction is recommended within the first 24 hours after surgery. Further follow-up should include regular tuning fork and nystagmus tests. If audiometric tests signal a worsening of the inner ear function or if the patient suffers from vertigo and/or shows spontaneous nystagmus, the ear canal packing should be removed to release tension and pressure from the tympanic membrane (and the prosthesis) and corticosteroids should be administered.

A small discharge of the ear is a rather normal postoperative event and usually disappears soon after removal of the ear packing. If the surgery only consists of repair of the ossicular chain (with an intact tympanic membrane), then the ear packing may be removed after 7–10 days. If the ossiculoplasty is combined with reconstruction of the tympanic membrane, the packing should remain in place for about three weeks to enhance epithelialization of the epithelial defect.

In the case of purulent discharge, however, with signs of an acute inflammatory process, the ear packing should be removed immediately and any secretion suctioned out of the ear canal. Thereafter, close observation of the patient and administration of local and systemic antibiotics is recommended. If symptoms do not resolve and if inner ear function decreases, revision surgery should be considered.

27.4 Complications

Surgery of the incudostapedial joint is associated with a number of intraoperative complications, most of which affect the postoperative hearing result. First, care should be taken not to exert excessive pressure when inserting the prosthesis onto the stapes's head given that this could damage the stapes or cause it to dislocate.[17] Second, the quality of the coupling of any prosthesis to the stapes on one side and to the incus or tympanic membrane on the other side directly relates to the postoperative hearing results. However, the coupling quality is not measurable intraoperatively and is thus subject to the surgeon's assessment. The only standardization of this attachment is offered by the clip mechanism described above.

When using biological autografts or allografts, osseous fixation to the bony wall of the tympanic cavity can develop, leading to fixation of the graft and functional problems. In addition, an auto-incus might also fuse to the stapes, which can be a problem in revision tympanoplasty as there is a high risk for stapes luxation when trying to free the incus from the stapes.

The main complication with cement ossiculoplasty is the loss of nearly all flexibility of the ossicular chain. As cement is considered to induce osteoneogenesis, a fixation to the surrounding bony walls of the tympanic cavity might also be possible. Moreover, inflammatory reactions have been observed when cement comes into contact with soft tissue. Foreign body reactions (granulation, bone erosion) have been observed with many of the different types of bone cement.[13] Last, but not least, certain doubts must be raised with regard to whether stable long-term results can be expected with use of cement in the bridging technique. In contrast to cement, bone is a living structure that is undergoing remodeling or continued resorption at the bony remnants, which may result in a loose contact where the bone and cement meet. In addition, resorption of cement has also been described.[18]

These complications illustrate a major advantage of the angular clip prosthesis, where ongoing resorption of the tip of the long process of the incus does not lead to an immediate loss of connection. Furthermore, the additional cartilage plate between the shaft of the angular clip prosthesis and the tympanic membrane provides an additional sound conduction (corresponding to a type III tympanoplasty), even in cases of progressive incus destruction.

27.5 Outcomes

Hearing outcome after any tympanoplasty is affected by a number of different biological, morphological, prosthesis-related, and surgeon-related factors.[19] Aeration of the middle ear, the quality of the mucosa, the presence of any scarring or adhesions, stiffening of the annular ligament, and acoustic quality of the tympanic membrane will all affect hearing. Because of these confounding factors, there are many limitations when comparing different reconstruction techniques, and meta-analyses are not convenient.

Some techniques show superior results in experimental temporal bone measurements, but these disappear when the clinical factors mentioned above are taken into account. An exemplary crucial factor is the aeration of the middle ear: The ideal prosthesis, even the native ossicular chain, will present with an air-bone gap (ABG) of 40 dB or more in cases of middle ear effusion. An analysis of results using the titanium angular clip prosthesis showed that the reduction of the ABG was consistently higher in patients with an aerated middle ear, displaying a type A tympanogram compared with a type B or C tympanogram (17 dB reduction versus 7 dB), with a postoperative air conduction of around 25 dB, compared with 43 dB in patients with type B/C tympanograms.[14]

In general, it should be noted that all reconstruction techniques for defects of the incudostapedial joint can potentially provide similar audiological results if the reconstruction is stable and if the material or prosthesis does not fixate or dislocate. However, as no surgical technique can restore all functions of the incudostapedial joint perfectly, it is not surprising that a complete closure of the ABG is almost never achieved.[20] Moreover, since the same defect can be reconstructed by several of the techniques described here, and as none of the techniques can currently be deemed to be evidence-based, it is ultimately the personal preference of the surgeon that decides which method will be used in an individual case.

27.6 Conclusion

For incudostapedial joint reconstruction, be it a bridging or an interposition technique, most clinical studies describe a postoperative ABG of 10–20 dB,[7,10,14,15,20] and, to date, none of the reconstruction techniques have proven to be superior. This is mainly because of the lack of objective measurement techniques for different forms of reconstruction[20] and the vast amount of variables, other than the reconstruction technique, that influence the postoperative hearing. If reconstruction techniques and prostheses are examined in temporal bone studies by laser Doppler vibrometry, and, thus, if only the surgeon and the technique are the relevant factors for the acoustic result, then the most crucial aspects of ossiculoplasty become clear: stable fixture of any hard material or prosthesis to the ossicular remnants, optimal contact to the tympanic membrane, and mobility of the stapes to drive the inner ear.

References

[1] Skinner M, Honrado C, Prasad M, Kent HN, Selesnick SH. The incudostapedial joint angle: Implications for stapes surgery prosthesis selection and crimping. Laryngoscope. 2003;113(4):647–653.

[2] Karmody CS, Northrop CC, Levine SR. The incudostapedial articulation: New concepts. Otol Neurotol. 2009;30(7):990–997.

[3] Hüttenbrink KB. The mechanics of the middle-ear at static air pressures: T*he role of the ossicular joints, the function of the middle-ear muscles and the behaviour of stapedial prostheses. Acta Otolaryngol Suppl. 1988;451:1–35.

[4] Tos M. Pathology of the ossicular chain in various chronic middle ear diseases. J Laryngol Otol. 1979;93(8):769–780.

[5] Wullstein HL. Funktionelle Operationen im Mittelohr mit Hilfe des freien Spalthauttransplantates. Arch Ohr-, Nas-, Kehlkheilkd. 1952;161:422–435.

[6] Zahnert T. Reconstructive methods in hearing disorders - surgical methods. GMS Curr Top Otorhinolaryngol Head Neck Surg. 2005;4:Doc02.

[7] Vishwakarma R, More YI, Joseph ST, Patel KB, Ramani MK, More RI. Incudostapedial joint arthroplasty using temporalis fascia/perichondrium ties. Am J Otolaryngol. 2009;30(3):171–175.

[8] Steinbach E, Karger B, Hildmann H. [Use of cartilage transplants in middle ear surgery. A histologic long-term study of cartilage implants] Laryngorhinootologie. 1992;71(1):11–14.

[9] Luers JC, Huttenbrink KB, Beutner D. The U-shaped cartilage for reconstruction of the incus' long process. Clin Otolaryngol. 2009;34(5):504–505.

[10] Somers T, Van Rompaey V, Claes G, et al. Ossicular reconstruction: hydroxyapatite bone cement versus incus remodelling: how to manage incudostapedial discontinuity. Eur Arch Otorhinolaryngol. 2012;269(4):1095–1101.

[11] Goldenberg RA, Emmet JR. Current use of implants in middle ear surgery. Otol Neurotol. 2001;22(2):145–152.

[12] Nikolaidis V. Traumatic dislocation of the incudostapedial joint repaired with fibrin tissue adhesive. Laryngoscope. 2011;121(3):577–579.

[13] Goebel JA, Jacob A. Use of Mimix hydroxyapatite bone cement for difficult ossicular reconstruction. Otolaryngol Head Neck Surg. 2005;132(5):727–734.

[14] Huttenbrink KB, Luers JC, Beutner D. Titanium angular clip: A new prosthesis for reconstruction of the long process of the incus. Otol Neurotol. 2009;30 (8):1186–1190.

[15] Smith J, Gardner E, Dornhoffer JL. Hearing results with a hydroxylapatite/titanium bell partial ossicular replacement prosthesis. Laryngoscope. 2002;112 (10):1796–1799.

[16] Hüttenbrink KB, Zahnert T, Wüstenberg EG, Hofmann G. Titanium clip prosthesis. Otol Neurotol. 2004;25(4):436–442.

[17] Hüttenbrink KB. Manipulating the mobile stapes during tympanoplasty: The risk of stapedial luxation. Laryngoscope. 1993;103(6):668–672.

[18] Hoffmann KK, Kuhn JJ, Strasnick B. Bone cements as adjuvant techniques for ossicular chain reconstruction. Otol Neurotol. 2003;24(1):24–28.

[19] De Vos C, Gersdorff M, Gérard JM. Prognostic factors in ossiculoplasty. Otol Neurotol. 2007;28(1):61–67.

[20] Neudert M, Zahnert T, Lasurashvili N, Bornitz M, Lavcheva Z, Offergeld C. Partial ossicular reconstruction: Comparison of three different prostheses in clinical and experimental studies. Otol Neurotol. 2009;30(3):332–338.

28 Autograft Ossicular Reconstruction

Patrick R. Axon and Venkata SPB Durvasula

Abbreviations used in this chapter:

MERI: Middle Ear Risk Index
MRI: magnetic resonance imaging
OOPS: Ossiculoplasty Outcomes Parameter Staging

28.1 Introduction

Autograft ossicular reconstruction was first described in 1957 by Hall and Rytzner.[1] The technique of using the patient's own tissue to reconstruct the ossicular chain seemed to the authors to be the most sensible approach to improve success rate and to avoid prosthesis rejection, which was a significant problem with alloplastic prostheses of the time. During the late 1950s and 1960s, the techniques for using a remodeled incus were refined and increasingly adapted to become the most popular method of ossicular reconstruction.[2] Over recent years, new alloplastic materials have become more popular because of their simplicity of design, reliability, and increasing stability in a well-reconstructed middle ear, but there are clear advantages of using autologous material, not least because of its ready availability and low cost.

28.2 Patient Selection

The two most common reasons for considering the reconstruction of the ossicular chain is the destruction of the ossicles caused by chronic middle ear disease and disarticulation of the ossicular chain as part of a surgical procedure to eradicate disease. Traumatic fracture of the long process of the incus or stapes superstructure rarely occurs, and, even more rarely, necrosis of the long process of the incus may occur for no clear reason, and always behind an intact and healthy tympanic membrane.[3]

On most occasions it is possible to retrieve at least the body of the incus to use for reconstruction because it is the long process of the incus, in isolation, that is most susceptible to erosion. The use of a refashioned incus or malleus cannot be guaranteed for a number of reasons that will be discussed later; therefore, it is sensible that the surgeon has other options available before embarking on reconstructive surgery. The decision to use an autograft is made during surgery after inspection of the autologous material at hand and the ossicular defect. The incus remnant might be unsuitable because cholesteatoma has demineralized the bone, leaving a ragged and soft residuum. This finding also raises the concern that recurrent cholesteatoma might occur because of unnoticed cholesteatoma within the bony remnant.[4,5] It is difficult to say whether this does occur, but common sense dictates that a badly damaged ossicle is unlikely to serve long-term hearing restoration and, therefore, should not be used.

Ossicular reconstruction should only be considered after eradicating the underlying disease and a plan has been made for repairing the tympanic membrane. Using the patient's own tissue to reconstruct has the inherent advantage of not being rejected, but that does not mean failure is easily avoided. It is common to operate on an ear that has persistent Eustachian tube dysfunction, and, therefore, retraction of the neotympanum must be considered. Cartilage is often employed to prevent tympanic membrane retraction in the presence of persistent negative middle ear pressure, and its uses are discussed in detail in Chapter 25. Suffice it to say that the surgeon must not only plan to deliver a high probability of hearing success, but also a tympanic membrane that will not retract around the refashioned ossicular chain, leading to recurrent disease or late hearing loss. This is one of the most difficult aspects of autograft ossicular reconstruction. The repositioned incus remnant often has an awkward shape that gets in the way of an effective cartilage tympanoplasty. The cartilage sliver must be tight against the malleus handle and scutum to avoid gaps through which the eardrum can retract.

Most autograft ossicular reconstruction techniques rely on placement of the refashioned incus between the stapes head and malleus handle. Stability and, therefore, success of such a reconstruction is reliant on a number of factors. The first is the dexterity and experience of the operating surgeon. This is not a simple technique. It requires considerable practice using cadaveric material, often after attending instructional courses and working with an experienced trainer.

The second factor is availability of a suitable incus remnant to refashion, taking into account the gap between the stapes head and malleus handle. The simplest reconstruction is one in which there is a relatively small gap between the stapes head and malleus handle and the latter lies more or less over the former. The stability of the reconstruction becomes increasingly compromised if the malleus handle lies more anterior or offset to a posteriorly placed stapes head. The more offset the two points of contact with the incus, the more unstable the reconstruction is likely to be. There are techniques described in Chapter 30 that enable repositioning of the malleus handle to reduce this gap, but surgeons should have a number of potential solutions and, once again, if one is inexperienced, then alternative alloplastic reconstruction techniques should be considered.

The third main factor that dictates success is the extent of ossicular destruction. It is often the case that the disease process only erodes the long process of the incus, but cholesteatoma or eardrum retraction can also erode the stapes superstructure. This leaves a much wider gap between the stapes footplate and malleus handle or tympanic membrane, and it is often impossible to find suitable material to bridge the gap unless a homograft incus or malleus is used.[6,7] The incus is rarely long enough because the long process is almost always eroded. Fashioning an ossicle replacement graft out of a cortical bone chip[8] has been described, but these are often quite large and produce an unstable arrangement. It is the authors' experience that these wide gaps have an unacceptable failure rate using autograft material, and alloplastic reconstructive techniques should be considered.

Patient selection, outlined above, is primarily for canal wall-up procedures. Many surgeons advocate canal wall-down surgery, which can result in a narrowed middle ear cleft so that the neotympanum lies close or even touches the stapes head. If the neotympanum is resting directly on the stapes, creating a Type III stapes columella arrangement, then nothing more needs to be done, although it is often sensible to strengthen the eardrum overlying the sinus tympani with a sliver of cartilage. If there is a small gap between the eardrum and stapes head, then cartilage might suffice or, alternatively, an incus remnant or the malleus head can be used as interposition autograft material. These are simple yet robust techniques that should always be considered if the opportunity arises.

28.3 Surgical Technique

In medicine, there are often a number of ways to tackle a problem, and the management of chronic middle ear disease is no exception. No matter which surgical approach is favored by a particular surgeon, it is likely that some form of ossicular reconstruction will be necessary. The authors favor a combined approach tympanoplasty with primary reconstruction of the ossicular chain. This allows a second attempt to reconstruct at second-look surgery if there is still a conductive hearing loss after the first procedure and will ensure that the middle ear cleft is maintained at its normal height.

The reconstructed eardrum sits in a position to enable the secure placement of the prosthesis. If the surgeon favors canal wall-down surgery, then the middle ear cleft is often narrower so that the position of the tympanic membrane is in closer proximity to the stapes head. The offset between the malleus handle and stapes head is magnified, so it often is more preferable to reconstruct from the stapes to the posterior pars tensa of the tympanic membrane. Whether opting for a canal wall-up or -down approach, the surgeon is not always presented with a constant anatomical arrangement. Thus, if autologous graft material is going to be used, then the surgeon will have to be flexible and use the design that best suits that ear.

28.3.1 Ossicular Reconstruction after a Canal Wall-Up Procedure

Stapes Superstructure Present

For the purposes of clarity, primary ossicular reconstruction should only be performed if it is known that macroscopic clearance of the disease has been achieved. There is no point, for example, in reconstructing the ossicular chain if there is concern that there might be residual cholesteatoma within the stapes superstructure. Some surgeons will wait until the second-look operation before reconstructing the ossicular chain, arguing that one can be confident that the procedure is performed in a disease-free ear without evidence of tympanic membrane retraction. If this is the decided course of action, then the incus remnant or malleus head must be stored in the mastoid cavity until it is required.[9] On the other hand, successful primary reconstruction in a postoperative stable ear can possibly avoid second-look surgery if there is a facility for non-echo planar magnetic resonance imaging (MRI).

The decision to reconstruct is made toward the end of the procedure once disease has been removed. It is rare not to reconstruct. The authors will only delay or avoid reconstruction if there is concern that the stapes is hypermobile (thus risking dislocation), if the footplate is partially eroded by cholesteatoma matrix, if it is impossible to be certain that all cholesteatoma matrix has been removed from the footplate, or if there is extensive middle ear tympanosclerosis fixing the stapes to its surrounding structures. On occasion there can be concern about persistent Eustachian tube dysfunction evidenced by an atelectatic adhesive otitis media and middle ear effusion. These cases can be particularly unrewarding as, even if it is possible to reconstruct the tympanic membrane using a robust palisade technique, ossicular reconstruction is rarely successful because of persistent middle ear effusion or fibrosis of the middle ear cleft.

Once the decision has been made to reconstruct, careful assessment of the residual ossicular arrangement can be made. The first step is to assess the stapes footplate. The authors always check the mobility of the stapes or whether there has been erosion of its superstructure. Sometimes the head of the stapes can be missing, but the crura are intact or that a crus of stapes has eroded, leaving a precarious arrangement that might require laser removal of the residual superstructure.

The next step is to assess the autologous material that will be used. The authors prefer the incus body over the malleus head because the incus has a thinner profile and so much of the design is already incorporated into its shape. The malleus head is a little bulky, and it can often rest on the promontory when placed between the stapes head and malleus handle.

The different methods of remodeling the incus are demonstrated in ▸ Fig. 28.1 and ▸ Fig. 28.2, and over time a surgeon will develop a technique that suits his or her particular practice. In addition, autograft reconstruction is not always the best choice, so most experienced surgeons will choose a technique and material that is best for a particular ear. The authors primarily use the incus when the malleus handle is not significantly offset to the stapes head and there is no evidence of persistent Eustachian tube dysfunction.

The incus remnant is scrubbed with a gauze swab to be certain that all cholesteatoma matrix has been removed, and then the body is carefully gripped with a mosquito forceps (▸ Fig. 28.3). The grip needs to be secure, and the incus should never be released until it is certain that it will not spring free. (There is nothing more disheartening than seeing the incus fly through the air and onto the floor!) A clean piece of drape should be used, and the microscope should be focused onto the incus that is held in the forceps. The mosquito forceps has a

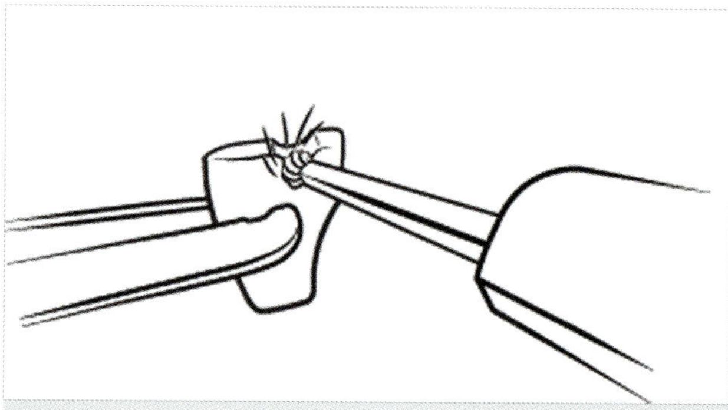

Fig. 28.1 Sculpting of incus using a diamond bur.

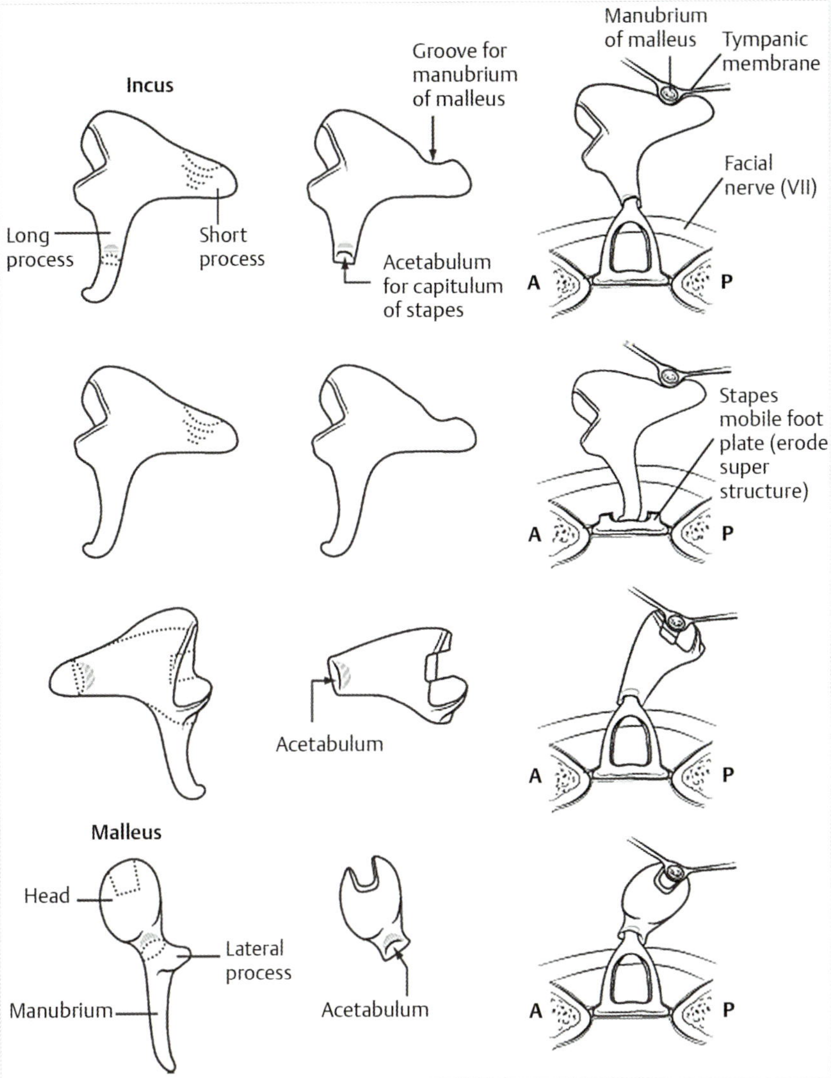

Fig. 28.2 Modifications for sculpting the incus and malleus. The authors prefer the modification shown in the third row. The modification in the second row is uncommon and is used more often with a homograft incus.

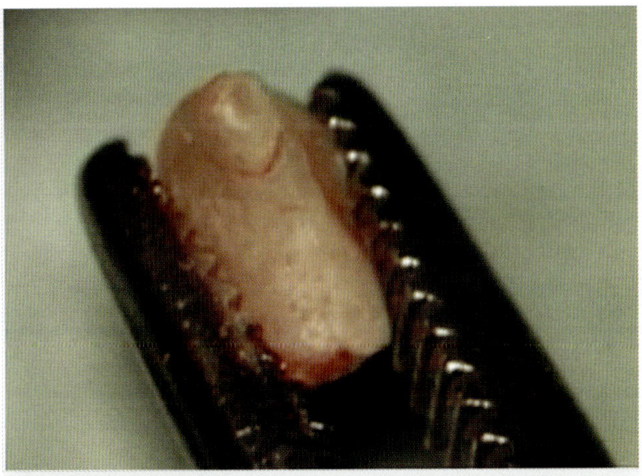

Fig. 28.3 Incus gripped between the jaws of a mosquito forceps with the short process uppermost.

gentle curve, and the part of the incus that requires drilling faces the convexity while the index finger supports the other side within the mosquito forceps concavity. An assistant drips saline onto the incus as the drill is gently worked across the surface, refashioning the incus remnant to its desired shape without burning the bone. The incus should never be held with fingers while drilling as there is a significant risk that the surgical gloves will quickly become wrapped around the bur's shaft. This is rather frightening and, once experienced, never repeated.

The authors' favorite incus design is one in which the short process sits on the stapes head and the disarticulated incudomalleal joint sits under the malleus handle. Any remnant of the eroded long process is removed, and a hole is drilled into the short process to accommodate the stapes head. To achieve the perfect fit, one must start with a large bur and gradually work with smaller, finer ones.

The short process is gently flattened with a 4- or 5-mm fine diamond bur. The surgeon should choose the largest and finest bur that he or she is comfortable with to reduce the risk of dislodging the incus from the mosquito forceps. A flat surface that is at least 2 mm in diameter is created, so that when the hole for the stapes head is drilled using a 1-mm fine diamond bur, there is at least 0.5 mm of healthy bone around its circumference (▶ Fig. 28.4). The hole for the stapes head lies opposite the disarticulated incudomalleal joint, which is the perfect shape to

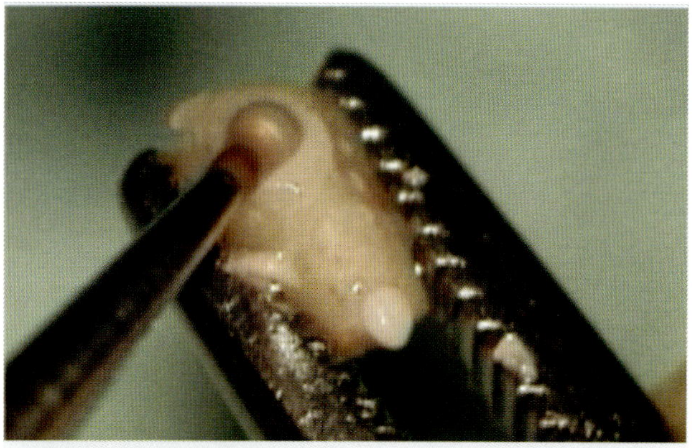

Fig. 28.4 Short process gradually reduced using a fine diamond bur so that the diameter of the flat surface is at least 2 mm. A 1-mm bur is then used to create a notch for the stapes head.

house the undersurface of the malleus handle. The refashioned incus is often tucked up against the tendon of the tensor tympani for further support. If it is too large, then more of the short process can be removed and the hole deepened for the stapes head.

Placing the refashioned incus into the perfect position can be challenging. An attempt should be made to have the main body of the incus facing posteriorly toward the stapedius tendon, so that when in position, it is not resting on the promontory. The incus is held with a fine sucker and positioned onto the head of the stapes first so that it is lying to the side, on the promontory (▶ Fig. 28.5). Using a needle and the sucker, one for each side of the incus, the incus is pivoted around the stapes head through 90 degrees so that the disarticulated incudomalleal joint sits snugly under the malleus handle (▶ Fig. 28.6). If successful, there is nothing more satisfying than a stable reconstruction where the three ossicles move as one.

Placing the short process on the stapes head is only possible if the malleus handle lies more or less above the stapes head. Pennington[10] described types Ia and Ib arrangements, to distinguish between a manubrium that is in vertical alignment to the stapes head, and type II, for a situation where the manubrium is more anterior and lateral to the stapes head, thus making the graft alignment offset. A type II arrangement means that the design described above will often pivot forward and become dislodged. In this situation one should consider using an allograft prosthesis, but if that is not available then an alternative autograft construction is required.

Drilling a hole into the long process remnant is more difficult because of its smaller diameter. One needs to be extremely careful not to breach its outer surface with the 1-mm given that the main strength in the offset incus arrangement is its support on the stapes head. A smaller bur can be used if available. A notch is then drilled across the opposite side of the short process that is deep enough to house the malleus handle (▶ Fig. 28.2). The position of the notch has to be perfect the first time. Widening the notch if it is incorrectly placed will only weaken the reconstruction. By using a similar technique to that described above, the autograft is eased into position. It will not feel as secure as the previous arrangement, and some surgeons will use a commercially available dissolvable sponge to help secure it in place. Both techniques benefit from an intact tensor tympani to act as a strut preventing the refashioned incus from slipping superiorly and also imparting some tension onto the arrangement. Dividing the tensor tympani to remove cholesteatoma makes ossicular reconstruction all the more difficult.

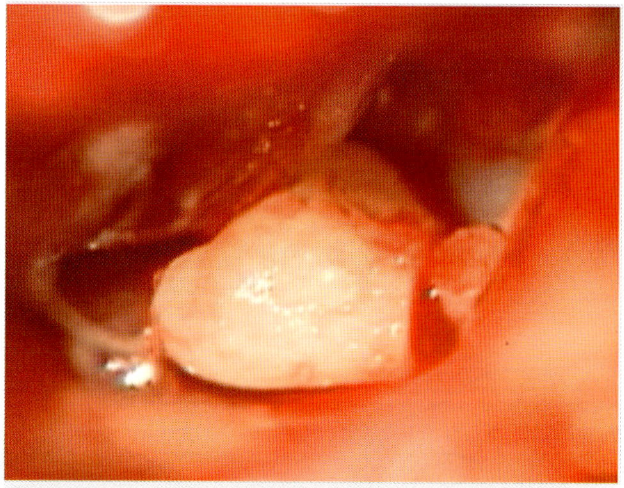

Fig. 28.5 Incus lying to the side on the promontory with the fashioned notch lying adjacent to the stapes head.

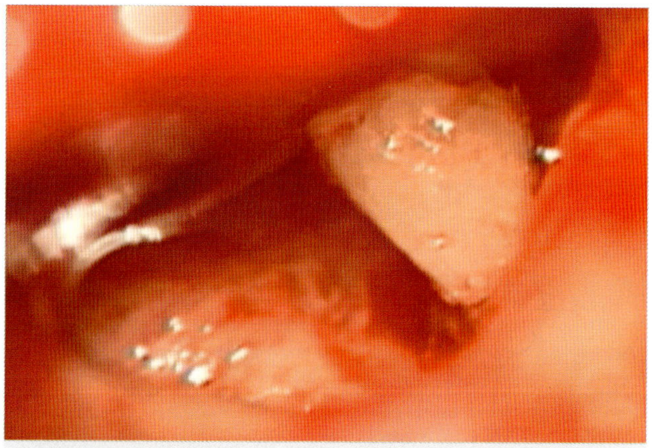

Fig. 28.6 Refashioned incus in place between the stapes head and malleus handle.

If there is no incus remnant, then the malleus head can be considered. The malleus head is more bulky and less forgiving, requiring considerably more refashioning to create the correct arrangement (▶ Fig. 28.2). In the authors' opinion, having to resort to a malleus head autograft in a canal wall-up procedure is far from ideal as the disease has been extensive enough to erode the whole incus.

Stapes Superstructure Absent

If the stapes superstructure is absent, then one is typically dealing with extensive and more aggressive disease. It is not only the increased gap between the footplate and malleus handle that adds to the difficulty of reconstruction, but also the lack of a secure post upon which to hang the reconstruction. The stapes footplate varies considerably in size and shape, occasionally disappearing out of sight in a tight ear. Once again, the surgeon needs to be confident that all cholesteatoma has been removed from its surface, and, as mentioned above, an eroded footplate should remain untouched. There is no glory in trying to reconstruct onto a paper-thin footplate resulting in footplate fracture and perilymph leak.

There are a number of articles and book chapters that describe the classical arrangement of an incus rotated so that the lenticular process rests on the stapes footplate and the notched body is stabilized under the malleus handle (▶ Fig. 28.2).[6] The perceived risk of Creutzfeld Jacob Disease transmission has made homograft use in this situation increasingly unacceptable. In addition, the authors have only seen two cases in many hundreds of operations whereby the stapes superstructure was eroded but the incus was in pristine condition for positioning. One alternative is to strip the entire malleus from the eardrum, enabling placement of the handle onto the footplate and the flattened end of the malleus under a sliver of cartilage used as an interposition graft against the posterior pars tensa of the tympanic membrane. The technique for stripping the malleus from an intact eardrum is made simpler if the malleus is still attached to the tensor tympani. Using a fine needle, it is possible to delicately strip the fibrous layer of the eardrum from the length of the malleus handle. The eardrum is densely adherent to the umbo, so a fine pair of microscissors is the best way to avoid perforating the drum. The umbo requires shortening to give a clean edge as does the malleus head. The amount of bone removed is dependent on the distance between the footplate and eardrum with cartilage interposition.

Cortical bone chips fashioned into a thin pillar has also been described, but these can be quite bulky and can rest on the adjacent structures, reducing the free movement of the reconstruction.[8]

28.3.2 Ossicular Reconstruction after a Canal Wall-Down Procedure

By their very nature, canal wall-down procedures result in loss of a large segment of scutum. The advantage of such an approach is ready access to the disease process; however, subsequent reconstruction has to take into account the loss of middle ear cleft height. A narrow middle ear cleft offers both advantages and disadvantages for subsequent ossicular reconstruction. A smaller gap between the stapes head and neotympanum is likely to increase the stability of the reconstruction. The main disadvantage is that as the tympanic membrane swings medially to meet the Fallopian canal or new canal wall, the malleus handle pivots away from the stapes head so that it is more offset. Placement of an autologous prosthesis between these two structures becomes less stable as the gap grows, and, therefore, the reconstruction might also require support from the posterior pars tensa of the tympanic membrane.[11] It has to be said that this is not usually a problem and, indeed, simply placing a refashioned incus remnant or malleus head containing a hole so that it can be placed securely on the stapes head with its lateral surface resting under the eardrum is often an adequate stable arrangement, delivering good closure of the air-bone gap.

Persistent Eustachian tube dysfunction cannot be ignored and one should always consider strengthening the tympanic membrane with cartilage, often using a palisade technique to reduce the risk of eardrum retraction. This will not always occur, but experience dictates that many cases do retract even if the preoperative middle ear cleft is fully aerated. The cartilage should be placed before fashioning the new ossicle so the distance of any gap that needs to be bridged can be calculated.

Pearls:

- Use only healthy ossicles and clean the ossicle remnant thoroughly with gauze to ensure cholesteatoma is removed.
- Check for mobility and health of the stapes superstructure before considering reconstruction. If there is no stapes superstructure, carefully inspect the footplate for thinning as footplate fracture can occur if there is excessive tension in the reconstruction.
- Prefer incus body over malleus head.
- It is easier to reconstruct vertically aligned malleus and stapes. The greater the gap between the two ossicles, the more unstable the reconstruction will become.
- Be careful when drilling the notch in the incus to house the stapes. If the drill cuts through the bony rim, the reconstruction will become unstable.

Pitfalls:

- Ossicular reconstruction in an ear that contains residual cholesteatoma will almost certainly lead to failure.
- If stapes superstructure is hypermobile, avoid reconstruction because this may result in dislocation.
- If revision surgery is necessary, beware that the autograft might have fused to the stapes superstructure, making disarticulation extremely difficult and increasing the risk of sensorineural hearing loss or even dead ear.
- Ossicular reconstruction without adequate care strengthening the posterior pars tensa with a cartilage will almost always lead to tympanic membrane retraction around the ossicular reconstruction.

28.4 Postoperative Care

After any form of reconstructive ear surgery, the reconstructed tympanic membrane and middle ear structures require support. There are a number of different methods that employ either dissolvable materials or wicks that are removed a couple of weeks after surgery. Most patients do not require any medication other than simple analgesia for a couple of days. Infected ears or ears that required extensive obliteration might require a course of antibiotics. Most patients can be discharged the same day, but an overnight stay might be required if extensive surgery was required. The authors will see a patient 2 weeks after surgery to remove the ear pack and then again 6 weeks later to clean the ear of any debris and formally check the hearing outcome. If possible, long-term follow-up is advised because only then will the surgeon be able to assess his or her surgical technique via personal experiences of both success and failure.

28.5 Outcomes

The recognition that so many factors can play a role in either the success or failure of ossiculoplasty has resulted in the development of a number of assessment and predictive tools. The Middle Ear Risk Index (MERI) describes the middle ear environment at the time of ossiculoplasty. This grading scheme, described by Kartush,[12] is a logical point system incorporating the Bellucci classification of middle ear disease,[13] the Austin classification for ossicular status,[14] as well as other middle ear factors thought to be significant in predicting outcome. Black reported his SPITE method of assessment, which divided prognostic factors into surgical, prosthetic, infection, tissue, and Eustachian.[15] Dornhoffer and Gardner developed the Ossiculoplasty Outcomes Parameter Staging (OOPS) Index that placed a risk value on factors, including the frequency of ear discharge, mucosal appearance, presence or absence of the malleus, whether canal wall-up or -down surgery was performed, and whether the operation was a primary or revision procedure.[16] Yung and Vowler in 2006 analyzed a number of potential prognostic factors and also found that the presence or absence of the handle of the malleus was the single most significant factor affecting long-term outcome.[17]

Literature in the past has been bedeviled by different methods of measuring success following hearing surgery. The Committee on Hearing and Equilibrium guidelines for the evaluation of results of treatment of conductive hearing loss recommended that authors adopt a 20-dB air-bone gap or better as an indication of good outcome.[18] Authors understandably want to publish patient series as soon as possible, especially if a new ossicular implant is under assessment. This unfortunately results in outcomes recorded over a period of months to years and being presented as an "average" follow-up with no clear indication of whether outcomes change over time. Some authors believe that success should only be judged after a minimum period of observation (e.g, 5 years)[19] but this does not allow for preliminary results, which are so important to stimulate the development of new techniques. It is our belief that longitudinal studies should be adopted to demonstrate short- and long-term outcomes using specific time points, such as 1 and 5 years post-reconstruction.

Pennington[10] described an incus interposition technique in 1973 achieving a 20-dB or better air-bone gap in 85% of 216 operated ears. He also commented that configuration of the incus had no effect on air-bone graft closure and that there was no evidence of incus resorption. Further, in order to consolidate his results, he published a 15-year report that included a series of 100 patients.[20] His results suggested that initial success was usually maintained, but if there was failure, then it occurred within the first 5 years as a result of middle ear atelectasis. If successful hearing was maintained to 5 years, then it was maintained long-term. Few subsequent studies have been published showing such good long-term results. Janzen[21] reported 77% of patients achieving a 20-dB or better postoperative air-bone gap in a series of 85 ears with 2 to 5 years of follow-up. Farrior and Nichols[22] found that the main factor for long-term success after autologous ossicle or cortical bone grafts was the presence or absence of the stapes. An absent stapes saw a 20-dB or better closure of the air-bone gap drop from 70% to only 28% at 10 years, mainly due to chronic Eustachian tube dysfunction causing collapse of the middle ear space. Siddiq and East[23] reported 70% closure to 20 dB or better after incus transposition at 9.2 years average follow-up. O'Reilly and colleagues[24] achieved hearing success in 66% of patients following autologous or homologous incus transposition although follow-up was only an average of 15.8 months.

Review of the literature would suggest that if hearing is maintained to 5 years then long-term success is likely. The main reason for long-term failure seems to be poor Eustachian tube function resulting in collapse of the middle ear space. The use of cartilage to prevent tympanic membrane atelectasis is crucial if Eustachian tube dysfunction is predicted. An autologous incus seems to remain viable long-term, and potential resorption should not be a reason to use alloplastic materials. Merchant and Nadol[25] performed histopathological studies on a series of ossicular implants and concluded that they maintain their morphologic structure, showing varying amounts of replacement of nonviable bone by new bone through a slow process of "creeping substitution."However, this same process may also serve as one of the chief disadvantages of autograft reconstruction in that it often results in fusion of the autograft and stapes superstructure, which can present problems if ever there is a need to remove the autograft from the stapes due to future disease considerations.

Despite relatively good outcomes, it is not surprising that the popularity of autograft reconstruction has slowly declined as interest in new and increasingly effective alloplastic prostheses have grown. This is evident in the survey by Goldenberg and Emmett,[2] who presented a clear change in the use of reconstructive materials used by surgeons over a short 10-year period. Their survey in 1999 showed that hydroxyapatite prostheses were the most common prostheses used by surgeons (82%), followed by autograft and homograft bone (72%), autograft and homograft cartilage (62%), and Plastipore (59%). A similar survey by the senior author in 1989 showed that 93% of surgeons used bone as a reconstructive material. The choice of reconstruction material has almost certainly changed again over the last decade and a half, particularly because titanium materials have now become so popular. It is, however, clear that because of the expense of alloplastic prostheses and the ready availability of the autograft material, using the patient's own tissue to reconstruct the ossicular chain will remain a cornerstone of otology and a necessary part of otologic training.

References

[1] Hall A, Rytzner C. Stapedectomy and autotransplantation of ossicles. Acta Otolaryngol. 1957;47(4):318–324.

[2] Goldenberg RA, Emmet JR. Current use of implants in middle ear surgery. Otol Neurotol. 2001;22(2):145–152.

[3] Kansu L, Yilmaz I, Akdogan V, Avci S, Ozluoglu L. Idiopathic necrosis: Analysis of 4 cases. Ear Nose Throat J. 2013;92(2):E10–E13.

[4] Sadé J. Epithelial invasion of intraossicular spaces. J Laryngol Otol. 1972;86(1):15–21.

[5] Ng SK, Yip WW, Suen M, Abdullah VJ, van Hasselt CA. Autograft ossiculoplasty in cholesteatoma surgery: Is it feasible? Laryngoscope. 2003;113(5):843–847.

[6] Silverstein H, McDaniel AB, Lichtenstein R. A comparison of PORP, TORP, and incus homograft for ossicular reconstruction in chronic ear surgery. Laryngoscope. 1986;96(2):159–165.

[7] Vercruysse JP, Offeciers FE, Somers T, Schatteman I, Govaerts PJ. The use of malleus allografts in ossiculoplasty. Laryngoscope. 2002;112(10):1782–1784.

[8] Mills RP. The use of cortical bone grafts in ossiculoplasty, II: Graft mass and hearing change at different frequencies. J Laryngol Otol. 1993;107(8):690–694.
[9] Gyo K, Hato N, Shinomori Y, Hakuba N. Storage of the incus in the mastoid bowl for use as a columella in staged tympanoplasty. Auris Nasus Larynx. 2007;34(1):5–8.
[10] Pennington CL. Incus interposition techniques. Ann Otol Rhinol Laryngol. 1973;82(4):518–531.
[11] Javia LR, Ruckenstein MJ. Ossiculoplasty. Otolaryngol Clin North Am. 2006;39(6):1177–1189.
[12] Kartush JM. Ossicular chain reconstruction. Capitulum to malleus. Otolaryngol Clin North Am. 1994;27(4):689–715.
[13] Bellucci RJ. Selection of cases and classification of tympanoplasty. Otolaryngol Clin North Am. 1989;22(5):911–926.
[14] Austin DF. Reporting results in tympanoplasty. Am J Otol. 1985;6(1):85–88.
[15] Black B. Ossiculoplasty prognosis: the spite method of assessment.* Am J Otol. 1992;13(6):544–551.
[16] Dornhoffer JL, Gardner E. Prognostic factors in ossiculoplasty: A statistical staging system. Otol Neurotol. 2001;22(3):299–304.
[17] Yung M, Vowler SL. Long-term results in ossiculoplasty: An analysis of prognostic factors. Otol Neurotol. 2006;27(6):874–881.
[18] Committee on Hearing and Equilibrium guidelines for the evaluation of results of treatment of conductive hearing loss. AmericanAcademy of Otolaryngology-Head and Neck Surgery Foundation, Inc. Otolaryngol Head Neck Surg. 1995;113(3):186–187.
[19] Yung M. Long-term results of ossiculoplasty: Reasons for surgical failure. Otol Neurotol. 2006;27(1):20–26.
[20] Pennington CL. Incus interposition. A 15-year report. Ann Otol Rhinol Laryngol. 1983;92(6 Pt 1):568–570.
[21] Janzen VD. Ossiculoplasty using a hemi-incus interposition. J Otolaryngol. 1984;13(4):211–212.
[22] Farrior JB, Nichols SW. Long-term results using ossicular grafts. Am J Otol. 1996;17(3):386–392.
[23] Siddiq MA, East DM. Long-term hearing results of incus transposition. Clin Otolaryngol Allied Sci. 2004;29(2):115–118.
[24] O'Reilly RC, Cass SP, Hirsch BE, Kamerer DB, Bernat RA, Poznanovic SP. Ossiculoplasty using incus interposition: Hearing results and analysis of the middle ear risk index. Otol Neurotol. 2005;26(5):853–858.
[25] Merchant SN, Nadol JB Jr. Histopathology of ossicular implants. Otolaryngol Clin North Am. 1994;27(4):813–833.

29 Ossiculoplasty with Synthetic PORPS and TORPS

John L. Dornhoffer

Abbreviations used in this chapter:

ABG: air-bone gap
HA: hydroxyapatite
OOPS: Ossiculoplasty Outcomes Parameter Staging
PORP: partial ossicular replacement prosthesis
TORP: total ossicular replacement prosthesis

29.1 Introduction

Several factors influence the results in ossiculoplasty, including the middle ear environment, the surgical technique, and the qualities of the prosthesis. There is no question that the first of these is the most important determinant of long-term hearing outcomes with ossiculoplasty in the chronic ear, but it is also the most difficult to understand for both novice and experienced ear surgeons. Prognostic features of the middle ear environment will be discussed later in this chapter in the context of results but should be considered early in the evaluation of a patient undergoing surgery for the chronic ear. By considering these during the preoperative assessment, patient stratification, realistic expectations, and informed consent are facilitated. The next most important factor influencing results is surgical technique, which will be the main focus of this chapter. By combining a fundamental understanding of middle ear mechanics and the consistent anatomical relationships that exist in even the diseased middle ear, the surgeon can have a direct impact on results. As long as good surgical technique is adhered to and care is taken to reinforce the reconstruction based on the middle ear environment, the qualities of the modern prosthesis are least important.

29.2 Patient Selection

When a patient is considered for tympanoplasty or ossiculoplasty, a thorough history, examination, and audiometric evaluation should be performed on both ears. Otoscopy and pneumatic insufflation under the binocular microscope, following careful removal of debris, provide a wealth of information. The results of the audiogram should always be correlated with the physical exam, including Weber and Rinne tuning fork tests, especially when a masking dilemma is present. If the audiogram and tuning fork exam do not agree, surgery should not be performed until this is reconciled.

A preoperative audiogram can be helpful in suggesting underlying pathology. Generally, a perforation will cause a conductive hearing loss of 5–40 dB, depending on its characteristics.[1] When the tympanic membrane is intact, a conductive hearing loss greater than 35–40 dB strongly suggests the possibility of ossicular chain dysfunction. Furthermore, the pattern of hearing loss may be typical of particular scenarios; for example, fixation of the lateral ossicular chain generally causes a prominent low-tone conductive hearing loss having an air-bone gap (ABG) that partially closes in the middle and high frequencies. In comparison, stapes fixation tends to affect the middle and high frequencies to a relatively greater degree.[2]

The status of the Eustachian tube will impact surgical outcomes, yet there is no consensus on the optimal way to reliably assess its function. Auto-inflation using the Valsalva or Toyenbee maneuver is helpful, albeit a non-physiologic test of tubal patency. Details of Eustachian tube assessment are outlined in Chapter 15. The clinical status of the contralateral ear likewise can provide insight into tubal maturity and function in the diseased ear.[3] As part of the Eustachian tube evaluation, the nose should be examined so that allergy, adenoiditis, and rhinosinusitis can be treated in an effort to promote optimized tubal function. Furthermore, aggressive medical treatment of infection involving the ear itself should be undertaken prior to surgery, including aural toilet and ototopical agent application.

Once patient assessment is complete, a few general rules should be applied to surgical candidacy. First, one should avoid elective surgery on an only-hearing ear as much as is reasonably possible. Second, when bilateral disease is present, surgery should be undertaken on the worse-hearing ear in the absence of any other compelling reason to do otherwise on account of underlying disease. Finally, special consideration should be given to the timing of surgery in the pediatric patient.

29.3 Qualities of the Prostheses

29.3.1 Materials

Numerous synthetic materials have been used in ossicular implants, such as porous high-density polyethylene, plastics, bioactive glass, stainless steel, gold, titanium, and hydroxyapatite (HA), the last two currently being most common in the United States and Europe. Promising short-term results continue to be published for most of these materials,[4] but the long-term histological fate is uncertain in many instances. Each of the two most common currently used materials, HA and titanium, has advantages and disadvantages. Hydroxyapatite is produced by molding, resulting in smooth edges and grooves that have benefit when placed against the tympanic membrane and notched under the malleus, compared with the sharp stamped edges of titanium. Titanium, however, is lighter and more malleable, which makes it possible to change the angle of the prosthesis to facilitate the conical shape of the drum and to create a cradle for secure fit to the stapes. There seems to be no clear acoustic advantage of one over the other, with the results dictated more by the technique used and experience of the surgeon.[5] A detailed discussion of biomaterials can be found in Chapter 8.

29.3.2 Prosthesis Design

Much has been discussed with regard to prosthesis design, including ideal weight, length, and general shape. However, most studies are performed with laser vibrometry in non-diseased cadaver bones, and whether or not these results can be extrapolated to the diseased ear is yet to be appreciated. The ideal weight of the prosthesis has been examined by a number of investigators. Some researchers suggest that a lighter prosthesis in the range of 3–4 mg functions more effectively[6] whereas others have suggested a weight between 10–35 mg to yield the best acoustic response with the vibrometer.[7] In the latter study, prostheses above this weight would cause low-frequency displacements to fall out of acceptable ranges, and prostheses below this weight would lead to high-frequency losses. Interestingly, the human incus normally weighs 30–40 mg. Realistically, prosthesis weight is probably not of critical importance in the diseased middle ear as long as it falls within these acceptable ranges. Cartilage is usually placed on top of the prosthesis head to present extrusion in most cases, and the added weight to the reconstruction appears to have no detrimental effect on the hearing result regardless of which material is used.

There are a myriad of prosthesis shapes available and an equal number of surgeons advocating one over the other. Suffice it to say that the goal of ossiculoplasty is to provide a reconstruction with immediate stability and long-term durability. It should comply with as many of the gain-benefit principles of ossicular acoustic mechanics as is practical. As such, the more stable the initial reconstruction, the higher likelihood of a good long-term outcome.

Most synthetic prostheses are divided into partial ossicular replacement prostheses (PORPs), to be used with an absent incus but present stapes superstructure, and total ossicular replacement prostheses (TORPs), which are used when both the incus and stapes superstructure are absent or in poor anatomical position. A PORP usually consists of a head to make contact to the tympanic membrane and/or malleus and a shaft or cradle to facilitate the stapes capitulum and superstructure. A TORP is similar in design but with a shaft or wire that runs directly to the footplate. Both PORPs and TORPS can be further subdivided into designs that are intended to directly impact the undersurface of the drumhead and those that are intended to engage the manubrium of the malleus.

Most ossicular prosthesis designs are inherently unstable in that they are top-heavy and will tend to tip unless adequately supported by the reconstruction technique. This effect can be negated somewhat with a design that is very light, such as titanium, or a head design that shifts the center of gravity over the shaft, as used in some molded HA designs. Short-term stability is likewise facilitated by effective 2-point (preferably bony) fixation. Thus, any design that incorporates the malleus should offer improved stability in that the prosthesis may be "locked" into place between the malleus manubrium and stapes. Furthermore, recent basic science research using infrared laser vibrometry as well as retrospective clinical studies on ossiculoplasty suggest that incorporating the malleus in the reconstruction provides increased acoustic gain.[8]

The primary goal of ossicular reconstruction is to maximally couple the stapes footplate to the tympanic membrane to reestablish the hydraulic lever effect, which is the most significant mechanism of acoustic gain of the middle ear mechanism. This gain results from the difference between the surface area of the tympanic membrane relative to that of the oval window (usually a ratio of nearly 21:1). Simply placing a prosthesis against the tympanic membrane by no means guarantees that the entire surface area will achieve coupling to the prosthesis, in contrast to placing the prosthesis to the malleus, which is optimally positioned for this purpose.

Flexibility of a prosthesis, allowing it to accommodate the conical shape of the eardrum and to be adjustable in length, would also be considered a relative benefit. As such, the choice of prosthesis is largely dependent on the philosophy of the surgeon but is dictated by the operative technique used.

These techniques can best be illustrated by addressing specific situations encountered in chronic middle ear surgery. The prostheses used in the examples to follow are a combination of HA and titanium of the author's design, but the surgical technique and anatomical relationships extrapolate to many other synthetic PORPs and TORPs being used today.

29.4 Surgical Technique

29.4.1 General Principles

Although it is generally possible to ascertain the need for ossiculoplasty during the preoperative evaluation based on the audiogram and physical exam, one should be prepared for this contingency in every middle ear surgical case. In addition, it should be considered routine practice to inspect the ossicular chain visually and mechanically every time the middle ear is entered. This can be performed with gentle palpation of the malleus, taking note of concomitant movement of the stapes and visualization of the round window reflex (movement of the membrane and fluid in the niche with palpation of the chain).

29.4.2 Incus Erosion

Due to its location relative to the common pathways of development of cholesteatoma and tympanic membrane atelectasis, as well as its rather tenuous blood supply suspended between the stapes and malleus, erosion of the long process of the incus is the most common ossicular defect. It can be encountered in roughly one-third of cases involving a chronic posterior tympanic membrane perforation due to a variety of factors, such as pressure necrosis, inflammation, and hydrolytic enzymes produced by cholesteatoma matrix.

Although an eroded incus is usually obvious during middle ear exploration, in some cases palpation is required to uncover the presence of a more subtle fibrous union between the stapes and incus. The key factor in this situation is the degree of bony contact remaining, which, if present to some reasonable degree, may compel the surgeon to leave the incus untouched. However, if contact is deficient and movement with palpation is incomplete, reconstruction is recommended.

There are basically two options for reconstruction when incus erosion is present. The first involves an attempt to reconstruct the incudostapedial joint with a Type II (modified) tympanoplasty as discussed in Chapter 27. All of the Type II reconstructive techniques share many of the same theoretical advantages and disadvantages. On the positive side, they reestablish the natural incudomalleal lever with minimal disruption of the normal anatomical relationships and native ossicular connections. The primary disadvantages relate to uncertain long-term durability as little is known about the pathophysiology and natural history of incus necrosis. If erosion is related to avascular necrosis, one may speculate that the remnant of the lenticular process, if used in ossicular reconstruction, may be subject to future loss. Given the relatively small acoustic gain afforded by preservation of the incudomalleal lever, Type II reconstruction of the diseased middle ear (2–3 dB) might not be worth the risk of possible revision.

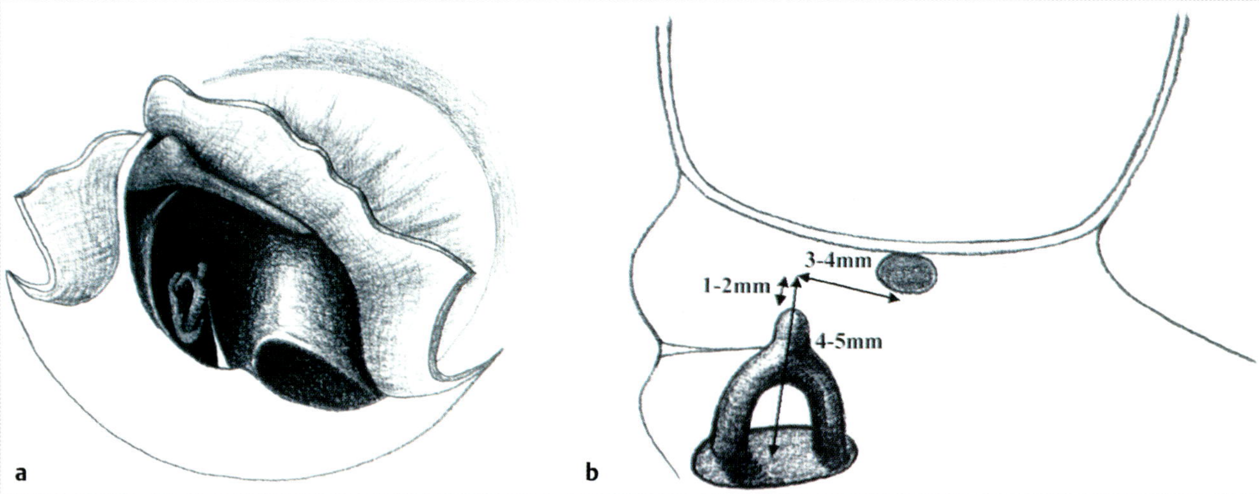

Fig. 29.1 Middle ear anatomy relevant to ossiculoplasty. (a) The tensor tympani tendon and the anterior malleal ligament anchor the malleus neck at the cochleariform process and anterior tympanic spine, respectively. These structures provide stability for tympanoplasty and ossiculoplasty procedures and should not be violated unless necessary. (b) The stapes capitulum is typically 2 mm in height below the undersurface of the neck of the malleus, which is the proper target for the ossicular reconstruction interface. This same site is approximately 3 mm in the lateral dimension from the capitulum; thus, 3 mm of reach is generally required for a sculpted ossicular graft or synthetic prosthesis.

The most commonly used reconstructive option for incus necrosis involves removal of the incus remnant and reconstruction between the stapes and malleus (or tympanic membrane), generally as a Type III minor columella mechanism. The fundamental anatomic principles governing this reconstruction are the same regardless of the graft or prostheses used. Some key relationships include the vertical height from the stapes capitulum to the plane of the neck of the malleus at the attachment of the tensor tympani tendon (2–2.5 mm) and the horizontal or translational distance from the capitulum to this same point (3–3.5 mm) (► Fig. 29.1). Although the malleus manubrium can become rotated medially as an effect of middle ear disease processes, especially along its distal aspect, in the author's experience, the malleus neck is spared from major rotational variation due to its anchoring attachments, which allow it to be used as a consistent prosthesis target in ossicular reconstruction. This is due to the fact that the axis of malleus medial rotation lies at the attachment of the fan-shaped anterior malleolar ligament to the anterior tympanic spine as well as the underlying tensor tympani tendon, which anchors the malleus to the cochleariform process. In the rare instance where the neck of the malleus is pathologically displaced to an extreme degree, it may be necessary to reposition it, as discussed in Chapter 30.

If the incus is deemed unusable or if the time and work involved with autograft preparation are not embraced, most surgeons opt for the use of a synthetic PORP. The recommended surgical technique utilizing a PORP as a minor columella is based on the principle that the vertical height to the malleus should be 2–2.5 mm and the horizontal reach should be 3–3.5 mm. Although many commercially prepared prostheses are produced with a wide range of lengths or are adjustable, if reconstruction is made to the malleus neck, adjustments are not often necessary. It has been the author's experience that similar consistency in measurements to what is encountered in stapes surgery is seen in incus replacement if the proper site at the malleus neck is utilized and the ligamentous malleus attachments have not been severely disrupted. Although it is sensible to confirm by measuring, a prosthesis with a vertical height of 2–2.5 mm and a horizontal reach of 3 mm can be used in the vast majority of cases as long as it is designed to engage the malleus handle and there is no stapes capitulum erosion or exaggerated inferior rotation onto the promontory. It is also the author's opinion that improper prosthesis sizing and failed reconstruction are much more likely if the surgeon attempts to measure the distance from the stapes capitulum to the estimated undersurface of the posterior-superior drumhead as opposed to utilizing the relatively consistent relationship between the stapes and malleus that is outlined above.

Another important point to consider when using a PORP is that many of them have broad heads that make contact with the tympanic membrane in addition to the malleus (in contrast to the "strut-like" structure of a sculpted incus autograft that spares tympanic membrane contact). Since the tympanic membrane is a conical structure and not a flat disk, it is desirable to use a prosthesis that can be bent approximately 30 degrees at the junction of the shaft and head to facilitate this shape (► Fig. 29.2). Doing so will encourage the superior edge of the prosthesis head under the malleus neck to become "locked" by the acute angle defined by the attachment of the tensor tympani tendon. In the end, the goal is to create a freestanding reconstruction that fixes to the tympanic membrane and stapes head, but not to other structures, such as the tympanic ring or cochlear promontory. A limited amount of absorbable packing can be used to achieve this end, but it should be noted that its use has been implicated with postoperative middle ear fibrosis, especially when denuded mucosa is present.

To combat synthetic prosthesis extrusion, a cartilage graft cap is recommended at the interface between the tympanic membrane and the adjacent prosthesis head. Although it has been suggested that this barrier may be optional with a prosthesis that features an HA head with smooth edges, cartilage is essential with sharper titanium prosthesis heads. As opposed to host incompatibility and lateral prosthesis migration beyond

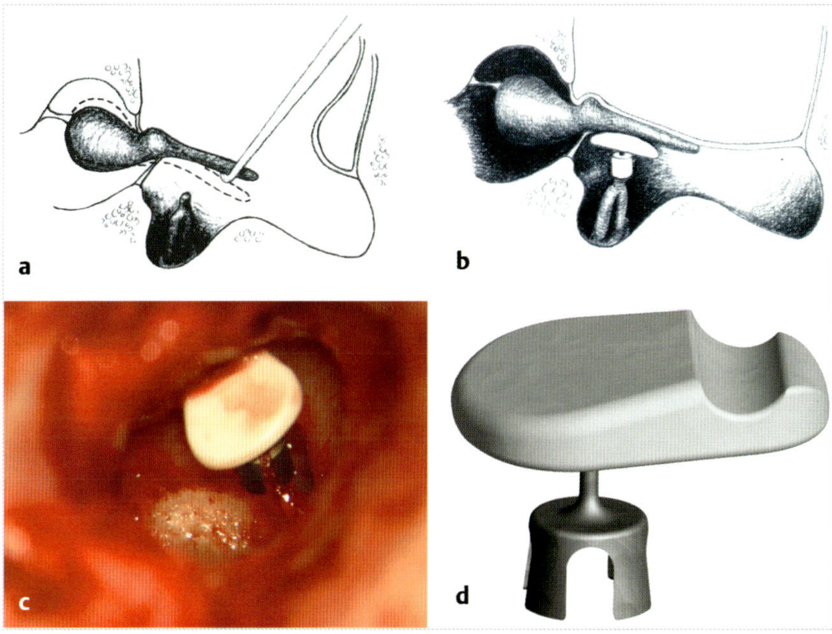

Fig. 29.2 Contour of prosthesis to malleus handle. (a) Although retraction can result in medial displacement of the umbo, the malleus neck orientation is relatively stable due to adjacent supporting ligaments. Thus, the malleus neck, not the handle, is the most constant target for ossiculoplasty. If required, the umbo can be lateralized with a blunt hook. (b) The prosthesis is manually contoured with a bend of 30 degrees at the interface of the shaft and head to fit properly under the malleus handle and tympanic membrane curvature. (c) Appearance of contoured PORP in proper stable position between the stapes capitulum and malleus neck. (d) Dornhoffer PORP with HA head and titanium shaft (Grace Medical, Memphis, Tennessee). The author asserts that, if properly shaped and applied, a prosthesis 2 mm in height can be used in nearly every single case.

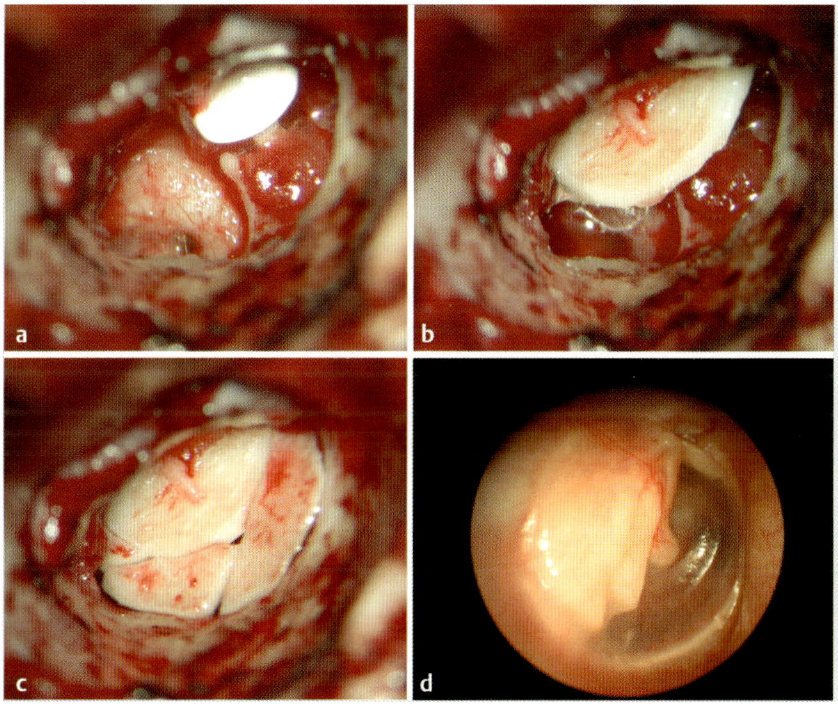

Fig. 29.3 Mosaic cartilage tympanoplasty with ossiculoplasty. (a) The PORP is set between the malleus neck and stapes capitulum. (b) A large crescent-shaped piece of cartilage is set directly upon the prosthesis. (c) Smaller crescent-shaped cartilage pieces are placed to form a "mosaic" of cartilage. (d) Postoperative appearance following cartilage mosaic underlay tympanoplasty (right ear).

the tympanic membrane, the pathophysiology of prosthesis extrusion with an appropriate-length prosthesis more often seems to involve postoperative medial retraction of the tympanic membrane around the prosthesis. Cartilage can be placed in conjunction with reconstruction of the posterior half of the tympanic membrane to prevent retractions or cholesteatoma formation. When the cartilage graft is reconstructed exactly in piecemeal fashion, it is known as the mosaic technique (▶ Fig. 29.3; see Chapter 25). It would also appear that the size of the cartilage between the prosthesis and eardrum has little effect on the hearing result; as long as the malleus is incorporated in the reconstruction, adequate coupling is ensured.

29.4.3 Incus and Stapes Absent

When both the incus and stapes superstructure are absent, common options for reconstruction include a Type III major columella mechanism or a Type IV tympanoplasty, the latter being suitable only in certain advanced cases of chronic ear disease involving a canal wall-down mastoidectomy. A synthetic TORP is typically what is used as a major columella. The same basic principles of reconstruction and recognition of anatomical consistencies discussed with the use of a PORP apply to a TORP. To account for the absence of the stapes superstructure, an additional 2–2.5 mm is added to the vertical height recommendation. Thus, the desired TORP dimensions will be approximately 4.5 mm in height, with 3 mm of reach to reconstruct to the malleus neck while maintaining the shaft oriented 90 degrees to the footplate.

One of the real challenges in this type of reconstruction relates to the lack of stability at the level of the footplate. Although the presence of the stapes superstructure offers no mechanism for acoustic gain, it does provide a convenient point for stable prosthesis fixation. The literature often shows superior hearing outcomes with a PORP versus a TORP, which is likely due to this difference in stability as opposed to acoustic advantage imparted by the presence of the superstructure. The same 30-degree angled interface with the neck of the malleus and tympanic membrane is utilized for lateral stability, as described earlier. However, this alone does not ensure a stable centered footplate contact point because the forces exerted by the tympanic membrane and malleus onto the TORP head encourage the shaft to displace. Several techniques have been introduced to counteract this phenomenon, including the use of footplate-stabilizing "shoes" made of titanium, HA, or cartilage (▶ Fig. 29.4). Related techniques that utilize small oval-shaped pieces of cartilage with a central hole have also been described.[9]

Although it is advisable to utilize the stapes superstructure when present, inferior rotation toward the promontory due to disease or previous surgery can make a minor columella reconstruction unsuitable. In such instances, a PORP or incus interposition may produce rocking of the stapes toward the promontory instead of the desired piston motion. A TORP placed on the footplate superior to the rotated superstructure is a more suitable alternative that tends to rotate the stapes superiorly into a more favorable position.[10] In other rare cases the superstructure may be deemed at risk of partial fixation if the adjacent middle ear structures are fibrotic or involved with tympanosclerosis, in which case careful removal of the superstructure and placement of a TORP may be desirable.[10]

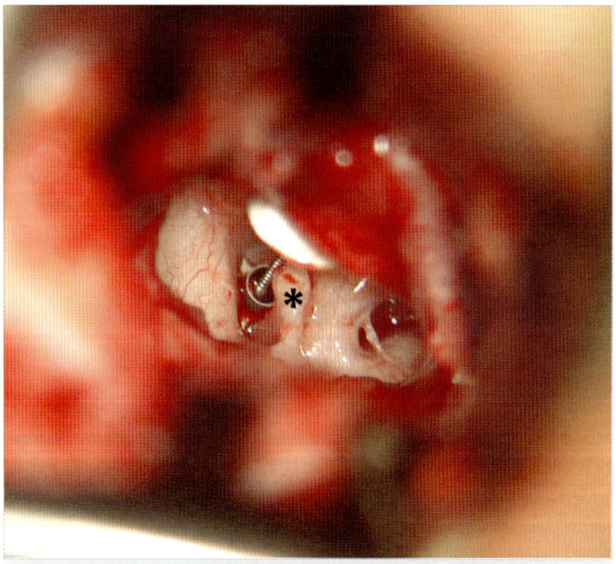

Fig. 29.4 TORP with footplate shoe for rotated stapes. When unfavorable inferior rotation of the stapes superstructure is present, a TORP is often preferable to maintain an approximate perpendicular orientation between the tympanic membrane and prosthesis shaft. In this case, the TORP is stabilized at the level of the footplate by a titanium shoe. The stapes capitulum is indicated by the asterisk.

29.4.4 Malleus Absent

The techniques previously described emphasize the use of the malleus for prosthesis stability and as an anatomical landmark for consistent length measurements; however, the malleus manubrium is not always present. Some otologists believe that the malleus is such a tremendous benefit in ossiculoplasty that techniques have been developed to create a "neo-malleus" from a piece of bone or a synthetic implant that is grafted into the tympanic membrane to be used later in staged ossicular reconstruction.[11] Nonetheless, several options do exist for single-stage tympano-ossicular reconstruction in the absence of a malleus manubrium.[10]

The most simple of these single-stage techniques is reconstruction directly between the drumhead and stapes superstructure with a Type III stapes columella mechanism (especially in a canal wall-down procedure). When a wider gap between the stapes and drumhead is present or when the superstructure is absent, the use of a PORP or TORP that directly contacts the drumhead (with or without the cartilage cap, depending on the prosthesis material used) is generally required. These techniques can be effective, but great care should be exercised in measuring the correct prosthesis length. It is recommended that the reconstructed drumhead be slightly tented by the prosthesis; however, a major reason for prosthesis extrusion, regardless of material, is excessive length. Because those cases involving an absent malleus harbor the potential for graft/prosthesis adherence to the undersurface of the reconstructed tympanic membrane and ossiculoplasty failure due to delayed lateralization of the capitulum or footplate as the reconstructed tympanic membrane heals and matures, many surgeons favor staged ossiculoplasty. One innovative way to accomplish this during the second stage is to perform an ossiculoplasty via the facial recess so that elevation of a tympanomeatal flap is avoided and a stable tympanic membrane measurement is afforded.[12]

Finally, an alternative single-stage technique favored by the author involves the creation of a "pseudo-malleus" by reconstructing the tympanic membrane with a composite perichondrium-cartilage island graft that forms a creased midline ridge to act in place of the manubrium (▶ Fig. 29.5). This is achieved by creating a circular cartilage island graft measuring 8–9 mm in diameter, with a 1-mm midline strip of cartilage removed from the perichondrium, bisecting the island into 2 half-circles. The anterior half-circle is inserted as an underlay below the tympanic ring inferiorly and anterior tympanic spine superiorly while supported medially with absorbable packing in the anterior mesotympanum. The posterior half-circle is then lifted to expose the posterior edge of the anterior island, which is placed near the position of the absent malleus handle. This pseudo-malleus ridge can then be used for ossicular reconstruction using the same length of prostheses described earlier.

29.4.5 Fixed Ossicular Chain

Tympanosclerosis involving the tympanic membrane and middle ear is common when significant otitis media has been present. When these chalky white plaques involve the tympanic membrane, little or no conductive loss is expected unless the ossicular chain is also affected. Hearing loss due to tympanosclerotic fixation can occur secondary to involvement with any component of the ossicular chain.

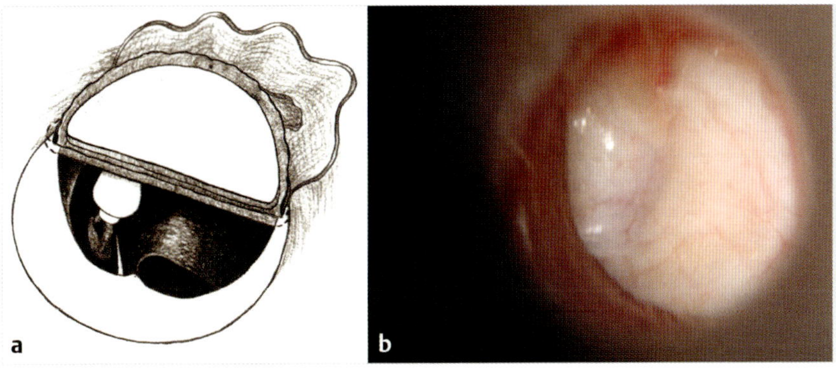

Fig. 29.5 Tympano-ossicular reconstruction without malleus. (a) When the malleus handle is absent, the folded ridge generated by opposing edges of a composite perichondrium-cartilage island graft can be used as a pseudo-malleus to support a prosthesis that has a notch intended for the malleus handle. (b) Postoperative appearance of tympanic membrane after total drum reconstruction using a composite perichondrium-cartilage island graft.

An isolated malleus head or incus fixation with a mobile stapes can be dealt with in two ways.[2] The most common technique involves disarticulation of the incudostapedial joint followed by removal of the incus and amputation of the malleus head just above the insertion of the tensor tympani. Rarely, the malleus head is so fixed that it must be left in place; thus, a 1-mm gap is drilled between the fixed head and the mobile remnant to prevent re-fixation. Reconstruction is then accomplished with a Type III minor columella, as described previously.

The second technique for correcting malleus fixation involves mobilization through an atticotomy by carefully releasing the point of fixation with a diamond drill burr. Although good results have been reported with this technique, great care must be taken not to contact the ossicular chain with the burr as high-frequency sensorineural hearing loss can result. Due to this and the risk of re-fixation with new bone growth, mobilization techniques are only recommended for low-complexity ossicular fixation. Stapes fixation from tympanosclerosis represents a more complicated problem that often requires a staged approach. This is covered in more detail in Chapter 31.

29.5 Postoperative Care

The packing is removed 7–10 days after the surgery and ototopical drops prescribed for 10 days. The patient is instructed to perform the Valsalva maneuver 3 times a day, starting 2 weeks after the surgery. The Otovent® (Abigo Medical, Sweden) has been used in children who are unable to perform this maneuver. The first postoperative audiogram is obtained 6–8 weeks post-surgery. If the patient is unable to perform the Valsalva maneuver or if the postoperative period is complicated by an effusion or retraction of the reconstructed tympanic membrane, a ventilation tube is placed 3–4 months after the surgery. Primary ventilation tube insertion is generally avoided.

29.6 Complications and Outcomes

Hearing outcomes with ossiculoplasty are more variable compared with Type I tympanoplasty, and long-term results are, on average, worse than short-term results.[13] This is likely because these procedures are more skill- and technique-dependent, are influenced by the inherent qualities of the prosthesis, and, on average, are associated with more advanced chronic ear disease. Traditionally, ossiculoplasty "success" has been roughly judged to be a pure-tone average ABG < 30 dB for a major columella

Table 29.1 Ossiculoplasty Outcomes Parameter Staging (OOPS) Index

Risk Factor		Risk Value
Middle Ear Factors		
Drainage	None	0
	Present > 50% of the time	1
Mucosa	Normal	0
	Fibrotic	2
Ossicles	Normal	0
	Malleus +	1
	Malleus -	2
Surgical Factors		
Type of surgery	No mastoidectomy	0
	Canal wall-up mastoidectomy	1
	Canal wall-down mastoidectomy	2
Revision surgery	No	0
	Yes	2

(TORP) and < 20 dB for a minor columella (PORP).[14] However, in the author's opinion, these benchmarks are only indicative of what is minimally acceptable without the need for revision and do not necessarily portray excellence in ossiculoplasty.

As mentioned in the Overview and Introduction for this surgical roundtable on ossiculoplasty, much has been discussed about the inherent qualities of a theoretically ideal ossicular replacement prosthesis, but assuming the material is biocompatible and is correctly placed, the qualities of the underlying middle ear environment have a far greater impact on hearing outcomes. As such, the results of ossiculoplasty must be reported in the context of the middle ear environment in which it is performed. Outcomes for the standardized technique of ossiculoplasty described in this chapter have been extensively reported in the literature, with typically excellent results.[15] Furthermore, this technique has been analyzed within the framework of middle ear risk, and this is has been published as the Ossiculoplasty Outcomes Parameter Staging (OOPS) index (▶ Table 29.1).[16] As depicted in ▶ Fig. 29.6, on average, an

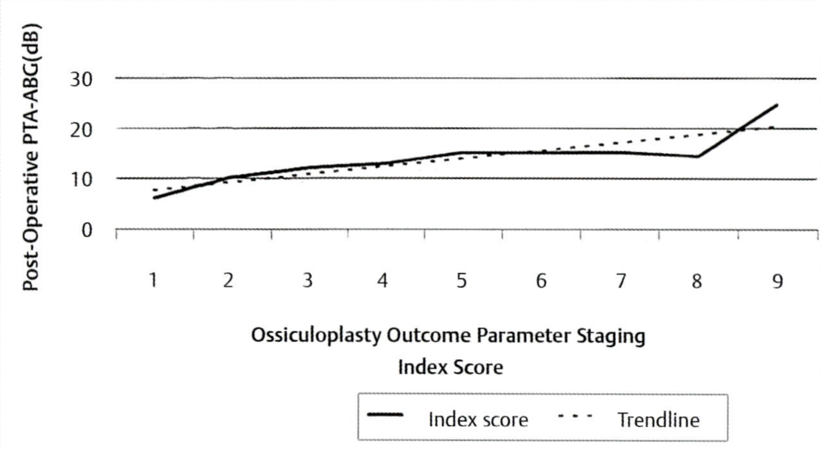

Fig. 29.6 Expected hearing outcomes based on the OOPS Index. Expected outcomes for the technique of ossiculoplasty described in this chapter are summarized by this graph, which plots the status of the middle ear environment against expected hearing outcomes.

expected postoperative ABG of approximately 10 dB is expected using this technique if the middle ear environment is ideal, compared with roughly a 20-dB ABG if the middle ear is extremely hostile. Furthermore, this standardized ossiculoplasty technique has been further validated by a second surgeon in a study that confirmed the short-term reproducibility of these results. An average postoperative ABG of 15.3 dB was noted to fall within the narrow expected hearing range that had been calculated based on underlying middle ear risk.[17]

Complications or failures of ossiculoplasty are generally divided into those caused by patient factors (prosthesis extrusion) and those related to surgical technique (prosthesis displacement). In a hostile middle ear environment with continued Eustachian tube dysfunction, even a well-executed ossiculoplasty, using a well-designed prosthesis is at risk of long-term failure. If the same pathologic process that made the surgery necessary in the first place is not alleviated, then the reconstructed tympanic membrane can retract around the prosthesis, leading to extrusion of the device. Methods utilized to minimize this risk would be to (1) treat the underlying Eustachian tube dysfunction/sinonasal disease prior to surgical intervention, (2) utilize the malleus when possible for bone-to-bone reconstruction, (3) use cartilage reconstruction techniques lateral to the prosthesis with good approximation to the posterior canal wall, and (4) consider long-term ventilation of the middle ear space with a tube in the postoperative period if effusion or retraction is seen to occur. Surgeon factors leading to successful ossiculoplasty have already been discussed, but in this author's experience, most surgical failures are related to a prosthesis that is too long or does not adequately couple with a malleus rather than one that is too short. For a PORP, a long prosthesis leads to inferior displacement of the device and also tends to push the superstructure toward the promontory, making revision tedious. For a TORP, a long prosthesis has the added risk of protrusion through the footplate, with resulting sensorineural hearing loss. These complications can be avoided by using a device of standard length, as described above, and by making sure the prosthesis is freestanding in the middle ear prior to placing the supporting absorbable packing. With a TORP, some type of footplate shoe or even a small piece of fascia can be very useful, not only for prosthesis stability, but also to spread out the surface area of the shaft over the footplate to prevent penetration.

References

[1] Mehta RP, Rosowski JJ, Voss SE, O'Neil E, Merchant SN. Determinants of hearing loss in perforations of the tympanic membrane. Otol Neurotol. 2006;27(2):136–143.

[2] Vincent R, Lopez A, Sperling NM. Malleus ankylosis: a clinical, audiometric, histologic, and surgical study of 123 cases. Am J Otol. 1999;20(6):717–725.

[3] Collins WO, Telischi FF, Balkany TJ, Buchman CA. Pediatric tympanoplasty: effect of contralateral ear status on outcomes. Arch Otolaryngol Head Neck Surg. 2003;129(6):646–651.

[4] Coffey CS, Lee FS, Lambert PR. Titanium versus nontitanium prostheses in ossiculoplasty. Laryngoscope. 2008;118(9):1650–1658.

[5] Yung M, Smith P. Titanium versus nontitanium ossicular prostheses-a randomized controlled study of the medium-term outcome. Otol Neurotol. 2010;31(5):752–758.

[6] Huttenbrink K. Middle Ear Mechanics in Research and Otosurgery. Dresden, Germany: Department of Oto-Rhino-Laryngology, University Hospital Carl Gustav Carus; 1997.

[7] Goode RL, Nishihara S. Experimental models of ossiculoplasty. Otolaryngol Clin. North Am. 1994;27(4):663–675.

[8] Bance M, Morris DP, Vanwijhe RG, Kiefte M, Funnell WR. Comparison of the mechanical performance of ossiculoplasty using a prosthetic malleus-to-stapes head with a tympanic membrane-to-stapes head assembly in a human cadaveric middle ear model. Otol Neurotol. 2004;25(6):903–909.

[9] Beutner D, Luers JC, Huttenbrink KB. Cartilage "shoe: a new technique for stabilisation of titanium total ossicular replacement prosthesis at centre of stapes footplate. J Laryngol Otol. 2008;122(7):682–686.

[10] Vincent R, Sperling NM, Oates J, Osborne J. Ossiculoplasty with intact stapes and absent malleus: The silastic banding technique. Otol Neurotol. 2005;26(5):846–852.

[11] Black B. Neomalleus ossiculoplasty. Otol Neurotol. 2002;23(5):636–642.

[12] Blevins NH. Transfacial recess ossicular reconstruction: Technique and early results. Otol Neurotol. 2004;25(3):236–241.

[13] Yung M, Vowler SL. Long-term results in ossiculoplasty: An analysis of prognostic factors. Otol Neurotol. 2006;27(6):874–881.

[14] Jackson CG, Glasscock ME III Schwaber MK, Nissen AJ, Christiansen SG, Smith PG. Ossicular chain reconstruction: the TORP and PORP in chronic ear disease. Laryngoscope. 1983;93(8):981–988.

[15] Dornhoffer JL. Hearing results with the Dornhoffer ossicular replacement prostheses. Laryngoscope. 1998;108(4 Pt 1):531–536.

[16] Dornhoffer JL, Gardner E. Prognostic factors in ossiculoplasty: A statistical staging system. Otol Neurotol. 2001;22(3):299–304.

[17] Gluth MB, Moore PC, Dornhoffer JL. Method and reproducibility of a standardized ossiculoplasty technique. Otol Neurotol. 2012;33(7):1207–1212.

30 The Malleus in Ossicular Reconstruction

Robert Vincent

Abbreviations used in this chapter:

ABG: air-bone gap
MRP: malleus replacement prosthesis
PORP: partial ossicular replacement prosthesis
TORP: total ossicular replacement prosthesis

30.1 Introduction

The presence or absence of a malleus affects the hearing results in ossiculoplasty, particularly in the absence of a stapes superstructure. Numerous authors have emphasized the importance of the malleus in successful ossiculoplasty,[1,2,3,4] and re-creation of the malleus has been used by several authors to enhance middle ear prosthesis stability.[5,6,7]

The presence of an anteriorly positioned malleus may also be a difficult situation for the otologist. In cases of an absent or a severely anterior malleus, the usual methods of ossiculoplasty presented in the literature have used reconstruction from the stapes head (or footplate) directly to the eardrum.[8,9] However, placement directly under the medial surface of the eardrum increases the possibility of both perforation and extrusion.[8,10] These ossicular reconstructions are frequently unstable because the lack of fixation by the malleus at the proximal end of the prosthesis can allow displacement at either the proximal or distal ends. Many authors believe that an acoustic benefit can be achieved by attaching the prosthesis to the manubrium of the malleus, as opposed to attaching it directly to the tympanic membrane, because of the catenary lever action of the malleus-tympanic membrane assembly.

Mounting evidence in the literature confirms the presence of the malleus as an important prognostic factor in ossiculoplasty, leading to better hearing results and lower rates of extrusion due to its role in preventing tympanic membrane lateralization.[11] De Vos, Gersdorff, and Gérard reiterated the absence of the malleus as an adverse prognostic factor because its presence not only gives stability to the reconstruction, but also acts as catenary lever, thereby contributing to acoustic gain.[12] However, it is not only the presence of the malleus, but also its position in relation to the stapes, that affects hearing outcomes. Vlaming and Feenstra demonstrated that the ideal reconstructive situation was when the malleus was positioned directly over the stapes. In practice, this anatomic configuration is very rarely seen but can be easily achieved with malleus relocation techniques.[13] The theory is that all of the force of vibration through a strut prosthesis would be converted into an efficient piston-like motion at the footplate.

When the malleus is malpositioned, ossiculoplasty is often unstable and mechanically inefficient, particularly if the malleus is angulated more than 45 degrees from the axis of the stapes superstructure or footplate.[14] Malleus relocation acts to reduce the angle to zero as the relocated malleus is positioned over the stapes head or footplate, allowing ideal placement of the prosthesis. In addition, this configuration allows an almost perpendicular direction of forces to the footplate, with optimal transfer of function and minimal dissipation of energy.

The Austin[15] classification of ossicular defects as modified by Kartush[8] provides a method for defining pre-reconstruction ossicular status. Presence of a malleus can be classified in Austin-Kartush Groups A (malleus and stapes intact and mobile) and B (malleus and stapes footplate present and mobile, stapes superstructure absent). An absent malleus can be classified in Austin-Kartush Groups C (malleus absent and stapes intact and mobile) and D (malleus and stapes superstructure absent, stapes footplate present and mobile). Our surgical technique of ossicular reconstruction will be presented for each of these four classifications.

30.2 Surgical Technique

30.2.1 Austin-Kartush Group A (Malleus and Stapes Intact and Mobile)

Reconstruction of the ossicular chain when the stapes and malleus are both present typically involves the use of a partial reconstruction prosthesis or incus autograft between the stapes head and the malleus handle or tympanic membrane, with or without supportive tissue to strengthen the tympanic membrane. Few authors advocate the use of a total reconstruction prosthesis from the footplate of a normal stapes to the malleus.[1,2,8,15]

Described here are two previously published original techniques: the malleus relocation technique[11] and the Silastic banding technique.[16] The malleus relocation technique allows for better placement of both partial (PORPs) and total ossicular replacement prostheses (TORPs). With the Silastic banding technique, a TORP is positioned from the stapes footplate to the relocated malleus despite the presence of a stapedial arch. The TORP is attached to the intact stapes superstructure with a band that allows for better prosthesis stability.

From 1991 to 2000, the author used a PORP positioned from the malleus to the stapes head in Austin-Kartush Group A cases. Since January 2000, the author has used a combined technique of malleus relocation and Silastic banding, and a TORP is inserted in all cases.

Malleus Relocation Technique

Entire separation of the malleus from the tympanic membrane is required (▶ Fig. 30.1; ▶ Fig. 30.2). Any remnant of the incus (even within the epitympanum) must be removed. The tensor tympani is sectioned as close as possible to its insertion into the malleus handle (▶ Fig. 30.3). Relocation of the malleus is performed using a strong 90-degree hook placed anterior to the neck of the malleus. Progressive posterior retraction of the malleus is applied until it comes to lie directly above the stapes capitulum or footplate (▶ Fig. 30.4). Subsequent anterior retraction of the malleus is avoided by overstretching the anterior malleal ligament, the position thereby being maintained by the superior ligament of the malleus, which is preserved (the

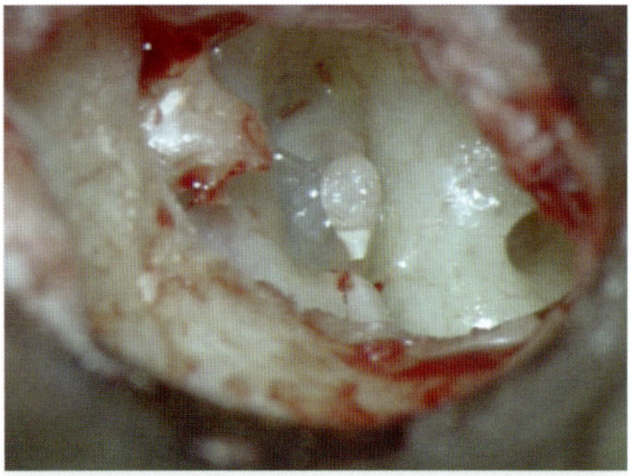

Fig. 30.1 Operative view of a right ear showing evidence of incus erosion, Austin-Kartush Group A. Both the stapes and malleus are mobile.

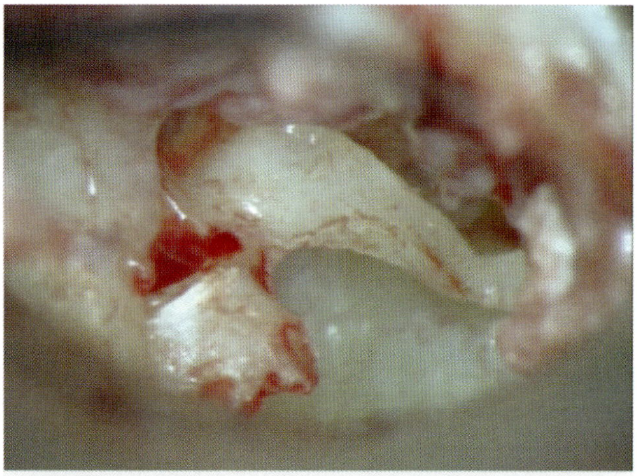

Fig. 30.2 The malleus is completely separated from the tympanic membrane.

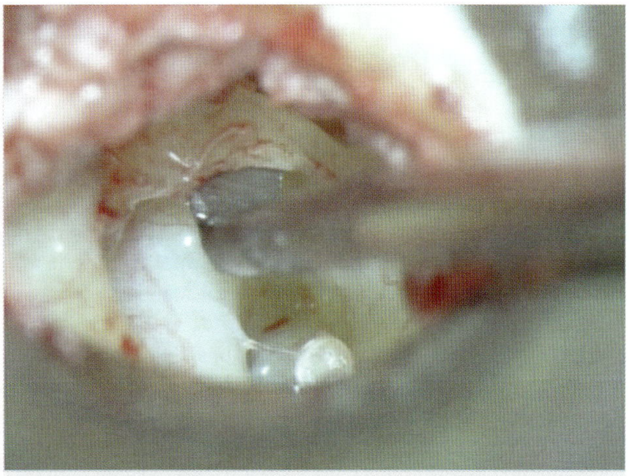

Fig. 30.3 The tensor tympani is sectioned as close as possible to its insertion into the malleus handle.

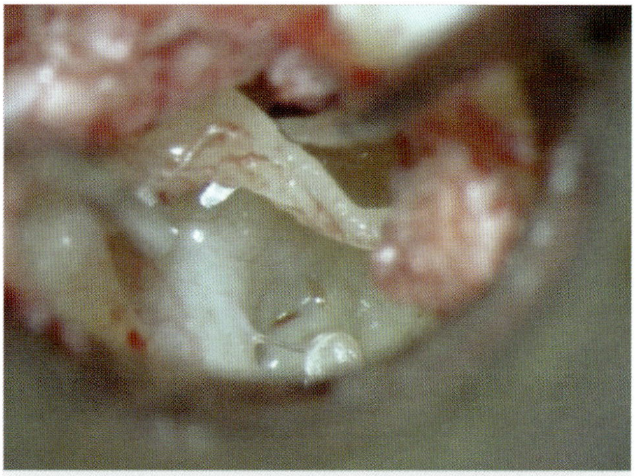

Fig. 30.4 Progressive posterior retraction of the malleus is applied until it comes to lie directly above the stapes capitulum or footplate.

malleus head is not removed). In the relocated position, the malleus should lie immediately over the stapes footplate (▶ Fig. 30.5). Precise measurement from the relocated malleus to the stapes capitulum or footplate can then be undertaken using a modified stapes-measuring rod (▶ Fig. 30.6).

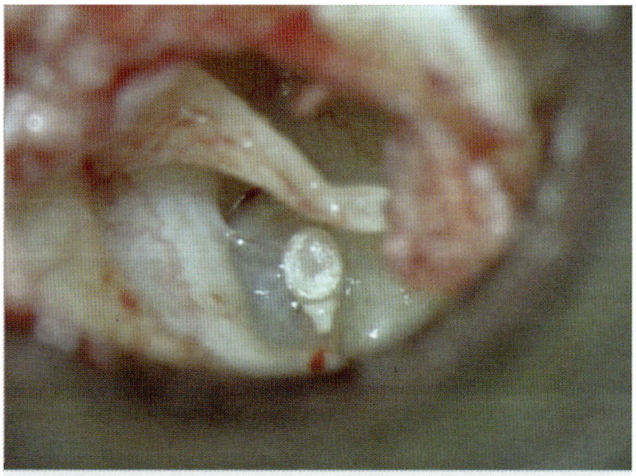

Fig. 30.5 The relocated malleus should lie immediately over the stapes footplate.

Silastic Banding Technique

A Silastic band is fashioned by creating a 1.2-mm disc from a thin sheet of Silastic using a specially designed punch (Medtronic-Xomed, Inc., Jacksonville, Florida). The center of the disc is then fenestrated with an 0.8-mm diameter punch (▶ Fig. 30.7). The band should fit snugly around the stapes neck. The stapedius tendon is divided as closely as possible to the pyramid because an attempt will be made to place the band beneath the stapedius tendon to avoid lateral displacement of the band. The prosthesis shaft is cut to the appropriate length and is introduced through the band (▶ Fig. 30.8). The shaft is introduced between the stapes and the Fallopian canal, with the distal end being lowered onto the center of the footplate

(▶ Fig. 30.9a). The head of the prosthesis is then introduced under the relocated malleus handle (▶ Fig. 30.9b). In its final position, the prosthesis head should rest directly under the malleus handle without undue tension, and the malleus neck should stay away from the superior wall of the external auditory canal.

The band is then gently pulled and positioned around the stapes capitulum, beneath the stapes tendon, which had been cut. By snugging the band down over the sectioned tendon, the prosthesis becomes firmly apposed to the stapes, allowing precise placement on the stapes footplate with sufficient rigidity (▶ Fig. 30.10). This assembly facilitates an almost perpendicular position of the prosthesis from the footplate to the malleus handle and tympanic membrane. By keeping the distal end of the prosthesis in proper position using the Silastic band, the tendency of the prosthesis to tip or migrate is virtually eliminated. This combined technique of malleus relocation and Silastic banding results in an increasingly stable and more functional ossicular arrangement (▶ Fig. 30.11).

30.2.2 Austin-Kartush Group B (Malleus and Stapes Footplate Present and Mobile, Stapes Superstructure Absent)

In cases of absent stapes superstructure with a mobile malleus, a TORP is interposed to restore the transfer function of the middle ear. The malleus-to-footplate prosthesis connects the malleus to the footplate. The malleus is relocated using the malleus relocation technique described above (▶ Fig. 30.12; ▶ Fig. 30.13).

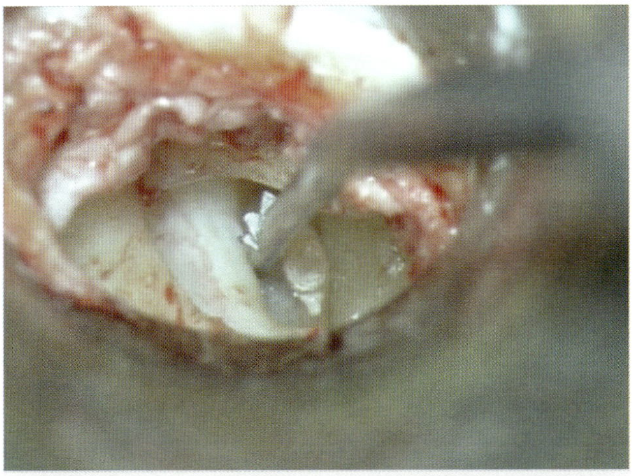

Fig. 30.6 Precise measurement from the relocated malleus to the stapes capitulum or footplate can be undertaken using a modified stapes-measuring rod.

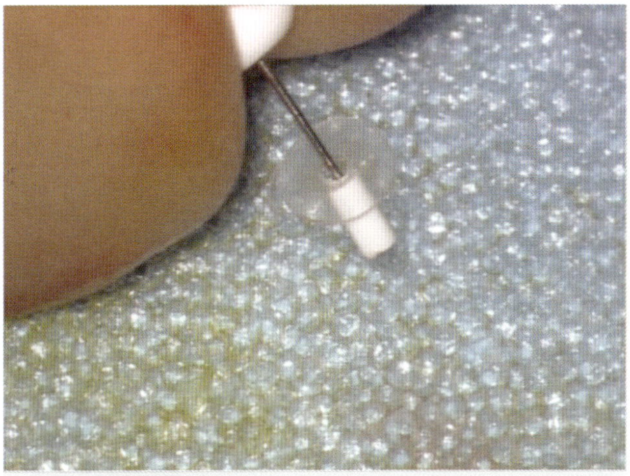

Fig. 30.8 The prosthesis shaft is cut to the appropriate length and introduced through the band.

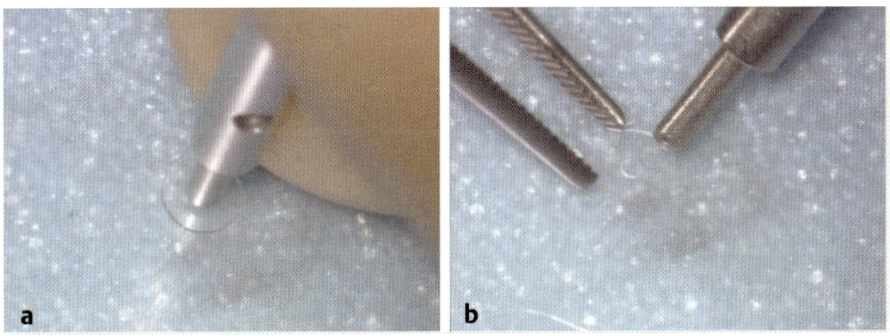

Fig. 30.7 (a) A Silastic band is fashioned by creating a 1.2-mm disc from a thin sheet of Silastic using a specially designed punch (Medtronic-Xomed, Inc., Jacksonville, Florida). (b) The center of the disc is then fenestrated with a 0.8-mm diameter punch.

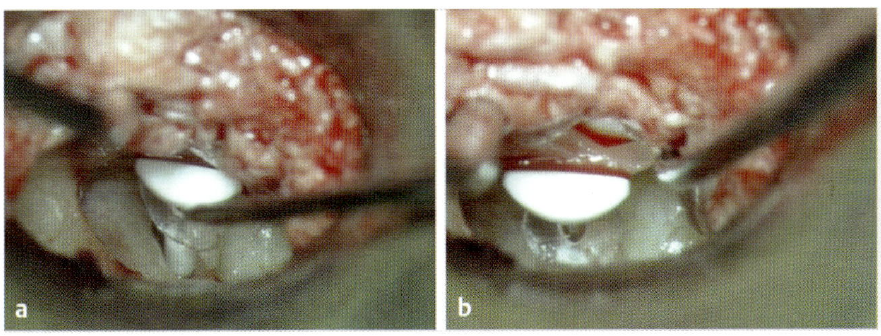

Fig. 30.9 (a) The shaft is introduced between the stapes and the Fallopian canal with the distal end being lowered onto the center of the footplate. (b) The prosthesis head is then introduced under the relocated malleus handle.

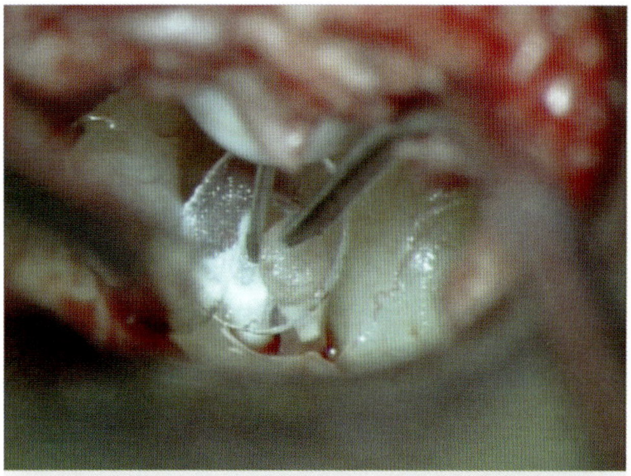

Fig. 30.10 The band is then gently pulled and positioned around the stapes capitulum.

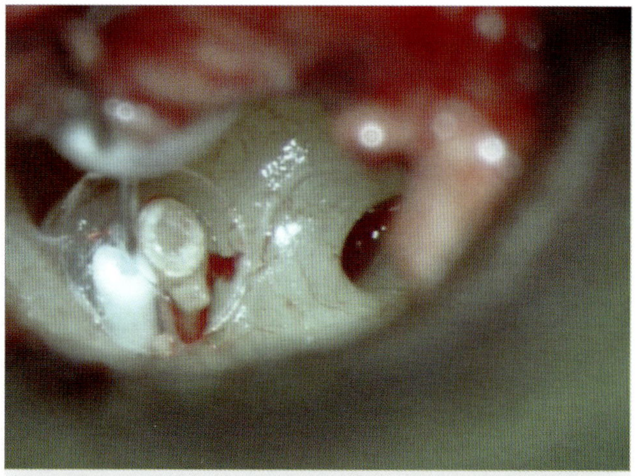

Fig. 30.11 Final view of surgical field, Austin-Kartush Group A. The prosthesis is in an almost perpendicular position from the footplate to the malleus handle and tympanic membrane and is kept in proper position by the band.

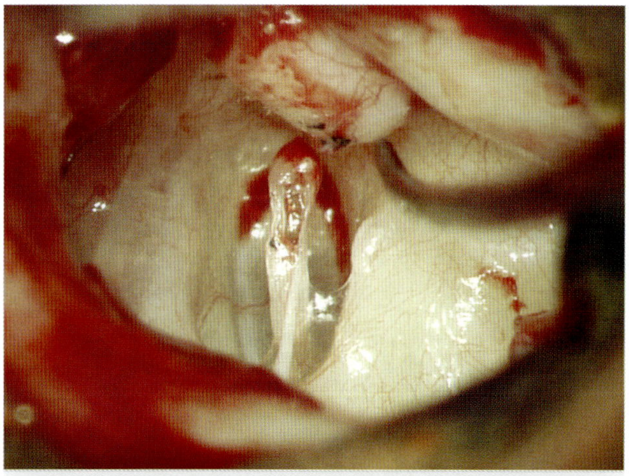

Fig. 30.12 Operative view of a left ear, Austin-Kartush Group B. Both the incus and stapes capitulum have been eroded. The eroded capitulum does not allow for the use of a PORP.

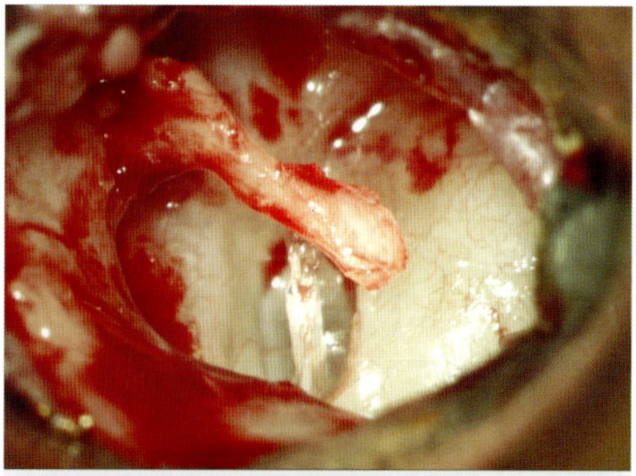

Fig. 30.13 The malleus is dissected free from the tympanic membrane and relocated in a position over the stapes footplate.

When the footplate appears to be very thin and fragile, it should be protected by an interposed vein graft. The technique of positionning the TORP is the same. The prosthesis is cut to the appropriate length as the shaft of the prosthesis must fit snugly onto the center of the footplate. The prosthesis head is then introduced under the relocated malleus handle (▶ Fig. 30.14). It is important to obtain a perpendicular position of the prosthesis from the footplate to the malleus handle.

30.2.3 Austin-Kartush Group C (Malleus Absent, Stapes Intact and Mobile)

Reconstruction of the ossicular chain when the stapes is present and the malleus is absent typically involves a PORP between the stapes head and tympanic membrane or graft surface.[8,9] However, these ossicular reconstructions are frequently unstable because the lack of fixation by the malleus at the proximal end of the prosthesis can allow displacement at either the proximal or distal ends. The Silastic banding technique is used by

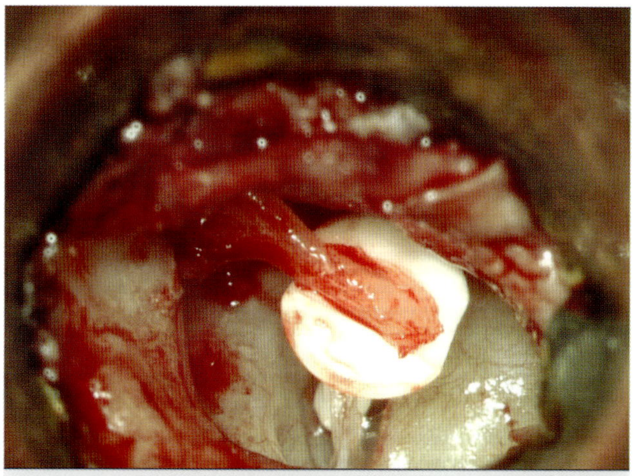

Fig. 30.14 Final view of surgical field, Austin-Kartush Group B. The prosthesis is cut to the appropriate length. The shaft of the prosthesis must fit snugly onto the center of the footplate. The prosthesis head is then introduced under the relocated malleus handle.

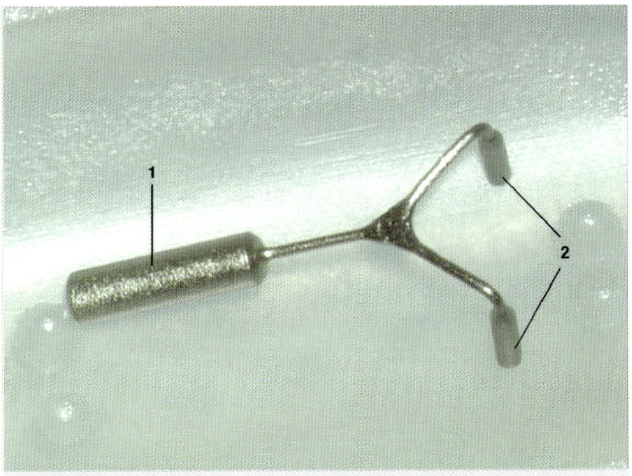

Fig. 30.15 Malleus Replacement Prosthesis (MRP). 1=0.8-mm diameter handle; 2=0.3-mm diameter posts that will be inserted in the external auditory canal.

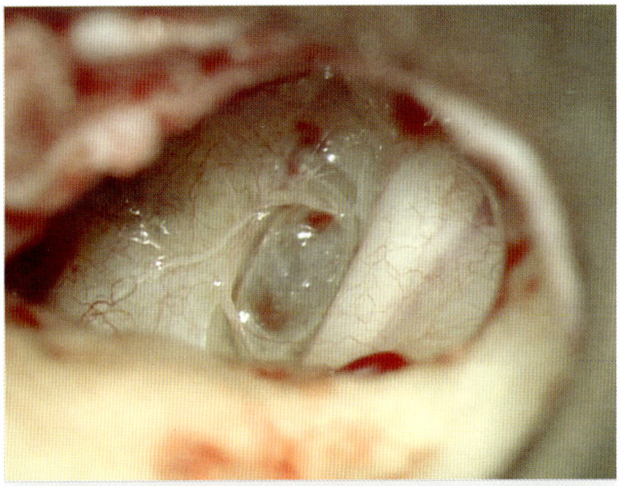

Fig. 30.16 Intraoperative view of a right ear with a mobile stapes footplate and absent lateral ossicular chain, Austin-Kartush Group D.

the author in all Austin-Kartush Group C cases, and a TORP is positioned from the stapes footplate to the tympanic membrane, despite the presence of a stapedial arch. The TORP is attached to the intact stapes superstructure. As previously described, the band allows for better prosthesis stability, thus eliminating tipping or migration. This configuration prevents prosthesis displacement and avoids contact with the promontory or the posterior canal wall. The Silastic banding technique also prevents undesirable contact with a dehiscent or overlying facial nerve. In many ears with an intact stapes superstructure, there is enough room between the horizontal segment of the facial nerve and the stapes superstructure to place the shaft of a TORP. We prefer this location because it provides a reliable vertical alignment of the prosthesis with the overlying tympanic membrane. However, if a dehiscent facial nerve is too close to the stapes superstructure, the shaft of the prosthesis is positioned on the other side, between the stapes and the promontory.

In general, determining the exact length of a prosthesis can prove to be difficult when the malleus is absent. This new technique achieves an almost perpendicular position of the prosthesis to the footplate and the tympanic membrane, allowing the use of an elongated stapes measuring rod (Xomed-Medtronic) for precise measurement within 0.5 mm, even in cases of lateralized tympanic membranes. The tympanomeatal flap is replaced in its anatomic position to verify the position of the head of the prosthesis beneath the under-surface of the tympanic membrane.

It is also possible to use a newly designed malleus replacement prosthesis (MRP) in Austin-Kartush Group C cases, which is combined with a TORP. This will be described in the Austin-Kartush Group D cases.

30.2.4 Austin-Kartush Group D (Malleus and Stapes Superstructure Absent, Stapes Footplate Present and Mobile)

In cases where the malleus and stapes are both missing, the author uses a newly designed titanium MRP, which was created in 2009 in collaboration with Heinz Kurz, Inc. (Dusslingen, Germany), to replace a missing malleus as an attempt to reduce the risk of prosthesis dislocation (▶ Fig. 30.15). Prior to the introduction of the MRP, the TORP head was universally placed in direct contact with the tympanic membrane (tympanic membrane-to-footplate assembly). The MRP is designed to be affixed to the bony ear canal to provide superior stabilization of a total or partial prosthesis coupled to it. A TORP is positioned from the MRP to the stapes footplate (MRP-to-footplate assembly) in all Austin-Kartush group cases (▶ Fig. 30.16).

The MRP is a titanium neo-malleus that is implanted underneath the tympanic membrane at any position in the bony rim of the external auditory canal. With the design of the MRP a new malleus handle is created, which can be used with any type of PORP or TORP by positioning the prosthesis under the neo-handle in a single- or two-stage procedure. The 0.8-mm diameter handle is attached via a Y-shaped titanium wire with two posts (diameter of 0.3 mm) that are intended to fix to the bony canal wall of the external auditory canal. These posts are inserted into two holes that are drilled with a 0.6-mm bur. The surgeon introduces the MRP and can connect almost any PORP or TORP due to the malleable MRP.

For placement of the MRP, two tunnels that are equal to the distance between the two posts of the MRP must be drilled through the external auditory canal wall (from side to side) with a 0.6-mm diamond bur (▶ Fig. 30.17). The drilling of the two tunnels requires highly regulated speed with constant irrigation to prevent burning or pressure necrosis of the bone. The choice of the position of these two tunnels is dictated by the status of the external auditory canal. In most cases they can be drilled approximately at 11 o'clock and 9 o'clock for a right ear and between 1 o'clock and 3 o'clock for a left ear, where 12 o'clock is positioned at the notch of Rivinus. Thus, the position of the titanium neo-handle of the MRP is slightly more posterior to a normal malleus handle. When there is not enough residual posterior-superior bony canal wall to allow for drilling out the tunnels, they can be drilled at approximatively 5 o'clock and 6 o'clock. In these cases, the position of the titanium neo-handle is more or less opposite but parallel to the position of a normal malleus handle.

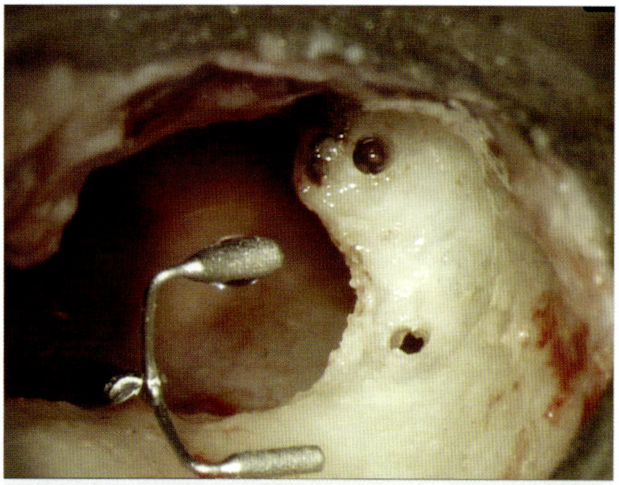

Fig. 30.17 Two tunnels are drilled through the external auditory canal from side to side with a 0.6-mm diamond dust bur to leave room for the two posts of the MRP. The tunnels shown were drilled at 9 o'clock and 11 o'clock.

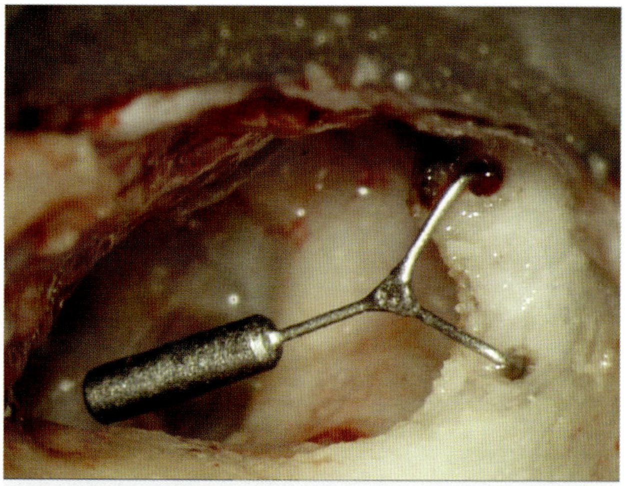

Fig. 30.18 The two posts of the MRP are inserted into the two tunnels, and the titanium handle is positioned over the stapes footplate.

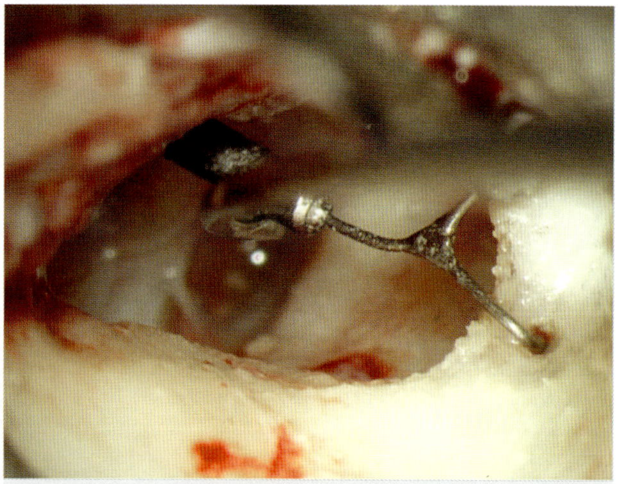

Fig. 30.19 While the MRP is kept in position by the two posts, the thin titanium link between the handle and the posts enables the surgeon to easily accomodate the position of the neo-handle to all anatomical conditions.

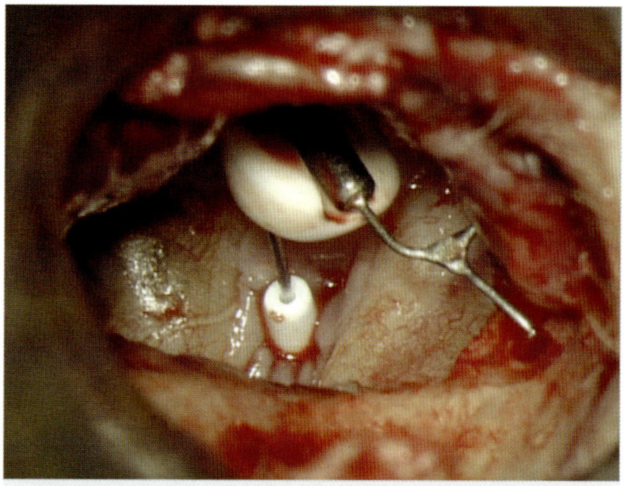

Fig. 30.20 Final view of surgical field showing the MRP handle, which is introduced within the groove of the TORP head.

The two posts of the MRP are inserted in the two tunnels, and the titanium handle is positioned over the stapes footplate (▶ Fig. 30.18). This configuration prevents MRP displacement and avoids contact between the neo-handle and the canal wall. While the MRP is kept in position by the two posts, the malleable titanium link between the handle and the posts enables the surgeon to easily accomodate the position of the neo-handle to all anatomical conditions (▶ Fig. 30.19). It is possible to slightly move the handle laterally, inferiorly, or superiorly. The foremost advantage of this prosthesis is that it keeps the neo-handle in a proper position overlying the stapes footplate in all cases.

The distance between the neo-malleus of the MRP and the stapes footplate is determined with an elongated stapes measuring rod. The TORP shaft is cut at the appropriate length, and the TORP is positioned from the handle of the MRP to the stapes footplate. The distal tip of the TORP shaft is centered on the stapes footplate, and the neo-handle of the MRP is easily introduced within the groove of the TORP head (▶ Fig. 30.20). A thin layer of tragal cartilage is interposed over the MRP in all cases, covering both the two posts and the neo-handle. When a tympanic membrane grafting is performed in combination with the MRP implantation, all fascia or perichondrium grafts are placed over the cartilage plate (lateral graft).

The MRP was developed to improve the postoperative hearing results in patients with an absent malleus who were undergoing ossiculoplasty that had been previously managed with columellae or the neo-malleus technique. Re-creation of the malleus has been used in the past.[6,7,17] Wehrs[6] suggested the use of a homologous drum and malleus, which usually requires staging for a stable reconstruction, in patients without an intact malleus. Black[7] introduced a technique of neo-malleus ossiculoplasty by using an autograft neo-malleus strut and an assembly rather than columella in cases in which the malleus was unavailable for assembly techniques.

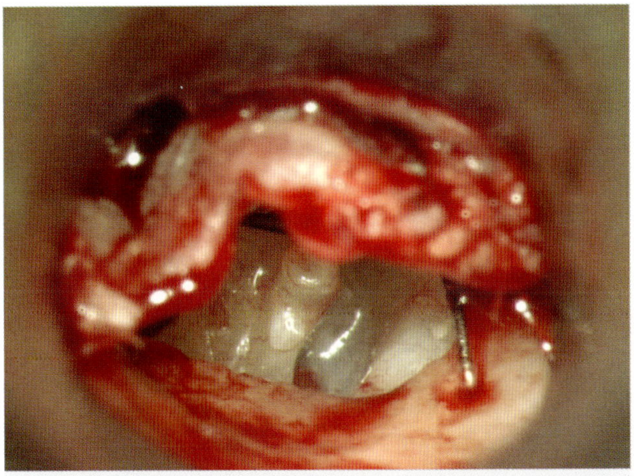

Fig. 30.21 Operative view of a left ear showing the handle of the MRP, which is positioned over the stapes footplate. The stapes is intact and the malleus is missing (Austin-Kartush Group C case).

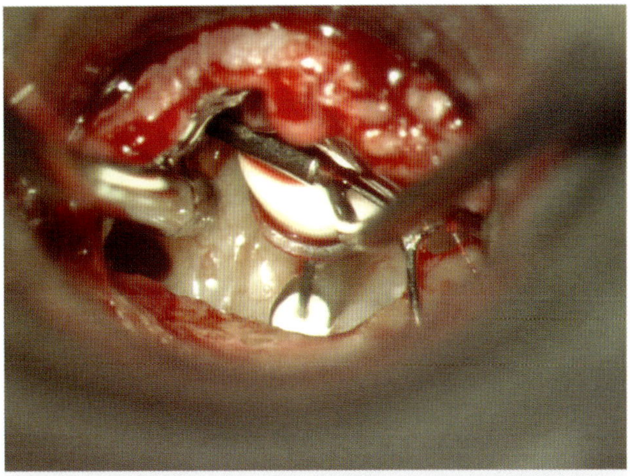

Fig. 30.22 The shaft of the TORP is positioned onto the center of the footplate, and the handle of the MRP is introduced within the groove of the head of the TORP.

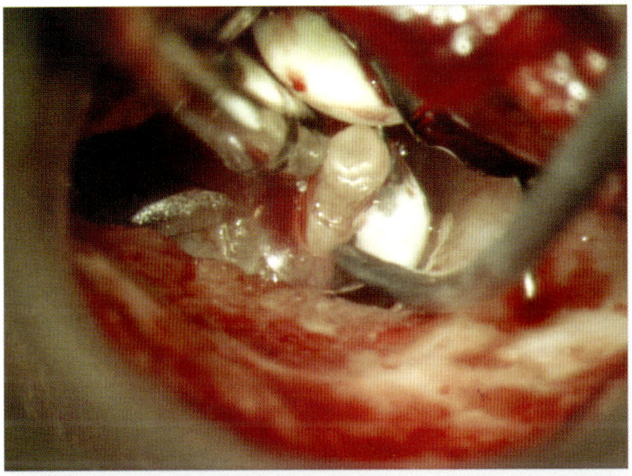

Fig. 30.23 The TORP is attached to the intact stapes superstructure with the Silastic band.

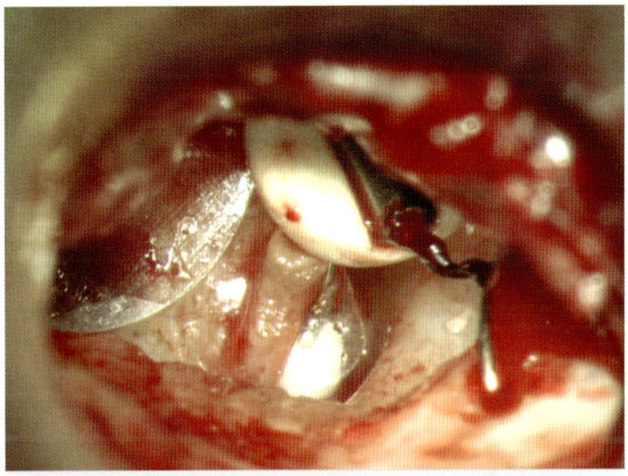

Fig. 30.24 Final view of surgical field after using the MRP, Austin-Kartush Group C. The Silastic banding technique achieves an almost perpendicular position of the TORP, which is positioned from the footplate to the MRP.

The MRP can be used in many other anatomical conditions when the malleus is missing, hypermobile, or eroded. For example, it is possible to insert the MRP in Austin-Kartush Group C cases. The combined technique of Silastic banding and MRP implantation increases the stability of the TORP, which is positioned from the MRP to the stapes footplate (▶ Fig. 30.21; ▶ Fig. 30.22; ▶ Fig. 30.23; ▶ Fig. 30.24).

30.3 Outcomes

Recently, the author compared hearing results in patients undergoing ossiculoplasty using either a PORP or TORP with Silastic banding and malleus relocation techniques in cases where the malleus and stapes were both present and mobile (Austin-Kartush Group A cases).[18] The postoperative hearing results for both groups are shown in ▶ Table 30.1. Overall hearing outcomes for the two groups in this study showed significantly superior results for the TORP group for air-bone gap (ABG) closure (68.9% and 86.9% closure of ABG to < 10 dB and < 20 dB, respectively) compared with the PORP group (54.3% and 70.4% closure of ABG to < 10 dB and < 20 dB, respectively) and postoperative mean ABG (8.9 dB for TORP group and 13.1 dB for PORP group). The mean gain in air-conduction thresholds also was significantly higher in the TORP group (16.2 dB versus 9.8 dB). We postulate that the reason for better hearing outcomes within the TORP group may be due to the favorable combination of malleus relocation, use of Silastic banding to secure the prosthesis, and footplate placement. This amalgamation results in an increasingly stable and more functional ossicular arrangement.

In 2005 the author published a prospective study of ossicular reconstruction using the Silastic banding technique in a consecutive series of 99 cases with an intact stapes superstructure and missing malleus (Austin-Kartush Group C cases).[16] Hearing results in 96 available postoperative cases are presented in ▶ Table 30.2. Overall, a postoperative ABG closed to within 10 dB was achieved in 61.5% of cases. An ABG < 20 dB was

Table 30.1 Postoperative overall hearing results in PORP and TORP groups

Variable	PORP (n=288)	TORP (n=283)	Mean or percentage difference (95% CI)	p-value
ABG < 10 dB (%)	54.3	68.9	14.6 (6; 23%)	< 0.001
ABG < 20 dB (%)	70.4	86.9	14.5 (10; 23)	< 0.001
Mean BC (dB)	28	25.5	2.5 (0.3; 4.8)	0.03
Mean AC (dB)	41.1	34.4	6.7 (3.7; 9.8)	< 0.001
Mean ABG (dB)	13.1	8.9	4.2 (2.2; 6.2)	< 0.001
Mean change in BC (dB)	-1.7	+ 0.3	-2.0 (-3.1; -0.9)	< 0.001
Mean change in AC (dB)	+ 9.8	+ 16.3	-6.4 (-9.0; -3.9)	< 0.001
Mean BC at 4 kHz (dB)	42.2	35.7	6.5 (3.1; 9.9)	< 0.001
Mean AC at 4 kHz (dB)	56.6	45	11.5 (7.8; 15.3)	< 0.001
Mean ABG at 4 kHz (dB)	14.3	9.3	5.0 (2.8; 7.3)	< 0.001
Change in BC at 4 kHz (dB)	-4.3	- 1.6	-2.7 (-4.5; 0.9)	0.003
Change in AC at 4 kHz (dB)	+ 2	+ 13.4	11.4 (8.3; 14.4)	< 0.001

BC, bone conduction; AC, air conduction; ABG, air-bone gap
Used with permission from Vincent R, Rovers M, Mistry N, Oates J, Sperling N, Grolman N. Ossiculoplasty in Intact Stapes and Malleus Patients: A Comparison of PORPs Versus TORPs With Malleus Relocation and Silastic Banding Techniques. Otol Neurotol 2011;32:616–25.

Table 30.2 Hearing results in 96 cases with the Silastic banding technique in Austin-Kartush Group C cases

Postop mean ABG (dB)		Postop ABG (%)			Postop Mean AC (dB)			Postop mean BC (dB)	
Preop	Postop	< 10 dB	10–20 dB	> 20 dB	Preop	Postop	Postop gain in AC > 20 dB	Preop	Postop
33.6	11.75	61.5	15.5	23	56.6	37.46	51	23	25.71

BC, bone conduction; AC, air conduction; ABG, air-bone gap
Used with permission from Vincent R, Sperling N, Oates J, Osborne J. Ossiculoplasty with Intact Stapes and Absent Malleus: The Silastic Banding Technique. Otol Neurotol. 2005;26:846–52.

Table 30.3 Literature Review of Austin-Kartush Group C Hearing Results

			Postop ABG (%)			
Series	Material	n	< 10 dB	0–20 dB	> 20 dB	Mean ABG (dB)
Austin 1976[19]	Partial autograft or homograft	23	12	39	61	27
Black 1991[20]	HA PORP	13	15	54	46	
Goldenberg 1994[9]	HA PORP	7	14	46	57	23
Moretz 1998[1]	HA PORP	6	0	10	90	24
	HA TORP	4	0	25	75	24
Vincent, Rovers, Mistry, Oates, and Sperling 2005[18]	HA TORP	96	66	77	23	12

BC, bone conduction; AC, air conduction; ABG, air-bone gap

obtained in 77% of cases. Postoperative improvement of air-conduction thresholds by at least 20 dB was found in 51% of cases. There was no case of postoperative sensorineural hearing loss. One case of extrusion of the prothesis was seen (1%). Our hearing results with this technique of Silastic banding in cases of a missing malleus compared favorably with the results reported by other authors in the same anatomic situation (▶ Table 30.3). The author has published the preliminary results of the MRP combined with a TORP in middle ear reconstruction in patients missing the malleus and stapes (Austin-Kartush Group D

Table 30.4 Austin-Kartush group D hearing results at 3-month follow-up according to TORP placement

Variable	TM-to-Footplate TORP placement (n=28)	MRP-to-Footplate TORP placement (n=29)	Mean or percentage difference (95% CI)	p-value
ABG ≤ 10 dB (%)	37.0	58.1	-21.1 (-44.5 to 2.3)	0.088
ABG ≤ 20 dB (%)	48.1	79.1	-30.9 (-53.4 to -8.5)	0.008
Mean BC, dB (SD)	31.1 (16.7)	25.2 (13.1)	6.0 (-1.2 to 13.1)	0.101
Mean AC, dB (SD)	54.4 (22.7)	37.7 (18.3)	16.8 (6.9 to 26.6)	0.001
Mean ABG, dB (SD)	23.3 (16.7)	12.5 (11.9)	10.8 (4.0 to 17.6)	0.002
Mean change in BC, dB (SD)	-0.3 (7.0)	+ 0.7 (6.2)	-1.0 (-4.2 to 2.2)	0.533
Mean change in AC, dB (SD)	+ 11.0 (15.5)	+ 21.3 (16.4)	-10.3 (-18.2 to -2.4)	0.011

BC, bone conduction; AC, air conduction; ABG, air-bone gap; SNHL, sensorineural hearing loss
Used with permission from Vincent R, Bittermann, A. J. N., Wenzel, G., Oates J, Sperling, N, Lenarz T, Grolman W. Ossiculoplasty in Missing Malleus and Stapes Patients: Experimental and Preliminary Clinical Results With a New Malleus Replacement Prosthesis With the Otology-Neurotology Database. Otol Neurotol 2013;34:83–90.

Table 30.5 Postoperative hearing results at 1 year according to TORP placement

Variable	TM-to-Footplate TORP placement (n=13)	MRP-to-Footplate TORP placement (n=19)	Mean or percentage difference (95% CI)	p-value
ABG ≤ 10 dB (%)	15.4	52.6	-37.3 (-67.1 to -7.4)	0.035
ABG ≤ 20 dB (%)	53.8	84.2	-30.4 (-62.0 to 1.3)	0.065
Mean BC, dB (SD)	37.9 (17.5)	26.8 (14.6)	11.1 (-0.5 to 22.8)	0.061
Mean AC, dB (SD)	60.4 (20.1)	39.7 (17.1)	20.7 (7.2 to 34.2)	0.004
Mean ABG, dB (SD)	22.5 (13.9)	12.9 (12.6)	9.6 (-0.1 to 19.3)	0.052
Mean change in BC, dB (SD)	-0.5 (5.2)	-1.5 (5.7)	1.0 (-3.0 to 5.1)	0.606
Mean change in AC, dB (SD)	+ 9.2 (14.6)	+ 19.9 (14.9)	-10.6 (-21.5 to 0.2)	0.055

BC, Bone conduction; AC, air conduction; ABG, air-bone gap; SD, standard deviations; dB, decibel (pure tone average); Means were calculated with 0.5, 1, 2, 4 kHz.
Used with permission from Vincent R, Bittermann, A. J. N., Wenzel, G., Oates J, Sperling, N, Lenarz T, Grolman W. Ossiculoplasty in Missing Malleus and Stapes Patients: Experimental and Preliminary Clinical Results With a New Malleus Replacement Prosthesis With the Otology-Neurotology Database. Otol Neurotol 2013;34:83–90.

Table 30.6 Literature Review of Hearing Results in Cases of Missing Malleus

Series	Austin-Kartush Group	Material	n	Postop ABG < 10 dB (%)	Postop mean ABG
Moretz[1]	C	PORP	6	0	24
	C	TORP	4	0	24
Vincent, Sperling, Oates, and Osborne [16]	C	TORP	96	66	12
Austin[19]	C	Partial autograft	23	12	27
Black[20]	C	PORP	13	15	-
Goldenberg[9]	C	PORP	7	14	23
Vincent, Bittermann, and Wenzel [21] at 3 mo	D	TORP + MRP	43	58.1	12.5
Vincent, Bittermann, and Wenzel [21] at 1 yr	D	TORP + MRP	19	52.6	12.9

ABG, air-bone gap
Data from Vincent R, Bittermann, A. J. N., Wenzel, G., Oates J, Sperling, N, Lenarz T, Grolman W. Ossiculoplasty in Missing Malleus and Stapes Patients: Experimental and Preliminary Clinical Results With a New Malleus Replacement Prosthesis With the Otology-Neurotology Database. Otol Neurotol 2013;34:83–90.

cases).[21] The results of this study indicated that superior postoperative hearing thresholds can be achieved using an MRP-to-footplate assembly, compared with a TM-to-footplate assembly in patients with an absent malleus undergoing ossiculoplasty. The postoperative air-conduction thresholds, after 3 months and 1 year, are significantly lower in patients treated with the MRP-to-footplate assembly (▶ Table 30.4; ▶ Table 30.5). ▶ Table 30.6 presents a literature review of hearing results in cases of a missing malleus.

References

[1] Moretz WH Jr. Ossiculoplasty with an intact stapes: Superstructure versus footplate prosthesis placement. Laryngoscope. 1998;108(11 Pt 2) Suppl 89:1–12.

[2] Dornhoffer JL, Gardner E. Prognostic factors in ossiculoplasty: A statistical staging system. Otol Neurotol. 2001;22(3):299–304.

[3] Albu S, Babighian G, Trabalzini F. Prognostic factors in tympanoplasty. Am J Otol. 1998;19(2):136–140.

[4] Black B. Ossiculoplasty prognosis: the spite method of assessment. Am J Otol. 1992;13(6):544–551.

[5] Fisch U, Schmid S. Total reconstruction of the ossicular chain. Otolaryngol Clin North Am. 1994;27(4):785–797.

[6] Wehrs RE. The homograft tympanic membrane after 12 years. Ann Otol Rhinol Laryngol. 1982;91(5 Pt 1):533–537.

[7] Black B. Neomalleus ossiculoplasty. Otol Neurotol. 2002;23(5):636–642.

[8] Kartush JM. Ossicular chain reconstruction. Capitulum to malleus. Otolaryngol Clin North Am. 1994;27(4):689–715.

[9] Goldenberg RA. Ossiculoplasty with composite prostheses. PORP and TORP. Otolaryngol Clin North Am. 1994;27(4):727–745.

[10] Shinohara T, Gyo K, Saiki T, Yanagihara N. Ossiculoplasty using hydroxyapatite prostheses: Long-term results. Clin Otolaryngol Allied Sci. 2000;25 (4):287–292.

[11] Vincent R, Oates J, Sperling NM, Annamalai S. Malleus relocation in ossicular reconstruction: managing the anteriorly positioned malleus: Results in a series of 268 cases. Otol Neurotol. 2004;25(3):223–230.

[12] De Vos C, Gersdorff M, Gérard JM. Prognostic factors in ossiculoplasty. Otol Neurotol. 2007;28(1):61–67.

[13] Vlaming MS, Feenstra L. Studies on the mechanics of the reconstructed humanmiddle ear. Clin Otolaryngol Allied Sci. 1986;11(6):411–422.

[14] Goode RL, Nishihara S. Experimental models of ossiculoplasty. Otolaryngol Clin North Am. 1994;27(4):663–675.

[15] Austin DF. Ossicular reconstruction. Otolaryngol Clin North Am. 1972;5 (1):145–160.

[16] Vincent R, Sperling NM, Oates J, Osborne J. Ossiculoplasty with intact stapes and absent malleus: The Silastic banding technique. Otol Neurotol. 2005;26 (5):846–852.

[17] Fisch U. Tympanoplasty, Mastoidectomy, and Stapes Surgery. New York: Thieme Medical Publishers, 1994.

[18] Vincent R, Rovers M, Mistry N, Oates J, Sperling N, Grolman W. Ossiculoplasty in intact stapes and malleus patients: A comparison of PORPs versus TORPs with malleus relocation and Silastic banding techniques. Otol Neurotol. 2011;32(4):616–625.

[19] Austin DF. Transcanal tympanoplasty: a 15-year report. Trans Sect Otolaryngol Am Acad Ophthalmol Otolaryngol. 1976;82(1):ORL30–ORL38.

[20] Black B. A universal ossicular replacement prosthesis: Clinical trials of 152 cases. Otolaryngol Head Neck Surg. 1991;104(2):210–218.

[21] Vincent R, Bittermann AJN, Wenzel G, et al. Ossiculoplasty in missing malleus and stapes patients: experimental and preliminary clinical results with a new malleus replacement prosthesis with the otology-neurotology database. Otol Neurotol. 2013;34(1):83–90.

31 Surgical Management of the Fixed Stapes in Chronic Ear Disease

Thomas E. Linder and Yannick Zaugg

Abbreviations used in this chapter:

ABG: air-bone gap
COM: chronic otitis media
CROS: contralateral routing of offside signaling
CT: computed tomography
DACS: Direct Acoustic Cochlear Stimulator
FTTP: Fisch Titanium Total Prosthesis
PORP: partial ossicular replacement prosthesis
TORP: total ossicular replacement prosthesis

31.1 Introduction

Surgical management of stapes fixation is well defined for otosclerosis and congenital stapes fixation, with respectable results.[1,2] However, the management of stapes fixation in chronic ear disease is more challenging, with far less predictable results. Whereas some surgeons find chronic ear disease a possible contraindication to ossiculoplasty in cases of stapes fixation, others believe that significant benefit can be achieved with surgery.[3,4,5]

The basic principles of treatment are restoration of footplate mobility or labyrinthine fenestration. Mobilization of the stapes is generally considered the first option and remains the technique of choice for several otologists.[3,5] If mobilization fails to improve hearing, some are reluctant to open the labyrinth because of the risk of inner ear damage[6] and propose a hearing aid instead. Still others choose labyrinthine fenestration as salvage surgery after insufficient mobilization attempts[3,5,7] or as a primary technique,[4,8,9] claiming that mobilization itself carries the same risks for the inner ear.

31.2 Patient Selection

The risks and benefits should be evaluated for each patient and depend on the underlying pathology, the estimated progression of the middle ear disease, the surgeon's experience, and the patient's expectations. All ossiculoplasty attempts have to be balanced against the benefits of conventional or implantable hearing aids. Continuous improvements in bone-conducting hearing devices and new methods for coupling active middle ear implants onto the round window membrane, even in case of stapes fixation, further compete with risky ossiculoplasties.

31.3 Causes of Stapes Fixation in Chronic Ear Disease

In chronic ear disease, there exist three main causes of stapes fixation. The most frequent etiology is tympanosclerosis, which was first reported by Zöllner in 1956.[10] In 1873 von Trölsch already described the characteristics of tympanic cavity sclerosis, named "Paukensklerose," which was further identified as a long-term sequela of chronic middle ear infections, with calcareous deposits within the tympanic membrane (myringosclerosis), tympanic cavity, and ossicular chain. In 1977, Shea reviewed his 1502 surgeries for chronic otitis media (COM) and found an incidence of stapes fixation in 112 patients, or 7.5% overall.[11] Within this subgroup, 62% were due to tympanosclerosis. In general tympanosclerosis affected 5% of his COM patients. The incidence of tympanosclerosis varies greatly (between 11% and 32%[12,13]), and not all patients present with stapes fixation. Such an oval window involvement was estimated by some authors to occur in 35% of patients with tympanosclerosis.[14] Since tympanoclerosis is an "end-stage" disease, the ear is usually dry and the non-affected mucosa can be quite healthy. Involvement of the tympanic cavity and the ossicles typically leads to severe hearing loss with an air-bone gap (ABG) of 40 dB or more.

Shea described another cause of stapes fixation, which he termed "postinflammatory osteogenic fixation."[11] Analyzing his 1502 middle ear surgeries for COM, he found 19 cases (1.2% overall) with a rigid stapes fixation as a consequence of chronic ear disease. He proposed that this was due to a new membranous bone growth along the stapediovestibular joint caused by an inflammatory reaction from either infection or trauma from vigorous footplate manipulation during previous surgeries. The ABGs ranged from 10–50 dB. Typically 80% of his patients had undergone previous middle ear surgery to correct the underlying suppurative otitis media.

Rarely, stapes fixation existing with COM can also be caused by concomitant otosclerosis or other occasional entities (Paget's disease, osteogenesis imperfecta, fibrous dysplasia, systemic inflammatory disease).

31.4 Preoperative Reflections: The Triple "A"

When facing a fixed stapes in chronic ear disease, and before choosing the surgical strategies, the following three factors should be taken into account.

31.4.1 Anticipation

Preoperative computed tomography (CT) scans infrequently detect stapes fixations; however, they do highlight the degree of pneumatization and ventilation of the middle ear and mastoid, and therefore provide an overall view of the middle ear pathology. That being said, neither CT scans nor the audiogram patterns can predict with reasonable sensitivity the non-otosclerotic fixation of the stapes. In case of previous surgery, an effort should be made to obtain the operating note of the previous surgeon, verifying the mobility of the stapes. However, one must keep in mind that concurrent granulation tissue at the time of first surgery may not allow proper assessment of stapes mobility, that partial fixation is even more difficult to evaluate, and that any progression of the middle ear disease may impair the footplate mobility after previous surgeries. Careful preoperative evaluation should anticipate the intraoperative findings and help in the planning of the surgical options.

31.4.2 Audible Range and Status of the Middle Ear

As in any ossiculoplasty, the condition of the ipsilateral hearing ear (type and degree of mixed hearing loss, speech discrimination score, high-frequency sensorineural impairment) and the condition of the contralateral ear determine how to estimate the benefit for the patient overall. In case of large asymmetry with poor cochlear reserve on the affected ear, surgery should be avoided. This is best anticipated by the Belfast rule of thumb: patients are likely to benefit from surgery if the air conduction threshold within the speech frequencies (500–4000 Hz) will be ≤ 30 dB or if the interaural difference is reduced to ≤ 15 dB.[15] The final result should also be plotted on the Glasgow Benefit Plot to account for bilateral hearing benefit.[16] In case these audiological goals cannot be anticipated, alternative methods may be more justified.

Equally important is the status of the middle ear: the presence of an acute infection at the time of stapes surgery increases the risk of sensorineural hearing loss.[17] Interestingly, pseudomonas infections harbor a much greater risk than other pathogens, such as *Haemophilus* or *Streptococcus pneumoniae*, at least in the animal model.[18] It seems safe to carry out a stapedotomy or malleostapedotomy in the setting of inactive or previously treated COM with an intact tympanic membrane.[19,20]

In summary, before planning any labyrinthine fenestration in COM, the middle ear must be dry and the eardrum closed. As the majority of patients in chronic ear disease (85% in a series of 775 patients by Asiri, Hasham, al Anazy, Zakzouk, and Banjar[12]) may still present with a tympanic membrane perforation, the fenestration should be performed in a second stage. Concomitant round window involvement with tympanoslerotic obliteration further reduces the chance of hearing improvement.

The status of the remaining ossicular chain and the type of previous or planned surgery is equally important: at least the presence of a mobile malleus in proper contact to the drum allows coupling of a prosthesis for reconstruction. If incus and malleus are absent, staged reconstructions with a neo-malleus and, later, a neo-malleus-vestibulopexy (malleostapedotomy) assembly may become an option. This may be further challenged by an open or closed cavity setting.

Many surgeons choose to avoid labyrinthine fenestration procedures in the background of poor Eustachian tube function because of concern related to subsequent prosthesis migration. Furthermore, in the absence of satisfactory middle ear ventilation, even the most well-conceived ossicular reconstruction is doomed to result in at least a 35–40 dB ABG.[21] With poor ventilation neither mobilization nor labyrinthine fenestration will provide good results. In all these instances, alternative methods should be proposed.

31.4.3 Alternatives

Conventional hearing aid amplifications are always an alternative in dry external ear canals with an intact drum, either in a closed or open cavity setting. Contralateral Routing of Offside Signaling (CROS) and Bilateral-CROS hearing aids, for use in cases of severe mixed and asymmetric hearing loss, have regained popularity since the reintroduction of wireless communication between the processors. The major competitors to ossiculoplasty remain the fitting of bone-anchored hearing devices or active middle ear implants coupled to the round window or to a cochleostomy/vestibulopexy approach.

31.5 Surgical Technique

Preconditions required to perform an ossiculoplasty are:

- Sterile middle ear cavity with an intact and healthy eardrum in a favorable position.
- Adequate ventilation of the middle ear space on long term.
- The presence of a malleus or reconstruction of a neo-malleus for prosthesis fixation is advisable.
- Expected outcome within the Belfast rule of thumb.
- Alternative hearing aids or implants have been discussed with the patient.
- Long-term follow-up (at least 5 years) is feasible, allowing surgeons to evaluate their own results and to improve their personal skills.

When the above conditions are filled, two main strategies are then available: stapes mobilization or labyrinthine fenestration. Most surgeons agree that stapes mobilization does not attempt to "rock" the stapes free, but, rather, to remove sclerotic plaques from the oval window niche using cold instruments (needle, hook, drill) and/or laser technology (Argon, KTP, Diode, or CO_2 laser systems). Rocking the stapes superstructure or the footplate itself may lead to fractures or refixation. Labyrinthine fenestration procedures include stapedectomy, stapedotomy, and lateral canal or vestibulum fenestration techniques. This situation is classified as Austin-Kartush Group F (see Chapter 1), or Fisch Class II_2 or III_3.[22,23]

31.5.1 Fixed but Intact Ossicular Chain

In case of tympanosclerosis with an intact ossicular chain, a primary attempt should be made to remove the plaques from the stapes arch and footplate in a posterior-anterior direction, allowing the stapes tendon to stabilize the footplate during dissection. Although controversial, we advise disconnecting the incudostapedial joint first to correctly assess the mobility of the incus/malleus complex and the stapes as separate entities. This approach also allows safer access to the oval window niche. Facial nerve monitoring is advisable since the plaques could cover a dehiscent facial nerve, and even careful removal with cold instruments or lasers may induce a facial nerve lesion. In case of additional incus and/or malleus fixation, mobilization of these other ossicles becomes part of the procedure, and incus interposition or prosthesis insertions may become necessary. A final ABG within 20 dB should be achieved in 60% to 80% of patients, and > 50% may even end up within 10 dB in cases of a previous intact ossicular chain.

In case of insufficient results or re-fixation of the ossicles, a fenestration procedure remains a good second-stage alternative.[5] The technique is described below. Others prefer not to attempt a stapes mobilization as a first option but to proceed

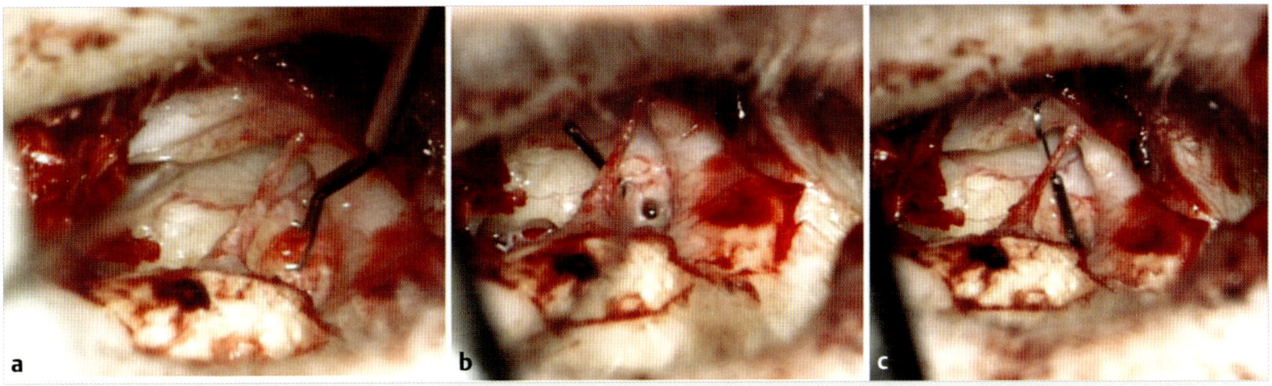

Fig. 31.1 Malleostapedotomy. (a) The length of the piston is measured. (b) Stapedotomy performed with a drill. (c) Introduction of the piston crimped to the malleus.

with an incus- or malleus-stapedotomy/stapedectomy procedure as their preferred choice.[4,8] In favor of a primary fenestration option is the fact that an intact ossicular chain is in the proper anatomic position and, therefore, favorable for the fixation of a piston perpendicular to the footplate.

31.5.2 Fixed Footplate and Incomplete Ossicular Chain

In case of a "fixed footplate–only" situation without a stapes superstructure, or in case of postinflammatory osteogenic fixation of the annular ligament without obvious tympanosclerotic plaques, footplate mobilization is not advisable. Even in cases of an intact superstructure but fixed footplate, any attempt to achieve a tympanoplasty Type III (open cavity setting) or any effort to place a partial ossicular replacement prosthesis (PORP) between the eardrum and the stapes will not provide any benefit. We found only 8 patients in our database of over 5000 files with such attempts. The postoperative hearing remained, as expected, unchanged. There was also no change in bone conduction. Tos, Lau, Arndal, and Plate also stated that any columella reconstruction inserted between a fixed footplate and the tympanic membrane revealed only unfavorable results, with hearing thresholds exceeding 40 dB.[3] Therefore, only a labyrinthine fenestration procedure may benefit these patients. There are two types of labyrinthine fenestrations, described below.

Malleostapedotomy or Staged Neo-malleus plus Neo-malleostapedotomy

In case of subtotal or total fixation of the stapes footplate, any reconstruction aims at connecting the sound conduction from the drum to the vestibule, necessitating the opening of the footplate. The stapes superstructure is not helpful and needs to be removed, leading to the Fisch Class III_3 or Austin-Kartush Type F basic situation.[22,23] These are all staged surgeries in a healthy middle ear environment. A calibrated opening into the stapes footplate is preferred over total stapedectomy to reduce the risk of inner ear damage.[24] In case of obliterative tympanosclerosis, a drill must be used to blueline the vestibule before entering. Once the blueline has been reached, the length of the piston is measured, the angulation determined, and the piston prepared

Table 31.1 Results of our malleostapedotomies in chronic ear disease with fixed stapes (0.5–3 kHz)

	(n=17)
Preop ABG (mean)	36.8 (dB)
Postop ABG (mean)	17.2 (dB)
Pts with ABG closure	
≤ 10 dB	18%
≤ 20 dB	71%

Preop, preoperative; Postop, postoperative; ABG, air-bone gap; n, number of patients; pts, patients

to fit perfectly. Next, the stapedotomy opening is completed and the piston introduced 0.5 mm into the vestibule and crimped to the malleus shaft just distal to the short process (▶ Fig. 31.1). The opening can be sealed using soft tissue and the patient's own blood. Even in the presence of an incus, we prefer to remove the incus to gain better access to the fixed and often obliterated footplate. Our results in 17 patients with malleostapedotomy verify a success rate of 18% of patients with an ABG ≤ 10 dB, 71% ≤ 20 dB, and only 1 patient with an ABG of more than 30 dB (▶ Table 31.1). These results are inferior to the overall results of malleostapedotomy in otosclerosis patients, indicating the less favorable middle ear condition in COM patients.[25]

In patients with a too anteriorly placed malleus, Vincent, Oates, Sperling, and Annamalai advised a malleus relocation technique to optimize its position perpendicular to the footplate and inserted a total ossicular replacement prosthesis (TORP) under the malleus, into a stapedotomy opening, covered by a vein graft. The authors also found the highest rate of failures (ABG > 20 dB in 32%) in Austin Group F.[26] Vincent, Bittermann, and Wenzel recently introduced a titanium malleus replacement prosthesis to overcome the difficulties in relocating a malpositioned patient-own malleus. The first results seem quite promising but have yet to focus on a mobile footplate situation.[27]

In a fixed footplate-only situation (absence of a malleus to attach the prosthesis for malleostapedotomy), Fisch, May, and Linder had already introduced a two-stage procedure of inserting first a titanium neo-malleus into the reconstructed ear drum and fixing a malleostapedotomy prosthesis 3–6 months later onto the neo-malleus and into a stapedotomy opening.[23] These multi-staged surgeries require a stable and well-ventilated middle ear situation and are technically very challenging. We do have very limited experience in a closed cavity situation. In open cavities with a well-ventilated middle ear space and the presence of a malleus over the fixed footplate, a malleostapedotomy can be performed in a similar fashion. These cases are very rare, for obvious reasons.

Stapedotomy/Stapedectomy and TORP Ossiculoplasty

Much more frequently encountered are patients with a fixed stapes-only situation, missing an incus and malleus, with a shallow middle ear space. In these cases, a stapedotomy/stapedectomy or TORP ossiculoplasty may be used. Labyrinthine fenestration for sound transfer into the inner ear can be performed as a calibrated opening, partial platinectomy, or total stapedectomy. The following challenges need to be addressed.

Safe Removal of the Fixed Footplate

Various techniques have been described to safely remove a fixed footplate. Most authors attempt to fracture the footplate centrally and carefully detach the anterior and posterior parts, lifting them laterally and avoiding mobilization and pressure waves onto the perilymph space underneath.

Graft and Type of Interposition

It is preferable to use a generously sized but thin graft (vein, perichondrium, fascia) to cover all corners of the oval window niche. Getting the graft well up on the tympanic facial nerve ridge superiorly and over the promontory inferiorly is important to avoid inserting the prosthesis too deeply into the vestibule. Cartilage struts or modified bony columellar reconstructions have been used in open and closed cavity situations. Others use hydroxyapatite, titanium, or other alloplastic TORP prostheses (▶ Fig. 31.2).

Stabilizing the Reconstruction

Once the proper length has been determined, a perpendicular position onto the oval window niche and underneath the drum has to be maintained. A cartilage disk can be used to keep the shaft of the prosthesis upright over the oval window, and another slice of thin cartilage is often required to prevent extrusion of the head of the prosthesis through the tympanic membrane. The adjustable L-shaped Fisch Titanium Total Prosthesis (FTTP, manufactured by Karl Storz GmbH, Tuttlingen, Germany) is the only alloplastic prosthesis that does not require interposing cartilage between the head of the protheses and the undersurface of the tympanic membrane because of the malleability of the very thin and flexible head (▶ Fig. 31.3).[28] We advise placing a 1-mm thick Silastic sheeting over the promontory in open cavities to avoid medialization of the TORP piston into the vestibule in case of tympanic membrane retraction over time.

A reasonable ABG of 15–25 dB can be expected, with a success rate of 70% within 20 dB.[8] Failures leading to an ABG above 30 dB are multifactorial and can be due to prosthesis migration, extrusion, displacement, or disconnection from either end. Worsening of bone conduction, total hearing loss, or induction

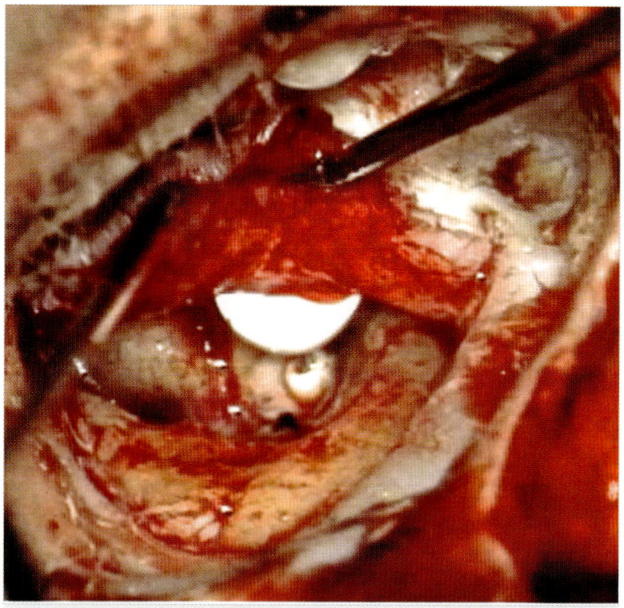

Fig. 31.2 Intraoperative view of a stapedectomy with perichondrium graft and TORP interposition.

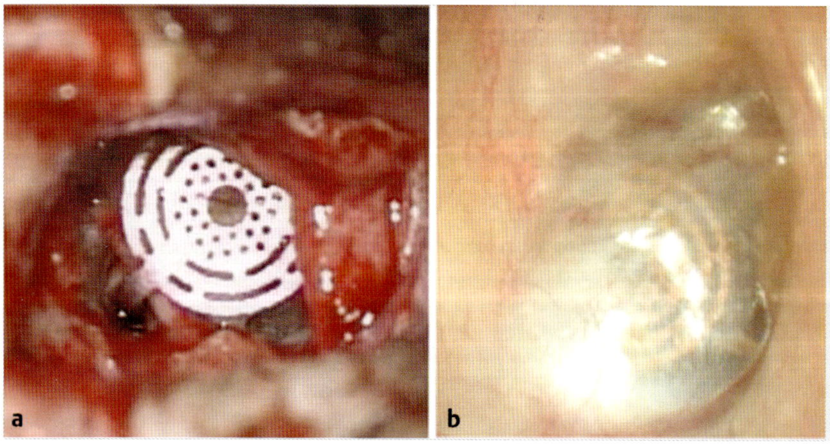

Fig. 31.3 Titanium total ossicular replacement prosthesis. (a) Intraoperative and (b) postoperative view of the FTTP (Karl Storz GmbH, Tuttlingen, Germany).

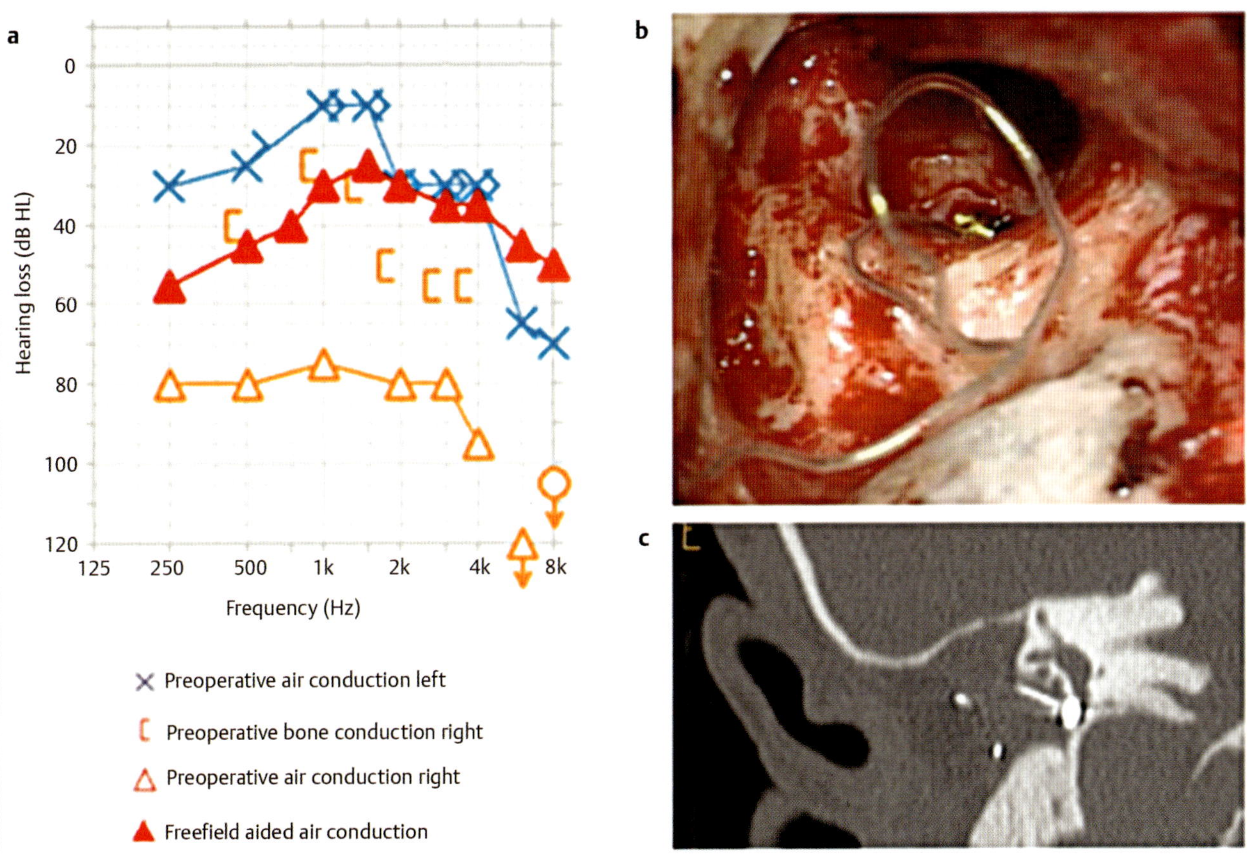

Fig. 31.4 Subtotal petrosectomy with round window vibroplasty. The Vibrant Soundbridge was placed in a 50-year-old patient with stapes fixation and chronic ear disease (7 years after a modified radical mastoidectomy). (a) Pre- and postoperative audiogram. (b) Intraoperative view. (c) Postoperative CT scan.

of severe tinnitus are rare but important risk factors that need to be carefully discussed with the patient prior to surgery.

31.5.3 Alternative Surgical Strategies

As outlined above, alternatives need to be considered in the overall approach to stapes fixation in chronic ear disease. Often in chronic ear disease there is a mixed hearing loss, and neither surgery nor a hearing aid alone offers sufficient rehabilitation to the patient. Bone conduction hearing implants provide reliably good results (see Chapter 43). As their auditory outcomes can be assessed without the need of implantation, a clinical trial should be offered to the patient. Active middle ear implants are also alternatives. They can be coupled onto the round window membrane or into a stapedotomy opening, such as with the Direct Acoustic Cochlear Stimulator (DACS) system (Cochlear Corporation, Sydney, Australia). Even in cases of a fixed stapes footplate, a round window vibroplasty using a Vibrant Soundbridge (Med-El Corporation, Innsbruck, Austria) can give a sufficient functional gain for optimal amplification (▶ Fig. 31.4).[29] A recent publication using this device described a stapedotomy approach to place a vibroplasty coupler through a cartilage disk into the vestibule, with good aided hearing results.[30] Therefore, all these alternatives should be discussed with the patient and should be part of the surgical strategy.

31.6 Complications and Outcomes

The risk of sensorineural hearing loss has been reported to be from 0% to 17% for stapes mobilization[5,31,32,33] versus 0% to 27% for labyrinthine fenestration (mainly 0% to 6% in a recent, larger series).[4,5,32,33,34] Quite surprisingly, the hearing improvement and the postoperative ABG seem not to differ between mobilization or fenestration procedures,[5,7,14] and the initial improvement for either group did not deteriorate during longer follow-up.[5] For some, results were better after stapedectomy than after mobilization,[34] and, for others, mobilization was more effective than stapedectomy.[24] For example Smyth[32] obtained closure of the ABG within 10 dB in 85% of patients with stapedectomy versus 54% with mobilization whereas Kinney[33] reported an ABG closure to within 10 dB in 57% of patients with mobilization versus 39% with stapedectomy.

Comparison between different studies regarding the outcome of stapes mobilization varies since the amount of sclerotic plaque removal is never described or quantified and the initial and final mobility of the stapes is judged clinically and depends on the experience of the surgeon. However, the best outcome seems to be achieved in an otherwise intact and mobile ossicular chain, and the worst outcome seems to occur with open cavities or modified radical mastoidectomies.[3]

31.7 Conclusion

The management of a fixed stapes in chronic ear disease will challenge every otologist. The cause of stapes fixation and the current and future status of the middle ear should be well analyzed. When the preconditions to perform an ossiculoplasty are fulfilled and alternative nonsurgical strategies have been discussed, the patient may opt for surgical correction. Although results are dependent on the residual ossicular status and the surgical skills of the otologist, favorable hearing outcomes are quite possible.

References

[1] Vincent R, Sperling NM, Oates J, Jindal M. Surgical findings and long-term hearing results in 3,050 stapedotomies for primary otosclerosis: A prospective study with the otology-neurotology database. Otol Neurotol. 2006;27(8) Suppl 2:S25–S47.

[2] Carlson ML, Van Abel KM, Pelosi S, et al. Outcomes comparing primary pediatric stapedectomy for congenital stapes footplate fixation and juvenile otosclerosis. Otol Neurotol. 2013;34(5):816–820.

[3] Tos M, Lau T, Arndal H, Plate S. Tympanosclerosis of the middle ear: late results of surgical treatment. J Laryngol Otol. 1990;104(9):685–689.

[4] Vincent R, Oates J, Sperling NM. Stapedotomy for tympanosclerotic stapes fixation: is it safe and efficient? A review of 68 cases. Otol Neurotol. 2002;23 (6):866–872.

[5] Teufert KB, De La Cruz A. Tympanosclerosis: Long-term hearing results after ossicular reconstruction. Otolaryngol Head Neck Surg. 2002;126(3):264–272.

[6] Tsuzuki K, Yanagihara N, Hinohira Y, Sakagami M. Tympanosclerosis involving the ossicular chain: mobility of the stapes in association with hearing results. Acta Otolaryngol. 2006;126(10):1046–1052.

[7] Giddings NA, House JW. Tympanosclerosis of the stapes: Hearing results for various surgical treatments. Otolaryngol Head Neck Surg. 1992;107(5):644–650.

[8] Querat C, Richard C, Martin C. Labyrinthine fenestration for tympanosclerotic stapes fixation. Eur Ann Otorhinolaryngol Head Neck Dis. 2012;129(6):297–301.

[9] Martin H, Martin C. [Typanosclerosis and labyrinthine trephination. Results] Ann Otolaryngol Chir Cervicofac. 1979;96(4–5):307–314.

[10] Tympanosclerosis ZF. J Laryngol Otol. 1956;70(2):77–85.

[11] Shea MC Jr. Postinflammatory osteogenic fixation of the stapes. Laryngoscope. 1977;87(12):2056–2065.

[12] Asiri S, Hasham A, al Anazy F, Zakzouk S, Banjar A. Tympanosclerosis: review of literature and incidence among patients with middle-ear infection. J Laryngol Otol. 1999;113(12):1076–1080.

[13] Austin DF. Reconstructive techniques for tympanosclerosis. Ann Otol Rhinol Laryngol. 1988;97(6 Pt 1):670–674.

[14] Emmett JR, Shea JJ. Surgical treatment of tympanosclerosis. Laryngoscope. 1978;88(10):1642–1648.

[15] Smyth GD, Patterson CC. Results of middle ear reconstruction: Do patients and surgeons agree? Am J Otol. 1985;6(3):276–279.

[16] Browning GG. Reporting the benefits from middle ear surgery using the Glasgow Benefit Plot. Am J Otol. 1993;14(2):135–140.

[17] Falcone MT, Gajewski BJ, Antonelli PJ. Hearing loss with stapedotomy in otitis media. Otolaryngol Head Neck Surg. 2003;129(6):666–673.

[18] Antonelli PJ, Briggs RD, Gerhardt KJ. Hearing preservation with labyrinthine ablation in otitis media. Laryngoscope. 2000;110(5 Pt 1):779–786.

[19] Lo TM, Zhang M, Young LJ, Antonelli PJ. Hearing loss with stapedotomy and treated otitis media. Otolaryngol Head Neck Surg. 2006;134(4):674–679.

[20] Gluth MB, Motakef S, Friedland PL, Atlas MD. Incus replacement malleostapedotomy in quiescent chronic otitis media with a mobile stapes footplate: an alternative to TORP in select cases. Otol Neurotol. 2011;32(2):242–245.

[21] Merchant SN, McKenna MJ, Mehta RP, Ravicz ME, Rosowski JJ. Middle ear mechanics of Type III tympanoplasty (stapes columella): II. Clinical studies. Otol Neurotol. 2003;24(2):186–194.

[22] Kartush JM. Ossicular chain reconstruction. Capitulum to malleus. Otolaryngol Clin North Am. 1994;27(4):689–715.

[23] Fisch U, May JS, Linder T. Tympanoplasty, Mastoidectomy, and stapes surgery. Thieme. Second edition 2008.

[24] Fisch U. Stapedotomy versus stapedectomy. Am J Otol. 1982;4(2):112–117.

[25] Rambousek A, Schlegel CH, Linder TE. From incus bypass to malleostapedotomy: technical improvements and results. J Laryngol Otol. 2012;126(10):995–1002.

[26] Vincent R, Oates J, Sperling NM, Annamalai S. Malleus relocation in ossicular reconstruction: Managing the anteriorly positioned malleus: Results in a series of 268 cases. Otol Neurotol. 2004;25(3):223–230.

[27] Vincent R, Bittermann AJN, Wenzel G, et al. Ossiculoplasty in missing malleus and stapes patients: Experimental and preliminary clinical results with a new malleus replacement prosthesis with the otology-neurotology database. Otol Neurotol. 2013;34(1):83–90.

[28] Fisch U, May J, Linder T, Naumann IC. A new L-shaped titanium prosthesis for total reconstruction of the ossicular chain. Otol Neurotol. 2004;25(6):891–902.

[29] Beltrame AM, Martini A, Prosser S, Giarbini N, Streitberger C. Coupling the Vibrant Soundbridge to cochlea round window: Auditory results in patients with mixed hearing loss. Otol Neurotol. 2009;30(2):194–201.

[30] Schwab B, Salcher RB, Maier H, Kontorinis G. Oval window membrane vibroplasty for direct acoustic cochlear stimulation: Treating severe mixed hearing loss in challenging middle ears. Otol Neurotol. 2012;33(5):804–809.

[31] Fischer M, Jahnke K. [Local antibiotic administration decreases risk of inner ear damage in effodation] Laryngorhinootologie. 2000;79(12):758–761.

[32] Smyth GD. Tympanosclerosis. J Laryngol Otol. 1972;86(1):9–14.

[33] Kinney SE. Postinflammatory ossicular fixation in tympanoplasty. Laryngoscope. 1978;88(5):821–838.

[34] Albu S, Babighian G, Trabalzini F. Surgical treatment of tympanosclerosis. Am J Otol. 2000;21(5):631–635.

Part 6

Roundtable on Tympanomastoidectomy

32 Overview and Introduction

John L. Dornhoffer and Michael B. Gluth

32.1 Introduction

The evolution of mastoidectomy has been a defining aspect of the development of modern otologic practice (see the historic review in Chapter 33). However, for a procedure that is often referred to as the most fundamental otologic surgical skill, there is surprisingly little clarity regarding how and when mastoidectomy should be applied in the chronic ear. The following roundtable chapters on mastoidectomy will outline the surgical steps involved with canal wall-up (also referred to in the field as intact-canal wall) and canal wall-down mastoidectomy techniques; additionally, there is a chapter on epitympanectomy that is quite relevant to this discussion as some surgeons perform epitympanectomy combined with or in lieu of other mastoidectomy approaches. It should also be noted that hybrid tympanomastoid surgical techniques (Part 7), which combine aspects of canal wall-up and canal wall-down surgery, are also relevant to this discussion; however, before considering these specific surgical techniques, the reader is urged to review this introductory discussion in which various historical indications for mastoidectomy are reviewed.

32.2 Chronic Oto-Mastoiditis

Because the middle ear cleft anatomically communicates with the mastoid air cell system, many cases of chronic suppurative otitis media are considered to be part of a spectrum of chronic oto-mastoiditis. Histopathology seems to support this general concept in that diseased mucosa, osteitis, and micro-abscess formation can be commonly observed in archived temporal bone specimens severely affected by chronic ear disease. Post-obstructive phenomena, such as cholesterol granuloma and air cell effusion, are regularly encountered as well. From a radiologic perspective, severely diseased chronic ears frequently demonstrate evidence of diffuse mastoid air cell opacification and indicators of mastoiditis, even when an ear has been made dry and temporarily stable from a clinical standpoint.

Given these associations, it has been standard practice for many otologic surgeons to perform mastoidectomy as a routine part of surgery intended to eliminate chronic tympanomastoid infection, typically alongside tympanic membrane repair. In fact, failure to thoroughly address mastoid air cell disease has been frequently asserted as a reason for surgical failure in both canal wall-up and canal wall-down scenarios. Some surgeons have even endeavored to identify particular air cell tracts that are most commonly associated with mastoidectomy failure, and many experienced otologists anecdotally recall cases where persistent mastoiditis seemed to have contributed to past surgical failure.[1,2]

Expert opinion and surgical tradition notwithstanding, a critical review of the literature does not appear to support the therapeutic role of mastoidectomy in chronic suppurative otitis media. In 2012, Albu et al. reported results of the only existing statistically powered prospective randomized trial comparing Type I tympanoplasty alone to tympanoplasty with canal wall-up mastoidectomy for ears with non-cholesteatoma chronic suppurative otitis media.[3] In this study, 282 ears that had been actively draining within 6 months prior to surgery were followed for 12 months. No statistically significant benefit was noted from the addition of mastoidectomy with respect to successful tympanic membrane repair or improvement of hearing. Of note, the two treatment arms in this study had been equally stratified according to the Middle Ear Risk Index (MERI), and they were equally matched in terms of perforation size, perforation location, preoperative hearing, age, and gender. In addition to this, in 2013 Eliades and Limb reported results of an exhaustive review and analysis of the existing literature pertaining to therapeutic mastoidectomy in chronic suppurative otitis media, which included 26 articles.[4] Following analysis of this data, they concluded "the available literature shows no additional benefit to performing mastoidectomy with tympanoplasty for uncomplicated tympanic membrane perforations."

Given these findings, it seems most likely that therapeutic mastoidectomy is perhaps useful only in select complicated cases, while the majority of ears appear capable of responding to closure of the middle ear space via tympanoplasty in combination with culture-directed systemic and/or oto-topical antibiotics. Situations where mastoidectomy may yet be possibly beneficial include refractory infection with antimicrobial-resistant pathogens, past surgical failures with radiologic evidence of extensive mastoid disease, or cases that involve an infectious complication, although there is insufficient evidence available to make strong recommendations for any of these indications.

32.3 Counteraction of Negative Middle Ear Pressure

The physiologic role of the mastoid and its air cell system in regulation of tympanomastoid gas pressure is not well understood. Contradictory opinions exist in the literature, with some advocating a vital role of healthy mucosa of the mastoid and epitympanum in maintaining postoperative tympanic gas homeostasis and others suggesting that mucosal gas absorption in these areas is partially responsible for recurrent tympanic membrane retraction and cholesteatoma.[5,6,7,8] In addition to the uncertain role of the mucosa, surgeons have for many years proposed canal wall-up mastoidectomy (with or without posterior tympanotomy) as a means of counteracting negative middle ear pressure. The theory behind this is that by expanding the volume of the tympanomastoid compartment via mastoidectomy, according to Boyle's Law, an effectual "volumetric pressure buffer" can be created that will help resist the acquisition of negative middle ear pressure.[9] This concept has been particularly championed in diseased ears having an underlying hypocellular and sclerotic mastoid, as these may be particularly prone towards selective epitympanic and mastoid dysventilation due to bottlenecked narrowing of the epitympanic diaphragm and aditus ad antrum.

Although the creation of a volumetric pressure buffer is an intellectually satisfying concept, evidence to support therapeutic mastoidectomy for this indication is also lacking to a degree, similar to what has been outlined above for chronic oto-mastoiditis. It is unclear whether this lack of evidence is due to an inherently flawed theory regarding the volumetric pressure buffer effect or if other complexities related to the design and execution of properly controlled clinical trials to test this hypothesis are in play. It also should be mentioned that maintaining patency of these surgically augmented communications between the middle ear and mastoid may be problematic as new bone formation and the development of adhesions may generate blockages.

32.4 Exposure of Cholesteatoma

No textbook on chronic ear disease would be complete without some discussion of the classic debate between canal wall-up mastoidectomy versus canal wall-down mastoidectomy. Although the reader will find opinions regarding the relative and controversial indications for these procedures in each chapter in this roundtable discussion on mastoidectomy, a basic decision-making scheme is depicted in ▶ Fig. 32.1, followed by a few of the editor's general opinions on this controversial topic.

32.4.1 It Is Highly Desirable to Avoid an Open Mastoid Cavity in Children

Canal wall-up mastoidectomy or one of the hybrid techniques that avoid creation of an open cavity is strongly recommended in children, and this can be achieved in the vast majority of cases.[10] Tolerance of the necessary office cleaning and examination is typically quite poor in the pediatric population; however, this ideal should not come at the expense of requiring a child to undergo numerous, repetitive failed closed tympanomastoid surgical procedures. If a surgeon is unable to fully expose and properly remove cholesteatoma without removing the canal wall and has not been trained in any of the hybrid techniques, then canal wall-down surgery must be done, and it must be done properly.

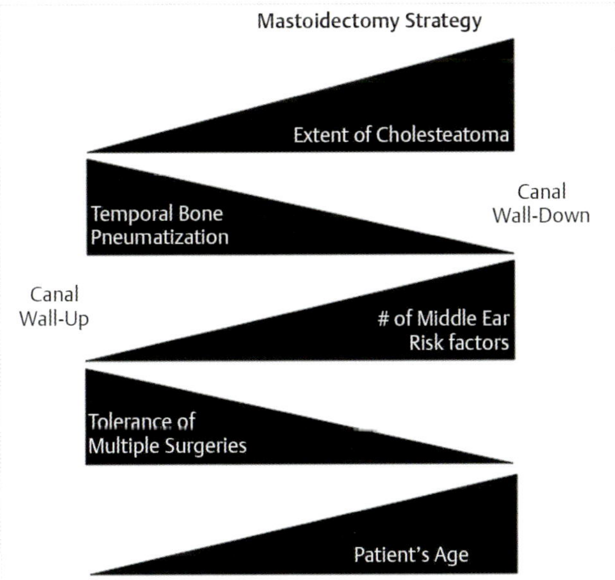

Fig. 32.1 General scheme for mastoidectomy decision-making. Although the decision between canal wall-up and canal wall-down mastoidectomy will vary from surgeon to surgeon, especially with the modern rise of hybrid canal wall reconstruction and mastoid obliteration techniques, a depiction is made of some of the general decision-making trends.

32.4.2 The Two Major Determinants in Deciding Between Canal Wall-Up versus Canal Wall-Down Surgery Should Be the Pneumatization of the Temporal Bone and the Extent of the Cholesteatoma

If the temporal bone is well pneumatized, it is almost always possible to achieve the required exposure with some combination of canal wall-up mastoidectomy, retrograde epitympanectomy, and extended posterior tympanotomy. This is fortunate because the consequences of taking the canal wall down in a pneumatized temporal bone are more substantial. Conversely, in a sclerotic temporal bone, adequate cholesteatoma exposure may be difficult due to anterior displacement of the sigmoid sinus or an extremely low-lying tegmen relative to the superior aspect of the bony external auditory canal wall. Fortunately, the impact of performing canal wall-down surgery in a sclerotic temporal bone should be limited since it is possible to create a small stable cavity that will typically act like an enlarged external auditory canal if properly shaped. In terms of disease extent, small cholesteatomas should almost always be amenable to removal via some type of canal wall-up technique whereas more extensive disease, especially when there is deep penetration into the anterior epitympanic cell, perilabyrinthine cells, supratubal recess, and protympanum, is more likely to require an open technique. The advantage of canal wall–down exposure related to disease in the sinus tympani is highly controversial.

32.4.3 Hearing Outlook Is Always Considered, but it Should Not be the Ultimate Factor that Determines Mastoidectomy Approach

Otologic surgeons commonly counsel patients that the foremost goal of cholesteatoma surgery is NOT to restore hearing, but instead to provide a clean, dry, and safe ear. We would be wise to internalize our own advice and not base the choice of mastoidectomy approach primarily on hearing outlook, for several reasons. First, the status of the canal wall is only one among numerous other factors that impact postoperative hearing. If the outlook for good hearing is already poor based on an abundance of negative middle ear risk factors, jeopardizing the quality of cholesteatoma dissection for purposes of a theoretic hearing benefit is not very sensible. Second, even though the literature suggests that, if all other factors are equal, hearing outcomes tend to be slightly better if the canal wall remains intact, it has also been shown that good hearing results are still possible with canal wall-down surgery if the reconstruction is carefully executed[11] (particularly with canal wall-down hybrid techniques that reconstruct the canal wall). Therefore, it is incorrect to assume that the prospects for good hearing will be abandoned if a canal wall-down approach is undertaken. Lastly, another factor that will impact hearing outcomes is the duration and severity of suppurative otitis media and extent of cholesteatoma insofar as these will result in more extensive damage to the ossicular chain and remodeling of the middle ear cleft when untreated over a long period of time. Thus, hearing benefits achieved by preserving the canal wall are likely forfeited by the collective disadvantage rendered if there is residual cholesteatoma, prolonged middle ear inflammation, and several additional tympanomastoid surgeries.

32.5 Exteriorization of Cholesteatoma

A final proposed indication for mastoidectomy, specifically canal wall-down surgery, is exteriorization of cholesteatoma. The concept here is to render particular areas of the tympanomastoid space heavily involved with cholesteatoma or at high risk for residual disease in continuum with the external auditory canal so that these areas can later be observed and cleaned in the office setting and further surgery can be avoided. Furthermore, by exteriorizing cholesteatoma, the surgeon hopes to avert future risk of developing severe disease-related complications, especially those that can occur within the intracranial compartment.

While otologic surgeons have utilized exteriorization for many years, there are several key aspects of this approach to cholesteatoma that deserve scrutiny. First, canal wall-down mastoidectomy in its most common form involves exteriorization of the mastoid and epitympanum while preserving the remaining portions of the middle ear cleft behind a reconstructed neo-tympanic membrane. Although this approach has the benefit of addressing cholesteatoma concerns in the key epitympanic region, it fails to exteriorize other common problem areas, such as the oval window niche, the sinus tympani, and the protympanum, where residual cholesteatoma is also known to commonly occur. Thus, if these areas are deemed to be at high risk for residual cholesteatoma, second-look surgery may still be required, even though the canal wall has been removed. Furthermore, this most common canal wall-down scenario has, in effect, required the surgeon to opt for the potential downside of an open mastoid cavity (if not obliterated) for the limited benefit of exteriorizing a large mastoid area, where residual cholesteatoma is in fact rarely encountered.

Unfortunately, the remedy to the above-described exteriorization dilemma is costly, as it involves more aggressive canal wall-down surgery. For example, a Type IV or Type V tympanoplasty procedure will exteriorize the round window niche, and a radical mastoidectomy will exteriorize the entire middle ear cleft. However, many surgeons are reluctant to perform aggressive canal wall-down surgeries such as these since both of these options also involve partial or full abandonment of tympano-ossicular reconstruction. In the case of the radical mastoidectomy, chronic accumulation of keratin debris within the resultant numerous, small exteriorized recesses of the middle ear cleft can be a lifetime nuisance.

A second aspect of exteriorization that deserves scrutiny is the notion that exteriorized cholesteatoma is definitively safe, especially when perilymph fistula is present. The case of perilymph fistula in an only-hearing ear has been a classic traditional indication for canal wall-down surgery under the premise that removing cholesteatoma matrix from a sizeable fistula will impart a greater risk to the inner ear than leaving it in place as part of an open cavity. However, the logic and evidence behind this practice is ambiguous. Not only will an exteriorized fistula often cause a high degree of caloric-effect vertigo, but it also places the inner ear at risk of subsequent damage due to suction trauma during requisite cavity cleaning (especially by another surgeon who has not been made aware of the fistula), noxious exposure to infectious and inflammatory elements of an unstable cavity, and potential accumulation of keratin debris within the bone divot that is commonly associated with a large labyrinthine defect. On the other hand, numerous reports now exist in the literature that suggest careful removal of cholesteatoma matrix from an open labyrinth should generally be considered safe, and the level of evidence to support this practice is at least on par with the practice of fistula exteriorization.[12] However, the safety of matrix removal probably depends on the size and location, with smaller fistulae and fistulae that spare the cochlea being best suited for safe dissection. Even if a surgeon opts for a canal wall-down approach, removal of matrix affords the ability to seal the fistula with a protective barrier, and if this is done carefully, preservation should be the expected outcome, similar to what has been reported with semicircular canal occlusion for other indications.

References

[1] Nadol JB Jr. Causes of failure of mastoidectomy for chronic otitis media. Laryngoscope. 1985;95(4):410–413.
[2] Pillsbury HC III Carrasco VN. Revision mastoidectomy. Arch Otolaryngol Head Neck Surg. 1990;116(9):1019–1022.
[3] Albu S, Trabalzini F, Amadori M. Usefulness of cortical mastoidectomy in myringoplasty. Otol Neurotol. 2012;33(4):604–609.
[4] Eliades SJ, Limb CJ. The role of mastoidectomy in outcomes following tympanic membrane repair: a review. Laryngoscope. 2013;123(7):1787–1802.
[5] Doyle WJ. The mastoid as a functional rate-limiter of middle ear pressure change. Int J Pediatr Otorhinolaryngol. 2007;71(3):393–402.
[6] Takahashi H, Honjo I, Naito Y, et al. Gas exchange function through the mastoid mucosa in ears after surgery. Laryngoscope. 1997;107(8):1117–1121.
[7] Magnuson B. Functions of the mastoid cell system: auto-regulation of temperature and gas pressure. J Laryngol Otol. 2003;117(2):99–103.
[8] Gantz BJ, Wilkinson EP, Hansen MR. Canal wall reconstruction tympanomastoidectomy with mastoid obliteration. Laryngoscope. 2005;115(10):1734–1740.
[9] Cinamon U, Sadé J. Mastoid and tympanic membrane as pressure buffers: A quantitative study in a middle ear cleft model. Otol Neurotol. 2003;24(6):839–842.
[10] Dornhoffer JL, Friedman AB, Gluth MB. Management of acquired cholesteatoma in the pediatric population. Curr Opin Otolaryngol Head Neck Surg. 2013;21(5):440–445.
[11] Berenholz LP, Rizer FM, Burkey JM, Schuring AG, Lippy WH. Ossiculoplasty in canal wall down mastoidectomy. Otolaryngol Head Neck Surg. 2000;123(1 Pt 1):30–33.
[12] Copeland BJ, Buchman CA. Management of labyrinthine fistulae in chronic ear surgery. Am J Otolaryngol. 2003;24(1):51–60.

33 Canal Wall-Up Techniques

Maroun T. Semaan, Cameron C. Wick, and Cliff A. Megerian

Abbreviations used in this chapter:

CT: computed tomography
CWD: canal wall-down
CWU: canal wall-up
ICW: intact-canal wall

33.1 Introduction

Variations of the mastoidectomy procedure are a prerequisite for the management of chronic ear disease. The canal wall-up (CWU, also known as intact-canal wall [ICW] or combined approach) mastoidectomy has been the mainstay of chronic ear management for the last 50 years. The CWU mastoidectomy preserves the posterior bony canal and reconstructs any canal defects with cartilage or autologous bone grafts. Historically, the CWU mastoidectomy accounts for 70% of mastoidectomy procedures performed for chronic ear disease.[1,2] This proportion is even higher in children with cholesteatoma.[3,4,5]

For centuries the role of mastoidectomy was limited to decompression for acute mastoiditis. The 18th century French surgeon Jean-Louis Petit (1674–1750) documented multiple mastoid trephinations in which he actively sought purulence before the infection developed its fatal intracranial sequelae.[6,7] Over the next 100 years, the operation was fraught with mixed results, often from questionable surgical indications and lack of specific technique. Anton Fredrich von Tröltsch (1829–1890) critically reviewed patient selection and laid the foundation for his protégée, Hermann Schwartze (1837–1910), to describe the surgical steps of a simple mastoidectomy with antrostomy.[6,8]

The "Schwartze" mastoidectomy sufficed for acute mastoiditis, but more extensive pneumatization was necessary for management of chronic ear disorders. Emanuel Zaufal (1837–1910) and Ludwig Stacke (1859–1918) in the 1890s introduced the radical mastoidectomy.[6,9] This technique and its demolition of the middle ear space left many patients with worse hearing and persistent otorrhea. Gustave Bondy (1870–1954) in 1910 popularized the modified radical mastoidectomy.[6,10] Bondy's insight that attic cholesteatomas could be exteriorized while preserving the ossicles and the pars tensa was a breakthrough in hearing preservation.

The radical and modified radical mastoidectomies were the mainstay of otologic surgery until the introduction of the otologic microscope and tympanoplasty techniques by Horst Wullstein (1906–1987) and F. Zollner in the 1950s.[11,12] Still, problems with reduced middle ear space and a damp environment often led to graft failure and poor hearing. This prompted William House (1923–2012), James Sheehy (1926–2006), and others to develop a procedure that preserved the natural position of the tympanic membrane and avoided the morbidity of a mastoid cavity. In 1963 the importance of an intact canal wall, development of the facial recess approach, and use of plastic sheeting to control adhesions led to the modern CWU mastoidectomy that remains largely unchanged today.[13]

33.2 Patient Selection

The most common indication for CWU mastoidectomy is management of chronic otitis media with or without cholesteatoma. The additional steps of opening the facial recess, extended facial recess, or lateral epitympanotomy allow disease to be eradicated from much of the mastoid and middle ear spaces. Whereas the decision to keep the canal wall intact often necessitates a "second look" on account of a higher recidivism rate, the benefit of less perioperative complications, less long-term maintenance, and improved hearing results are significant.[2,14,15,16] Additionally, the CWU method has been the procedure of choice for children to avoid the life-long morbidity of an open cavity.[4]

Access to the round window via the facial recess makes the CWU mastoidectomy an intricate part of cochlear implantation. Skeletonization of the vertical segment of the facial nerve, tegmen mastoideum, and tegmen tympani may facilitate repair of a facial nerve injury or encephalocele.[16,17] Mastoidectomy has been used for tympanoplasty with the notion that a well-aerated mastoid cavity will improve graft viability and hearing results. Recent reviews have not supported a global improvement in tympanoplasty results with mastoidectomy.[18] The senior authors still include a mastoidectomy as part of the tympanoplasty if the ear is fraught with chronic disease or otorrhea or if there is concern for cholesteatoma.

When House, Sheehy, and others first described the CWU mastoidectomy, they did so with the understanding that an obligatory second procedure 6–12 months after the original operation, termed a "second-look" procedure, would be performed. This second operation may be performed via either the transcanal or postauricular approach, often based on the extent of disease found at the original surgery. Multiple reports have indicated that cholesteatoma is not infrequently left in the mastoid cavity or along the tegmen, which cannot be accessed or inspected through the transcanal approach.[5,19] Therefore, at our institution we regularly utilize the postauricular approach for its ability to recognize persistent disease in the mastoid and epitympanum. Furthermore, an extended facial recess approach affords the possibility of performing ossiculoplasty through the recess without necessitating canal incisions.

Even with sound surgical technique, sometimes the extent of disease or patient anatomy is not amenable to the CWU approach. Clinical scenarios requiring a canal wall-down (CWD) procedure include extensive canal wall destruction from the disease process, a far anterior sigmoid sinus, low-lying tegmen, or severely sclerotic bone, all of which can limit exposure of the epitympanum to access disease in the anterior supralabyrinthine/supratubal area. Other considerations for a CWD mastoidectomy are patients at high risk of perioperative anesthetic morbidity, disease in the only-hearing ear, persistent disease overlying a labyrinthine fistula, and patient refusal to undergo a second-look procedure.

Like all mastoidectomy procedures the goals of surgery in order of importance are to (1) extirpate all disease, (2) create a dry/safe ear, and (3) preserve/restore hearing.[4,5,20,21]

Pearls and Pitfalls

- Mastoidectomy Goals: disease extirpation, creation of a dry/safe ear, hearing preservation/restoration by maintaining an air-containing mucosa-lined middle ear space.
- CWU Indications: chronic otitis media with or without cholesteatoma, second-look procedures with or without ossiculoplasty, middle ear access via the facial recess (i.e., cochlear implantation), treatment of tympanic and jugulotympanic paragangliomas if a limited excision is planned. Two-stage procedures are indicated with extensive mucosal disruption requiring placement of Silastic sheeting (mucosal disease), uncertainty of cholesteatoma removal (residual disease), and a fixed stapes (ossicular disease).
- CWU Contraindications: extensive disease, only-hearing ear, unfavorable anatomy, unreconstructible bony canal defect, persistent disease overlying a labyrinthine fistula, patient refusal to follow-up or undergo a second-look procedure.

33.3 Preoperative Evaluation

Preoperative evaluation begins with a thorough examination of the head and neck and includes use of an otomicroscope to identify ear pathology. Active infection should be treated, reserving cultures only for recalcitrant cases. Particular attention should be paid to the health of the paranasal sinuses and Eustachian tube function. Management of comorbid conditions should be addressed. Patients are counseled on smoking cessation, which includes a frank discussion on poorer tympanoplasty results, a five-time increase in postoperative complications, and a higher recurrence rate.[22,23] Non-contrasted, high-resolution computed tomography (CT) of the temporal bone is not required for every case but may be of particular value for revision cases, severe disease, and craniofacial abnormalities, or when there is concern for labyrinthine fistula. Further considerations related to the management of chronic suppurative otitis media in the office setting are covered in Chapter 16.

33.4 Surgical Technique

33.4.1 Canal Incisions

For cases that necessitate elevation of the tympanic membrane and/or tympanoplasty, the procedure begins with preparation of the external auditory canal. With an otomicroscope, an ear speculum is placed and the canal is injected with a mixture of local anesthetic and a vasoconstrictive agent in a slow, steady manner to avoid blebs and hematomas. Using a round knife or a Rosen knife, the medial canal cut is made from 12 o'clock to 6 o'clock approximately 2–4 mm lateral and parallel to the annulus. Using a sickle knife or Beaver blade, the medial incision is extended laterally out to the bony-cartilaginous junction, facilitating the later folding of the canal skin. If a total drum replacement is anticipated (onlay or lateral graft tympanoplasty), then the medial cut is omitted. The anterior canal skin is removed and an anterior canalplasty is completed. This exposes the anterior tympanomeatal angle and creates a bony shelf that supports the onlay graft.

33.4.2 Postauricular Incision

A curvilinear incision is made just posterior to the postauricular sulcus, from the superior helical root to the mastoid tip. In children the incision may be stopped short of the mastoid tip to avoid an aberrantly superficial facial nerve. In a supraperiosteal plane, tissue is elevated anteriorly toward the external auditory canal.

A self-retaining retractor is placed at the superior aspect and elevated to splay the loose areolar tissue of the temporalis fascia. A scalpel dissects through the loose areolar tissue until the temporal fascia is identified. An appropriately sized piece of this fascia is elevated off of the temporalis muscle and excised with scissors in preparation for tympanic membrane reconstruction. A 1-cm strip of temporal fascia at the inferior aspect of the muscle is preserved to facilitate closure. The harvested fascia is prepped on the back table and allowed to dry for later tympanoplasty. In the absence of adequate temporalis fascia, tragal perichondrium, false fascia, and even acellular dermal implants (e.g., Alloderm, LifeCell, New Jersey) can be used for reconstruction.

The mastoid periosteum is incised in an inverted 7 or C-shaped anteriorly based flap. The flap extends from the linea temporalis superiorly to the mastoid tip inferiorly. Using a periosteal elevator, the temporalis muscle is elevated to expose the linea temporalis. Additional surface landmarks, such as the spine of Henle and Macewen's triangle, are appreciated as the bony canal is approached. With the ear retracted anteriorly, the posterior canal skin is delicately raised and the canal cuts are identified. The vascular strip is secured behind a self-retaining retractor. The mastoid cortex, posterior bony canal wall, and tympanic membrane are now in view (▶ Fig. 33.1). In revision cases, caution and palpation are advised at all steps to detect dehiscences of the sigmoid sinus, dura, or facial nerve.

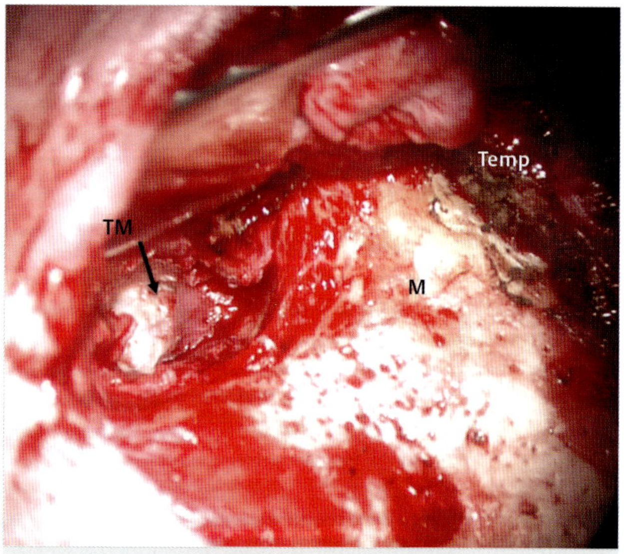

Fig. 33.1 Soft tissue elevation. After canal incisions, elevation of the periosteal flap, and retraction of the vascular strip, the surface landmarks of the mastoid and the tympanic membrane are exposed. M, mastoid; Temp, temporalis muscle; TM, tympanic membrane.

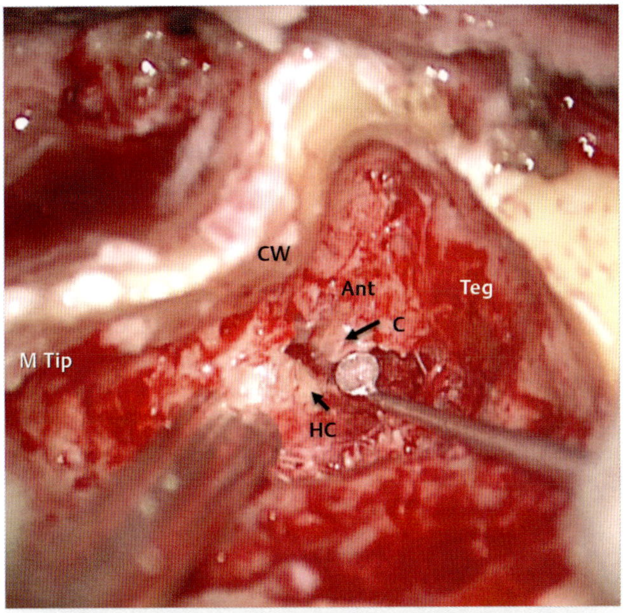

Fig. 33.2 CWU mastoidectomy. At completion of the mastoidectomy the antrum should be opened and the posterior canal wall, tegmen, horizontal semicircular canal, and sigmoid sinus well defined. Cholesteatoma is visible in the antrum. Ant, antrum; C, cholesteatoma; CW, canal wall; HC, horizontal semicircular canal; M tip, mastoid tip; Teg, tegmen.

33.4.3 Complete Mastoidectomy

Dissection of the cortical surface of the mastoid begins with a large cutting burr. The first cut begins at the zygomatic root and extends posteriorly along the linea temporalis to the sinodural angle. The second cut is perpendicular to the first cut and defines the posterior canal wall. It begins at the zygomatic root and extends inferiorly to the mastoid tip. The third cut connects the previous two with a line from the mastoid tip to the sinodural angle. This creates a triangle with an island of cortical bone that can be quickly removed. The apex of the triangle (anterior-superior direction) is the spine of Henle, which approximates the underlying horizontal semicircular canal and antrum.

The mastoid cavity is then systematically enlarged with progressive saucerization and identification of underlying structures. The deepest portion of the dissection is always anterior-superior to facilitate opening of the antrum and identification of the horizontal semicircular canal. To open the antrum, Körner's septum (a remnant of the petrosquamous suture line) must be removed, which leads to a central mastoid air cell and the underlying dense otic capsule bone. Once the antrum has been opened, the tegmen and sigmoid sinus are better defined. Care must be taken when defining these structures because there is wide variation in tegmen height, position of the sigmoid sinus, and pneumatization of the mastoid cavity. The cells lateral to the horizontal canal and inferior to the mastoid tip can be removed (▶ Fig. 33.2). Anatomical knowledge of the vertical portion of the facial nerve is critical to gauge the amount of bone removal. The surgeon should be aware that the vertical segment travels in a more lateral position as the nerve approximates the stylomastoid foramen.

Exposure of the antrum is facilitated by aggressively thinning the posterior canal wall and exenteration of the zygomatic root. At the conclusion of these steps, the antrum should be opened, allowing identification of the horizontal canal and short process of the incus. Care must be taken to avoid drilling on the incus. Primary acquired cholesteatoma often extends posteriorly towards the antrum and may extensively involve the mastoid, obliterating the view of the typical mastoid landmarks. The astute surgeon should be mindful of a horizontal canal fistula and avoid manipulation of the incus unless incudostapedial separation has been confirmed. Often, matrix is left overlying the fistula and removal is deferred until the completion of the cholesteatoma removal to avoid inadvertent penetration or injury to the endosteum. After removal of the matrix, or should the endosteum be violated, avoiding suctioning and promptly covering the fistula with a piece of fascia will protect the inner ear neuroepithelial structures.

33.4.4 Facial Recess (Posterior Tympanotomy)

Access to the middle ear from the mastoid is dependent on proper opening of the facial recess and is an essential component of the CWU approach. The facial recess is an inverted triangle defined superiorly by bone of the fossa incudis, posterior-medially by the facial nerve, anterior-laterally by the chorda tympani, and inferiorly by the takeoff of the chorda tympani from the facial nerve. At times, an air cell tract in this recess extends parallel to the vertical segment of the facial nerve.

Opening of the facial recess begins with recognition of the previously noted landmarks. Drilling of the recess starts, typically with a 2-mm diameter diamond burr, at the superior portion, where a ligament extending from the short process of the incus may be identified. The short process of the incus "points" to the expected opening of the facial recess. Continuous irrigation avoids charring of bone and thermal injury to the nerve. A small strip of bone overlying the short process of the incus, termed the incus buttress, is preserved to protect inadvertent contact between the drill and ossicles, which may cause unnecessary labyrinthine trauma and sensorineural hearing loss. With the incus buttress defined, the course of the facial nerve can be better appreciated as the second genu of the nerve is located inferior and medial to the horizontal semicircular canal. Appropriate thinning of the posterior canal wall is critical for this to occur. The chorda tympani lies immediately beneath the annular ligament. In the diseased ear, cholesteatoma may invade the facial recess and extend towards the sinus tympani and round window niche. Elevation of the dome of the cholesteatoma (or retraction pocket) allows identification of the incudostapedial joint (▶ Fig. 33.3). If incus removal is planned or necessary, separation of the joint protects the inner ear structures from mechanical injury while manipulating the disease or removing the incus to expose the epitympanum. Removal of the incus allows exposure of the malleus and posterior epitympanum.

33.4.5 Extended Facial Recess

If the dome of the cholesteatoma extends inferiorly beyond the chorda tympani, or the chorda tympani is resected during

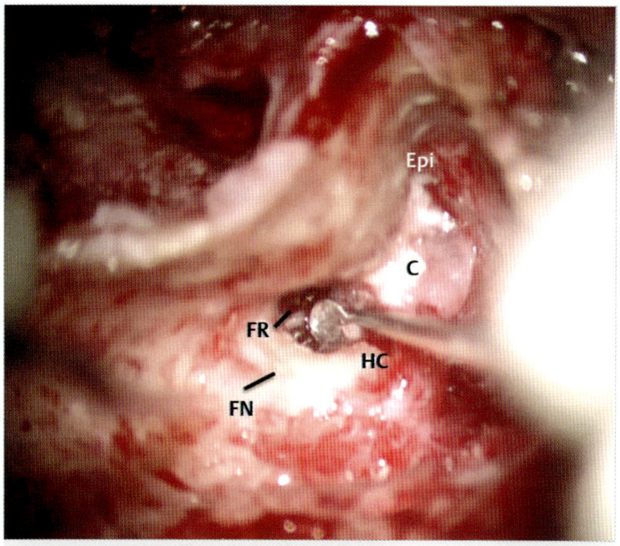

Fig. 33.3 Facial recess. The facial recess is opened to expose the mesotympanum. A Rosen knife introduced through the facial recess demonstrates elevation of the dome of the cholesteatoma from the stapes superstructure. C, cholesteatoma; Epi, epitympanum; FN, facial nerve; FR, facial recess; HC, horizontal semicircular canal.

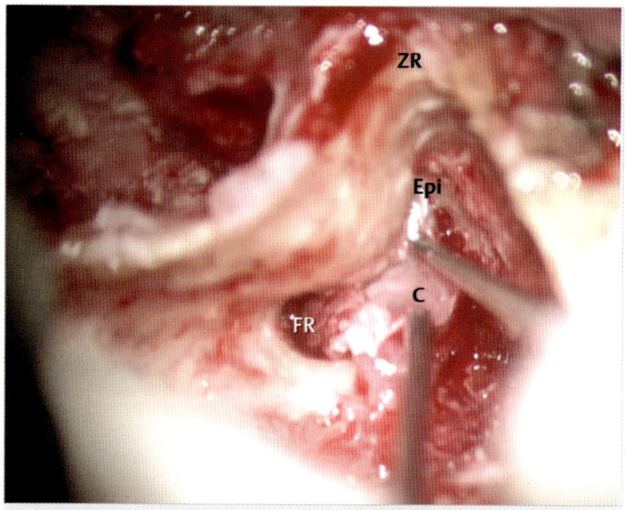

Fig. 33.4 Lateral epitympanotomy. Removal of the incus and malleus head along with resection of the zygomatic root and thinning of the superior canal wall opens the epitympanum and allows further cholesteatoma resection. C, cholesteatoma; Epi, epitympanum; FR, facial recess; ZR, zygomatic root.

middle ear work, extending the facial recess by sacrificing the chorda tympani (extended facial recess approach) provides an improved view of the mesotympanum, in particular, the round window niche area, the hypotympanum, and the uppermost aspect of the sinus tympani. Newer endoscopic techniques may also benefit from the increased exposure.[24] This approach is best suited for cholesteatoma with posterior-inferior extension towards the facial recess and sinus tympani area but may also be applied to other benign middle ear pathology, like glomus tympanicum, glomus jugulare, or adenomas.[25]

33.4.6 Epitympanic Approaches (Lateral Epitympanotomy)

To expose the epitympanum the antrum is fully opened by aggressively thinning the superior canal wall and resecting the zygomatic root (▶ Fig. 33.4). Bone lateral to the epitympanum is gradually removed using small diamond burrs. Care is taken to avoid drilling on an intact ossicular chain or violating the tegmen plate. The skull base may gradually drop as dissection is carried anteriorly, resulting in a narrower dissection. For complete exposure of the epitympanum, the incus is discarded after separation of the incudostapedial joint, and the malleus head is removed with a malleus head nipper. Drilling may continue far anterior until the temporomandibular joint capsule is encountered and skeletonized. Removal of the cog, a bony overhang from the tegmen tympani that separates the epitympanum into anterior and posterior compartments, exposes the anterior epitympanum and supratubal recess area. Due to cholesteatomas's proclivity for retraction into the anterior epitympanum, it is essential to expose this space as omission of this step often leads to persistent disease. The retraction pocket often causes destruction of the superior bony canal (attic) (▶ Fig. 33.5).

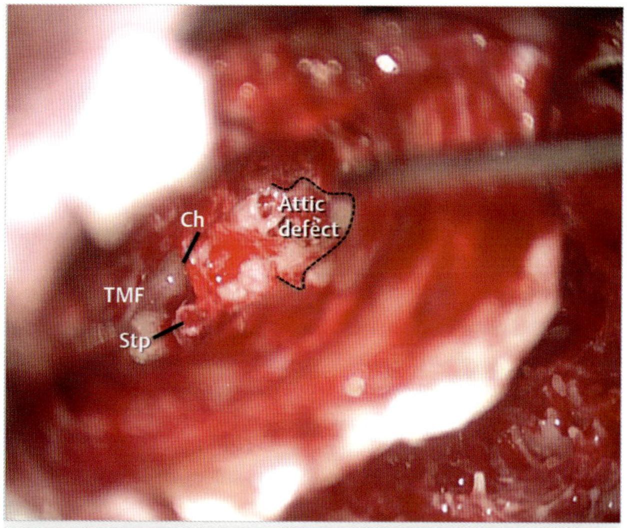

Fig. 33.5 Canal defect. The posterior canal wall remains intact while the tympanic membrane is elevated to reveal a bony defect in the superior canal (attic). Ch, chorda tympani; Stp, stapes; TMF, temporalis muscle fascia.

The extended facial recess and lateral epitympanotomy approaches have enabled the CWU mastoidectomy to reach nearly all aspects of the epitympanum, mesotympanum, and hypotympanum (▶ Fig. 33.6). With this increased exposure, the surgeon is offered a greater chance at complete disease resection while preserving the canal wall (▶ Fig. 33.7).

33.5 Closure and Postoperative Care

The fascia graft with or without ear cartilage is used to perform a tympanoplasty (▶ Fig. 33.8; ▶ Fig. 33.9). The vascular strip and ear canal skin are repositioned, and the canal is packed (▶ Fig. 33.10). The periosteum is closed in a water-tight fashion,

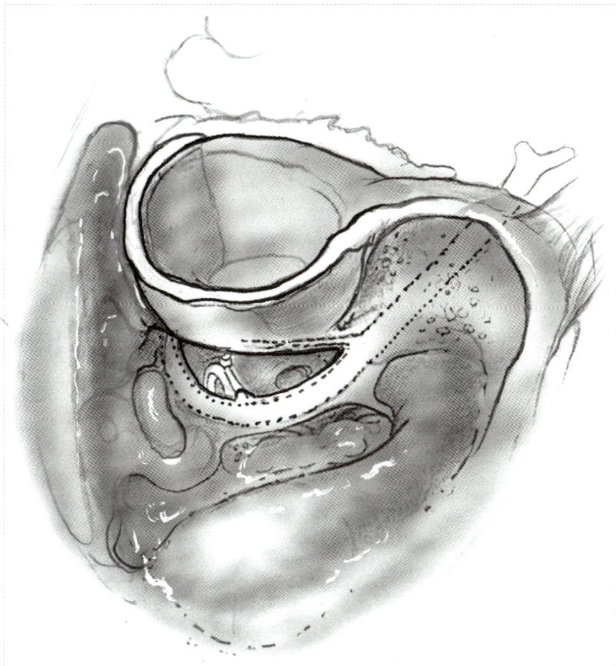

Fig. 33.6 CWU mastoidectomy with posterior tympanotomy. This figure demonstrates the full extent of posterior exposure provided with CWU mastoid surgery. Posterior access such as this is coupled with a transcanal view to afford a "combined approach" tympanomastoidectomy. A posterior tympanotomy is created by opening the facial recess and by identifying the mastoid segment of the facial nerve distal to its second genu. The incus bone and the incus buttress have been removed. The malleus head has been amputated. The tegmen tympani is skeletonized with eggshell-thin bone as drilling is extended far anterior into the zygomatic root toexpose the anterior epitympanum and entrance into the supratubal recess.

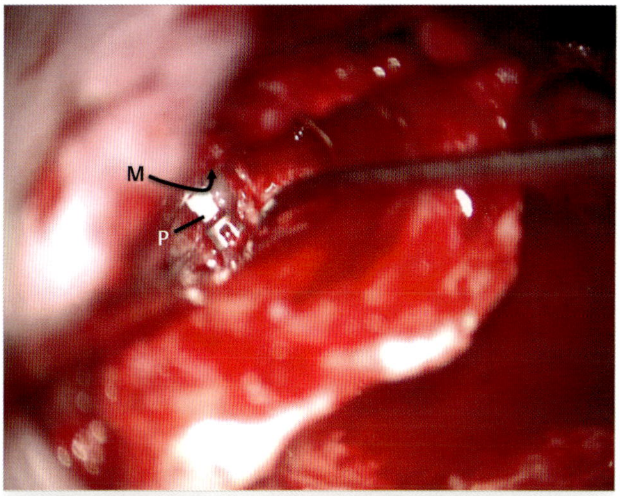

Fig. 33.7 Primary ossiculoplasty. With an intact canal wall, if the middle ear is disease-free, then ossicular chain reconstruction may be attempted even at the time of the initial cholesteatoma resection. Pictured is an elevated tympanic membrane through which an Alto Wedge prosthesis (Grace Medical, Memphis, Tennessee) has been placed to span the manubrium of the malleus to the capitulum of the stapes. M, manubrium; P, prosthesis.

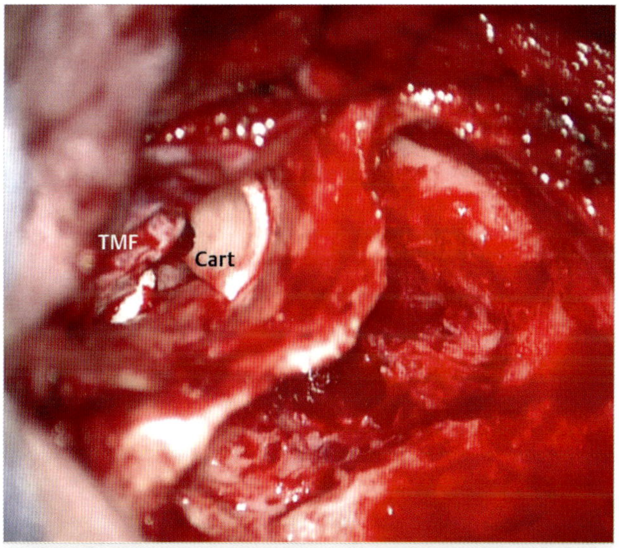

Fig. 33.8 Canal defect reconstruction. Conchal cartilage spans the attic defect. This improves the strength of the tympanoplasty, which prevents retraction pockets and decreases recurrent cholesteatoma. Cart, cartilage; TMF, temporalis muscle fascia.

followed by a subcutaneous closure of the postauricular incision. Adhesive strips, a cotton-ball, and a mastoid dressing are applied. The procedure is by and large performed on an outpatient basis. Postoperative management and surveillance are similar to other mastoidectomies or otologic procedures.

33.6 Complications

Complications are an unfortunate inevitability when performing surgery, but diligent technique and forthright preoperative counseling can limit the physical and emotional impact that they cause. Mastoidectomy risks include: anesthesia; bleeding; infection; ear numbness; dizziness; otorrhea; hearing loss; tinnitus; temporomandibular joint pain; vascular injury; taste disturbance; and facial nerve and dural injury. A few selected complications are discussed below, but most serious complications are less than 1%.[26]

33.6.1 Facial Nerve Injury

A thorough understanding of the course of the facial nerve through the temporal bone is a requisite of any otologic surgeon, and the many important relationships between the nerve and temporal bone landmarks have previously been described.[5,27] Revision cases, extensive disease, and patients with congenital anomalies are particularly challenging, but the astute surgeon should always be mindful of an unanticipated aberrant course or dehiscence.[28] The horizontal segment as it approaches the second genu is the most common site of iatrogenic injury (55%), followed by the vertical segment (32%).[29] A common error for novice or infrequent mastoid surgeons during a CWU mastoidectomy is to skeletonize the middle fossa insufficiently. This error can lead to approaching the antrum via an inferior trajectory that places the second genu of the facial nerve and horizontal semicircular canal at risk.

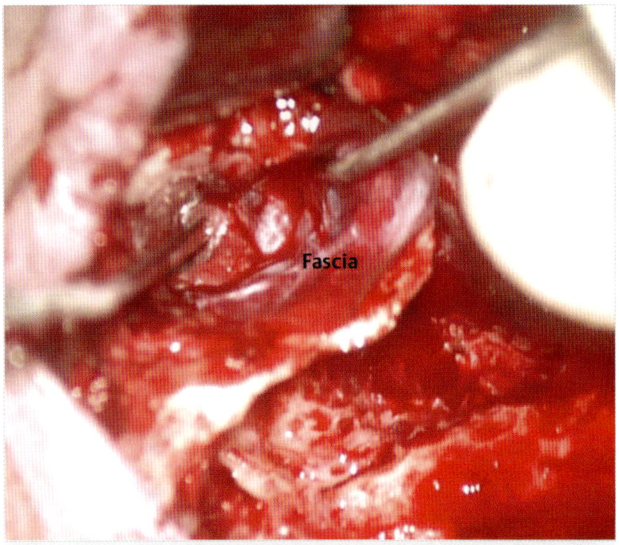

Fig. 33.9 Tympanoplasty. Temporalis muscle fascia is draped over the reconstructed attic defect and intact bony canal wall.

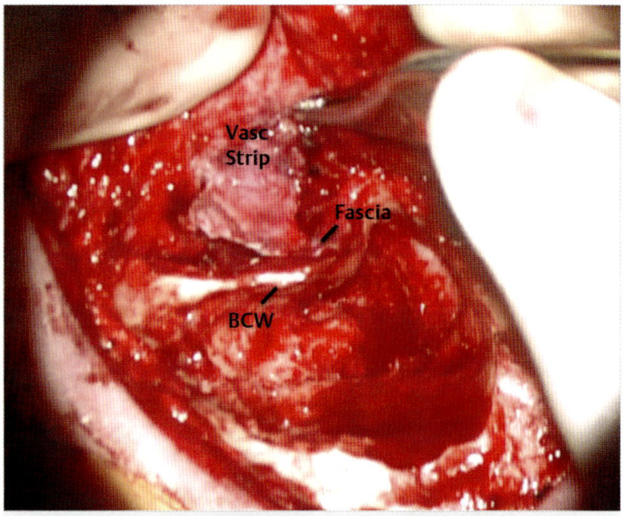

Fig. 33.10 Closure. The vascular strip is repositioned in the canal, taking care not to invert any epithelial edges. The vascular strip overlies the fascia securing it to the canal. BCW, bony canal wall; Vasc Strip, vascular strip.

33.6.2 Hearing Loss

There are multiple etiologies of hearing loss after mastoidectomy. The need to remove ossicles creates an obvious conductive hearing loss, but other factors, such as middle ear adhesions, tympanic membrane perforation, middle ear effusion, and failed ossiculoplasty, may also contribute. The greatest risk of sensorineural hearing loss comes from drilling on the ossicular chain or removal of cholesteatoma overlying a labyrinthine fistula. Maintaining an intact incus buttress or disarticulating the incudostapedial joint protects the cochlea against incidental drill contact. Patients with cholesteatoma have a 10% risk of labyrinthine fistula formation, with the horizontal canal being the most commonly affected.[30] Fistulas into the cochlea may also exist and carry a significantly higher rate of sensorineural hearing loss (35% versus 3%).[5,30,31,32]

33.6.3 Canal Defects

Defects of the bony canal wall can be attributed to pathologic or iatrogenic etiologies, both of which may jeopardize the advantages of an intact wall. Full-thickness bony defects should be repaired, particularly if the defect is greater than 5 mm.[4] Cholesteatoma-induced osteolysis can be attributed to pressure necrosis and enzymatic dissolution from cytokine-induced inflammation, particularly matrix metalloproteinases.[33] Cholesteatoma has a propensity for scutum destruction (anterior epitympanum) but may also erode through other canal wall locations. Retrospective studies have demonstrated bony canal erosion in 60% of first-stage CWU procedures, the majority of which were at the scutum (87%).[34] We typically repair both pathologic and iatrogenic canal defects with conchal or tragal cartilage. Other methods of reconstruction with bone pate, temporalis fascia, and titanium mesh have also been advocated.[35,36]

If the canal wall bone is rendered too thin or is subjected to excessive burning by the drill, there is a risk of delayed canal wall bone atrophy. This phenomenon has been recognized in 4.8% to18% of CWU cases and may occur with or without the presence of recurrent cholesteatoma.[37,38] The clinical significance of delayed canal wall atrophy varies depending on the size of the defect and whether a retraction pocket forms. Specific assessment of the posterior canal wall should be part of the postoperative otologic surveillance, otherwise this complication can be missed.

33.7 Outcomes

Generally, there are two reasons for failure: recurrent disease and residual disease. Residual, or persistent, disease is defined by residual epithelial cells in the middle ear cleft that lead to formation of a cholesteatoma. En-bloc resection without disruption of the cholesteatoma sac ensures complete removal. However, in extensive disease an en-block resection is often not possible. In some series, up to 75% of CWU tympanomastoidectomies performed for the treatment of active chronic otitis media with cholesteatoma are staged for mucosal or "residual" reasons. In addition, 10% to 15% of CWU procedures performed for active chronic otitis media without cholesteatoma are staged for "mucosal" reasons. Recurrent disease is defined by the recurrence of the anatomical condition that leads to the cholesteatoma formation. Use of cartilage tympanoplasty and careful reconstruction of attic and canal wall defects helps avoid recurrence of the retraction pocket. In addition, addressing causes of Eustachian tube dysfunction (allergies, adenoidal hypertrophy, etc.) decreases recurrence. Tympanostomy tube placement may have a role.

Placement of a thick silicone sheeting in the middle ear avoids adhesion formation and improves the likelihood of maintaining an air-containing mucosa-lined middle ear space. The later is a *sine qua none* for optimal hearing restoration. A silicone sheet, introduced through the facial recess between the stapes and tympanic graft, creates a separation and prevents the formation of middle ear adhesions (▶ Fig. 33.11). In addition, the silicone sheeting provides protective coverage of important structures (dehiscent facial nerve) and may serve as a temporary stapes columella, resulting in some hearing improvement (▶ Fig. 33.12). If disease is cleared at the second-look operation, an ossiculoplasty through the extended facial recess can be performed (▶ Fig. 33.13). This avoids canal cuts and their associated delayed healing and complications.

Recidivism is the tendency to relapse into a previous condition; in this context it incorporates both recurrent and residual disease. Cholesteatoma management is compared with the CWD recidivism rate of 5% to 15%.[2,15,21] After the first stage of a CWU mastoidectomy, a recidivism rate of 15% to 35% is anticipated.[2,13,15,36] Disease can be found in a variety of locations but frequently persists along the tegmen, epitympanum, or sinus tympani.[2,15,19] Analyses of recurrent disease have asserted that residual diseased air cells at the sinodural angle and tegmen to be of particular importance.[19,39] This is why the senior authors often use a postauricular approach for the second-look surgery so that the entire mastoid cavity can be reexamined. Recidivism rates after the second CWU operation frequently drop to 3.2%to 8.4%.[2,13,15]

A factor for the reduced recidivism rate of the CWD approach may be the ease of disease removal from areas like the sinus tympani. Maneuvers such as opening the facial recess, an extended facial recess, or release of the scutum often provide adequate visualization of disease in the mesotympanum and hypotympanum, but the narrow corridors may make instrumentation more difficult. The additional use of endoscopes may also complement visualization during a CWU mastoidectomy.

Hearing results have consistently been superior with CWU compared with CWD procedures.[40,41,42] Although not the primary goal of operating on a chronically diseased ear, this does significantly impact the patient's quality of life. A long-term air-bone gap of less than 20 dB was seen in 59% of CWU compared with 45.7% of CWD mastoidectomies.[41,42] Improved hearing can be expected when the stapes and malleus handle are intact.[41]

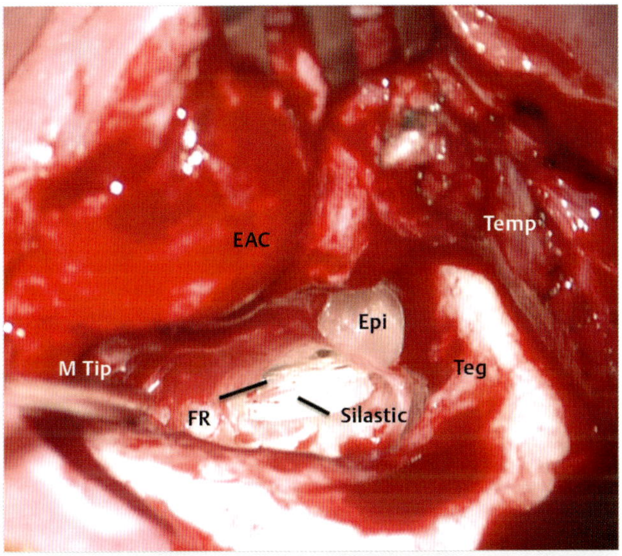

Fig. 33.11 Silicone sheeting. If extensive middle ear disease is present, silicone sheeting placed through the facial recess can prevent adhesions and allow better healing of the neo-tympanic membrane and/or canal defect reconstruction. Pictured is a piece of Silastic (Dow Corning, Midland, Michigan) in the facial recess. EAC, external auditory canal; Epi, epitympanum; FR, facial recess; Temp, temporalis muscle; Teg, tegmen; M Tip, mastoid tip.

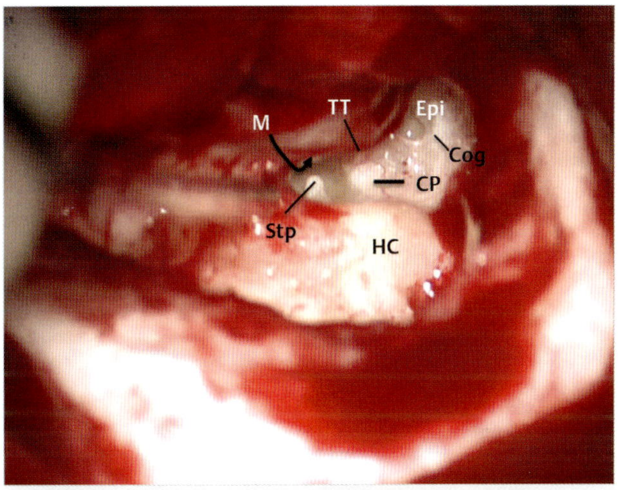

Fig. 33.12 Postauricular approach for a second-look surgery. The postauricular approach can be used for second-look procedures. It has the advantage of identifying residual cholesteatoma along the tegmen or in the mastoid cavity. CP, cochleariform process; Epi, epitympanum; HC, horizontal semicircular canal; M, malleus; Stp, stapes; TT, tensor tympani; Cog, cog, divides the epitympanum into anterior and posterior divisions.

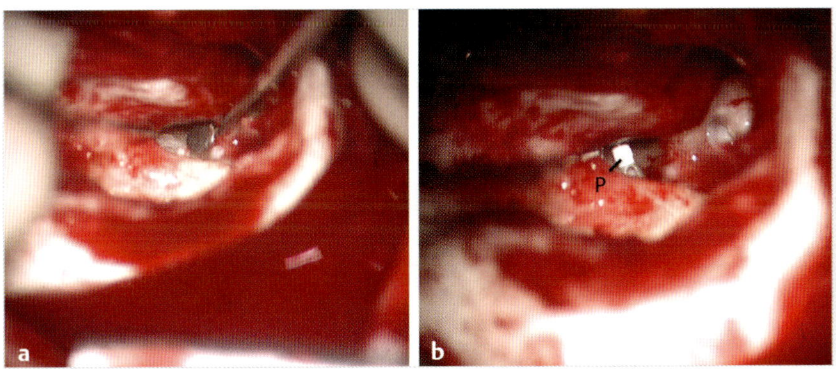

Fig. 33.13 Ossiculoplasty via facial recess. Ossicular reconstruction can be performed through the facial recess. If done at the time of a second-look procedure, it may prevent the need for making a canal incision and elevation of the tympanic membrane. (a) A Rosen knife is used to measure the distance between the manubrium of the malleus and the capitulum of the stapes. (b) An Alto Wedge prosthesis (Grace Medical, Memphis, Tennessee), seen through the facial recess, reconstructs the ossicular chain. P, prosthesis.

References

[1] Sheehy JL, Robinson JV Cholesteatoma Surgery at the Otologic Medical Group. Cholesteatoma surgery at the otologic medical group: Residual and recurrent disease. A report on 307 revision operations. Am J Otol. 1982;3(3):209–215.

[2] Syms MJ, Luxford WM. Management of cholesteatoma: Status of the canal wall. Laryngoscope. 2003;113(3):443–448.

[3] Committee on Conservation of Hearing of the American Academy of Ophthalmology and Otolaryngology. Standard Classification for Surgery of Chronic Ear Infection. Arch Otolaryngol Head Neck Surg. 1965;81:204–205.

[4] Bennett M, Warren F, Haynes D. Indications and technique in mastoidectomy. Otolaryngol Clin North Am. 2006;39(6):1095–1113.

[5] Syms CA, Syms MJ, Sheehy JL. Mastoidectomy – Intact Canal Wall Procedure. In: Brackmann D.E., Shelton C., Arriaga M.A. Otologic Surgery, 3rd Ed. Philadelphia, PA: Elsevier; 2010:195–207.

[6] Sunder S, Jackler RK, Blevins NH. Virtuosity with the Mallet and Gouge: the brilliant triumph of the "modern" mastoid operation. Otolaryngol Clin North Am. 2006;39(6):1191–1210.

[7] Petit J-L. Traité des maladies chirurgicales, et des operations qui leur conviennent. Nouv. Edition. Paris: 1790.

[8] Schwartze H, Eysell C. Uber die kunstliche eroffnung des warzenfortsatzes. Arch Ohrenheilkd. 1873;7:157–162.

[9] Stacke L. Indicationen betreffend de Excision von Hammer und Amboss. Arch Ohrenheilkd. 1890;31:201–215.

[10] Bondy G. Totalaufmeisselung mit Erhaltung von Trommelfell und Gehorknochelchen. Monatsschr Ohrenheilk. 1910;15–23.

[11] Wullstein H. Theory and practice of tympanoplasty. Laryngoscope. 1956;66 (8):1076–1093.

[12] Zollner F. The principles of plastic surgery of the sound-conducting apparatus. J Laryngol Otol. 1955;69(10):637–652.

[13] Sheehy JL, Patterson ME. Intact canal wall tympanoplasty with mastoidectomy. A review of eight years' experience. Laryngoscope. 1967;77(8):1502–1542.

[14] Park KT, Song JJ, Moon SJ, Lee JH, Chang SO, Oh SH. Choice of approach for revision surgery in cases with recurring chronic otitis media with cholesteatoma after the canal wall up procedure. Auris Nasus Larynx. 2011;38(2):190–195.

[15] Wilson KF, Hoggan RN, Shelton C. Tympanoplasty with intact canal wall mastoidectomy for cholesteatoma: long-term surgical outcomes. Otolaryngol Head Neck Surg. 2013;149(2):292–295.

[16] Brown JS. A ten year statistical follow-up of 1142 consecutive cases of cholesteatoma: the closed vs. the open technique. Laryngoscope. 1982;92(4):390–396.

[17] Semaan MT, Gilpin DA, Hsu DP, Wasman JK, Megerian CA. Transmastoid extradural-intracranial approach for repair of transtemporal meningoencephalocele: A review of 31 consecutive cases. Laryngoscope. 2011;121 (8):1765–1772.

[18] Eliades SJ, Limb CJ. The role of mastoidectomy in outcomes following tympanic membrane repair: a review. Laryngoscope. 2013;123(7):1787–1802.

[19] Megerian CA, Cosenza MJ, Meyer SE. Revision tympanomastoid surgery. Ear Nose Throat J. 2002;81(10):718–720, 722, 725–726 passim.

[20] Arriaga MA. Mastoidectomy – Canal Wall Down Procedure. In: Brackmann D. E., Shelton C., Arriaga M.A. Otologic Surgery, 3rd Ed. Philadelphia, PA: Elsevier; 2010:209–220.

[21] Jackson CG, Glasscock ME III Nissen AJ, Schwaber MK, Bojrab DI. Open mastoid procedures: contemporary indications and surgical technique. Laryngoscope. 1985;95(9 Pt 1):1037–1043.

[22] Becvarovski Z, Kartush JM. Smoking and tympanoplasty: Implications for prognosis and the Middle Ear Risk Index (MERI). Laryngoscope. 2001;111 (10):1806–1811.

[23] Dornhoffer JL. Retrograde mastoidectomy with canal wall reconstruction: A follow-up report. Otol Neurotol. 2004;25(5):653–660.

[24] Haberkamp TJ, Tanyeri H. Surgical techniques to facilitate endoscopic second-look mastoidectomy. Laryngoscope. 1999;109(7 Pt 1):1023–1027.

[25] Jackson CG. The infratympanic extended facial recess approach for anteriorly extensive middle ear disease: a conservation technique. Laryngoscope. 1993;103(4 Pt 1):451–454.

[26] Weber PC. Iatrogenic complications from chronic ear surgery. Otolaryngol Clin North Am. 2005;38(4):711–722.

[27] Litton WB, Krause CJ, Anson BA, Cohen WN. The relationship of the facial canal to the annular sulcus. Laryngoscope. 1969;79(9):1584–1604.

[28] Sheehy JL. The facial nerve in surgery of chronic otitis media. Otolaryngol Clin North Am. 1974;7(2):493–503.

[29] Green JD, Jr, Shelton C, Brackmann DE. Iatrogenic facial nerve injury during otologic surgery. Laryngoscope. 1994;104(8 Pt 1):922–926.

[30] Sheehy JL, Brackmann DE. Cholesteatoma surgery: Management of the labyrinthine fistula—a report of 97 cases. Laryngoscope. 1979;89(1):78–87.

[31] Dornhoffer JL, Milewski C. Management of the open labyrinth. Otolaryngol Head Neck Surg. 1995;112(3):410–414.

[32] Smith JA, Danner CJ. Complications of chronic otitis media and cholesteatoma. Otolaryngol Clin North Am. 2006;39(6):1237–1255.

[33] Semaan MT, Megerian CA. The pathophysiology of cholesteatoma. Otolaryngol Clin North Am. 2006;39(6):1143–1159.

[34] Gyo K, Yanagihara N. Defects in the bony wall of the mastoid bowl: A study based on staged intact canal-wall tympanoplasty. Am J Otol. 1991;12(6):403–406.

[35] Althaus SR. Tympanomastoid surgery: A technique for repairing posterior osseous canal wall defects with autologous temporalis fascia and bone pâte. Otolaryngol Head Neck Surg. 1985;93(2):227–229.

[36] Bacciu A, Pasanisi E, Vincenti V, Di Lella F, Bacciu S. Reconstruction of outer attic wall defects using bone paté: Long-term clinical and histological evaluation. Eur Arch Otorhinolaryngol. 2006;263(11):983–987.

[37] Weinberg J, Sadé J. Posterior wall atrophy. A late silent complication of the combined approach tympanoplasty operation. Am J Otol. 1982;3(4):315–317.

[38] Sanna M, Gamoletti R, Bortesi G, Jemmi G, Zini C. Posterior canal wall atrophy after intact canal wall tympanoplasty. Am J Otol. 1986;7(1):74–75.

[39] Nadol JB Jr. Causes of failure of mastoidectomy for chronic otitis media. Laryngoscope. 1985;95(4):410–413.

[40] Kaylie DM, Gardner EK, Jackson CG. Revision chronic ear surgery. Otolaryngol Head Neck Surg. 2006;134(3):443–450.

[41] Wilson KF, London NR, Shelton C. Tympanoplasty with intact canal wall mastoidectomy for cholesteatoma: Long-term hearing outcomes. Laryngoscope. 2013;123(12):3168–3171.

[42] Vartiainen E. Ten-year results of canal wall down mastoidectomy for acquired cholesteatoma. Auris Nasus Larynx. 2000;27(3):227–229.

34 Epitympanectomy

Joseph Chen and Jafri Kuthubutheen

Abbreviations used in this chapter:

CSF: cerebrospinal fluid
CT: computed tomography
MRI: magnetic resonance imaging

34.1 Introduction

The epitympanum is an important anatomical region in otologic surgery, particularly in the treatment of cholesteatoma and chronic suppurative otitis media. Its relevance in the treatment of lesions that extend or impact on the structures within the epitympanum cannot be overemphasized. These include tympanosclerosis, glomus tumor, facial schwannomas, neoplastic lesions from the external auditory canal (such as squamous cell carcinoma), and meningoencephaloceles, among others.

The epitympanum is bounded laterally by the scutum, the malleus, and the pars flaccida. The tegmen tympani serves as its roof and the tympanic diaphragm and tensor canal its floor. It communicates with the incudal fossa posteriorly. The facial nerve and the ampullae of the lateral and the superior semicircular canals are the most important structures within this space medially.[1] Anteriorly, the tegmen tympani courses inferiorly to the level of the tympanic diaphragm and attaches to the tensor tympani bony canal. There are several variations in the anterior epitympanic region, depending upon the size of the cog (the bony plate extending from the tegmen), the space anterior to the cog (often called the epitympanic sinus), the length of the tensor fold, and the size of the supratubal recess superior to the Eustachian tube.[2] At the medial wall of the anterior epitympanum, the facial nerve may be dehiscent due to disease or from an anatomical variation. We have shown the most consistent landmark leading into the epitympanum is the cochleariform process. The facial nerve curves in a consistent fashion posterior-superiorly around the cochleariform process within 2 mm. Past this point, the cochleariform process is on average 7.81 mm from the nerve at the geniculate ganglion. As it deviates from the cochleariform process superior-medially, the facial nerve makes a mean angle of 30 degrees from the tensor tympani tendon.[3]

34.2 Patient Selection

Epitympanectomy can be performed alone or in combination with more extensive temporal bone dissections. It is useful in the context of limited disease, particularly when encountering a sclerotic temporal bone that requires a more strategic approach. Of course, such a determination can only be made through the use of a computed tomography (CT) assessment. Atticotomy is a term often used synonymously with epitympanectomy. However, in our opinion, atticotomy implies a procedure designed to access the posterior portions of the epitympanic space, whereas an epitympanectomy includes exposure of the anterior epitympanic space and the supratubal recess.

An epitympanectomy can be performed as the sole procedure or in combination with a mastoidectomy. Accessing the epitympanum directly through the ear canal (endaural), through a posterior corridor (canal wall-up), or when the facial ridge is lowered (canal wall-down) depends on those clinical decisions relative to the disease, its extent, and the degree of temporal bone pneumatization. By far the most common indication for an epitympanectomy is removal of a pars flaccida retraction pocket or cholesteatoma.

The preoperative workup should be conducted with a thorough history, microscopic examination of the ear, audiologic testing, and high-resolution CT scanning of the temporal bones. Magnetic resonance imaging (MRI) may be performed if the diagnosis of a cholesteatoma is in doubt, particularly in evaluating recidivism. It is also useful in the diagnosis and in defining the extent of a meningoencephalocele. Although the true extent of the disease may only be confirmed intraoperatively, a CT scan is integral in the process of informed consent, vis-a-vis complications, and in planning the surgical approach. The feasibility of middle ear reconstruction, posterior canal preservation, or the need for a postauricular incision is part of this decision process.

34.3 Surgical Technique

There are two primary approaches to an epitympanectomy: endaural and postauricular. Both utilize a two-handed technique with a standard surgical microscope and are familiar approaches to the ear used commonly for tympanoplasty, mastoidectomy, and cochlear implantation. Each technique has advantages and disadvantages (▶ Table 34.1). The endaural approach results in a smaller and less cosmetically visible scar but allows a smaller lateral working space. A postauricular approach requires a larger incision but allows a more lateral working space. A well-placed postauricular incision can also be cosmetically acceptable, and a previous postauricular approach may steer a surgeon towards using the same incision.

Accessing the epitympanic space through a postauricular approach usually aims to preserve the canal wall. It requires identifying the mastoid antrum and continuing the dissection anteriorly between the canal wall and the tegmen tympani to remove the bone lateral to the epitympanic space. This can then

Table 34.1 Endaural versus postauricular approaches

	Endaural	Postauricular
Advantages	• Smaller skin incision • Surgical approach through meatoplasty	• Greater lateral working space • Access to temporalis fascia • Meatoplasty skin easily sutured
Disadvantages	• Smaller lateral working space • Separate incision for temporalis fascia • More difficult meatoplasty skin suturing	• Larger skin incision

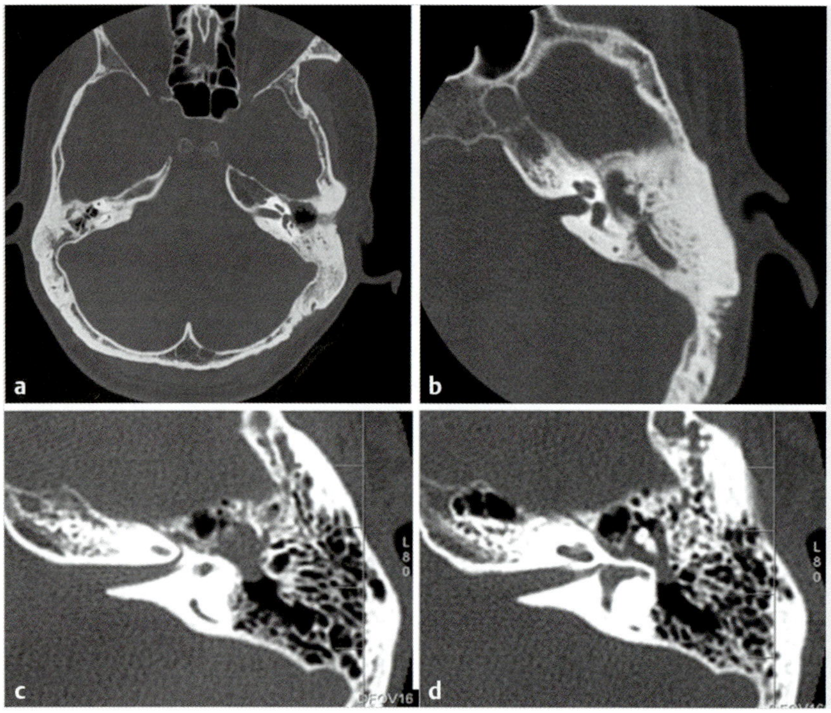

Fig. 34.1 (a) Axial view CT temporal bone of a sclerotic mastoid. There is bony sclerosis and minimal mastoid air cell pneumatization bilaterally. The right sigmoid sinus is dominant and anteriorly displaced. (b) Close up axial view CT temporal bone scan, left. At the level of the tympanic facial nerve, there is opacification of the epitympanum and mastoid antrum with significant bony sclerosis (c) Axial view CT temporal bone scans, left. The temporal bone is well pneumatized. There is an epitympanic cholesteatoma surrounding the body of incus and malleus head. The top figure represents a plane just superior to the tympanic facial nerve in the same patient.

be combined with an endaural dissection to remove the disease in a so-called combined approach. The endaural approach, our preferred technique, requires stepwise removal of the scutum and variable amounts of the canal wall to expose the epitympanum. The benefit of this is that the exposure required is tailored to the extent of the disease, with less surgical time and overall morbidity. A partial or complete epitympanectomy may be performed depending upon the volume of disease. Complete epitympanectomy requires the removal of the incus and head of the malleus and complete removal of the lateral epitympanic bone to expose all the boundaries of the epitympanum. The endaural approach also allows for harvesting of reconstructive material, such as temporalis fascia (through the superior extension of the incision) or cartilage and perichondrium (from the tragus or the concha).

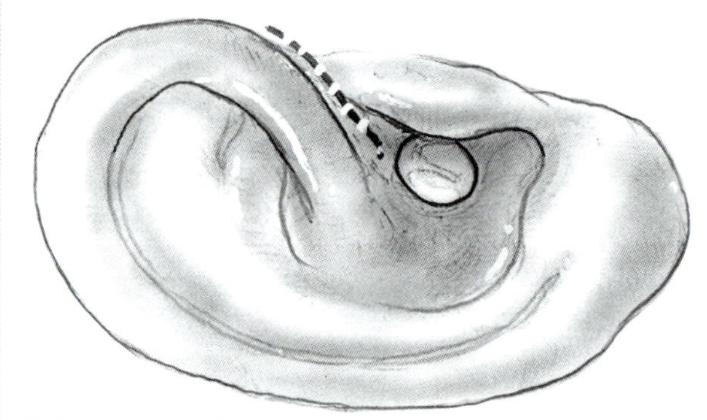

Fig. 34.2 Endaural incision, right. The incision is made from the 12 o'clock position to the groove between the tragal cartilage and the root of the helix.

34.3.1 Stepwise Surgical Technique

Here we demonstrate the stepwise surgical technique of an epitympanectomy via an endaural approach for a limited cholesteatoma in a sclerotic temporal bone. A typical CT scan of a sclerotic temporal bone is shown in ▸ Fig. 34.1a and ▸ Fig. 34.1b. For comparison, ▸ Fig. 34.1c and d show an epitympanic cholesteatoma in a well-pneumatized temporal bone.

Preparation

Once the patient has been prepped and draped, local anesthetic with epinephrine is used to infiltrate the terminal incisure, conchal bowl, and the external auditory canal. Shaving is not needed.

Endaural Incision and Meatoplasty

A #15 blade is used to mark out an incision between the tragus and root of the helix (▸ Fig. 34.2). This is carried down into the bony ear canal at the 12 o'clock position. A Lempert periosteal elevator is used to expose the bone beneath. A transverse incision is then made just deep to the conchal cartilage, along the posterior wall of the canal from the 12 o'clock to the 6 o'clock position (▸ Fig. 34.3). Sharp dissection of the skin to undermine the conchal bowl cartilage and root of the helix is performed to remove this tissue to create an appropriately sized meatus (▸ Fig. 34.4; ▸ Fig. 34.5; ▸ Fig. 34.6; ▸ Fig. 34.7). Because this maneuver provides the exposure for the operation, the size of the meatoplasty will depend upon how much dissection is needed. An aggressive dissection and bony exposure is usually required. Two double-pronged endaural retractors (Fisch endaural retractors with anti-reflective coating, Karl Storz GmbH & Co KG, Tuttlingen, Germany) are used both in an anterior-posterior position as well as in a superior-inferior position (▸ Fig. 34.8; ▸ Fig. 34.9). Performing a meatoplasty early means it need not be done at completion of the surgery, where

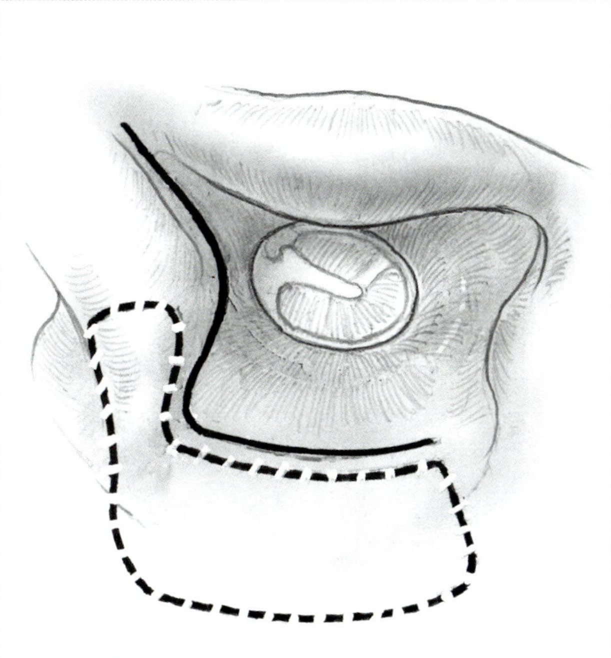

Fig. 34.3 Lateral meatal skin incision and meatoplasty, right. This incision is made transversely just medial to the concha from 6–12 o'clock and connects to the endaural incision. The dotted line indicates the position of the underlying conchal cartilage and slip of incisural cartilage.

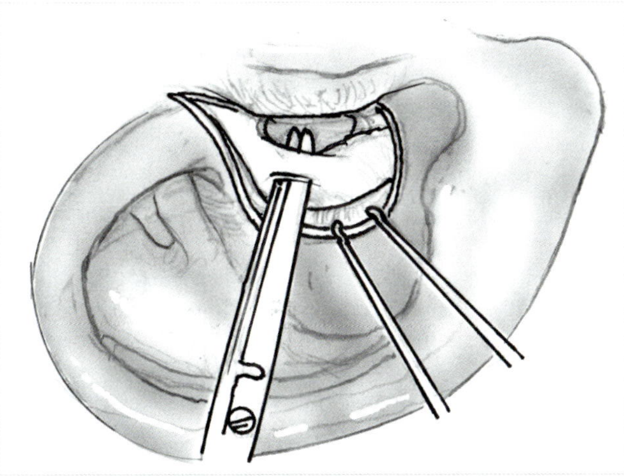

Fig. 34.5 Meatoplasty (cont.), right. The distal tip of the incisural cartilage is dissected free from the overlying skin using a curved iris scissors passing under the slip of cartilage.

bleeding can obscure the surgical field. Tragal cartilage and temporalis fascia can also be harvested at this stage. Undermining the meatal flap is also advised at this stage to help preserve meatal skin for reconstruction.

Treatment of the External Canal Skin

A more medially placed incision parallel to the lateral canal incision is made (▶ Fig. 34.10; ▶ Fig. 34.11). The resultant inferiorly based skin flap can be used to reconstruct the lining of the canal or the mastoid cavity if required. A duckbill or round knife is then used to elevate the medial canal skin down to the bony annulus. Care must be taken to elevate the tympanomeatal flap superior to the incisura angularis; it can be transected superiorly and rolled inferiorly. The meatal skin can be protected

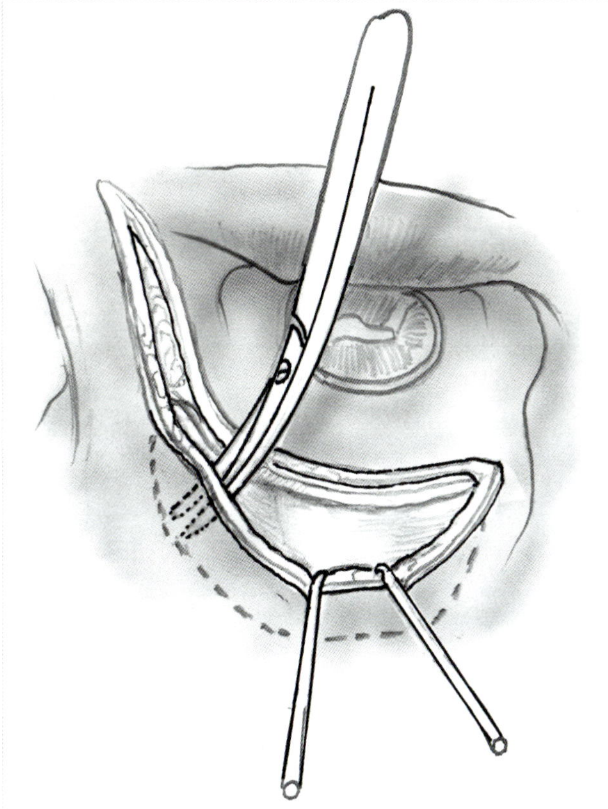

Fig. 34.4 Meatoplasty, right. Dissection begins by finding a plane between the conchal and incisural cartilages and the overlying skin.

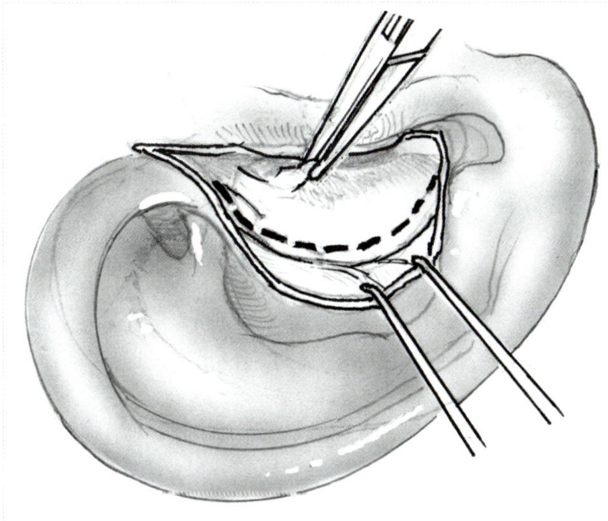

Fig. 34.6 Meatoplasty (cont.), right. The cartilage is then grasped with a forceps and removed with an 11-blade along the dotted line.

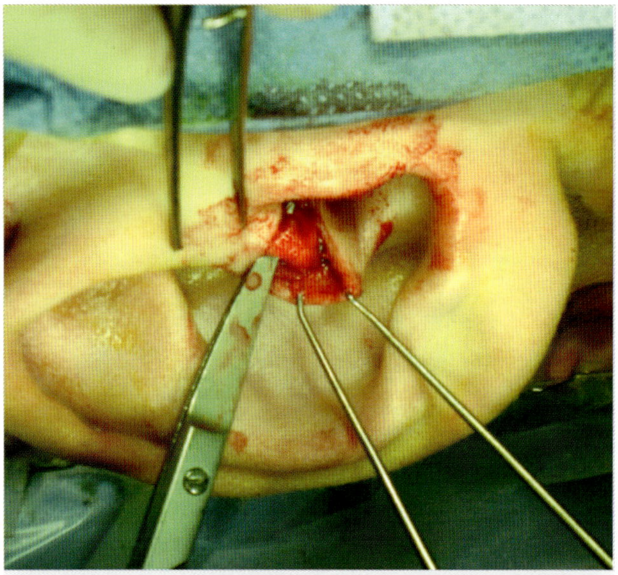

Fig. 34.7 Meatoplasty (cont.), right. Intraoperative photo showing dissection of the incisural cartilage

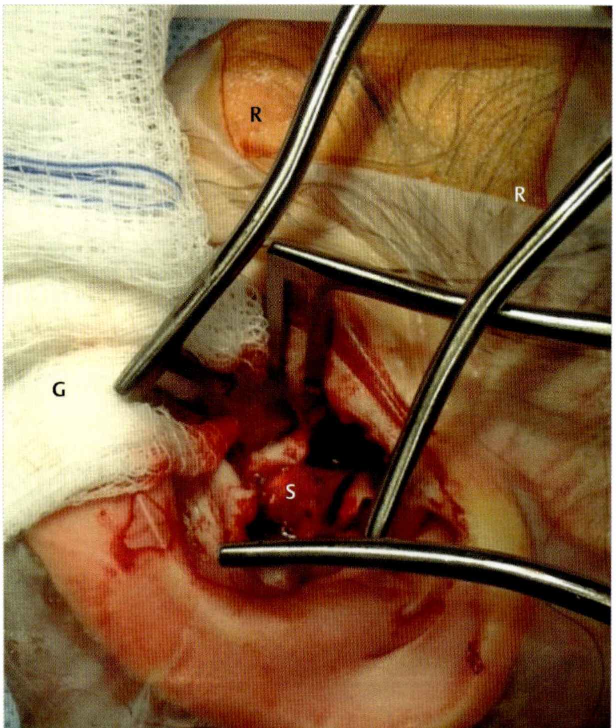

Fig. 34.9 Retractor placement, left. Intraoperative photo showing placement of the endaural Fisch retractors (R) at right angles to each other. The inferior skin is protected by gauze (G) and further soft tissue of the conchal bowl (S) can be removed to expose the underlying bone.

using an aluminum strip fashioned from disposable materials, such as a suture package (▶ Fig. 34.12). Elevation of the flap may reveal the neck of the cholesteatoma, which can be transected to reveal the entrance to the sac.

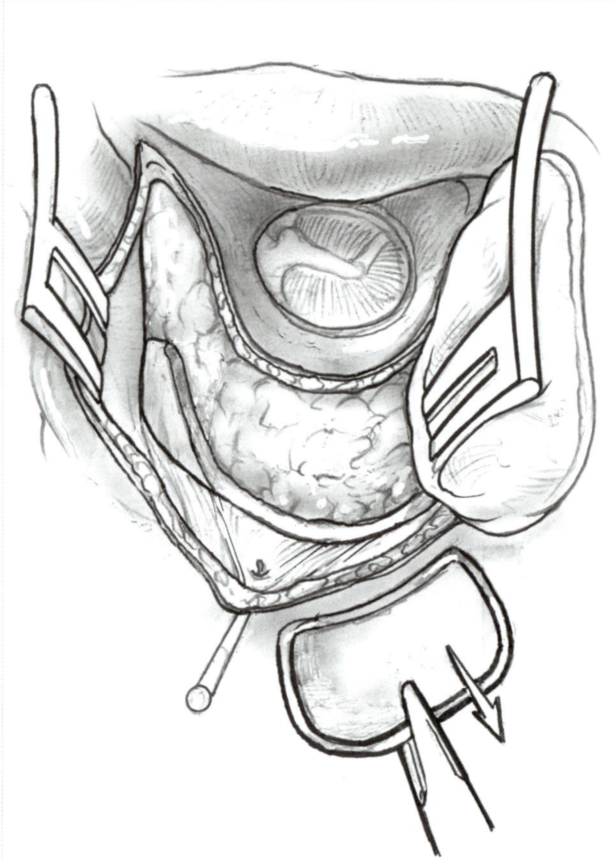

Fig. 34.8 Retractor placement, right. Once cartilage of the conchal bowl and incisure are removed (and saved for later use), Fisch retractors are placed. Further soft tissue may need to be removed to expose the lateral temporal bone surface. Gauze is used to protect the inferior skin.

Bone Removal

Before drilling begins, it is imperative that adequate bony exposure is achieved to include the root of the zygoma, the spine of Henle, and the mastoid cortex (depending on disease volume and the size of the antrum). Drilling usually begins with a 3-mm cutting burr. The degree of bone removal is dictated by the extent of disease. The smaller surgical field of view, compared with that of a postauricular approach, is compensated for by a more direct anterior access to the epitympanum. Following the matrix of the cholesteatoma and gradual debulking to reveal more medial structures permit a safe and controlled approach for fully dissecting this region. If the ossicular chain is thought to be intact, great care needs to be taken to avoid drilling over the body of the incus as it has a lateral orientation, usually 2–3 mm lateral to the free edge of the scutum.

The initial landmarks encountered are the chorda tympani nerve, the body of the incus (if present), and the neck of the malleus. Frequently these landmarks are absent because of bony resorption from the disease state. The extent of the disease can now be compared with the CT findings in the context of its location relative to the ossicular chain, the semicircular canals, and the anterior mesotympanum. The tegmen tympani is a reliable and consistent landmark in a sclerotic mastoid or if

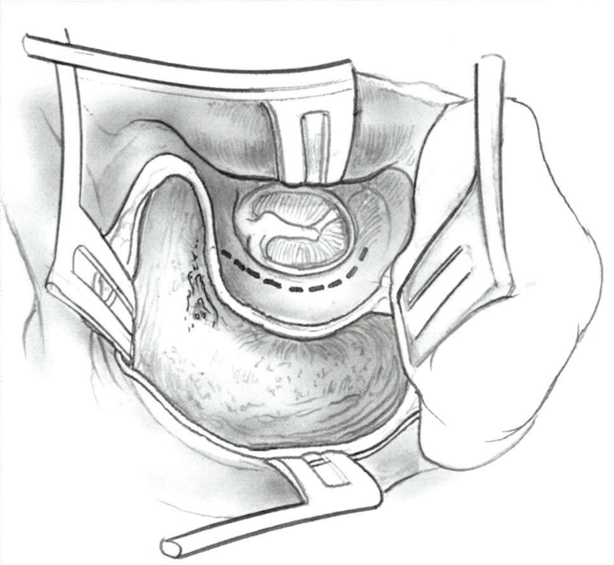

Fig. 34.10 Bone exposure, right. Diagram showing the complete bony exposure before drilling can commence. The spine of Henle is usually visible. A more medially placed skin incision parallel to the lateral canal incision is made (dotted line). This inferiorly based meatal skin flap is elevated, rolled inferiorly and protected by an aluminum strip for later use in reconstructing the cavity.

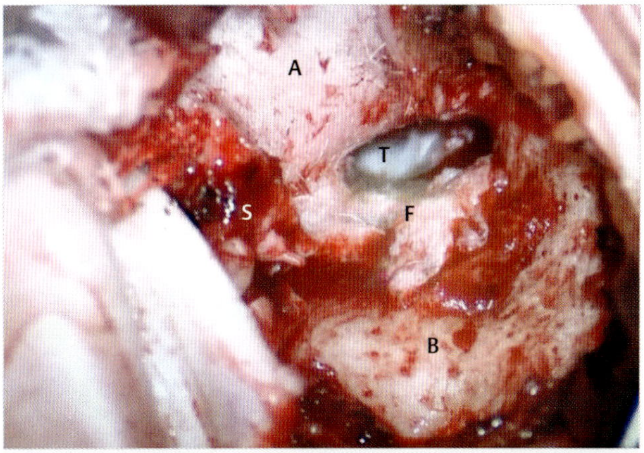

Fig. 34.11 Bone exposure, left. Intraoperative photo corresponding to Fig. 34.10. F, Inferior skin flap; T, tympanic membrane; A, anterior canal wall skin; B, lateral temporal bone; S, lateral skin flap.

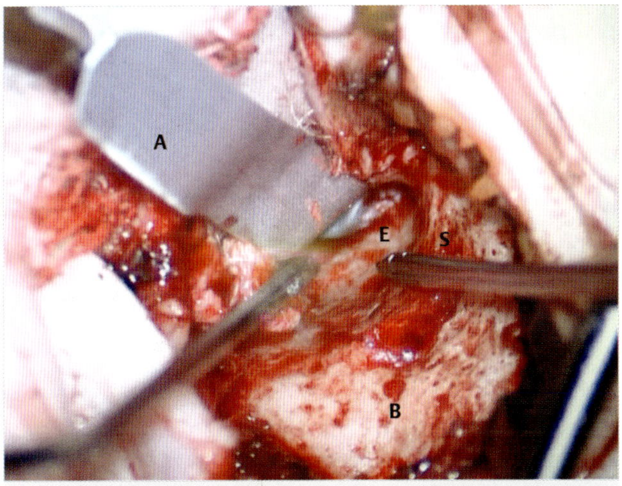

Fig. 34.12 Bone exposure, left. Intraoperative photo showing the aluminum strip in position and prior to bony removal. A, aluminum strip; S, spine of Henle; E, elevation of canal wall skin up to cholesteatoma neck; B, exposure of bone of the mastoid cortex.

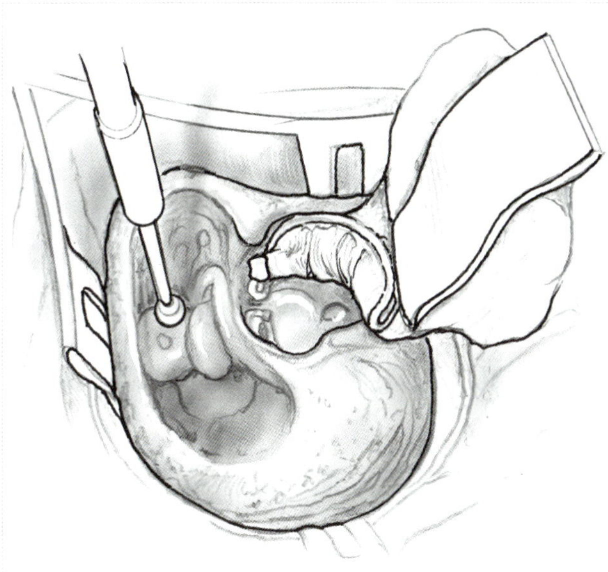

Fig. 34.13 Epitympanectomy, right. The tympanic membrane has been elevated anteriorly to expose the middle ear. The incus and malleus head have been removed to leave the stapes superstructure intact. The scutum has been drilled away to expose the epitympanic space, underlying semicircular canals and part of the fallopian canal. An aluminum strip is used to protect the inferior skin flap.

other landmarks are visually indistinct. Removal of an eroded incus and the head of the malleus early will improve visibility in more extensive disease. A good understanding of the three-dimensional anatomy of the facial nerve relative to the cochleariform process, the lateral semicircular canal, the cog, and the remnant of the stapes will provide a margin of safety.[3] The posterior limit of the dissection should at least extend to the mastoid antrum for an epitympanectomy or further back if disease removal requires it. The anterior limit should expose and drill away the cog to clear the epitympanic sinus or supratubal air cell tract if present (▶ Fig. 34.13).

Disease Removal

It is common for disease removal to occur simultaneously with exposure, especially when there is extensive granulation tissue or cholesteatoma obscuring the view. Disease removal with gentle suctioning (size #17 suction or smaller) and a variety of instruments, including a cupped micro-forceps, Fisch dissector, round knife, and Rosen needle, are routinely used depending upon the underlying structure. Special considerations need to be taken in managing a dehiscent facial nerve, exposed dura, and a lateral canal fistula. Meticulous dissection with variable pressure under direct visualization with adrenaline-soaked cottonoids is preferred.

34.3.2 Management of the Ossicular Chain

There are two main issues to consider when managing the ossicular chain in an epitympanectomy. The first is whether to remove or keep the ossicles and the second is whether the ossicular chain should be reconstructed. The ultimate goal of an epitympanectomy is to remove disease and, therefore, the ossicular chain is usually a secondary consideration. It is better to have an ear free of disease than to risk incomplete disease removal or recurrence by leaving all or part of the ossicular chain.

The most common ossicle to be involved in epitympanic disease is the incus, followed by the head of the malleus. The malleus handle may be foreshortened and medially displaced if there is coexisting mesotympanic disease, and, likewise, the stapes may also be eroded or absent in the presence of mesotympanic disease. The most common scenario, however, is an eroded incus or absent incus. The decision to reconstruct the ossicular chain depends on the status of the middle ear, the stapes superstructure, and the malleus. Primary ossicular reconstruction is best delayed until it is clear the disease has been eradicated. The ossicular chain may be left intact in the presence of tympanosclerosis or non-cholesteatoma disease if this can be removed without damaging the ossicles. An epitympanic retraction can also usually be removed while leaving the ossicular chain alone. This is best done under high magnification with the aid of a Fisch dissector or Rosen needle to ensure no residual epithelium is left.

34.3.3 Reconstruction of the Canal Wall Defect

Following an epitympanectomy, there may be a defect in the medial canal wall, the size of which will depend upon how much exposure was required to remove the disease. The decision to reconstruct the defect depends on its size, the degree of temporal bone pneumatization, the presence of granulation tissue, and the status of the ossicular chain. Small, minimal defects can be left without reconstruction and covered with fascia or perichondrium as part of the tympanoplasty. A sclerotic mastoid bone is associated with a low-lying tegmen tympani and, therefore, a small epitympanum, which can be treated in the same manner. Larger defects that expose the body and short process of the incus, the head of the malleus, and the aditus ad antrum require reconstruction to prevent retraction of a simple fascia or soft tissue repair. Cartilage is the favored material and can be harvested from the tragus or the conchal bowl (if more tissue is required). The cartilage with adjacent perichondrium should be suspended from the medial wall or the ossicles to allow for ventilation of the middle ear space (▶ Fig. 34.14). The defect should be measured (with a disc elevator or Fisch dissector) and the defect carved. A more irregular defect can be sized with a cutout from the suture pack, which can then be traced onto the cartilage. When the epitympanectomy is performed in the setting of a canal wall-down mastoidectomy, we do not reconstruct the canal wall.

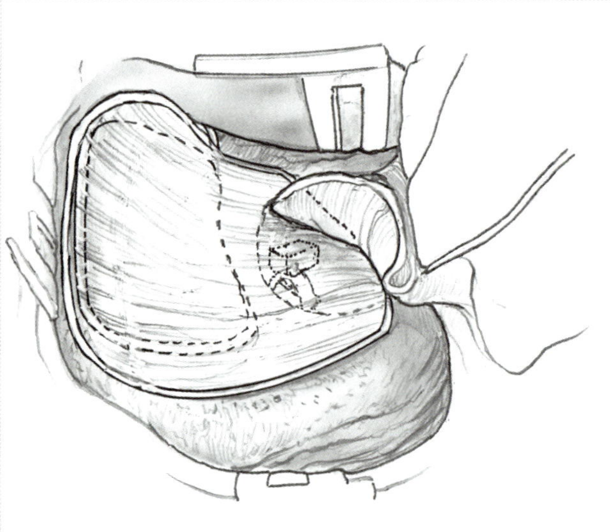

Fig. 34.14 Epitympanectomy defect reconstruction, right. Reconstruction of the epitympanectomy defect using a combination of temporalis fascia layered over a cartilage graft in an underlay fashion. A type III tympanoplasty using cartilage between the head of the stapes and the tympanic membrane is shown.

34.3.4 Surgical Pearls and Pitfalls

One should have a low threshold for sacrificing the chorda tympani nerve, especially if it is involved in disease or if it impairs visualization. It is important not to touch the ossicles when removing the medial canal wall bone with either a drill or curette to minimize transmitted vibrations. The stapes should also be counter-stabilized with cottonoids when peeling disease away to minimize lateral stapes movements and provide a blood-free zone. One should always be vigilant for hidden complications, such as a tegmen dehiscence or a semicircular canal fistula, which may not be visible on a CT scan or which may have developed while the patient was awaiting surgery. Cerebrospinal fluid (CSF) leaks should be repaired when they are discovered with a trilaminar repair combination of absorbable gelatin sponge, fascia, or perichondrium and bone pate. When removing cholesteatoma in the medial epitympanum, the possibility of erosion of the superior semicircular canal and facial nerve canal needs to be considered, especially around the anterior border of the canal.

34.4 Postoperative Care

Routine postoperative care includes dry-ear precautions for at least 4 weeks and ototopical antibiotic ear drops (such as ciprofloxacin and dexamethasone). Patients should be seen in the office for limited microdebridement and wound inspection 2 weeks following surgery. Subsequent visits will depend upon the status of the ear. Most of the healing has usually occurred by 8 weeks, and subsequent follow-up will need to be done clinically and supplemented with radiological testing as appropriate. Second-look tympanotomies should be performed when the canal wall is left up or if there is a high suspicion of recurrent or residual disease. This is usually done at 6–9 months following the initial procedure. Audiologic testing should be done at 3 months following surgery to allow for any middle ear effusion to settle and avoid an artifactual conductive hearing loss.

34.5 Complications

The most common complication in epitympanectomy is injury to the chorda tympani nerve, but, as stated earlier, one should have a low threshold for sacrificing this nerve. Stapes dislocation can occur due to poor attention to stabilization when dissecting disease from the ossicles or, more commonly, from disarticulating the incudostapedial joint. If the stapes has been partially dislocated, further manipulation should be ceased. Another complication that can occur is a defect in the tegmen tympani. This should be repaired with bone pate, or, if a CSF leak has occurred, with a trilaminar repair as mentioned above. Less common complications include injury to the facial nerve in the tympanic segment or genu, which can occur from lack of appreciation of the landmarks during posterior epitympanectomy. This can be avoided by remaining superior to the chorda-facial junction and watching the medial end of the burr when drilling the medial canal wall. Disease recidivism is always a potential long-term complication, particularly when the canal wall is preserved. This should be managed by close postoperative clinical surveillance and routine second-look tympanotomy (especially for cholesteatoma). MRI is an emerging technique for monitoring disease recurrence, but it has its disadvantages. An ossiculoplasty may be combined with a second-look procedure if the hearing is inadequate.

References

[1] Proctor B. Surgical anatomy of the ear and temporal bone. Stutgart: Thieme, 1989.

[2] Tos M. Manual of middle ear surgery. Mastoid Surgery and Reconstructive Procedures Volume 2. New York, Stutgart: Thieme; 1995.

[3] Wong D, Chen J. Surgical anatomy of the epitympanum and supralabyrinthine Spaces. Am J Otol. 1996;17:193–196.

35 Canal Wall-Down Mastoidectomy

Michael B. Gluth and Marcus D. Atlas

Abbreviations used in this chapter:

BMRM: Bondy modified radical mastoidectomy
CSF: cerebrospinal fluid
CWD: canal wall-down
CWU: canal wall-up
DW MRI: diffusion-weighted magnetic resonance imaging
MRM: modified radical mastoidectomy
PORP: partial ossicular replacement prosthesis
RM: radical mastoidectomy
TORP: total ossicular replacement prosthesis

35.1 Introduction

Canal wall-down (CWD) mastoidectomy is a surgical procedure that, in its most common application, involves removal of the superior and posterior bony external auditory canal wall such that a continuous open cavity is formed consisting of the external auditory canal lumen, epitympanum, and open mastoid cavity (▶ Fig. 35.1).[1] This procedure is employed primarily for the indication of cholesteatoma as a means to obtain wide exposure and access to the tympanomastoid air cell tracts for disease removal; however, it also provides the benefit of exteriorizing areas that are involved with cholesteatoma so that they can be monitored in the office setting without concern for cholesteatoma recurrence or intracranial complication.

There are three main subtypes of CWD procedures:

1. The *radical mastoidectomy* (RM) exteriorizes the entire tympanomastoid compartment, often with plugging of the Eustachian tube. The middle ear cleft is allowed to epithelialize without an attempt at reconstruction of the tympano-ossicular mechanism; thus, resulting hearing is poor.
2. The *modified radical mastoidectomy* (MRM) usually exteriorizes only the epitympanum and the mastoid cavity. The tympano-ossicular mechanism is reconstructed in some form such that a middle ear space is preserved, albeit with a smaller volume. MRM is by far the most common form of CWD mastoid surgery and one that affords the possibility of good hearing. Some surgeons believe that this procedure should be termed *CWD mastoidectomy with tympanoplasty*, reserving the designation MRM only for Bondy's procedure (discussed below); however, this point is not universally agreed upon. It is important to recognize that MRM is fundamentally different from the epitympanectomy techniques that are described in Chapter 34 of this book.
3. The *Bondy modified radical mastoidectomy* (BMRM) may be applied to those small lateral epitympanic cholesteatomas present in a scenario with three distinct features: the mesotympanum is spared, the ossicular chain is intact, and the canal wall is drilled down. After removal of the bony canal wall, the cholesteatoma is either marsupialized into the open cavity, with the medial aspect of the sac left in place on the ossicular chain, or removed completely, followed by placement of a fascia graft directly onto the incus body and malleus head. As a result, the mastoid cavity and lateral aspect of the epitympanum are exteriorized, with the ossicular chain and majority of the middle ear space preserved. Although BMRM is rarely performed, hearing results are typically excellent (▶ Fig. 35.2).

35.2 Patient Selection

The indications for CWD surgery are controversial, differing from surgeon to surgeon.[2,3,4,5] Some advocate CWD surgery for all cases of cholesteatoma due to a superior track record with respect to lower rates of residual and recurrent cholesteatoma compared with canal wall-up (CWU) mastoidectomy. Other surgeons favor CWD surgery in the sclerotic temporal bone or when complications of cholesteatoma due to bone erosion are present, such as labyrinthine fistula, facial nerve involvement, or dura involvement. CWD surgery may also be indicated in a patient who is not deemed to be a good candidate for second-look surgery following CWU mastoidectomy due to poor health or suspect patient compliance.[6]

In the authors' view, the primary indication for CWD mastoid surgery is quite simply to provide access for definitive cholesteatoma removal. The underlying disease extension, the patient's temporal bone anatomy, and the surgeon's experience and training will influence this decision.

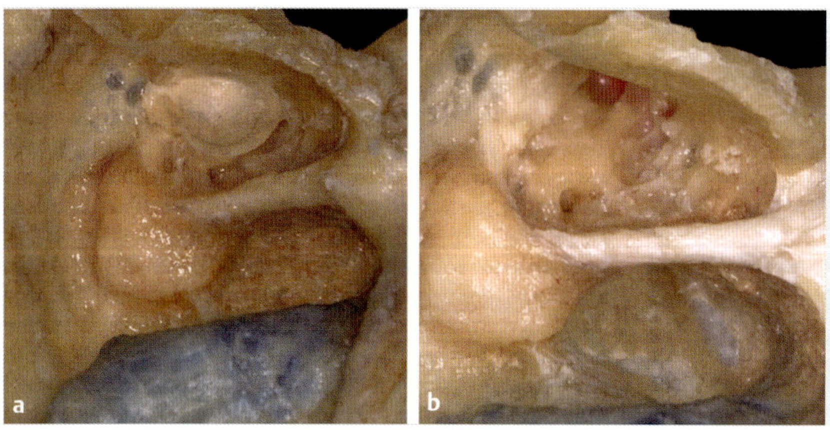

Fig. 35.1 CWD mastoidectomy. (a) The MRM (right ear) is a CWD mastoidectomy procedure that involves exteriorizing the epitympanum and mastoid cavity in continuum with the external auditory canal while preserving a middle ear space by reconstructing the tympano-ossicular mechanism. (b) In contrast, the RM exteriorizes the entire tympanomastoid space without tympano-ossicular reconstruction. (Used with permission from Atlas M, Eisenberg R. A Guide to Temporal Bone Dissection. 2nd Ed. Perth: Lions Ear 2004.)

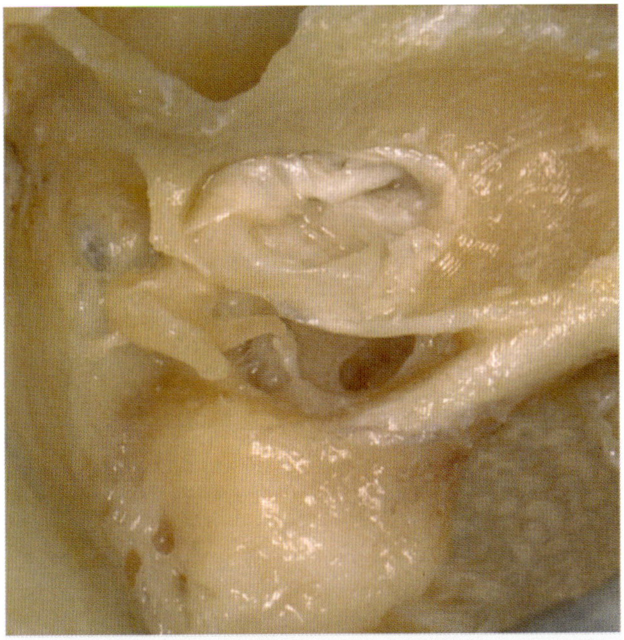

Fig. 35.2 Bondy modified radical mastoidectomy (BMRM). The BMRM (right ear) is a CWD mastoidectomy procedure that involves exteriorizing the lateral epitympanic space and mastoid cavity while preserving the ossicular chain. This is achieved by either marsupializing the cholesteatoma, with the portion of the sac in contact with the ossicular chain left in place, or by removing the cholesteatoma sac and placing a fascia graft onto the lateral aspect of the ossicular chain. (Used with permission from Atlas M, Eisenberg R. A Guide to Temporal Bone Dissection. 2nd Ed. Perth: Lions Ear 2004.)

Removal of the canal wall facilitates a panoramic view of the epitympanum and particularly augments exposure to the supralabyrinthine air cells, the anterior epitympanic region, the supratubal recess, and the protympanum by opening the surgical angles that define the posterior-to-anterior surgical vantage point. Whether or not CWD surgery provides improved access to the posterior mesotympanum (particularly the sinus tympani) is controversial. In a randomized trial in cadaveric temporal bones, Hulka et al. found improved visualization of this region with CWD exposure as opposed to CWU exposure.[7]

In the authors' opinion, visualization of the posterior mesotympanum may be achieved with a CWU approach in a way that is comparable to CWD surgery if the surgeon purposefully drills the scutum and posterior canal wall bone sufficiently enough to view the entire pyramidal process and ponticulus (often as far as the mastoid segment of the facial nerve), and if the surgeon assumes a far anterior vantage point. However, it is also the authors' opinion that, although visualization of this key area may be comparable, actual surgical dissection of the posterior mesotympanum is much easier with a CWD approach due to the fact that wide lateral access of instruments into the middle ear is better afforded, thereby facilitating deft cholesteatoma dissection. Also, drilling away the bone anterior to the mastoid segment of the facial nerve, a maneuver that opens the view into the vestibule of the sinus tympani, is much more effective with CWD exposure. It should also be noted that access to and removal of disease from the sinus tympani is impacted by its size and by the degree of pneumatization in this region.

35.3 Surgical Technique

The aim of cholesteatoma surgery is to create a safe, dry, and hearing ear. A safe ear is free of recurrent and residual cholesteatoma. A dry ear has an intact migrating epithelium that is waterproof. Hearing is dependent on many factors, but the mastoid cavity may need to be able to accommodate a hearing aid, especially if there is a mixed hearing loss. Successful CWD surgery achieves all of these aims; however, this is heavily dependent on a surgeon's ability to construct an ear that resists retention of keratin debris and moisture as these lead to foreign body reactions, aural polyp, granulation tissue, and microbial overgrowth.[8,9]

Assessment and management of the mastoid cavity in the clinic setting, including a discussion of cavity instability, is covered in Chapter 14. A common fundamental mistake among novice cholesteatoma surgeons is to consider CWD surgery as essentially the same as CWU mastoidectomy with the simple addition of bony canal wall removal. This error often leads to a cavity that is designed to fail (▶ Fig. 35.3). Consistently good outcomes in CWD mastoidectomy require an understanding that an optimal CWD technique requires several additional steps after cholesteatoma removal that not only generate proper shape and contour, but also match the caliber of the external auditory meatus with the size of the cavity.[10]

35.3.1 Canal Wall-Down Cholesteatoma Exposure

A desired aim in cholesteatoma surgical exposure is to view the entire lateral aspect of the cholesteatoma sac before proceeding with removal, as this will maximize the chance of complete removal while avoiding piecemeal dissection. For primary acquired epitympanic cholesteatoma, this involves isolation of the neck of the cholesteatoma sac at the junction with the tympanic membrane by progressively removing adjacent canal wall bone starting at the eroded scutum. As the origin of the sac is clearly delineated, it can then be amputated from the remnant tympanic membrane, which will facilitate elevation of a tympanomeatal flap, middle ear exploration, and confirmation that the incudostapedial joint has been eroded or disarticulated (to avoid iatrogenic noise-induced hearing loss during the drilling phase).

35.3.2 Mastoidectomy and Epitympanic Dissection

Keeping the goal of wide lateral sac exposure in mind, a stepwise approach to CWD mastoidectomy drilling then begins. First, the tegmen mastoideum, sigmoid sinus, and digastric ridge are broadly skeletonized. In doing so, the central mastoid air cell tract is drilled, Korner's septum is penetrated, and the mastoid antrum is entered. The mastoid segment of the facial nerve is then carefully identified under copious irrigation using the horizontal semicircular canal and digastic ridge as useful landmarks. The superior and posterior canal wall bone is then progressively removed, including elimination of the facial recess and chorda tympani nerve. Dissection then proceeds with skeletonization of the tegmen tympani and drilling into the

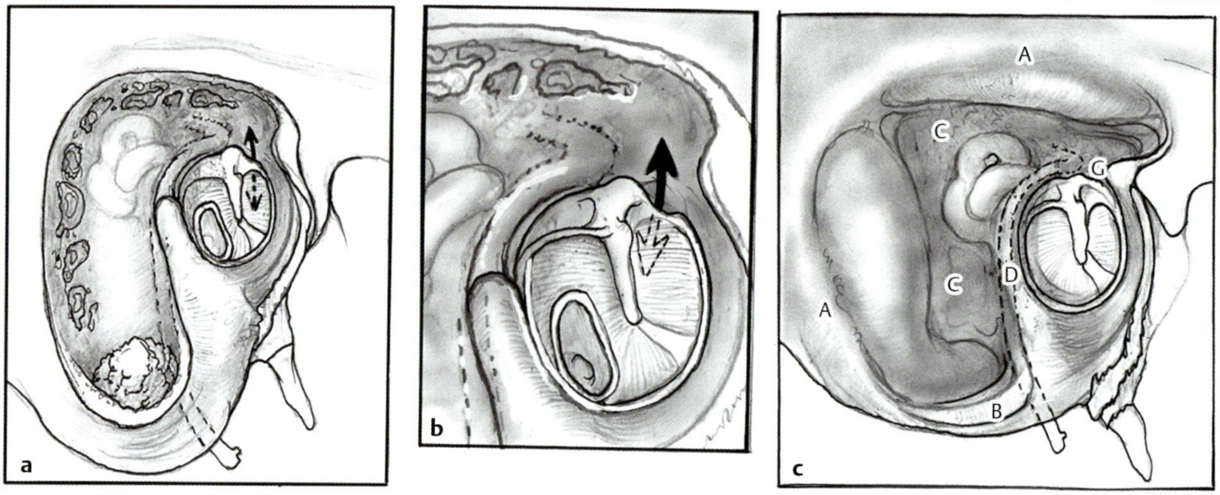

Fig. 35.3 An unfavorable versus a properly formed canal wall-down mastoidectomy. (a) In the unfavorable cavity note the steep non-saucerized edges, the potholes from residual air cells, the intact open mastoid tip with debris, the uncontoured tympanic bone forming a kidney-shaped cavity, the high facial ridge. A, steep non-saucerized edges; B, potholes from residual air cells; C, intact open mastoid tip with debris; D, uncontoured kidney-shaped tympanic bone; E, high facial ridge; (b) Also note the tympanic membrane perforation, and the unsealed communication between the mesotympanum and the exteriorized epitympanum. F, tympanic membrane perforation; G, unsealed communication with epitympanum. (c) In contrast, the properly formed canal wall-down mastoidectomy features saucerized edges, a mastoid tip that has been amputated from the digastric muscle, air cells that have been drilled away until the smooth posterior and middle fossa dural plates are exposed, a completely lowered facial ridge, a inferior tympanic bone that has been rendered concave having a smooth junction with the mastoid, an intact tympanic membrane, and an intact seal between the epitympanum and the mesotympanum. A, saucerized edges; B, mastoid tip amputated from digastric muscle; C, cells drilled away up to smooth dural plate; D, facial ridge lowered; E, tympanic bone smoothly fractured with junction of mastoid; F, intact tympanic membrane; G, middle ear sealed from epitympanum.

zygomatic air cells to complete removal of the entire lateral epitympanic wall.

One of the major advantages of a CWD approach compared with CWU surgery is the ability to widely open the anterior epitympanic communication into the supratubal recess, as this is a critical site of cholesteatoma invasion (▸ Fig. 35.4). This involves identification of the cog, amputation of the malleus head, and drilling open the anterior epitympanic bone into the prominent anterior epitympanic air cell (epitympanic sinus). In doing so, the mucosal fold of the tensor tympani is taken down, and the supratubal recess is rendered widely continuous with the epitympanum. If necessary, the dissection can then proceed inferiorly with removal of the anterior tympanic spine and anterior-superior tympanic ring to expose the protympanum.

During dissection in this region it is commonplace for many surgeons to indiscriminately cut the tensor tympani tendon and/or to remove the malleus. Although this step is unavoidable in many cases, the authors' bias is to endeavor to preserve the entire manubrium and at least a single ligamentous anchoring malleus attachment (among the anterior malleal ligament or tensor tendon) when the extent of cholesteatoma makes this reasonably feasible. Benefits of partial malleus preservation include the following: 1) aiding wound healing as the umbo is the epicenter of tympanic membrane keratinocyte proliferation[11]; 2) serving as an anchor for the drumhead to prevent lateralization; and 3) acting as a stabilizing focus during ossiculoplasty. In most cases, it is possible to obtain excellent exposure while preserving the tensor tendon by releasing the anterior malleal ligament, elevating the anterior-superior tympanic membrane annulus, retracting the malleus and attached remnant drumhead posteriorly, and drilling away the exposed anterior tympanic spine.

The final stage of cholesteatoma exposure involves removal of bone from the anterior border of the facial nerve within the tympanic cleft. This final maneuver will improve access to the posterior mesotympanic wall, including the vestibule of the sinus tympani. Once cholesteatoma is removed, attention is then given to extirpate all diseased air cells, with particular attention given to the perilabyrinthine, retrosigmoid, and retrofacial groups.

35.3.3 Lowering the Facial Ridge

After the process of CWD cholesteatoma removal is complete, a raised ridge of bone may remain partially overlying the mastoid segment of the facial nerve. Incomplete lowering of this facial ridge has been shown to have perhaps the greatest negative effect on mastoid cavity stability than any other surgical error (▸ Fig. 35.5).[12] A high facial ridge is defined as having bone overlying the facial nerve that is 2 mm or greater in thickness although lowering the ridge less than this is commonly desired.[13] The effect of a high ridge is to create a steep "cliff" within the cavity that promotes posterior accumulation of debris and hinders centrifugal epithelial migration.

To properly lower the facial ridge, the mastoid segment of the facial nerve is clearly identified from the second genu to the distal fanned-out aspect of the Fallopian canal that constitutes the stylomastoid foramen. If present, any residual chorda tympani nerve is then identified by drilling away any remnant bone lateral to the facial nerve (facial recess). In doing so, the process

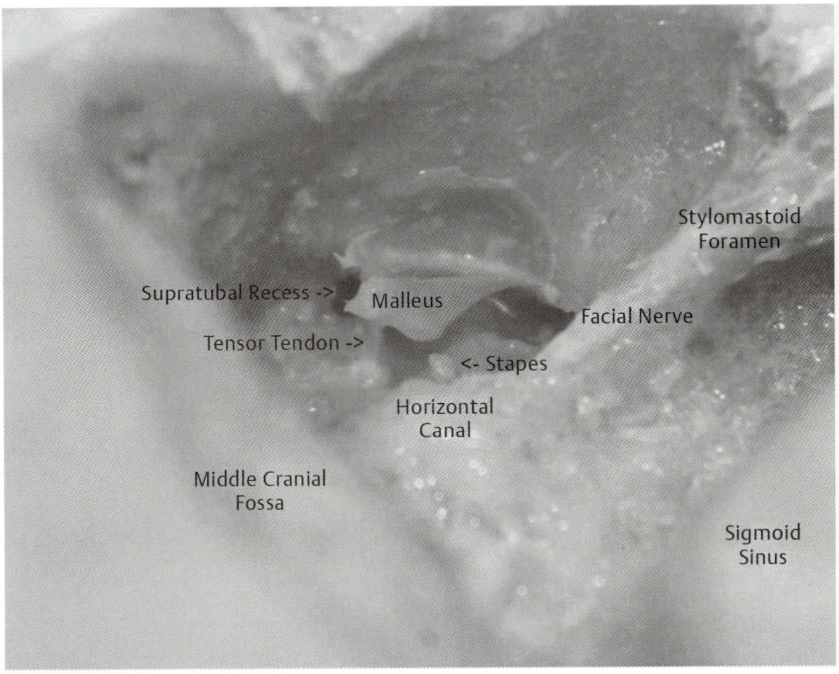

Fig. 35.4 Exposing the anterior epitympanum and supratubal recess. One major advantage of CWD mastoid surgery is enhanced exposure of the anterior epitympanum. Often, this requires release of the residual tympanic membrane and malleus from the anterior tympanic spine to allow drilling of the anterior-superior aspect of the tympanic ring and smooth contouring of the anterior buttress, which constitutes the transition from the native external auditory canal bone to the epitympanum.

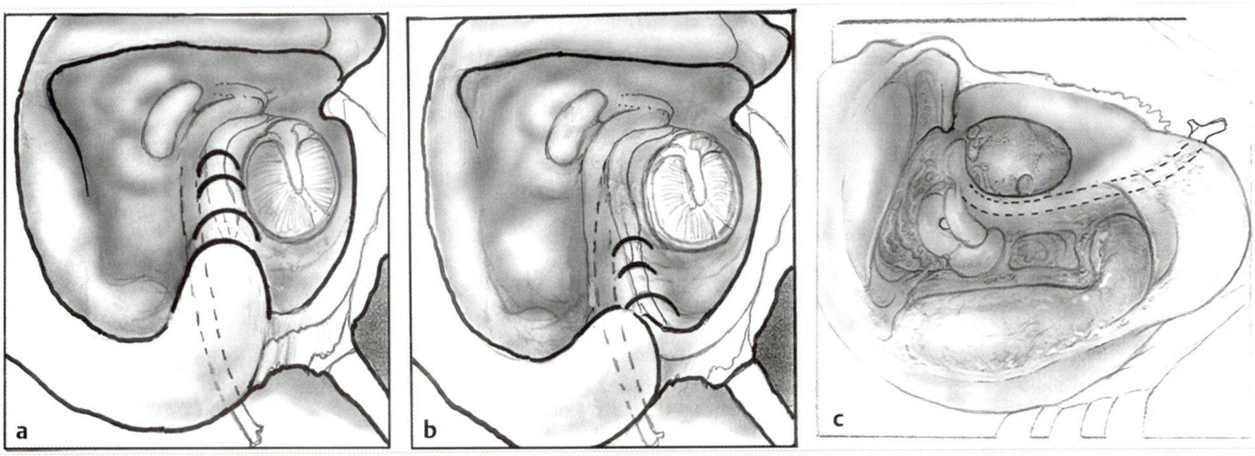

Fig. 35.5 Lowering the facial ridge. The facial ridge is lowered by removing the bone lateral to the mastoid segment of the facial nerve. A high facial ridge (a) is compared with a low ridge (b). Proper lowering of the facial ridge (radical mastoidectomy) is achieved by skeletonizing the nerve with a thin residual rim of bone (< 2 mm) from the second genu to the chorda tympani-facial nerve junction (c). In doing so, progressive removal of the chorda tympani nerve will act as a helpful guide. As part of this process, the tympanic bone anterior to the nerve is rendered concave having a smooth junction with the mastoid cavity.

of lowering the ridge is executed by following and removing the chorda tympani remnant until passage just distal to the chorda-facial junction is complete. This point usually lies just inferior to the tympanic annulus.

35.3.4 Contouring the Tympanic Bone Junction with the Mastoid Cavity

The tympanic bone is a vital part of the petrous temporal bone that should be given particular attention during CWD surgery. The anterior and inferior external auditory canals include the tympanic bone and must be removed to create a concave smooth junction with the adjacent mastoid. The non-contoured tympanic bone has been described as a "kidney shape" that, similar to a high facial ridge, has been shown to impart a major negative impact on the likelihood of mastoid cavity stability.[12]

To achieve proper contour, drilling of the tympanic bone is undertaken anterior and lateral to the distal aspect of the facial nerve (▶ Fig. 35.6). Typically, there is a convex, pyramid-shaped segment of tympanic bone that must be rendered concave to create a junction into the mastoid cavity. The apex of such a pyramid acts as the midline hilum of an imaginary kidney or bean and should be eliminated. As with lowering of the facial ridge, this step is performed under copious irrigation with an extra-course diamond burr.

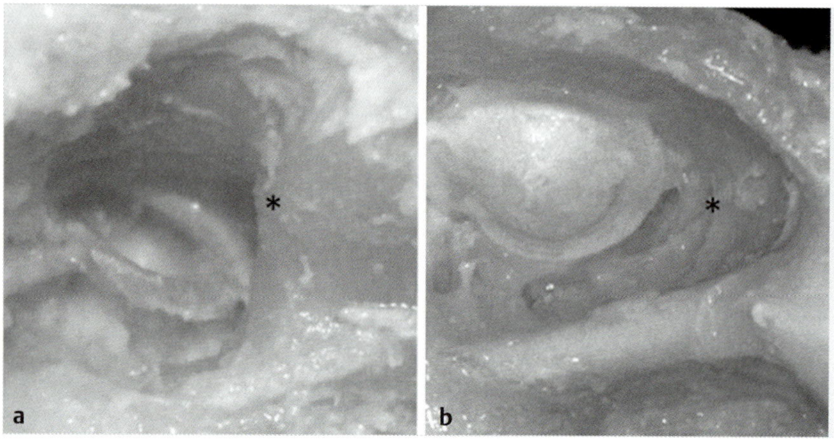

Fig. 35.6 Contouring the tympanic bone. (a) Drilling of the tympanic bone inferior to the tympanic ring and anterior to the facial nerve is necessary to eliminate the "kidney shape" of the resultant cavity and to provide a smooth junction between the native external auditory canal and mastoid cavity. (b) The prominent convex point at the apex of the undrilled native tympanic bone (asterisk) must be rendered convex and saucerized.

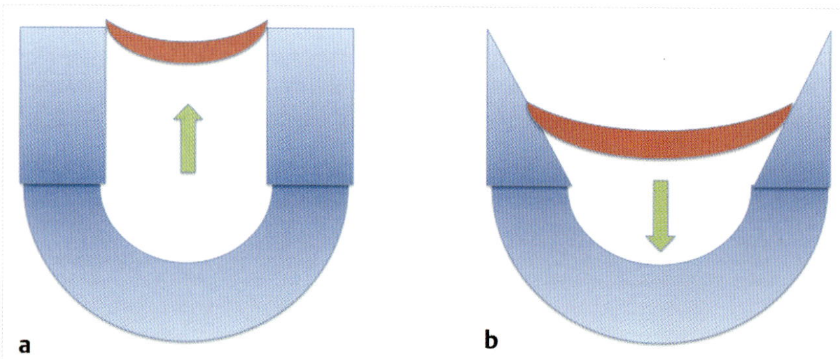

Fig. 35.7 Mastoid cavity saucerization. By beveling the edges of the cavity (blue), the lateral soft tissues (red) are invited to collapse inward, which acts to reduce cavity volume.

35.3.5 Elimination of Cavity Irregularities

To minimize irregularities that may potentially retain epithelial debris, it is highly desirable to remove as many air cells as possible down to the smooth bony plate overlying the middle and posterior fossa dura and sigmoid sinus. It should be noted that while doing so, the surgeon should not indiscriminately "polish" the bone throughout the cavity without minding proper irrigation as this will result in burned devitalized bone within the cavity that is prone to osteitis, infection, and delayed healing.

Because it may not be practical to eliminate every single air cell within the mastoidectomy cavity, particularly the supralabyrinthine air cell tract, it is useful to apply a soft tissue lining to fill these irregularities. This can be augmented with densely pressed bone pate if deemed safe from the perspective of cholesteatoma involvement. Fascia, thin vascularized flaps, and split-thickness skin grafts have been described for this purpose, each of which should be thin enough to avoid hiding cholesteatoma recurrence within involved areas of the cavity.

After the above steps have been completed, there are two general schemes that may be followed to complete CWD mastoidectomy. The choice of which scheme to follow may be impacted by the degree of mastoid pneumatization.

35.3.6 Scheme for a Pneumatized Temporal Bone

Thoroughly drilling a pneumatized temporal bone will usually result in a large cavity that includes a wide-open mastoid tip. The effect of an open mastoid tip will be a gravity-dependent sewer or "sump" effect that will retain moisture and debris postoperatively and, therefore, should be eliminated. To reduce cavity volume in a pneumatized temporal bone, two particular steps are considered, as detailed below.

Saucerization

To invite inward collapse of soft tissue and resultant partial cavity auto-obliteration, the edges of the mastoid cavity should be widely beveled superiorly over the lateral aspect of the middle fossa dura and posteriorly over the lateral edge of the sigmoid sinus, with removal of all retrosigmoid air cells. The effect of saucerization may be understood by considering the hypothetical example of a hole that is dug into the ground and then covered by a wet piece of canvas. If the edges of such a hole are then beveled, broad inward collapse of the canvas will greatly reduce the volume of the hole (▶ Fig. 35.7).

Mastoid Tip Amputation

Amputation of the mastoid tip not only will eliminate much of the above-mentioned sump effect, but also will further promote cavity auto-obliteration (▶ Fig. 35.8a). In particular, tip removal has the desired effect of allowing the posterior border of the cavity to rotate and reorient such that the anterior face of the sigmoid sinus will then become the posterior boundary of the cavity and the digastric ridge/muscle will serve as the inferior border. In a well-pneumatized temporal bone, the distance from the anterior edge of the sigmoid to the anterior wall of the native external auditory canal is roughly 2 cm, with a similar

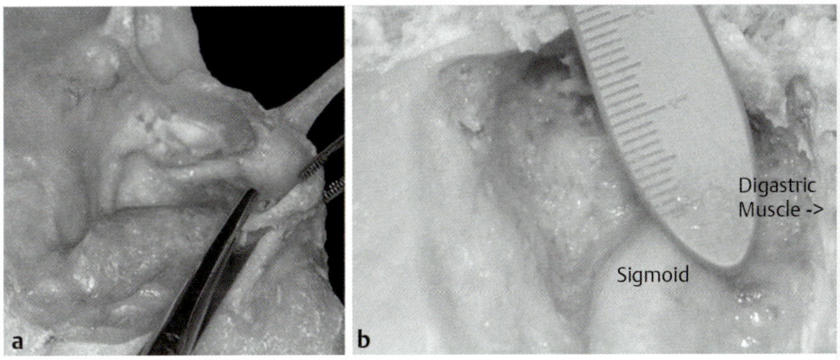

Fig. 35.8 Amputation of the mastoid tip. (a) The mastoid tip is amputated from the digastric muscle. When performing this step, rotational pressure is placed on the tip such that the fractured aspect of the tip is rotated away from the adjacent facial nerve. (b) Removal of the mastoid tip will greatly reduce mastoid cavity volume by shifting the posterior boundary of the cavity to the anterior wall of the sigmoid sinus. Even in a well-pneumatized mastoid cavity, the distance from the anterior edge of the sigmoid sinus to the anterior wall of the native external auditory canal is a mere 2 cm. The saucerized retrosigmoid aspect of a mastoid cavity will auto-obliterate. (8a is used with permission from Atlas M, Eisenberg R. A Guide to Temporal Bone Dissection. 2nd Ed. Perth: Lions Ear 2004.)

measurement typical for the vertical dimension up to the middle fossa (▶ Fig. 35.8b). Thus, even without mastoid cavity obliterative techniques, an ideal cavity should be no larger than approximately 2 cm x 2 cm if properly drilled.

The technique for mastoid tip amputation first involves exposure of the digastric muscle within the previously identified digastric ridge. This is safely achieved by aggressively drilling the retrosigmoid aspect of the inferior mastoid tip. Once the digastric muscle is exposed, drilling proceeds anteriorly along the digastric, progressively moving towards the facial nerve. In doing so, the digastric ridge provides a projection of the level of depth of the facial nerve within the stylomastoid foramen (▶ Fig. 35.9).

The final stage of tip amputation involves passage through the tympanic bone anterior and lateral to the stylomastoid foramen until parotid fascia is encountered. At this point, the tip can be manually released, but this must be done by applying inferior pressure on the lateral aspect of the tip edge so as to rotate the released medial bony edge adjacent to the stylomastoid foramen away from the facial nerve. Lifting and rotating the tip away from the digastric muscle and sharply dissecting it from the sternocleidomastoid attachments with scissors complete this final step.

35.3.7 Scheme for a Sclerotic Temporal Bone

In the case of a severely sclerotic temporal bone, the mastoid may be extremely hypocellular to the point of consisting of only a single antral air cell. In such a case, the mastoid tip comprises marrow and solid bone. Thus, rather than widely saucerizing the cavity and amputating the mastoid tip, some surgeons prefer to contour the cavity by drilling only what is needed to generate what amounts to a small circular tympanomastoid compartment that functionally should act as an enlarged bony ear canal.

To achieve this, the appropriate desired circumference is estimated according to the size of the attic and antral cell defect that is created during cholesteatoma exposure and removal of diseased mucosa. Once the facial ridge has been completely lowered (still recommended in a sclerotic temporal bone), the tympanic bone is then contoured inferiorly in continuum with drilling of the mastoid to the necessary extent that completes a circular cavity. In most instances, this does not require wide exposure of the sigmoid sinus, but this will vary if the sinus is displaced far anteriorly. It is typical for the facial nerve to nearly bisect a small round cavity such as this (▶ Fig. 35.10).

35.3.8 Reconstruction of the Tympano-Ossicular Mechanism

A dry cavity is much more likely to occur if the tympanic membrane is intact to provide barrier separation between the Eustachian tube and the exteriorized mastoid and epitympanum.[14] Modified radical mastoidectomy involves a tympanoplasty that causes rotation of the superior and posterior annulus medially, such that the tympanic and mastoid segments of the facial nerve then act as the boundaries of the neo-tympanic membrane. The result of this rotation is a reduction of the middle ear volume and relocation of the drumhead to closer proximity to the promontory, oval window niche, and sinus tympani. Although most cases of tympanoplasty with MRM preserve sufficient middle ear volume to avoid a major negative impact on middle ear acoustics (at least 0.7 mL, but ideally ≥ 1 mL),[15] the acoustic tolerance of any subsequent acquired retraction is dramatically impaired. As such, although tympanoplasty typically involves underlay grafting with temporalis fascia (Chapter 23), it is highly desirable in MRM to robustly reinforce the tympanic membrane with cartilage (Chapter 25).

Another unique consideration in MRM is the additional need to close the communication between the exteriorized anterior epitympanum and mucosalized mesotympanum. Failure to do so will result in a "pseudo-perforation," effectively creating an open Eustachian tube. This can be achieved by covering with fascia; in addition, this communication may also be filled with a small plug of free muscle, pending the status of cholesteatoma involvement. In cases where there is extensive loss of healthy canal wall skin and native tympanic membrane epithelium, split-thickness skin grafts are useful in promoting timely healing (Chapter 48). Overlay skin grafting is particularly useful when reconstructing the anterior drumhead and tympanomeatal angle when both a subtotal perforation and exposed anterior canal wall bone are present.

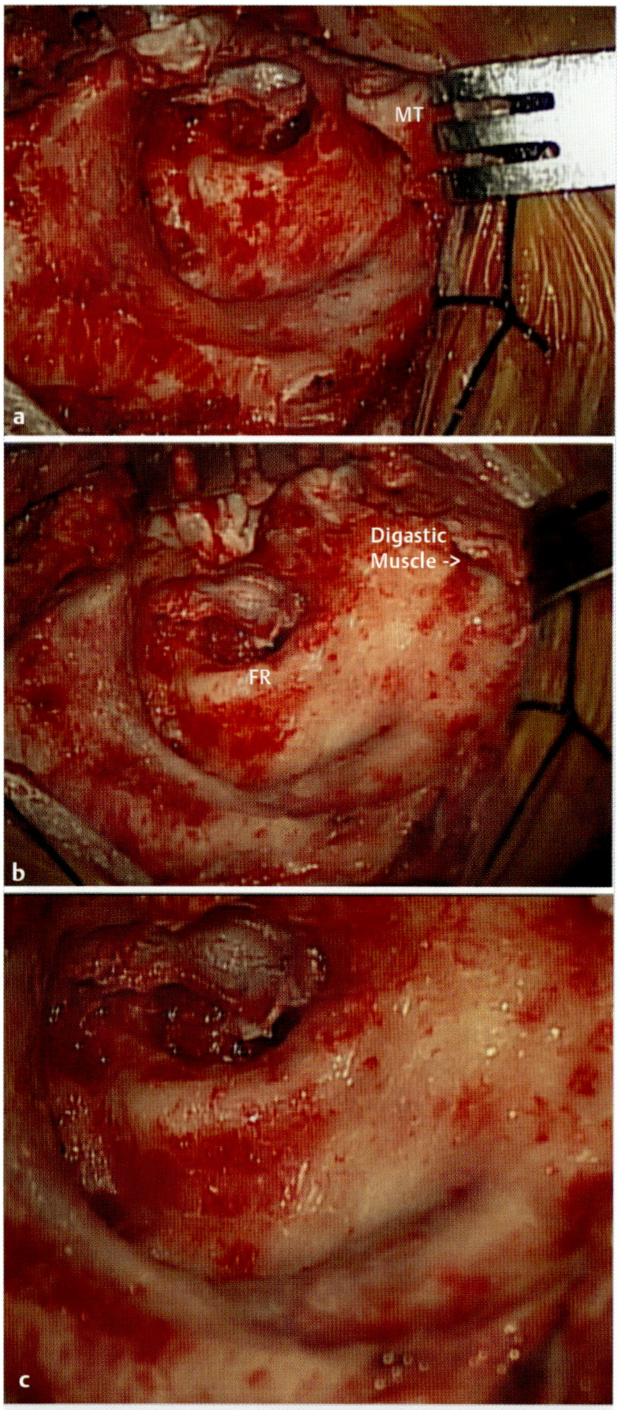

Fig. 35.9 Intraoperative view of CWD mastoidectomy. Shown is an intraoperative view of CWD mastoidectomy before (a) and after (b) amputation of the mastoid tip (MT) and saucerization of the inferior tympanic bone. The facial ridge (FR) has been lowered. (c) Note the smooth and saucerized appearance of the cavity after all diseased air cells have been removed and after the cavity has been properly contoured.

In some cases, it is wise to complete tympano-ossicular reconstruction in a staged manner, particularly if a second-look procedure is required due to concern for residual mesotympanic cholesteatoma, if the outlook for single-stage ossiculoplasty is poor, or if the middle ear environment is hostile. This process involves placement of thin (0.005 mm) nonreinforced silicone sheeting within the mesotympanum that extends up to the Eustachian tube orifice. This sheeting is intended to promote generation of a stable middle ear mucosal envelope that is favorable for ossicular reconstruction and to minimize the development of adhesions between the undersurface of the reconstructed drumhead and cochlear promontory. During the second stage, the sheeting is removed and ossicular reconstruction is executed.

The most simplified form of ossicular chain reconstruction in MRM involves a direct Type III stapes columella type mechanism. If the facial ridge has been completely lowered and the stapes suprastructure is intact without excessive inferior rotation, this is very simple to achieve by simply applying cartilage directly onto the stapes capitulum. When doing so, acoustic benefit is maximized by using a round piece of cartilage that is at least 4 mm in diameter, compared with grafting fascia directly onto the capitulum or using a smaller piece of cartilage.[16,17]

For cases where additional length is required to bridge the gap between the tympanic membrane and stapes, several options are available. If cartilage is used, plates can be stacked one upon another, or the shaft (with prosthesis head removed) of a titanium partial ossicular replacement prosthesis (PORP) can be partially embedded into a thick cartilage plate and then the cradle can be set upon the suprastructure. Alternatively, thin disk-type prostheses have been especially designed for this CWD scenario. If the malleus head is free of cholesteatoma, another option is to sculpt an autograft, which is placed upon the stapes to directly engage the undersurface of the tympanic membrane in a minor columella type reconstruction.

If the surgeon desires to reconstruct the ossicular chain with a full synthetic prosthesis, the techniques described in Chapter 29 can be used. The stabilizing effects of the malleus are particularly desirable in MRM ossiculoplasty because the middle ear space is reduced; however, the prosthesis may need to be shortened slightly (especially a total ossicular replacement prosthesis [TORP]), compared with CWU surgery, and the resultant gap between the superior margin of the neo-tympanic membrane and adjacent exteriorized medial epitympanic wall will need to be filled with cartilage or soft tissue to avoid a large unsupported "step-off" in this area.

If the entire malleus and stapes suprastructure are both absent, obtaining a good hearing result in the CWD scenario by simply placing a TORP between the footplate and neo-tympanic membrane is possible using the techniques described in Chapter 29, but these are difficult to consistently achieve. Surgeons should also keep in mind that the option of Type IV tympanoplasty, wherein the oval window niche is exteriorized while shielding the round window behind the neo-tympanic membrane within a small middle ear space (cavum minor), will provide better hearing results than the near-maximal conductive hearing loss that will result from performing tympanoplasty with no ossiculoplasty at all.[18] The minimum resultant air-bone gap following Type IV tympanoplasty is 20 dB in the best-case healing situation, with a 30–40 dB gap being typical.

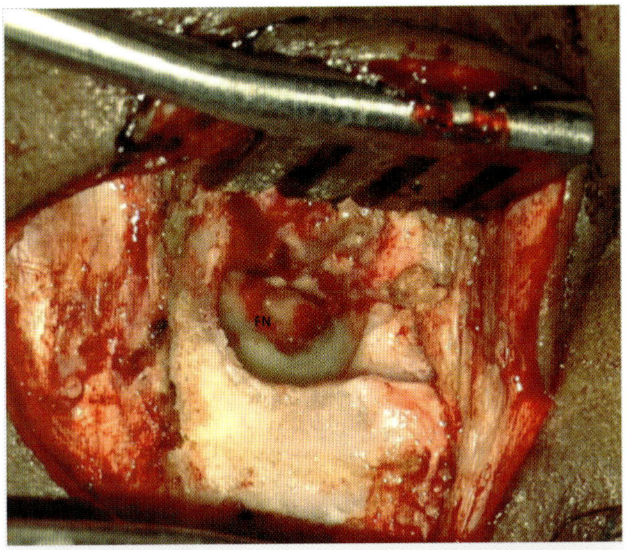

Fig. 35.10 CWD mastoid contouring for a severely sclerotic temporal bone. If there are no mastoid air cells, it is possible to create a small cavity with the need for limited drilling. Once the epitympanum and single antral air cell have been exposed, the surgeon completes a rounded cavity while lowering the facial ridge. If smoothly contoured, the result will amount to a widened bony ear canal. Typically, the facial nerve (FN) will bisect such a cavity. This technique is not recommended in most ears because some degree of mastoid pneumatization is usually present.

35.3.9 Meatoplasty

The final stage in CWD mastoid surgery is creation of an appropriately sized meatoplasty.[19] Various techniques of meatoplasty are discussed in Chapter 20. It is important to recognize that meatoplasty requirements are impacted by the size of the underlying cavity and that a "one size fits all" mentality in creating a very large meatus in every single case is not ideal. While a large meatoplasty is generally favored, if excessive, this can lead to a cosmetic defect and increase caloric-effect vertigo. Thus, for example, if a sclerotic mastoid results in a particularly small cavity or if mastoid cavity obliteration is performed, meatoplasty requirements should be modest. Ideally, the surgeon will make an accounting of the visualization of the posterior cavity recess to assist in determining appropriate meatoplasty sizing.

35.4 Postoperative Care

Prior to surgery, patients must be instructed that postoperative care will be an essential part of the surgical process. In general, a properly crafted mastoid cavity will tend to achieve durable stability, but only if it is allowed to completely epithelialize in the first place postoperatively.

At the conclusion of the procedure, the mastoid cavity and external auditory meatus are packed with ribbon gauze that is coated with antimicrobial ointment (the authors favor mupirocin ointment for its activity against methicillin-resistant *Staphylococcus aureus*). If split-thickness skin grafts are applied, a thin (0.005 mm) piece of non-reinforced silicone sheeting may be placed directly over the skin grafts to act as an interface with the ribbon gauze to prevent graft trauma during gauze placement and removal. Typically, patients are treated with a postoperative course of oral antibiotics directed at preoperatively or intraoperatively cultured pathogens.[20]

Packing is typically left in place for 2 to 3 weeks before removal in the office for adults or in the operating room under mask anesthesia for children. Debris and secretions are suctioned at this stage and an assessment of cavity healing is made. Typically, if healing is advanced, due to extensive residual canal wall epithelium, and pus and granulation tissue are scarce at this stage, the cavity is left open and the patient is instructed to apply a large volume (8–10 drops) of otic drops that contain a combination of antibiotic and corticosteroid twice daily for 10 days. However, if pus and granulation are prominent at the first visit, the cavity is re-packed with ribbon gauze heavily coated with steroid and antibiotic-containing ointment. In both instances, patients are serially examined at 10- to 14-day intervals until advanced stages of healing and epithelialization are achieved (▶ Fig. 35.11).

35.5 Complications

There are a few negative aspects to CWD surgery and some particular scenarios that merit discussion. First, if there is widespread exposure of the dura and/or sigmoid sinus or if there is broad dehiscence of the facial nerve, uncovered exteriorization of these structures within a mastoid cavity is ideally avoided. Protection and coverage of these vital structures can be achieved by performing mastoid cavity obliteration, ideally with vascularized soft tissue (Chapter 41).[21] If the surgeon is unfamiliar with obliterative techniques or if the cavity is not deemed safe for obliteration, it may be wise to perform subtotal petrosectomy and blind sac closure of the external auditory canal (Chapter 42), with planned second-look surgery or postoperative imaging for disease surveillance.

Second, maintenance of a CWD mastoid cavity in the pediatric population is often problematic due to a lack of the requisite patient cooperation for essential postoperative in-office cleaning and inspection; thus, unless dealing with a sclerotic temporal bone, it is generally favorable to avoid CWD surgery in children or, when possible, to combine it with a mastoid obliteration procedure.[22] A particular problem in children is extensive cholesteatoma in a highly pneumatized temporal bone occupying many of the cells of the tympanomastoid space. Although access is best achieved with CWD surgery, extensive obliteration over potential residual disease should be avoided and a second-look procedure or surveillance with diffusion-weighted imaging magnetic resonance imaging (DW MRI) should be considered.

If postoperative mastoid cavity instability occurs (discussed in detail in Chapter 14), there will be chronic otic discharge, poor hearing aid tolerance, and a need for frequent office visits with application of ototopical medications. An open mastoid cavity can also result in caloric-effect vertigo due to outward exposure of the lateral semicircular canal to temperature change via air current or water exposure. Likewise, these symptoms may also suggest the need for judicious mastoid cavity obliteration.[23]

Finally, all of the intraoperative complications possible with CWU mastoidectomy also apply to CWD surgery, namely, facial nerve injury, labyrinthine injury, noise-induced hearing loss,

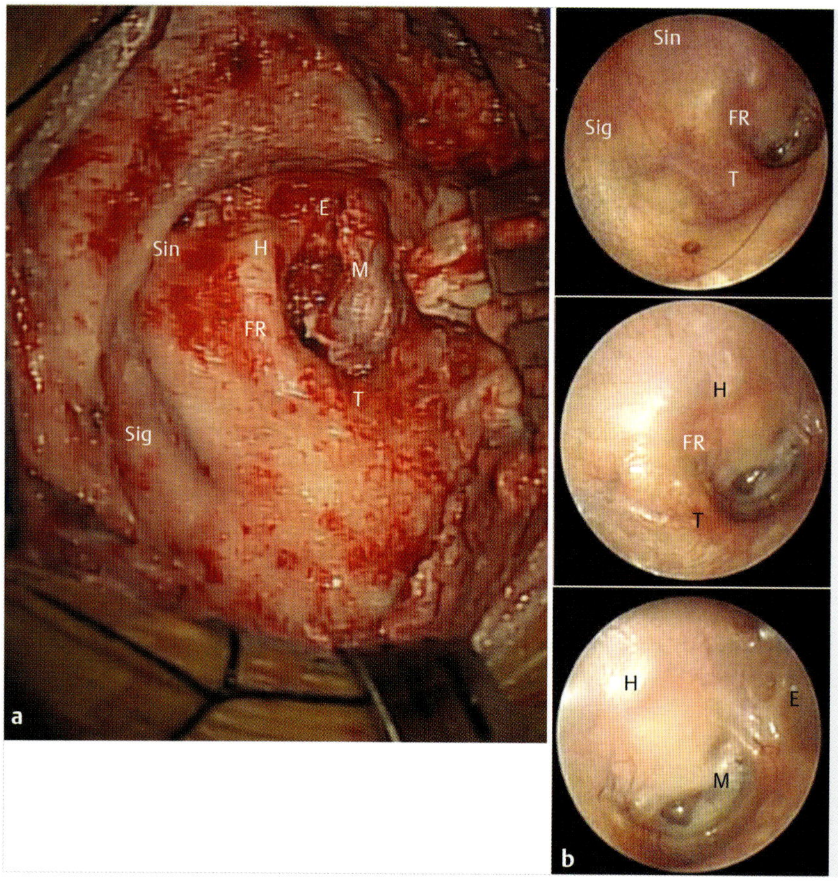

Fig. 35.11 Anatomic correlation between intraoperative view (a) and a healed mastoid cavity (b) in an MRM. This cavity is smoothly contoured and has healed such that retention of debris, the primary cause of mastoid cavity instability, is unlikely to occur. There is no high facial ridge, kidney shape, prominent "pot holes," or open mastoid tip. The tympanic membrane has been robustly reconstructed with cartilage and the epitympanum has been exteriorized. Sin, sinodural angle; Sig, sigmoid sinus; H, horizontal semicircular canal; T, tympanic bone; FR, facial ridge; M, malleus; E, epitympanum.

cerebrospinal fluid (CSF) leak, bleeding from one of the great vessels, and taste disturbance.

35.6 Outcomes

There are three aspects to consider for assessment of CWD surgical outcomes: cholesteatoma control, cavity stability, and hearing.

Impressively low long-term rates of residual or recurrent cholesteatoma after CWD surgery have been reported, ranging from 2% to17%.[2,24,25,26,27] In general, these outcomes are superior to what has been reported with CWU surgery, and many consider CWD mastoidectomy to be the gold-standard cholesteatoma operation. However, not all surgeons consider these superior outcomes in cholesteatoma control, compared with CWU surgery, and the potential ability to complete surgery in a single stage as justification for the associated possible negative side effects of having an open cavity. Furthermore, the development of hybrid tympanomastoid approaches (see Part 7, Roundtable on Hybrid Tympanomastoid Surgical Techniques) and progress in the techniques used for mastoid cavity obliteration have further clouded the discussion of what is the ideal approach to cholesteatoma.

In expert hands, the vast majority of CWD cavities (up to 90%) should be generally stable over the long term if the steps promoted in this chapter are followed (▶ Fig. 35.11).[10] However, this ideal is rarely achieved by novice otologic surgeons and 10% to 60% of cavities have been reported to be intermittently or permanently unstable in most case series.[12,14,28,29] Given the potential wide variability in application of CWD surgical technique, comparison of results between surgeons is difficult.

When viewed in the best-case theoretic scenario, the creation of a CWD mastoid cavity and reduction of middle ear volume associated with MRM should not have an appreciable negative effect on hearing outcomes based on laboratory studies of middle ear acoustics.[15] However, in practice, the collective long-term postoperative effects of chronic ear variables, such as tympanic membrane retraction, middle ear fibrosis, and retained middle ear secretions, seem to impart a greater negative impact on the CWD than on the CWU scenario. As such, although excellent hearing outcomes have been reported for CWD surgery,[24,30,31] there seems to be a trend in the literature towards slightly worse hearing outcomes, even when outcomes are statistically corrected to account for worse disease severity.[32] That being said, it is quite incorrect to presume that opting for CWD surgery involves an abandonment of hope for a good hearing outcome. Because long-term hearing outcomes in tympanomastoid surgery are far more dependent upon the underlying condition of the middle ear than anything else,[33] a bias towards CWU over CWD surgery based solely on the perception of slightly improved hearing outcomes is not logically justified.

References

[1] Atlas M, Eisenberg R. A Guide to Temporal Bone Dissection. 2nd Ed. Perth: Lions Ear & Hearing Institute; 2004.

[2] de Zinis LO, Tonni D, Barezzani MG. Single-stage canal wall-down tympanoplasty: Long-term results and prognostic factors. Ann Otol Rhinol Laryngol. 2010;119(5):304–312.

[3] Osborn AJ, Papsin BC, James AL. Clinical indications for canal wall-down mastoidectomy in a pediatric population. Otolaryngol Head Neck Surg. 2012;147 (2):316–322.

[4] Syms MJ, Luxford WM. Management of cholesteatoma: Status of the canal wall. Laryngoscope. 2003;113(3):443–448.

[5] Smyth GD. Canal wall for cholesteatoma: up or down? Long-term results. Am J Otol. 1985;6(1):1–2.

[6] Garap JP, Dubey SP. Canal-down mastoidectomy: Experience in 81 cases. Otol Neurotol. 2001;22(4):451–456.

[7] Hulka GF, McElveen JT Jr. A randomized, blinded study of canal wall up versus canal wall down mastoidectomy determining the differences in viewing middle ear anatomy and pathology. Am J Otol. 1998;19(5):574–578.

[8] Black B. Mastoidectomy elimination. Laryngoscope. 1995;105(12 Pt 2) Suppl 76:1–30.

[9] Youngs R. Temporal bone histopathology of open mastoidectomy cavities. J Laryngol Otol. 1993;107(6):569–573.

[10] Wormald PJ, van Hasselt CA. A technique of mastoidectomy and meatoplasty that minimizes factors associated with a discharging mastoid cavity. Laryngoscope. 1999;109(3):478–482.

[11] Santa Maria PL, Redmond SL, Atlas MD, Ghassemifar R. Histology of the healing tympanic membrane following perforation in rats. Laryngoscope. 2010;120(10):2061–2070.

[12] Wormald PJ, Nilssen EL. The facial ridge and the discharging mastoid cavity. Laryngoscope. 1998;108(1 Pt 1):92–96.

[13] Gluth MB, Metrailer AM, Dornhoffer JL, Moore PC. Patterns of failure in canal wall down mastoidectomy cavity instability. Otol Neurotol. 2012;33(6):998–1001.

[14] Sadé J, Weinberg J, Berco E, Brown M, Halevy A. The marsupialized (radical) mastoid. J Laryngol Otol. 1982;96(10):869–875.

[15] Whittemore KR Jr Merchant SN, Rosowski JJ. Acoustic mechanisms: Canal wall-up versus canal wall-down mastoidectomy. Otolaryngol Head Neck Surg. 1998;118(6):751–761.

[16] Mehta RP, Ravicz ME, Rosowski JJ, Merchant SN. Middle-ear mechanics of Type III tympanoplasty (stapes columella): I. Experimental studies. Otol Neurotol. 2003;24(2):176–185.

[17] Merchant SN, McKenna MJ, Mehta RP, Ravicz ME, Rosowski JJ. Middle ear mechanics of Type III tympanoplasty (stapes columella): II. Clinical studies. Otol Neurotol. 2003;24(2):186–194.

[18] Merchant SN, Rosowski JJ, Ravicz ME. Middle ear mechanics of type IV and type V tympanoplasty: II. Clinical analysis and surgical implications. Am J Otol. 1995;16(5):565–575.

[19] Mirck PG. The M-meatoplasty of the external auditory canal. Laryngoscope. 1996;106(3 Pt 1):367–369.

[20] Gluth MB, Tan BY, Santa Maria PL, Atlas MD. Unique microbiology of chronically unstable canal wall down tympanomastoid cavities: considerations for surgical revision. J Laryngol Otol. 2013;127(5):458–462.

[21] Singh V, Atlas M. Obliteration of the persistently discharging mastoid cavity using the middle temporal artery flap. Otolaryngol Head Neck Surg. 2007;137(3):433–438.

[22] Dornhoffer JL, Friedman AB, Gluth MB. Management of acquired cholesteatoma in the pediatric population. Curr Opin Otolaryngol Head Neck Surg. 2013;21(5):440–445.

[23] Beutner D, Helmstaedter V, Stumpf R, et al. Impact of partial mastoid obliteration on caloric vestibular function in canal wall down mastoidectomy. Otol Neurotol. 2010;31(9):1399–1403.

[24] Kos MI, Castrillon R, Montandon P, Guyot JP. Anatomic and functional long-term results of canal wall-down mastoidectomy. Ann Otol Rhinol Laryngol. 2004;113(11):872–876.

[25] Palva T. Surgical treatment of chronic middle ear disease. II. Canal wall up and canal wall down procedures. Acta Otolaryngol. 1987;104(5–6):487–494.

[26] Chang CC, Chen MK. Canal-wall-down tympanoplasty with mastoidectomy for advanced cholesteatoma. J Otolaryngol. 2000;29(5):270–273.

[27] Vartiainen E. Ten-year results of canal wall down mastoidectomy for acquired cholesteatoma. Auris Nasus Larynx. 2000;27(3):227–229.

[28] Males AG, Gray RF. Mastoid misery: quantifying the distress in a radical cavity. Clin Otolaryngol Allied Sci. 1991;16(1):12–14.

[29] Youngs R. The histopathology of mastoidectomy cavities, with particular reference to persistent disease leading to chronic otorrhoea. Clin Otolaryngol Allied Sci. 1992;17(6):505–510.

[30] De Corso E, Marchese MR, Sergi B, Rigante M, Paludetti G. Role of ossiculoplasty in canal wall down tympanoplasty for middle-ear cholesteatoma: hearing results. J Laryngol Otol. 2007;121(4):324–328.

[31] Berenholz LP, Rizer FM, Burkey JM, Schuring AG, Lippy WH. Ossiculoplasty in canal wall down mastoidectomy. Otolaryngol Head Neck Surg. 2000;123(1 Pt 1):30–33.

[32] Dornhoffer JL, Gardner E. Prognostic factors in ossiculoplasty: A statistical staging system. Otol Neurotol. 2001;22(3):299–304.

[33] Demir UL, Karaca S, Ozmen OA, Kasapoglu F, Coskun HH, Basut O. Is it the middle ear disease or the reconstruction material that determines the functional outcome in ossicular chain reconstruction? Otol Neurotol. 2012;33 (4):580–585.

Part 7

Roundtable on Hybrid Tympanomastoid Surgical Techniques

36 Overview and Introduction

John L. Dornhoffer and Michael B. Gluth

36.1 Introduction

Otologic surgeons have traditionally been required to judge the relative advantages of improved surgical exposure and superior cholesteatoma control afforded by canal wall-down (CWD) surgery against the benefits of preserved natural anatomy, avoidance of an open cavity, and improved hearing associated with canal wall-up surgery (CWU), also known as intact-canal wall (ICW) surgery. At issue is the exposure of the critical anatomic regions for cholesteatoma removal: the epitympanum and associated supratubal recess and the mesotympanum. These are the two areas associated with most recurrent disease.[1] Primary acquired cholesteatomas typically begin as retraction pockets in the pars flaccida (epitympanic cholesteatoma) or posterior pars tensa (mesotympanic cholesteatoma), so adequate exposure of these areas is paramount.

CWU surgery, especially in cases with poorly developed zygomatic root cells and a low tegmen, can provide very limited exposure of the epitympanum and posterior mesotympanum, leading to blind and piecemeal removal of the cholesteatoma, which contributes to the high recidivism rate. Because of these shortcomings, second-stage surgery is frequently recommended 9–12 months after the initial CWU tympanomastoidectomy.[2,3,4] A review of the literature shows a wide variation in the reported recurrence rates with this technique.[2,3] As pointed out so aptly by Smyth,[1] long-term results with CWU cholesteatoma can be very humbling, with recurrence rates of 15% to 50%, even after staging. Nyrop and Bonding's 10-year follow-up of CWU cases in Copenhagen showed that 70% required a later CWD surgery.[5]

The CWD technique creates an open cavity after removal of the bony posterior canal wall, providing excellent exposure for cholesteatoma removal. The epitympanum, cog, and supratubal recess are widely exposed, facilitating complete removal of the cholesteatoma sac and lowering the recurrence rate to 5–10%.[6,7] The main disadvantages of this technique are related to the necessity for periodic cleaning of the mastoid cavity.[6,7] Subsequent bowl infections can occur, especially when the cavity becomes wet, causing significant lifestyle changes, particularly in the pediatric age group.[7] In addition, the hearing results are frequently worse due to the shallow middle ear cleft.[6,7]

36.2 Evolution of Hybrid Techniques

There has been a trend toward the development of surgical techniques that involve temporary removal of the canal wall, offering the exposure of CWD surgery for cholesteatoma extirpation, followed by reconstruction of the canal wall defect using autologous (bone, cartilage) or alloplastic (hydroxyapatite cement, titanium) graft materials to capture the advantage of the CWU situation.[8,9,10,11,12,13,14] Four techniques are presented in this surgical roundtable: retrograde mastoidectomy with canal reconstruction, canal wall removal with subsequent mastoid obliteration, soft-wall canal reconstruction, and retrograde removal with synthetic wall reconstruction. Although these techniques differ in the way the canal wall is reconstructed, they all share the common philosophy of removal of all or a portion of the canal wall for disease extirpation.

Although these newer hybrid techniques show promising early results, a few obstacles stand in the way of their routine acceptance. First and foremost, long-term follow-up and patterns of failure must be assessed and recognized. Patterns of failure are divided into recurrent and residual disease. Recurrent disease (or recurrent retraction pockets leading to cholesteatoma) is determined largely by how the tympanic membrane, scutum, and/or canal wall are reconstructed. Residual disease, on the other hand, is due to disease that is left behind and is dictated to a large extent by the exposure offered during the intervention to allow complete removal. Especially with these newer hybrid techniques, it will be critical to differentiate between the two patterns of failure. One would anticipate that residual disease would be lowered by the improved exposure offered by these techniques, but the complexity of canal wall reconstruction could have an influence on recurrent cholesteatoma.

The second obstacle to the routine acceptance of these hybrid approaches is that some of these techniques can be difficult to learn and to properly execute, especially for a novice surgeon who has not been directly trained. These hybrid techniques represent not only new surgical skills, but also a break from the traditional philosophy of CWU versus CWD surgery. As such, dissemination of some of these techniques into the otologic surgical community may be slow. It will be interesting to see if the improved exposure afforded by these newer techniques will influence long-term cholesteatoma eradication and ultimately represent the "best of both worlds."

References

[1] Smyth GD. Cholesteatoma surgery: The influence of the canal wall. Laryngoscope. 1985;95(1):92–96.

[2] Hirsch BE, Kamerer DB, Doshi S. Single-stage management of cholesteatoma. Otolaryngol Head Neck Surg. 1992;106(4):351–354.

[3] Austin DF. Single-stage surgery for cholesteatoma: an actuarial analysis. Am J Otol. 1989;10(6):419–425.

[4] Schuring AG, Lippy WH, Rizer FM, Schuring LT. Staging for cholesteatoma in the child, adolescent, and adult. Ann Otol Rhinol Laryngol. 1990;99(4 Pt 1):256–260.

[5] Nyrop M, Bonding P. Achievement of stable ears in cholesteatoma surgery: Long-term results of three surgical techniques. Paper presented at: Fourth International Conference on Cholesteatoma and Mastoid Surgery, 1993;Niigata, Japan.

[6] Cody DT, McDonald TJ. Mastoidectomy for acquired cholesteatoma: Follow-up to 20 years. Laryngoscope. 1984;94(8):1027–1030.

[7] Smyth GD. Surgical treatment of cholesteatoma: the role of staging in closed operations. Ann Otol Rhinol Laryngol. 1988;97(6 Pt 1):667–669.

[8] Black B. Mastoidectomy elimination: obliterate, reconstruct, or ablate? Am J Otol. 1998;19(5):551–557.

[9] Grote JJ. Reconstruction of the middle ear with hydroxylapatite implants: long-term results. Ann Otol Rhinol Laryngol Suppl. 1990;144:12–16.

[10] Magnan J, Chays A, Pencroffi E, Locatelli P, Bruzzo M. Canal wall prosthesis—new devices. Rev Laryngol Otol Rhinol (Bord). 1995;116(1):19–21.

[11] Wullstein SR. Osteoplastic epitympanotomy. Ann Otol Rhinol Laryngol. 1974;83(5):663–669.

[12] Wiet RJ, Harvey SA, Pyle MG. Canal wall reconstruction: A newer implantation technique. Laryngoscope. 1993;103(6):594–599.

[13] Zini C, Quaranta N, Piazza F. Posterior canal wall reconstruction with titanium micro-mesh and bone patè. Laryngoscope. 2002;112(4):753–756.

[14] McElveen JT Jr Chung AT. Reversible canal wall down mastoidectomy for acquired cholesteatomas: Preliminary results. Laryngoscope. 2003;113(6):1027–1033.

37 Retrograde Technique for Management of Cholesteatoma

John L. Dornhoffer

Abbreviations used in this chapter:

CT: computed tomography
PORP: partial ossicular replacement prosthesis
TORP: total ossicular replacement prosthesis

37.1 Introduction

The retrograde technique of cholesteatoma exposure attempts to combine the favorable attributes of canal wall-down and canal wall-up tympanomastoidectomy. The rationale behind this technique is to create a temporary canal wall–down situation by following the cholesteatoma's growth back from its origin in the tympanic membrane toward the mastoid. This removes the superior aspect of the canal wall to completely expose the critical epitympanum and supratubal recess for disease extirpation. The canal wall is then reconstructed with auricular cartilage from the concha cymba that is securely inset into grooves drilled into the remnant canal wall buttresses. Primary ossicular reconstruction serves as a scaffold for the posterior drum reconstruction, both of which are performed as a single-stage surgery. To prevent recurrent disease, the mosaic cartilage technique is employed to reconstruct the tympanic membrane in close approximation to the reconstructed canal wall. If the anterior drum is also involved, then total cartilage reconstruction is performed with the island technique.

37.2 Patient Selection

The assessment of a patient with cholesteatoma should start at the nose and end at the ear. As most acquired cholesteatomas are believed to be related to some form of Eustachian tube dysfunction, which in turn may be related to sinonasal disease, the patient history should begin here and treatment initiated if indicated. In a child, one should address previous surgical intervention, such as pressure equalizing tubes, adenoidectomy, and allergy or sinus surgery. In adults, sniffing behavior should be assessed as well as sinonasal disease and smoking history. Any vertigo should be noted, which could indicate the possibility of a labyrinthine fistula. The patient should be asked to perform the Valsalva maneuver, with the response in both ears recorded. The physical exam should begin with the opposite ear to determine if the condition is bilateral, perhaps due to more pervasive Eustachian tube dysfunction, and to determine the shape of the normal canal, which can be helpful in the examination of the diseased ear as the latter could show distorted landmarks.

The origin of the cholesteatoma should be noted so that the pattern of cholesteatoma spread can be anticipated. Primary acquired cholesteatomas typically begin as retraction pockets in the pars flaccida (epitympanic cholesteatoma) or posterior pars tensa (mesotympanic cholesteatoma). One should anticipate more extensive involvement of the anterior epitympanum and supratubal recess with epitympanic cholesteatoma, but because the disease enters the mastoid lateral to the incus, the facial nerve and sinus tympani are usually involved less extensively or only later in the course of the disease. Mesotympanic cholesteatoma, on the other hand, involves the facial nerve and sinus tympani very early in the course of the disease, and a more difficult dissection should be anticipated.

A complete audiogram should be performed, including speech discrimination testing. The findings should be supported by the tuning fork exam using at least the 512-Hz fork. A significant sensorineural component to the hearing loss could suggest labyrinthine fistula, especially when associated with any balance disturbance.

Although a computed tomography (CT) scan is not absolutely essential, it can be very helpful with the retrograde technique and is recommended. The CT scan allows development of the mastoid to be noted, but, more importantly, the position of the tegmen tympani can be visualized. The lateral portion of the temporal lobe can be displaced quite inferiorly in some cases, which can make retrograde drilling more challenging, necessitating use of a smaller burr. The extent of the cholesteatoma can usually be ascertained with a CT scan, especially in adult cases, which usually show an expansile mass and destruction of the bony septae. However, even with CT, the extent of involvement in the mastoid can be underestimated, especially in pediatric cholesteatoma where well-developed air cells can be invaded by numerous "octopus tentacles" of cholesteatoma without obvious destruction of the septae.

37.3 Surgical Technique

37.3.1 Cholesteatoma Removal

The mastoid cortex is widely exposed through a traditional postauricular skin incision. A tympanomeatal flap is then developed, and the middle ear is entered inferiorly, away from the cholesteatoma, to determine the extent of disease in the middle ear. As this technique involves extensive drilling in close proximity to the lateral aspect of the head of the malleus and the body of the incus, it is necessary to visualize the incudostapedial joint and the integrity of the lenticular process of the incus as an initial step. Except in cases of very limited retraction pockets, the incudostapedial joint is disarticulated to avoid trauma to the inner ear from the subsequent drilling. A canalplasty is performed posteriorly until air cells can just be visualized through the intact cortical bone of the ear canal. This improves the view of the posterior mesotympanum and facilitates subsequent drilling of the superior canal wall as the cholesteatoma is followed throughout the epitympanum and into the antrum. A prominent tympanosquamous suture and spine are taken off at this point to increase exposure of the pars flaccida.

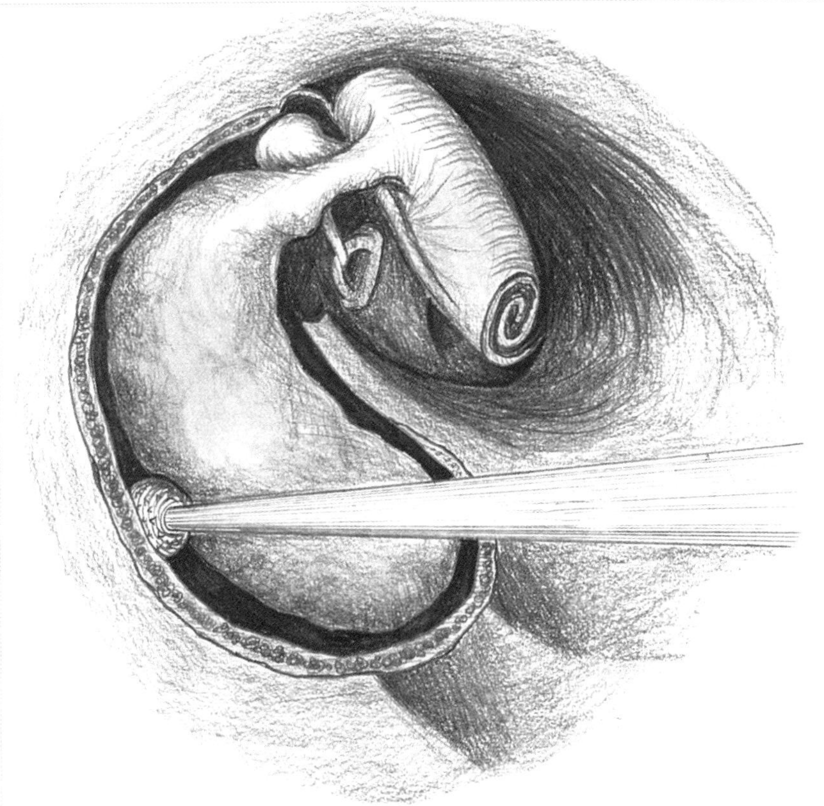

Fig. 37.1 Cholesteatoma is followed back posteriorly, with exposure of the entire sac at its origin from the tympanic membrane.

Drilling for cholesteatoma removal begins on the canal side with a 3-mm to 4-mm cutting bur or a rough-cut diamond bur at the upper posterior quadrant of the posterior canal wall, leaving a thin layer of bone at the scutum to protect the neck of the cholesteatoma, which is removed later with a smooth diamond bur. This drilling differs from a traditional atticotomy in that it extends all the way to the lateral external canal as a groove, with exposure of the tegmen tympani. Anatomical landmarks that can be used to gauge the proper extent of canal wall removal would be the area between the anterior tympanic spine and, inferiorly, the approximate exit of the chorda tympani from the bone (9 o'clock to 1 o'clock in a right ear).

There are two important points to keep in mind during this portion of the drilling. One is that if more than 30% of the canal wall is removed, reconstruction becomes difficult. The most common mistake is to initiate drilling at too inferior a point relative to the anterior tympanic spine, underestimating the extent of anterior-superior involvement. Subsequent drilling to expose the supratubal recess then leaves a larger canal wall defect than initially expected. Therefore, it is always better to initiate drilling superior at the anterior tympanic spine, as approximated by the short process of the malleus. The other important point to remember is that the tegmen at the lateral external canal frequently is more inferior than the more medial tegmen at the level of the epitympanum, so care must be taken to avoid injury to the dura laterally. As mentioned previously, a pre-operative CT can be very helpful to predict the height of the tegmen on the coronal view.

As bone removal continues posteriorly, the antrum is opened and the extent of the cholesteatoma can be appreciated. The goal is to remove only the bone necessary to expose the back edge of the sac, and a complete mastoidectomy is not necessary. Some recent evidence suggests that preserving the mucosa in the mastoid might improve subsequent middle ear/mastoid aeration.[1] With a small cholesteatoma in a sclerotic mastoid, the surgeon may frequently find the cholesteatoma extends only to the antrum, so minimal drilling is needed. The sac is followed back as posteriorly as is necessary until normal air cells or cholesterol granuloma is encountered behind the sac. This technique differs from that described by Tos,[2] in which a small cavity is created should extensive cholesteatoma be encountered. Instead, the sac is followed toward the mastoid tip, referred to as "turning the corner," leaving the inferior two-thirds of the posterior canal wall intact to facilitate reconstruction (▶ Fig. 37.1). This modification allows the removal of extensive cholesteatoma in a well-aerated mastoid, as frequently found in children, thus avoiding a canal wall-down situation.

The diamond bur is then used to remove the thin bone over the cholesteatoma sac, taking care not to violate the sac. The posterior edge of the sac is identified, and this is dissected upward out of the mastoid cavity, following a posterior-to-anterior direction. This allows visualization of any fistula of the bony labyrinth (horizontal semicircular canal). When the mastoid portion of the cholesteatoma has been dissected free, the incus is removed, followed by the head of the malleus, to complete the exposure (▶ Fig. 37.2). At this point, the sac remains intact, and its neck entering the retraction in the tympanic membrane can be visualized and resected from this area, leaving a small defect in the tympanic membrane.

The exposure for cholesteatoma removal is very similar to that of a canal wall-down situation and allows a nice

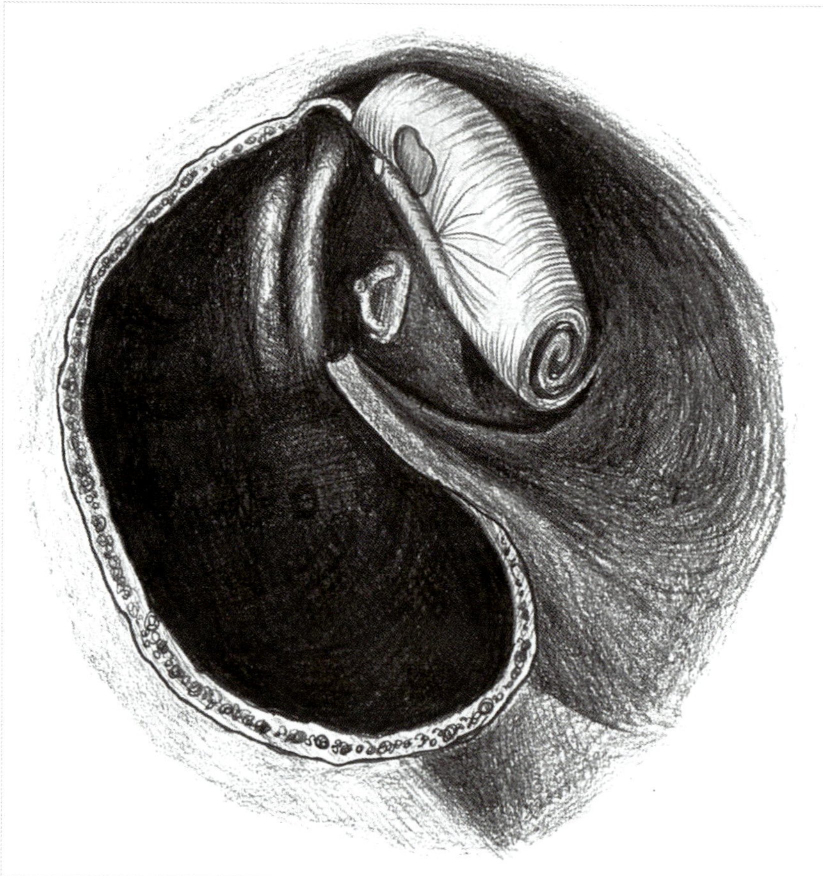

Fig. 37.2 The sac is resected, including the incus and head of malleus.

progression of disease removal, with direct visualization of the horizontal canal, facial nerve, and oval window/stapes area. If necessary, one can drill the cog to follow disease in the supratubal recess. If disease extends anteriorly into the protympanum, it is possible to gain increased exposure by cutting the tensor tympani tendon. If possible, the tendon is left intact to facilitate and secure the ossicular reconstruction.

37.3.2 Reconstruction

Although removal of the cholesteatoma is important to reduce residual disease, reconstruction is equally important to prevent recurrence of retraction pockets. Primary ossicular reconstruction is performed in all ears, even when second-look surgery is planned, because the prosthesis acts as a scaffolding to support the cartilage reconstruction of the tympanic membrane and maintain the middle ear space during the healing phase.

To reconstruct the canal wall, a 1-mm to 2-mm diamond bur is used to form grooves in the bone at the tegmen superiorly and in the inferior aspect of the remaining posterior canal wall. The superior groove at the zygomatic root is very important and must be drilled properly to ensure a good fit. The groove should be 1–2 mm wide and 2 mm deep and should be oriented parallel to the inferior canal to avoid torsion of the graft. Medially, the groove and subsequent reconstruction should extend down to and just posterior to the anterior tympanic spine and anterior malleal ligament so that it will approximate the cut edge of the malleus precisely. The inferior groove should be drilled carefully because the canal is frequently thin due to a combination of the canalplasty and subsequent mastoidectomy. Often a shelf, as opposed to a groove, is drilled here.

Autologous cartilage appears to be the ideal material for canal wall reconstruction. A piece of cartilage is harvested from the cymba of the conchal bowl to reconstruct the posterior canal wall. Because of its appropriate curvature, cartilage from the cymba is ideal for this purpose, and it usually has a uniform thickness of 1 mm. Generally, the cartilage will be 1–2 mm wider than the bony defect, allowing the canal wall reconstruction to snap into place under a little tension. While learning this technique, foil templates can be helpful to judge the size of the cartilage, which is cut like a trapezoid. The medial fit of the canal wall reconstruction is the most critical, and it is essential that a good fit between the cartilage and the residual bony canal wall be achieved and that the superior edge of the cartilage reconstruction be placed medially so that it closely approximates the handle of the malleus (▶ Fig. 37.3).

A hydroxyapatite/titanium hybrid prosthesis is typically used for ossicular reconstruction, and an attempt is made to utilize the malleus in the reconstruction. It has been shown that incorporation of the malleus in ossicular reconstruction provides an acoustic gain, possibly due to its cantenary lever action or improved acoustic coupling in the tympanic membrane.[3] Likewise, the presence of the malleus with an intact anterior malleal ligament offers improved prosthesis stability by allowing precise length adjustments and ultimate fit, leading to optimal hearing results.[4] When the malleus handle and suspensory ligaments are present, a partial ossicular replacement prosthesis (PORP), which is 2 mm in length, and a total ossicular replacement prosthesis (TORP), cut to 4.0–4.5 mm, can be consistently used for precise reconstruction when the notch of the prosthesis is placed just inferior to the insertion of the tensor tympani (▶ Fig. 37.4).

After precise ossicular reconstruction is performed, the posterior half of the tympanic membrane is reconstructed with pieces of cartilage using the mosaic technique (as described in Chapter 25). With this technique, the tympanic membrane is put together like a jigsaw puzzle: a half moon-shaped piece is placed on top of the prosthesis first, abutting the malleus handle, followed by the scutum piece; any spaces left between these two plates and the canal wall are reconstructed with slivers of cartilage cut to fit precisely in these areas (▶ Fig. 37.5). The trifurcation of the malleus handle, canal reconstruction, and tympanic membrane reconstruction has proven to be critical for recurrence prevention, so small chips of cartilage are very important in this area. Likewise, if the drilling proceeds superior to the anterior malleal ligament, care should be taken to reinforce this small area with cartilage. The reconstruction is then covered with perichondrium or fascia and the tympanic membrane remnant, if available. No space is left between the canal wall and reconstructed tympanic membrane to prevent cholesteatoma or retraction pocket recurrence. The anterior half of the tympanic membrane is typically not reconstructed with cartilage to allow postoperative surveillance and tube insertion, if necessary. The canal is then packed with antibiotic ointment, and a Pope Oto-Wick (Medtronic, Jacksonville, Florida) is placed in the ear canal; this packing material is removed 10 days post-surgery.

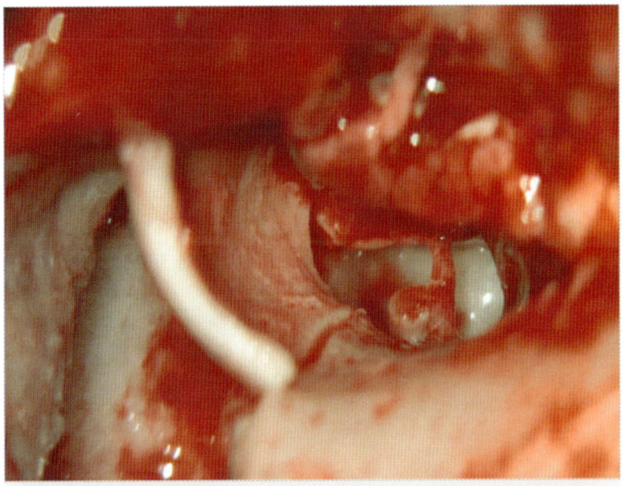

Fig. 37.3 Canal wall defect reconstructed with cymba cartilage, with close proximity to the cut edge of the manubrium.

37.4 Postoperative Care

The patient is instructed to perform the Valsalva maneuver three times a day, starting 2 weeks after the surgery. The Otovent (Abigo Medical, Askim, Sweden) has been used in children who are unable to perform this maneuver. The first postoperative audiogram is obtained 6–8 weeks post-surgery. If the patient is unable to perform the Valsalva maneuver or if the postoperative period is complicated by an effusion or retraction of the reconstructed tympanic membrane, a ventilation tube is placed 3–4 months after the surgery. Primary ventilation tube insertion is generally avoided.

For the most part, the retrograde mastoidectomy allows removal of the cholesteatoma sac in one piece with direct exposure, so second-look surgery is only performed in those cases where the cholesteatoma sac was violated and had to be removed piecemeal. The area of the sinus tympani is the most

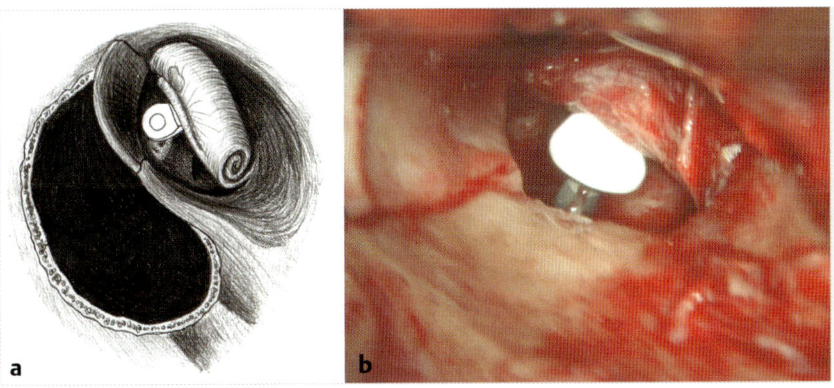

Fig. 37.4 (a) Schematic showing reconstruction of the ossicular chain after canal reconstruction. (b) Interoperative picture demonstrating reconstruction.

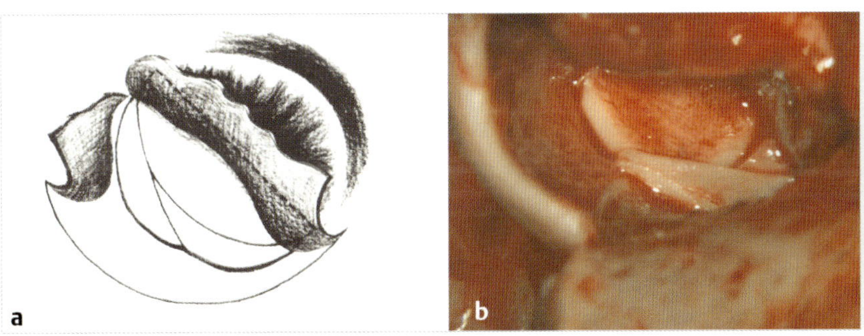

Fig. 37.5 (a) Schematic showing reconstruction of the posterior tympanic membrane with the mosaic technique. (b) Interoperative picture demonstrating precise fit between reconstruction of the tympanic membrane and canal wall reconstruction.

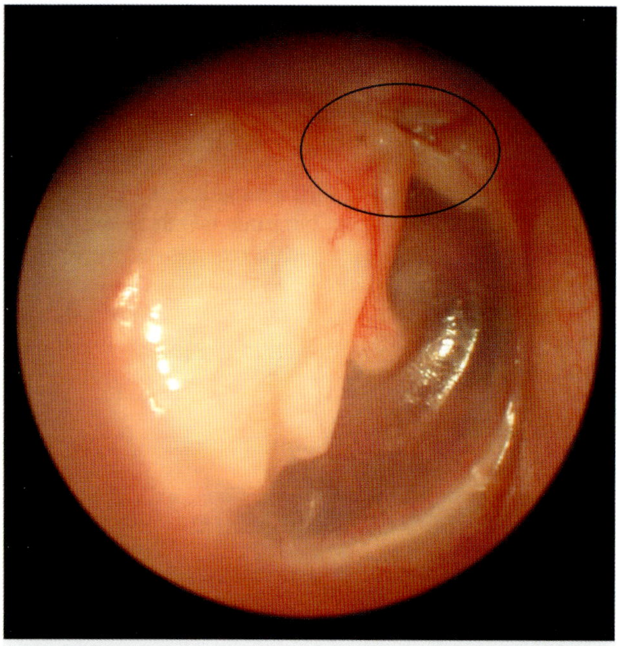

Fig. 37.6 Postoperative picture after the retrograde technique. Area in ellipse demonstrates "high-risk" area reinforced with additional pieces of cartilage.

problematic region as exposure here is difficult even with the retrograde mastoidectomy.

37.5 Complications

Although removal of the canal wall allows excellent exposure for complete removal of the cholesteatoma, leading to very low incidence of residual disease, reconstruction of the canal wall and posterior tympanic membrane is challenging, and there is a definite learning curve. Most recurrences have been noted during the initial 2-year follow-up, and the area between the canal wall and tympanic membrane cartilage reconstruction has been identified as a high-risk site. Because of this, much greater care is now taken to reinforce this area with chips of cartilage (▶ Fig. 37.6). The effect of this modification is felt to be positive, and the last 10 years have seen a reduction in recurrences in this area. We have experienced no cases of facial nerve injury or worsening of the sensorineural hearing level.

37.6 Outcomes

As of this writing, the retrograde technique has been used at our institution as the primary surgery for cholesteatoma removal for 20 consecutive years, resulting in an experience with more than 2000 ears. Short-term (2-year)[5] and longer-term (8-year)[6] results have been reported, indicating a dramatic reduction in recurrence rates and in need for a second surgery compared with our experience with canal wall-up surgery.[7] We no longer perform canal wall-down surgery as a primary surgery unless more than 50% of the canal wall is destroyed by disease or exterioration is needed because of large labyrinthine or cochlear fistulae, where the matrix cannot be safely removed.

In our longer-term study,[6] we examined the results of 46 patients (representing 50 ears undergoing this procedure) who had an average 7-year follow-up. Second-look surgery was performed in 4% for questionable incomplete removal of disease in the sinus tympani or footplate area. One of these patients had residual disease at the footplate. We found recurrent cholesteatoma in 8 ears (6 adult and 2 pediatric), representing a recurrence rate of 16%. The site of the original cholesteatoma was evenly divided between the epitympanum and the mesotympanum. However, of the recurrent cholesteatomas, 63% had originally been mesotympanic and 37% had originally been epitympanic, suggesting a higher recurrence rate for mesotympanic cholesteatomas. It is possible that mesotympanic cholesteatomas result from more pervasive Eustachian tube dysfunction compared with epitympanic cholesteatomas, the latter of which may reflect anatomical or structural blockage of the antrum, which could be more easily corrected with surgical removal of the disease.

The site of recurrence after reconstruction was typically in the epitympanic area (6 of 8 ears), just above the malleus handle, between the canal wall reconstruction and the tympanic membrane reconstruction. All 6 of these ears were revised, with removal of the previously inserted canal wall cartilage to expose the recurrent retraction, removal of the retraction, and reinsertion of the canal wall with reinforcement of the epitympanum.

The negative impact of smoking on long-term results was apparent in our longer-term study.[6] If one includes as complications the presence of recurrent disease, need to intubate the ear postoperatively, occurrence of a perforation, and need for a second-look surgery due to poor hearing results, the long-term complication rate of smokers was 79% (15 of 19 ears), compared with 16% (5 of 31 ears) for nonsmokers, making overall complications in smokers five times that seen in nonsmokers.

Long-term hearing results with the retrograde mastoidectomy technique have been encouraging, and compare favorably with those reported for staged ossiculoplasty.[8] In our longer-term study, there was a slight trend toward worsening hearing compared with the earlier follow-up, especially in the pediatric group, but the decrease was not significant, and the original gain from the preoperative level was maintained.[6] The type of ossicular reconstruction (PORP versus TORP) had no apparent impact on hearing results. Because there may have been a trend for those patients experiencing no complaints to disregard long-term follow-up (all but one of the 14 patients who had not been recently seen were doing well), it is possible that our longer-term data are biased toward worse outcomes. However, whether patients did not return for follow-up because they were doing well or because they were doing poorly is impossible to know with any degree of certainty.

References

[1] Kanemaru S, Umeda H, Yamashita M, et al. Improvement of eustachian tube function by tissue-engineered regeneration of mastoid air cells. Laryngoscope. 2013;123(2):472–476.

[2] Tos M. Mastoid Surgery and Reconstructive Procedures. Vol 2. New York: Thieme Publishers;1995.

[3] Dornhoffer JL, Gardner E. Prognostic factors in ossiculoplasty: A statistical staging system. Otol Neurotol. 2001;22(3):299–304.

[4] Dornhoffer JL. Hearing results with the Dornhoffer ossicular replacement prostheses. Laryngoscope. 1998;108(4 Pt 1):531–536.

[5] Dornhoffer JL. Retrograde mastoidectomy with canal wall reconstruction: a single-stage technique for cholesteatoma removal. Ann Otol Rhinol Laryngol. 2000;109(11):1033–1039.

[6] Dornhoffer JL. Retrograde mastoidectomy with canal wall reconstruction: a follow-up report. Otol Neurotol. 2004;25(5):653–660.

[7] Stern SJ, Fazekas-May M. Cholesteatoma in the pediatric population: Prognostic indicators for surgical decision making. Laryngoscope. 1992;102(12 Pt 1):1349–1352.

[8] Glasscock ME III. Results in cholesteatoma surgery. Paper presented at: First International Conference on Cholesteatoma, 1977; Birmingham, Alabama.

38 Canal Wall Removal and Replacement with Obliteration

Rick F. Nelson and Marlan R. Hansen

Abbreviations used in this chapter:

CWR: canal wall reconstruction
MRI: magnetic resonance imaging

38.1 Introduction

The major advantages of the canal wall reconstruction (CWR) procedure are that it provides the improved exposure to eradicate disease afforded by canal wall-down techniques and, when reconstructed, it provides a near-normal middle ear space, eliminates the need for routine bowl cleanings, allows patients to swim, and, aesthetically, does not require a large meatoplasty. Recurrence rates are low with CWR because blocking the attic physically prevents retraction of the tympanic membrane and obliterating the mastoid removes gas-absorbing mucosa.[1]

38.2 Patient Selection

Canal wall reconstruction is indicated for patients with cholesteatoma that extends into the epitympanum or mastoid and is not amenable to transcanal procedures such as tympanoplasty or atticotomy. Both congenital and acquired cholesteatomas in patients of any age can be treated with this technique. Canal wall reconstruction can be used to treat recurrent cholesteatoma in patients with prior mastoidectomy as long as the canal wall is intact and the lateral portion of the canal wall has not been lowered. Canal wall reconstruction can also be used to treat disease in patients with facial paralysis, labyrinthine fistula, encephalocele, or extensive scutal erosion. The inability to remove cholesteatoma from the mastoid air cells, such as in severe mastoid cholesteatosis, represents the major contraindication for the CWR technique.

38.3 Surgical Technique

38.3.1 Patient Preparation

The patient is given perioperative antibiotics to cover pseudomonas infection (typically piperacillin-tazobactam and ciprofloxacin). Pediatric patients are not given fluoroquinolones. Penicillin-allergic patients are given clindamycin and ciprofloxacin. The area posterior and superior to the auricle is shaved about 2 cm into the hairline. A C-shaped incision just inside the hairline is marked and injected with approximately 10 mL of 1% lidocaine with 1:100,000 epinephrine.

38.3.2 Incision and Collection of Bone Pate

The incision is made inside the hairline and carried down to the level of the temporalis fascia superiorly. The postauricular skin is carried forward in this plane, leaving the mastoid periosteum down. An anteriorly based musculoperiosteal (Palva) flap is incised along the temporal line and curved down to the mastoid tip. The Palva flap is elevated off the mastoid cortex. However, if there is a cortical mastoid defect from prior surgery or from cholesteatoma, this step is delayed until bone paté is collected. The temporalis muscle and the posterior musculoperiostium are elevated. Bone paté is obtained by drilling the occipital and temporal cortex with a large cutting burr and suctioning the paté through a screen collector attached to the suction (Otomed Corporation, Lake Havasu City, Arizona). Paté collection is limited to the cortical bone and stops if the mastoid air cells are entered or when there is approximately 10 mL of paté. The paté is soaked in 50,000 units bacitracin diluted with 10 mL of Ringer's solution until needed at the reconstructive portion of the case.

38.3.3 Mastoidectomy

Next, an intact canal wall cortical mastoidectomy with facial recess is performed. The posterior canal wall should not be lowered (medialized) or violated. Cholesteatoma and diseased air cells in the sinodural angle, mastoid tip, and retrofacial areas are removed. The facial recess is opened inferiorly, leaving the facial nerve covered with bone to protect it, as the saw blade will start in the facial recess. The incus and head of the malleus are removed.

The patient is then rotated toward the surgeon, and the external canal skin is elevated off the posterior, superior, and inferior ear canal down to the annulus. The annulus is elevated, and the tensor tympani tendon is cut. The canal skin and anterior drum remnant are pushed anteriorly.

38.3.4 Canal Wall Cuts

A microsagittal saw is used to cut out the posterior canal wall in a manner that, when reconstructed, will prevent it from collapsing into the mastoid. There are two cuts superiorly at 90 degrees to each other (▶ Fig. 38.1). The first cut runs posterior to anterior and parallel to the tegmen/temporal lobe. The second cut is perpendicular to the first, starting in the external canal and running toward the tegmen/temporal lobe. The inferior cut is a compound miter (angled and beveled) starting in the inferior facial recess and running laterally (▶ Fig. 38.1). It is important to bevel the cut from medial to lateral and posterior to anterior so that when the canal wall is replaced, it does not collapse back into the mastoid.

The posterior canal wall segment is removed and any skin or mucosa is removed with a gauze sponge or diamond drill. The wall is set aside for later reconstruction.

38.3.5 Eradication of Disease

Now with the posterior canal wall removed, the visualization is that of a canal wall-down mastoidectomy. Cholesteatoma is completely removed from the mastoid and middle ear. The cog is drilled to expose the anterior epitympanic space, and cholesteatoma is removed.

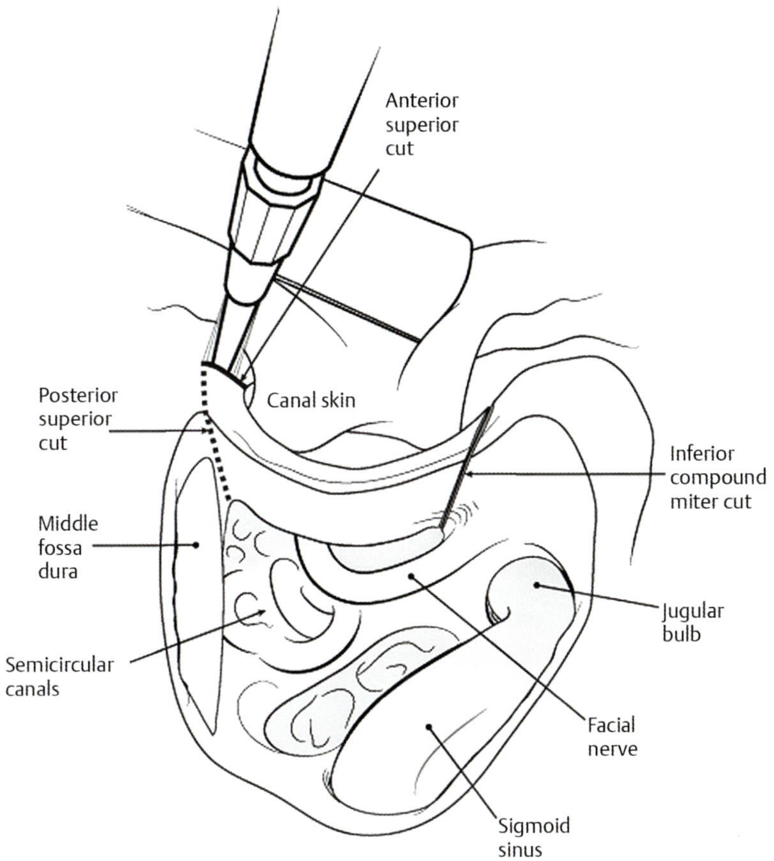

Fig. 38.1 Canal wall cuts. First, the posterior-superior cut is parallel to the middle fossa dura and bony tegmen. The second cut (anterior-superior) is made at a 90-degree angle to the tegmen. Finally, the inferior compound miter cut is made from medial to lateral. This beveled and angled cut prevents the replaced canal bone from falling into the mastoid after reconstruction.

38.3.6 Tympanoplasty with Temporalis Fascia and Silastic Spacer

Reconstruction begins by placing a teardrop-shaped piece of 0.04-inch reinforced medical grade silcone sheeting (Bentec Medical, Woodland, California) into the middle ear with the point extending into the Eustachian tube (▶ Fig. 38.2). This functions to hold space for reconstruction during a second-look procedure. The Silastic spacer rests on top of the stapes superstructure (if present) but does not extend posteriorly into the facial recess. In a patient without a stapes superstructure, an additional wedge-shaped piece of Silastic is placed onto the footplate, resting underneath the first piece of Silastic.

A large piece of temporalis fascia is harvested. The graft must be large enough to extend beyond the margins of the posterior canal wall cuts (▶ Fig. 38.2). The fascia is placed medial to the anterior drum remnant. Absorbable gelatin sponge is placed lateral to the anterior drum remnant. The fascia is reflected along the posterior canal wall skin and extends past the bony-cartilaginous junction.

38.3.7 Replacement of Posterior Canal Wall and Blocking the Epitympanum

The posterior canal wall bone is replaced (▶ Fig. 38.3). Large calvarial or mastoid tip bone chips are harvested with a mallet and chisel. These are trimmed and placed in the epitympanum, extending from the anterior epitympanum posteriorly to the posterior aspect of the lateral semicircular canal (▶ Fig. 38.3). Another bone chip is used to obliterate the facial recess.

38.3.8 Obliteration of the Mastoid with Bone Pate

The mastoid cavity is completely filled with bone paté, and dry gauze is used to compress the paté in place and wick off excessive bacitracin solution. The Palva flap is sutured posteriorly with 3–0 Vicryl suture to help prevent collapse of the posterior external canal meatus.

38.3.9 Packing of Ear Canal and Closure

Next, the patient is rotated back toward the surgeon. A Cottle speculum is used to displace the posterior canal wall skin onto the bony posterior canal wall. More absorbable gelatin sponge is used to secure the graft medially. The external ear canal is then packed with 0.5-inch iodoform strip gauze soaked in bacitracin ointment. In selected patients, such as those with extensive infection or inflammation associated with the cholesteatoma, a small Penrose drain is placed laterally to the Palva flap. The postauricular skin is closed with dermal 3–0 Vicryl sutures and Monocryl or nylon.

38.4 Postoperative Care

Patients are discharged with oral ciprofloxacin (in adults), amoxicillin/clavulanic acid (in adults allergic to fluoroquinolones

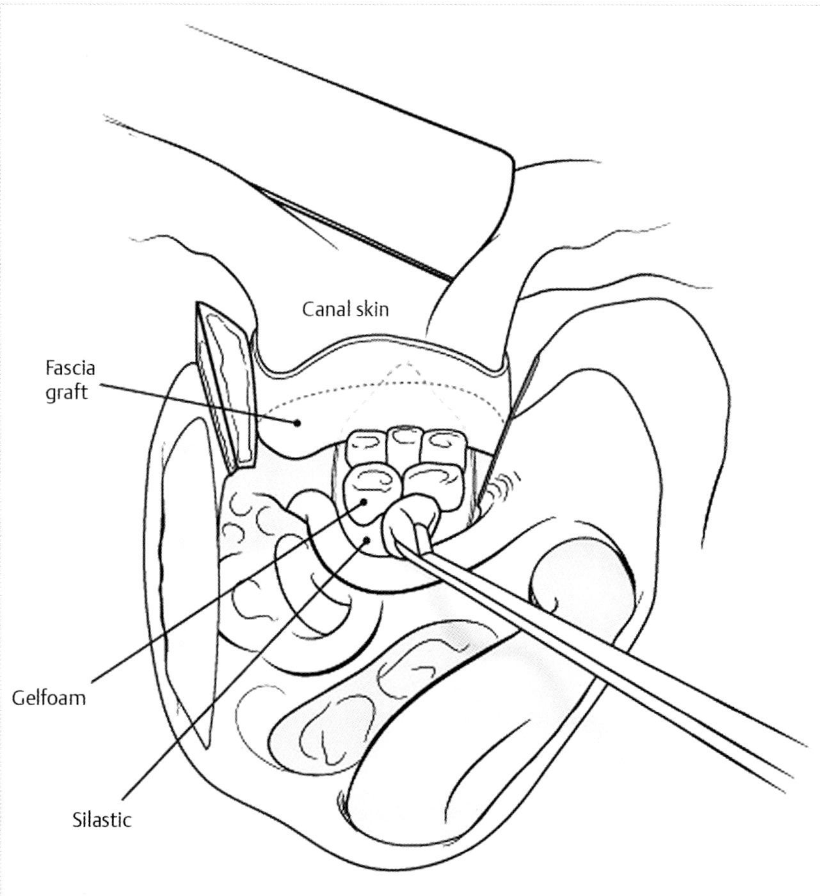

Fig. 38.2 Middle ear reconstruction. A 0.04 Silastic spacer is placed in the middle ear. A large piece of temporalis fascia is placed under the anterior annulus remnant. The fascia continues laterally along the posterior canal skin.

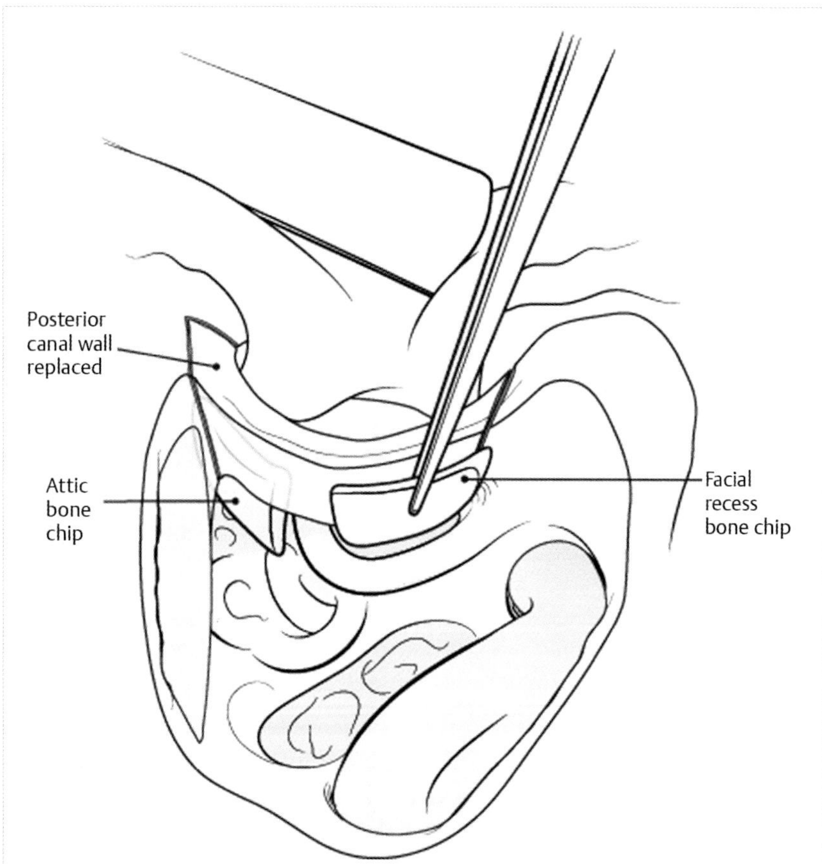

Fig. 38.3 Canal wall reconstruction. The posterior canal bone is replaced. Bone chips are used to block the attic and facial recess. The mastoid is obliterated with bone paté.

or patients < 18 years of age), or clindamycin (in patients allergic to fluoroquinolones and penicillin) to complete a 7-day course. In cases deemed at high risk for infection, particularly those with extensive perioperative infection, intravenous antibiotics are continued for 24–48 hours postoperatively. If placed, the Penrose drain is removed on the first postoperative day. The iodoform pack is removed 1 week postoperatively, and the postauricular sutures are removed.

The patient uses ofloxacin-based ear drops after the pack is removed until follow-up at 1 month. At this point the ear is examined and cleaned. The tympanic membrane is tested for mobility. A second-look tympanoplasty with ossiculoplasty is performed at 6–12 months. During the second surgery, the middle ear is examined for residual cholesteatoma and ossicular reconstruction with a cartilage graft is performed.

38.5 Complications

Canal wall reconstruction can have similar complications to other mastoidectomy procedures, such as tympanic membrane perforation. Attention to placement of the fascia graft can reduce this risk. If perforation does occur, the tympanic membrane can be repaired at the time of the second-look procedure.

Wound infection is also a risk with CWR. This occurs about 5% of the time and often is associated with *Pseudomonas aeruginosa* infection. Limiting paté collection to cortical bone without entering diseased mastoid air cells significantly reduces the risk of postoperative infection. Further, soaking the paté in bacitracin solution should help prevent infection. In some patients, placement of a Penrose drain in the wound can prevent fluid collection and postoperative wound infections. Finally, treatment with antibiotics can reduce the risk of postoperative infections.

Retraction of the tympanic membrane can lead to recurrence of cholesteatoma. In the CWR procedure, placement of large bone chips in the epitympanum to block this space prevents the membrane from retracting back into the mastoid. Then, if there is retraction of the tympanic membrane into the middle ear, it will likely be self-cleaning and the ear will be safe.

38.6 Outcomes

In 2013, the surgeons at the University of Iowa published their results from 285 CWR procedures in patients ranging in age from 2 to 80 years.[2] The average follow-up was over 4 years, and only 2.6% of patients required conversion to a canal wall-down procedure or closure of the ear (subtotal petrosectomy) for recurrent cholesteatoma. The postoperative infection rate was about 5%. Most patients underwent second-look ossiculoplasty, and the average postoperative air-bone gap was 23 dB. Patients should be advised that Eustachian tube function and aeration of the middle ear play a large role in the degree of conductive loss after cholesteatoma surgery.

To date, no cases of residual cholesteatoma in the obliterated mastoid cavity have been identified. Magnetic resonance imaging (MRI) with HASTE sequence is helpful for surveying for cholesteatoma in any case where there is concern for potential residual or recurrent cholesteatoma in the obliterated mastoid cavity.

38.7 Conclusion

Canal wall reconstruction tympanomastoidectomy provides an excellent intraoperative exposure for removal of cholesteatoma without the disadvantages of a canal wall-down mastoidectomy. The long-term cholesteatoma recurrence rate is low, and the procedure can be performed in children. Most patients have a safe and dry ear that is self-cleaning.

References

[1] Gantz BJ, Wilkinson EP, Hansen MR. Canal wall reconstruction tympanomastoidectomy with mastoid obliteration. Laryngoscope. 2005;115(10):1734–1740.

[2] Walker PC, Mowry SE, Hansen MR, Gantz BJ. Long-term results of canal wall reconstruction tympanomastoidectomy. Otol Neurotol. 2014;35(6):954–960.

39 Soft-Wall Canal Reconstruction

Haruo Takahashi

Abbreviations used in the chapter:

CT: computed tomography
SWCR: soft wall canal reconstruction

39.1 Introduction

Although there are numerous procedures for external auditory canal wall reconstruction after its removal during cholesteatoma surgery, the soft-wall canal reconstruction (SWCR) technique, first reported by Smith et al in 1986,[1] is now quite popular (especially in Japan) due to its characteristic features and clinical versatility. The process of SWCR comprises canal wall-down mastoidectomy followed by reconstruction of the external auditory canal wall defect using only soft tissues, such as a remnant of the external auditory canal wall skin and a piece of temporalis fascia (▶ Fig. 39.1).

39.2 Patient Selection

Any patient undergoing removal of all or part of the external auditory canal wall may be a candidate for SWCR. Additionally, SWCR can be used in cases of non-inflamed ears, such as surgery for facial decompression, cochlear implantation, and ossiculoplasty for congenital or traumatic ossicular disruption.[6]

Contraindications to this procedure would be cases that require reconstruction of both the anterior and posterior canal wall using free skin grafts, such as surgery for lateralization of the eardrum. In those cases, if all the directions of the ear canal (360 degrees) were reconstructed by a soft tissue, stricture and shrinkage would ensue.

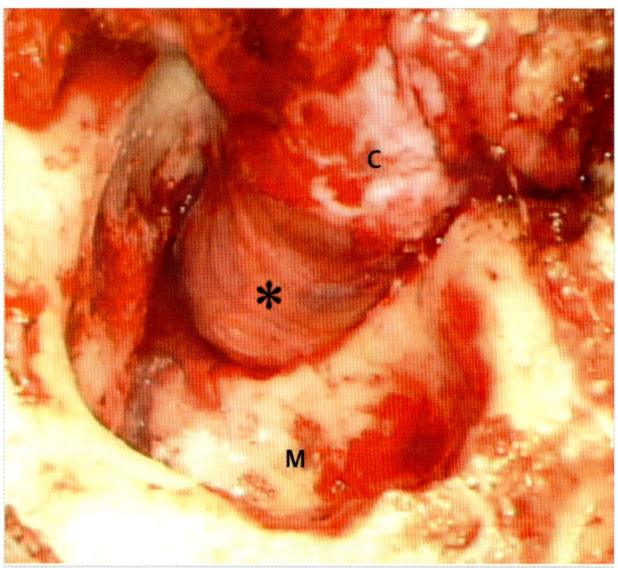

Fig. 39.1 Intraoperative view of SWCR (right ear). Defects in the posterior canal wall skin (C) and tympanic membrane are reconstructed only with a piece of temporalis fascia (asterisk). M, mastoid cavity.

The generally recognized advantages of SWCR include a wide surgical view, similar to that of the canal wall-down procedure; less required time and effort for fitting and trimming of material, unlike hard-tissue reconstruction; and a shorter time for wound healing as the area of the open wound is far smaller than with the canal wall-down procedure. Also, SWCR uniquely allows the status of the underlying mastoid mucosal function to naturally determine the ultimate contour of the healed ear canal as the soft wall either remains in a canal wall-up configuration or gradually retracts into a radical cavity canal wall-down configuration.

39.3 Surgical Technique

39.3.1 General Approach

SWCR is performed after removing the portion of the superior and posterior external auditory canal wall required for satisfactory cholesteatoma exposure and after removal in combination with either an epitympanectomy or canal wall-down mastoidectomy, as determined by the surgeon. A piece of temporalis fascia is harvested in the typical fashion, pressed thin, and appropriately sized and shaped. The size and shape absolutely depend on the underlying defect of the eardrum and ear canal wall after cholesteatoma removal, but typically this involves a rough size of 1.5 cm^2 and a rounded shape. The fascia is then placed to account for the canal wall defect on the extra-luminal aspect of the external auditory canal wall. The fascia is usually fixed with fibrin glue, but this is not necessary if it is of sufficient size to widely cover the defect. The residual preserved canal wall skin is then re-draped overlying the fascia, and the canal wall is packed with 2–3 small pieces of antibiotic-soaked gauze through the outer canal.

39.3.2 SWCR with Mastoid Obliteration

If the drilled mastoidectomy cavity is deemed excessively large, mastoid obliteration using bone paté and/or other material in combination with SWCR is recommended in order to avoid a problematic cavity should the soft wall ultimately retract (▶ Fig. 39.2a). The space between the mastoidectomy cavity and the soft posterior wall will typically shrink gradually and the soft wall retracts, forming a smoothly shaped posterior wall (▶ Fig. 39.2b).[7]

39.3.3 Second-Stage Surgery and Silicone Sheeting

In the event that a second-stage surgery is deemed necessary, a large silicone sheet can be used to cover the Eustachian tube up into the mastoid cavity in lieu of mastoid obliteration (▶ Fig. 39.3). This has been shown to facilitate recovery of mastoid aeration even after mastoidectomy.[8]

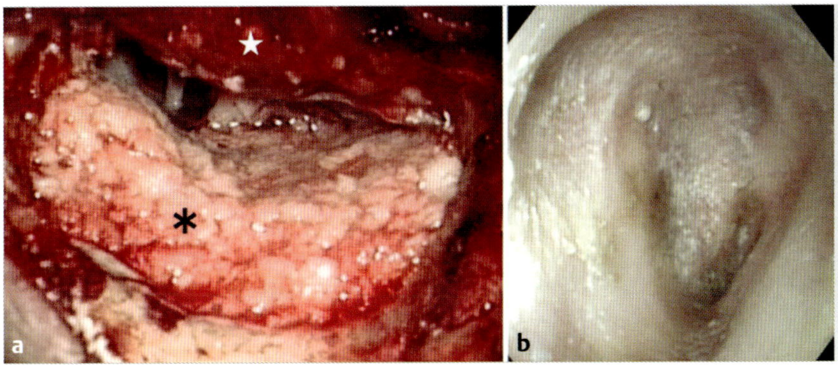

Fig. 39.2 Intraoperative views of mastoid obliteration combined with SWCR on the right ear (a) and postoperative otoscopic view (b). After SWCR (star), the mastoid was obliterated with bone paté (asterisk), and the space between them gradually shrinks to form a smoothly shaped posterior wall after surgery.

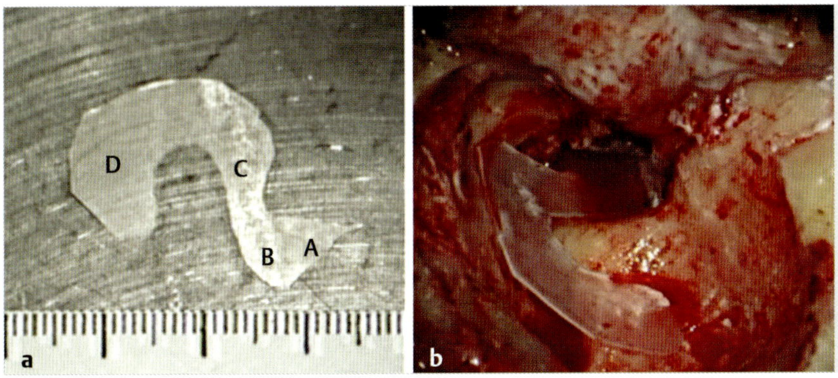

Fig. 39.3 Whole view (a) and intraoperative view (b) of a large-sized silicone sheet extending from the Eustachian tube (A), tympanum (B), epitympanum (C), and mastoid (D).

39.3.4 Application of SWCR for Non-Inflamed Ears

In cases that do not involve cholesteatoma and chronic ear disease, most of the intact mastoid and epitympanic mucosa can be preserved. Thus, the bony posterior wall can be removed with a high degree of confidence that mastoid aeration will recover in the early postoperative period and that the soft canal wall will not retract. It is actually easier to preserve the mastoid and epitympanic mucosa during surgery in these ears than in those with chronic otitis media because the middle ear is usually clean and does not have to be eradicated. For example, in such instances, a transmeatal atticotomy can be confidently extended to a transmeatal antrotomy and then further extended to a canal wall-down procedure, if needed, without hesitation. Similarly, a transmastoid facial recess approach can be expanded in the lateral direction to encompass the entire bony posterior external auditory canal wall if necessary. With any of these approaches, the soft wall will not retract after surgery if the canal skin and most of intact mastoid and epitympanic mucosa can be preserved.

39.4 Postoperative Care

Packing is kept in place usually for 3-6 days. After removal of packing, all we should do is to use eardrops containing both antibiotics and steroids for 3 days. Patients are followed up at 1, 3, 6, and 12 months after surgery and once every year for 5 years after that.

39.5 Complications

One possible disadvantage of SWCR is difficulty with post-surgical inspection and care of an open mastoid cavity that may result if the soft posterior wall retracts, especially if this cavity is large relative to the small size of the external auditory meatus. To avoid this, the surgeon may opt to make an incision in the soft posterior wall medially up to the edge of the tympanic membrane, opening the skin; however, the result will typically be an open mastoidectomy cavity instead of a SWCR, and the ear will lack the advantage of rapid healing. Alternatively, the M-meatoplasty, first reported by Mirck,[9] is the author's preferred technique to deal with this possible complication, due to the ability to selectively open the lateral aspect of the meatus while relatively sparing the deep part of the meatal wall, thereby allowing inspection of the ear while preserving the advantages of SWCR. The technique of M-meatoplasty is described in detail in Chapter 20.

Other possible complications, such as graft failure, necrosis, or incomplete canal wall closure, are similar to standard canal wall-up mastoidectomy procedures in their incidence. Antibiotic eardrops often successfully prevent infection on necrotic fascia, leading to natural healing, and placement of antibiotic-soaked absorbable packing may often cause natural closure of the defect. Finally, although the soft wall may hide residual cholesteatoma, its incidence is usually low given that this procedure includes a wide surgical view, similar to that of the canal wall-down mastoidectomy procedure.

39.6 Outcomes

As already alluded to, two distinct patterns can be observed postoperatively regarding the behavior of the soft posterior canal wall. In some ears, the reconstructed soft wall retracts to form a space similar to an open mastoidectomy cavity; however, in other ears, the canal wall remains in the original position, similar to a canal wall-up procedure. When viewing this phenomenon from the standpoint of middle ear ventilation and pressure regulation, interesting features have been noted. When the mastoid and possibly the epitympanic mucosa are preserved even partially during surgery, the soft wall typically remains in position without retraction. However, if mastoid mucosa is sacrificed via mastoidectomy, the soft wall usually retracts (▶ Fig. 39.4, ▶ Fig. 39.5). Thus, whether or not the soft posterior canal wall retracts appears to be strongly correlated with whether or not the mastoid mucosa was removed during surgery (▶ Fig. 39.6). Subsequent retraction also seems highly related to postoperative recovery of mastoid aeration, which also depends on the surgical treatment of the mastoid (▶ Fig. 39.7).

A hypothesis to explain this pattern of soft wall behavior is related to some of the presumed physiologic properties of mastoid mucosa. When preserved during surgery, the ventilatory (gas exchange) and mucociliary clearance functions of the mastoid mucosa may contribute to recovery of mastoid aeration in

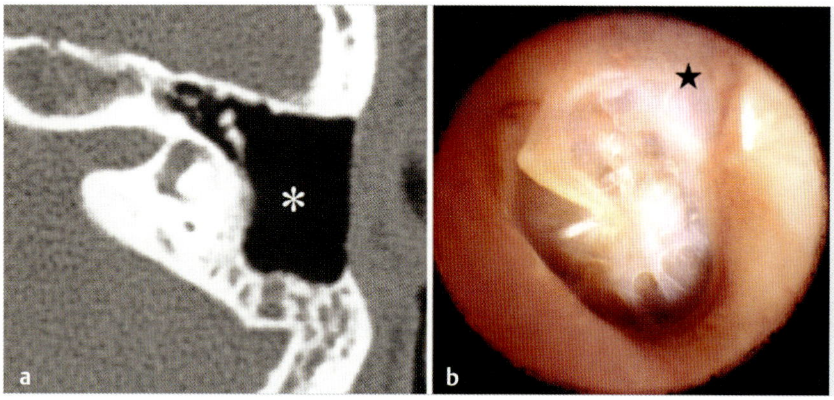

Fig. 39.4 Computed tomography (CT) scan (a) and clinical appearance (b) 6 months after surgery for attic cholesteatoma in a 21-year-old female patient. Mastoid mucosa was preserved during surgery, and mastoid aeration recovered clearly (asterisk), with the soft posterior wall (star) keeping a proper position without retraction.

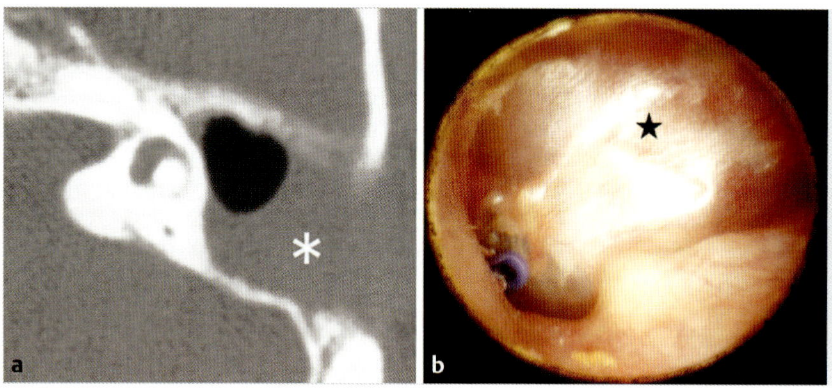

Fig. 39.5 CT scan (a) and clinical appearance (b) 5 months after surgery for attic cholesteatoma in a 47-year-old male patient. A mastoidectomy was performed during surgery, and mastoid aeration did not recover (asterisk), with the soft posterior wall (star) retracting to form a large cavity. It is interesting to note that this retraction occurred despite insertion of a tympanostomy tube during surgery.

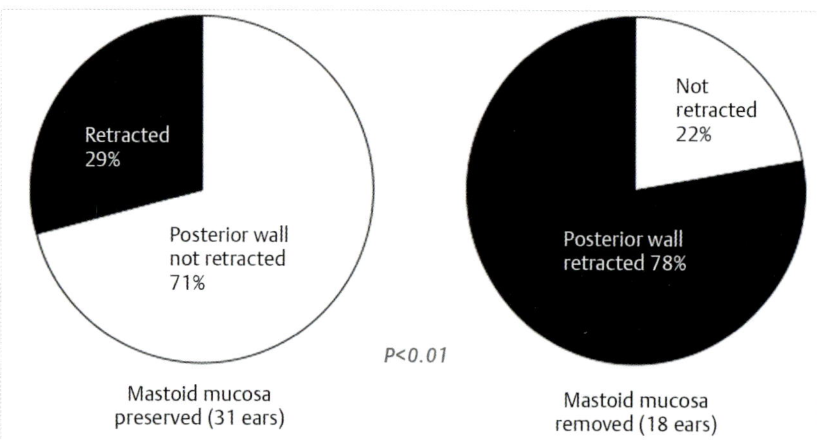

Fig. 39.6 Correlation between the treatment of mastoid mucosa during surgery (mastoidectomized or not) and retraction of the soft posterior canal wall.

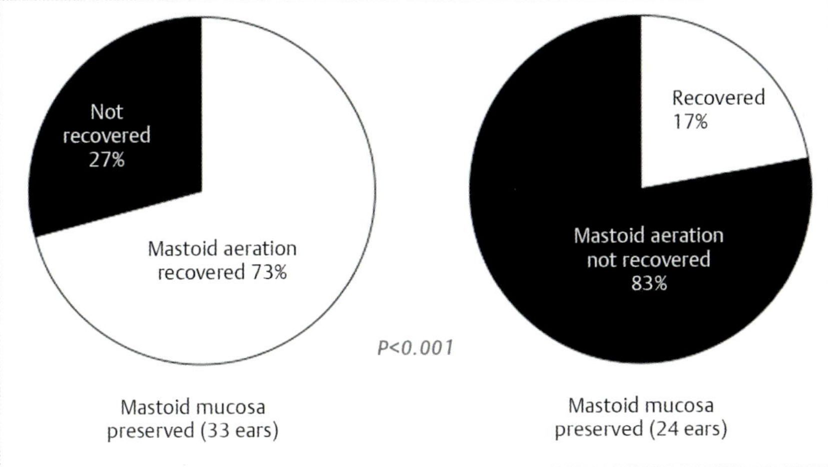

Fig. 39.7 Correlation between the treatment of mastoid mucosa during surgery and recovery of mastoid aeration after surgery.

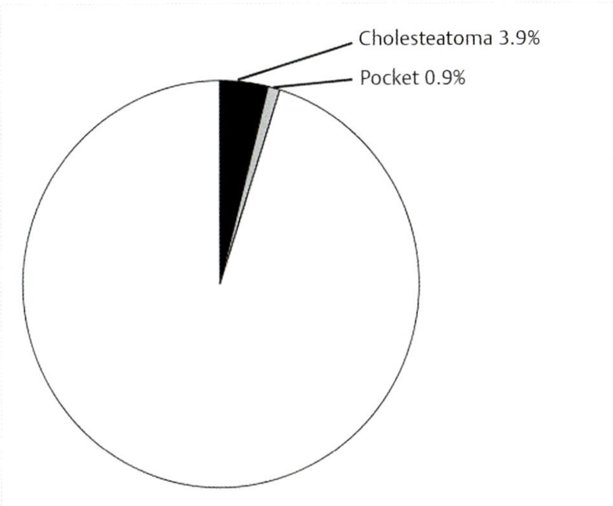

Fig. 39.8 Incidence of recurrent cholesteatoma after SWCR. Fresh cholesteatoma, 205 ears.

the early postoperative period. However, when mastoid mucosa is sacrificed during mastoidectomy, these beneficial properties may be lost and, therefore, mastoid aeration does not easily recover. As a result, negative pressure forms within the mastoid cavity, the soft wall retracts, scar tissue is formed, and an open mastoid cavity is created.

Therefore, we may say that SWCR allows the mastoid cavity itself to determine its ultimate post-surgery configuration according to its residual functions. This is why, with SWCR, the most stable form of the mastoid compatible with its function is typically obtained, and unpleasant occurrences such as attic retraction or recurrent cholesteatoma do not frequently occur (▶ Fig. 39.8). Consequently, SWCR allows surgeons to avoid the dilemma of having to choose between a canal wall-up or canal wall-down technique as the middle ear will naturally settle the question.

In instances where the soft posterior wall retracts, it is uncommon to encounter a retraction pocket with a small entrance into a cavity with large volume; rather, the entire soft wall generally will retract, and there is little risk of recurrent cholesteatoma formation. Furthermore, the soft wall has been found to be quite durable, generally avoiding necrosis or perforation due to the robust vascularization of the posterior external auditory canal wall skin. In contrast to other techniques that involve the rigid reinforcement of the external auditory canal wall with nonviable tissue or synthetic materials, SWCR does not impose an additional burden on the vascularization of the posterior external auditory canal skin.

39.7 Illustrative Case

A 61-year-old woman with facial palsy underwent facial decompression surgery due to poor recovery. Since she also had a narrow facial recess, about one-fourth of the posterior-

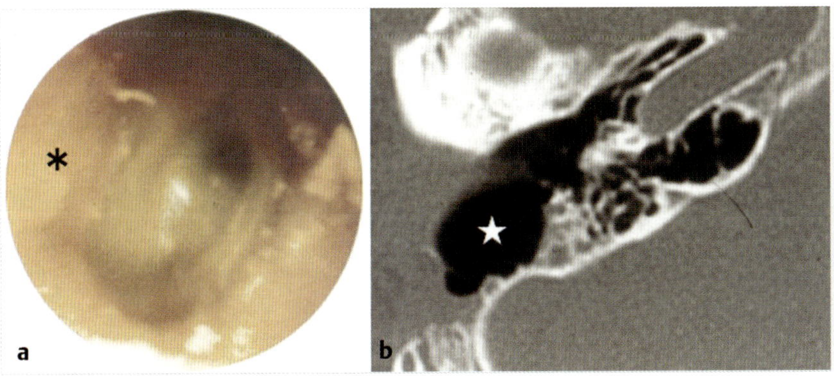

Fig. 39.9 Postoperative findings of the eardrum (a) and CT (b) of a female patient undergoing facial decompression, during which a part of the bony posterior canal wall was removed and was not reconstructed by hard tissue. Four years after the surgery, the tympanic membrane and posterior external auditory canal wall were observed to be in the proper position (star), without retraction, with complete recovery of aeration in the mastoid demonstrated by CT (asterisk).

superior portion of the bony external auditory canal wall was removed during the surgery in order to obtain a wider surgical view. The majority of the normal air cells and mucosa were preserved in the epitympanum and mastoid. The defect of the posterior external auditory canal wall was reconstructed only with soft tissue, and the skin of the posterior external auditory canal wall was preserved. Four years after the surgery, the tympanic membrane and posterior external auditory canal wall were observed to be in the proper position, without retraction, with complete recovery of aeration in the mastoid as demonstrated by CT (▶ Fig. 39.9).

References

[1] Smith PG, Stroud MH, Goebel JA. Soft-wall reconstruction of the posterior external ear canal wall. Otolaryngol Head Neck Surg. 1986;94(3):355–359.

[2] Hosoi H, Murata K. Tympanoplasty with reconstruction of soft posterior meatal wall in ears with cholesteatoma. Auris Nasus Larynx. 1994;21(2):69–74.

[3] Takahashi H, Honjo I, Naito Y, Miura M, Tanabe M, Hasebe S. Cause of posterior canal wall retraction after surgery from the viewpoint of mastoid conditions. Am J Otol. 1998;19(2):131–135.

[4] Takahashi H, Hasebe S, Sudo M, Tanabe M, Funabiki K. Soft-wall reconstruction for cholesteatoma surgery: Reappraisal. Am J Otol. 2000;21(1):28–31.

[5] Haginomori S, Nonaka R, Takenaka H, Ueda K. Canal wall-down tympanoplasty with soft-wall reconstruction using the pedicled temporoparietal fascial flap: technique and preliminary results. Ann Otol Rhinol Laryngol. 2008;117(10):719–726.

[6] Takahashi H, Honjo I, Hasebe S, Sudo M, Tanabe M. Soft-wall reconstruction of posterior canal wall for surgery of noninflamed ears: a preliminary report. Am J Otol. 1999;20(1):31–35.

[7] Takahashi H, Iwanaga T, Kaieda S, et al. Mastoid obliteration combined with soft-wall reconstruction of posterior ear canal. Eur Arch Otorhinolaryngol. 2007;264(8):867–871.

[8] Kazama K, Takahashi H, Kaieda S, et al. Effect of a large-sized silicone sheet upon recovery of mastoid aeration after mastoidectomy. Otolaryngol Head Neck Surg. 2008;138(6):738–742.

[9] Mirck PGB. The M-meatoplasty of the external auditory canal. Laryngoscope. 1996;106(3 Pt 1):367–369.

40 Canal Wall Reconstruction Using the Titanium Mesh Cage

Konrad Schwager

Abbreviations used in this chapter:

HA: hydroxyapatite
TORP: total ossicular replacement prosthesis

40.1 Introduction

As mentioned in Chapter 36, there has been a trend in the development of hybrid techniques that combine the advantages of canal wall-down and canal wall-up surgery for cholesteatoma. Many of these techniques start by following the disease from its origin in the epitympanum into the mastoid by drilling the posterior canal wall in a retrograde or in-out type fashion. If the mastoid is sclerotic, the resulting small open cavity is an excellent solution and reconstruction of the middle ear is undertaken. However, in situations where there is a well-aerated mastoid, the canal wall-down procedure may result in a large cavity with many postoperative care problems, so reconstruction of the canal wall is undertaken in these situations.

To reach the goal of anatomical and functional reconstruction of the canal wall after safe cholesteatoma removal, the use of biomaterials in many cases is necessary. There are several options, including cortical bone, reimplanted posterior canal wall, cartilage, and alloplastic materials. In theory, a patient's own tissue should be the best material for reconstruction, and, originally, the reimplantation of the temporarily removed posterior wall or the use of cortical bone seemed to be adequate. However, because of the nutritional requirements of the devascularized bone, the results of bony reconstruction were not encouraging.

Due to its bradytrophic nature, cartilage has been used in all types of tympanoplasty reconstructions and is a well-established tissue for the reconstruction of the posterior wall. Excellent wound healing is possible, even under adverse situations, because of cartilage's low needs for nutrition. However, the adhesion forces in the diseased middle ear can cause it to retract into the cavity, so combining it with other alloplastic materials is being investigated, including cements such as hydroxyapatite (HA)[1] and ionomeric cement,[2] solid ceramic cements,[3,4] and metals such as titanium. The latter can be formed into a "cage" and combined with cartilage plates for reconstruction.[5]

This chapter highlights the advantages and disadvantages of these biomaterials (see Chapter 8 for a further discussion), while featuring a technique of canal wall reconstruction using the titanium mesh cage.

40.2 Alloplastic Materials

40.2.1 Ionomeric Cement

The hybrid bone substitute ionomeric cement is derived from its application in dental medicine. This is a glass-based material that is available in a preformed design, but it is also available as a moldable consistency for the reconstruction of the posterior canal wall. This material has an excellent compatibility with bone,[2] but epithelialization is problematic. Even if the cement is covered with a soft tissue (Palva) flap, a high rate of nonepithelialized posterior wall results. Thus, a failure rate in up to one-third of patients has occurred, and the recommendation for this material was reduced for selected cases only.[2]

40.2.2 Hydroxyapatite (HA)

Pure HA is a demineralized bone matrix that has been used as a material for ossicular replacement prostheses since the 1980s. Two types are in use: high-density HA and regular HA. Preformed canal-shaped implants are individually adapted using the drill.[3] Also nonrigid implants have been used, which are composite flexible HA sheets consisting of a polymer in combination with HA.[6] For epithelialization purposes, periosteal flaps or temporalis fascia flaps have been proposed.[7,8] Proper epithelialization could be achieved in 60% to 80% of patients.[9,10] Histographic studies in animals showed no inflammatory response or foreign body reaction using HA cement.[1] Micrographic scans of explanted specimens in humans showed biodegradation by osteoclasts. In an experimental setting, demineralized bone matrix that naturally consists of HA was used for mastoid obliteration and posterior canal wall reconstruction. Wound healing was uneventful, but the material was not rigid enough to withstand retraction and adhesive forces.[11]

40.2.3 Bioactive Ceramics

Bioactive glass ceramic was first introduced as biomaterial for ossicular replacement prostheses. The material has good body acceptance but is degraded by osteoclasts and macrophages, causing instability in ossiculoplasty. In a series of 20 patients with a posterior wall reconstructed with bioactive glass ceramic, four patients suffered from consistent otorrhea, leading to the removal of the material.[4]

40.2.4 Polymeric Materials

Mersilene (Ethicon, Inc., Cincinnati, Ohio) is a polyester nonabsorbable fiber suture that has been used in a net configuration for reconstruction of the posterior canal wall. Proplast, a combination of carbon fibers and polytetrafluoroethylene, is a stable material with a porous surface designed to help connective tissue ingrowth, which should help to integrate the material. However, both of these materials have shown low tissue integration rates, and healing disturbances were reported in 30% to 50% of patients. Histological studies showed a high number of giant foreign body cells as obvious signs of nonacceptance.[12,13]

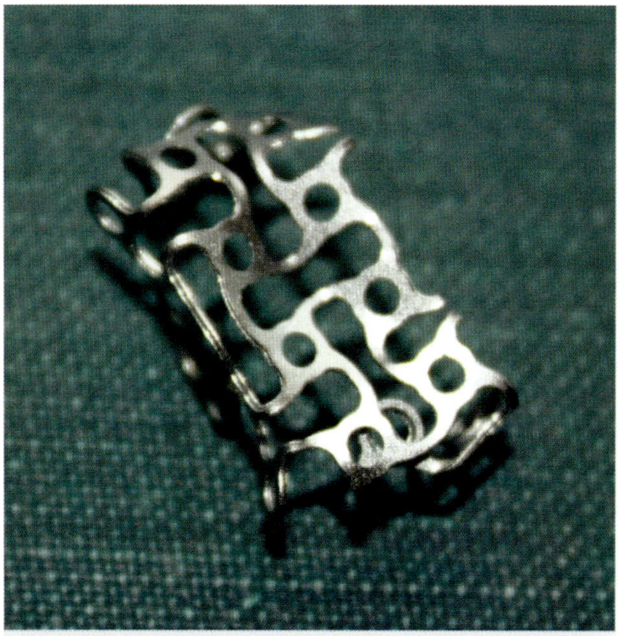

Fig. 40.1 Preformed titanium mesh cage.

40.2.5 Titanium

Titanium, with its tissue interactive surface of titanium dioxide, is a well-known material widely used in osteosynthesis and for replacement of bone. It has seen wide usage for construction of artificial joints in orthopedic surgery. Because of its stability and the possibility of creating delicate structures, it is an excellent material for ossicular replacement prostheses. In addition, due to its demonstrated biocompatibility,[14] titanium has gained popularity for canal reconstruction in the form of solid plates[15] and in mesh form.[16]

Titanium has also been combined with HA for reconstructing the posterior canal wall. A titanium net covered with a porous HA coating was fixed with screws to the mastoid tip and zygomatic root. In a small number of patients, good results could be achieved.[17]

The desire to restore the original anatomical situation by reconstructing the posterior wall and, to some extent, the mastoid cell system, led to the concept of the titanium cage. Titanium mesh is bent to form a cage-like structure to imitate the mastoid cells and to stabilize and support the posterior meatal wall. This cage is placed in the antrum and mastoid and additional fixation is not necessary. The cage is covered with cartilage plates and chips. Nutritional support reaches the cartilage through the openings of the cage. Wound healing and epithelialization are shown to be uneventful. The advantage of the cage over a pure canal seems to be the anatomical restoration of the mastoid. Wound healing disturbances have not been observed.[5]

40.3 Patient Selection

Patients with cholesteatoma in a well-pneumatized mastoid are candidates for mastoid reconstruction with the titanium cage as are patients who failed primary cartilage reconstruction of the posterior wall because of massive adhesion or cartilage retraction. Cholesteatoma in a poorly pneumatized mastoid should be treated with an open cavity technique as a first choice.

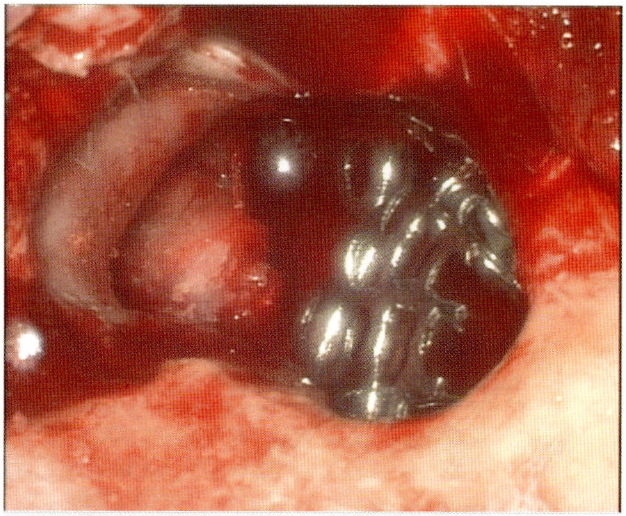

Fig. 40.2 Titanium mesh cage in situ following canal wall-down cholesteatoma surgery.

40.4 Surgical Technique

Canal wall reconstruction using the titanium mesh cage begins with a postauricular incision for exposure of the mastoid and external bony canal wall. The middle ear is entered and the ossicular chain is examined and disarticulated if still intact. The growth pattern of the cholesteatoma is noted. A canalplasty is performed until the mastoid air cells are just visible through thin bone and drilling is then commenced in the posterior-superior direction, following the cholesteatoma back from the middle ear into the aditus ad antrum and mastoid. Drilling is continued until the back edge of the cholesteatoma is seen or cholesterol granuloma is encountered behind the sac.

A decision regarding reconstruction is then made based on the size of the resulting cavity. As mentioned earlier, if the mastoid is sclerotic, then middle ear reconstruction is completed. A meatoplasty is made commensurate with the size of the cavity. On the other hand, if the cavity is large, canal reconstruction is performed.

Initially, reconstruction of the posterior canal wall was performed with cartilage plates supported by a titanium total ossicular replacement prosthesis (TORP) acting as a scaffolding. Because of some failures due to collapse of the cartilage reconstruction into the mastoid cavity, the technique was changed by reinforcing the cartilage reconstruction with titanium mesh. A 1-mm thick titanium mesh (Synthes Corporation, Tuttlingen, Germany) is used to build a size-adapted cage to rebuild the posterior canal wall, including the mastoid (▶ Fig. 40.1). The major part of this cage is created to support and stabilize the soft tissue reconstruction of the posterior wall. Other parts are bent as "legs" that are placed within the cavity (▶ Fig. 40.2). Thus, the titanium cage is rigid enough to keep a space open for aeration, while allowing passage through the antrum.

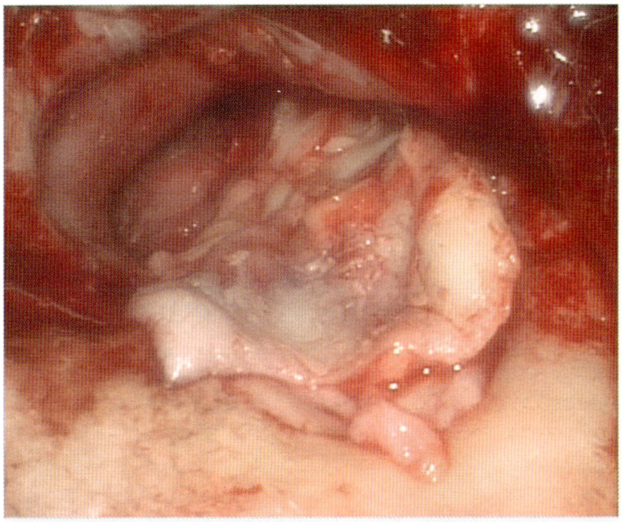

Fig. 40.3 Reconstructed posterior wall, Ti-cage covered with cartilage chips and temporary removed skin.

The portion of the titanium cage that supports the posterior canal wall is covered with cartilage chips of various sizes obtained from the patient, followed by the preserved skin of the auditory canal (▶ Fig. 40.3). The material for tympanoplasty in most cases is cartilage, and a titanium ossicular replacement prosthesis (Kurz Corporation, Dusslingen, Germany) is used for ossiculoplasty. Meticulous attention should be paid to close all gaps between the cartilage pieces to have a good layer that can easily be epithelialized. Regional flaps, as described for other reconstruction techniques, are not necessary. The ear canal and tympanic membrane are covered with Silastic sheets, and the canal is packed with absorbable gel packing soaked in vibromycin solution.

40.5 Postoperative Care

Patients are evaluated in the clinic at 3 weeks post-surgery, at which time the packing is removed. The patients are instructed to perform the Valsalva maneuver at this time. An audiogram is performed 6–8 weeks after surgery, and the patients are followed thereafter on a yearly basis.

40.6 Outcomes

In a clinical study this technique was performed in a total of 12 patients.[5] The average follow-up was 45.3 months. In one patient cholesteatoma was found during a planned second-look procedure. In all patients the reconstruction remained covered with cartilage and epithelialized within 3 months. None of the reconstructed walls necrosed, and no complications were recognized related to the inserted material. All recurrences were related to the condition of the underlying disease, rather than to the reconstructive material. The postoperative audiograms showed air-bone gaps ranging from 5 to 26 dB at 500, 1000, and 2000 Hz.

40.7 Conclusion

Canal wall reconstruction using cartilage plates supported by a titanium cage designed at the time of surgery for the specific defect appears to offer a durable option for canal wall reconstruction. By constructing both the mastoid cell system and canal wall, the titanium cage technique helps to facilitate tissue ingrowth and epithelialization of the reconstructed canal. Although the results are short-term, no exposure of the titanium has been seen, and functional results are acceptable. As in all cases of cholesteatoma, long-term follow-up of a larger group of patients will be necessary to determine the durability of the reconstruction.

References

[1] Dornhoffer J, Simmons O. Canal wall reconstruction with Mimix hydroxyapatite cement: Results in an animal model and case study. Laryngoscope. 2003;113(12):2123–2128.

[2] Geyer G, Helms J. Ionomer-based bone substitute in otologic surgery. Eur Arch Otorhinolaryngol. 1993;250(5):253–256.

[3] Wiet RJ, Harvey SA, Pyle MG. Canal wall reconstruction: A newer implantation technique. Laryngoscope. 1993;103(6):594–599.

[4] Della Santina CC, Lee SC. Ceravital reconstruction of canal wall down mastoidectomy: Long-term results. Arch Otolaryngol Head Neck Surg. 2006;132(6):617–623.

[5] Schwager K, Zirkler J. Reconstruction of the mastoid using a titanium cage. Otol Neurotol. 2014;35(8):1463–1465.

[6] Zanetti D, Nassif N, Antonelli AR. Surgical repair of bone defects of the ear canal wall with flexible hydroxylapatite sheets: A pilot study. Otol Neurotol. 2001;22(6):745–753.

[7] Black B. Mastoidectomy elimination: obliterate, reconstruct, or ablate? Am J Otol. 1998;19(5):551–557.

[8] Lenis A. Hydroxylapatite canal wall reconstruction in patients with otologic dilemmas. Am J Otol. 1990;11(6):411–414.

[9] Grote JJ. Results of cavity reconstruction with hydroxyapatite implants after 15 years. Am J Otol. 1998;19(5):565–568.

[10] Gyllencreutz T. Reconstruction of the ear canal wall using hydroxylapatite with and without mastoid obliteration and by obliteration with bone chips. Acta Otolaryngol Suppl. 1992;492:144–146.

[11] Leatherman BD, Dornhoffer JL, Fan CY, Mukunyadzi P. Demineralized bone matrix as an alternative for mastoid obliteration and posterior canal wall reconstruction: Results in an animal model. Otol Neurotol. 2001;22(6):731–736.

[12] Gammert C, Eitschberger E. [Artificial mesh in the reconstruction of the posterior auditory canal wall (author's transl)] HNO. 1978;26(3):100–103.

[13] Shea JJ, Jr, Malenbaum BT, Moretz WH, Jr. Reconstruction of the posterior canal wall with Proplast. Otolaryngol Head Neck Surg. 1984;92(3):329–333.

[14] Schwager K. Titanium as an ossicular replacement material: results after 336 days of implantation in the rabbit. Am J Otol. 1998;19(5):569–573.

[15] Magnan J, Chays A, Pencroffi E, Locatelli P, Bruzzo M. Canal wall prosthesis—new devices. Rev Laryngol Otol Rhinol (Bord). 1995;116(1):19–21.

[16] Sudhoff H, Brors D, Al-Lawati A, Gimenez E, Dazert S, Hildmann H. Posterior canal wall reconstruction with a composite cartilage titanium mesh graft in canal wall down tympanoplasty and revision surgery for radical cavities. J Laryngol Otol. 2006;120(10):832–836.

[17] Magliulo G, D'Amico R, Forino M. Reconstruction of the posterior auditory canal with hydroxyapatite-coated titanium. J Otolaryngol. 2001;30(6):330–333.

Part 8

Special Topics and New Horizons in Surgery for Chronic Ear Disease

41 Mastoid Cavity Obliteration

John L. Dornhoffer and Michael B. Gluth

Abbreviations used in this chapter:

IMP: inferior musculoperiosteal
MRI: magnetic resonance imaging
MTA: middle temporal artery
PORP: partial ossicular replacement prosthesis
TORP: total ossicular replacement prosthesis

41.1 Introduction

An unstable canal wall-down mastoidectomy cavity has the potential to impart a major negative impact on a patient's quality of life due to the collective burden of chronic otorrhea, frequent office visits, expensive pharmacotherapy, and occasional discomfort.[1,2,3,4] In the pediatric population, where tolerance of office examination and aural toilet may be poor, this is a particular dilemma.[5] Even in the best cases, a cavity that is stable from a chronic infection standpoint can still require occasional cleaning, cause caloric-effect vertigo, and inhibit optimal hearing aid fitting. Given this reality, mastoid obliteration offers many advantages and the potential to eliminate some of the undesirable aspects of the canal wall-down scenario.[6,7,8,9,10,11]

A review of the literature portrays a rate of mastoid cavity instability that roughly ranges from 10% to 60%, with apparent heavy dependence on the skill of the surgeon in executing a sound canal wall–down mastoidectomy technique, such as what is detailed in Chapter 35.[2,3,4,6,12] Even if a particular surgeon is averse to performing primary canal wall-down mastoid surgery, encountering and at times revising such cavities is an inevitable part of an otologic practice. Thus, familiarity with canal wall–down mastoidectomy and mastoid obliteration techniques should be viewed as a valuable tool within an otologic surgeon's skill set.

41.2 Patient Selection

Candidates for mastoid obliteration include both adults and children undergoing either primary or revision canal wall-down mastoidectomy surgery. The general obliterative scheme utilized and extent of obliteration will vary depending on factors such as the nature of the underlying cholesteatoma, temporal bone pneumatization, and degree of infection. In general, obliterative techniques are frowned upon in areas deemed at high risk of cholesteatoma recurrence; however, such risk often does not particularly apply to the mastoid because cholesteatoma within the mastoid is rarely difficult to expose and definitively remove. This point is highlighted by the fact that recurrent cholesteatoma within the mastoid cavity during second-stage canal wall-up surgery is rare.[13]

If temporal bone pneumatization is limited, it is quite common to achieve a small self-cleaning cavity without the need for mastoid obliteration. However, combined mastoid and epitympanic obliteration in these cases may still be deemed advantageous as a means of repositioning the height of the tympanic membrane at the level of the native tympanic ring, thereby preserving normal middle ear volume and facilitating a successful ossiculoplasty. When infection is severe or factors are present that negatively impact healing, such as diabetes, radiation, immunosuppression, or tobacco use, mastoid obliteration is particularly advantageous given that patients with these conditions may be at high risk of developing an unstable cavity.[1]

41.3 Surgical Technique

41.3.1 Obliteration Schemes

The first step made by the surgeon is deciding which areas to obliterate. In the typical situation where the mastoid is deemed to be at low cholesteatoma risk, the mastoid is obliterated with application of filler and a liner in sequence. When doing so, the purpose of the filler is not only to eliminate cavity volume, but also, more importantly, to fill cavity irregularities and to provide a smoothly contoured platform upon which to apply a liner that will subsequently epithelialize.

If epitympanic cholesteatoma risk is also deemed low, the obliteration scheme can be expanded to include the epitympanum to re-create the natural annulus height. In the uncommon situation where the mastoid cavity is felt to be at high risk, such as infiltrative cholesteatosis involving the perilabyrinthine air cells, the obliterative scheme is limited by sparing part of the mastoid cavity or by applying only a thin liner alone without the use of fillers.

The technique of canal wall-down mastoidectomy may slightly differ in a pneumatized versus a sclerotic temporal bone, which may also impact the approach taken toward obliteration. In a pneumatized bone, the general scheme often will involve lowering the edges of the cavity via wide saucerization and amputation of the mastoid tip, which results in a broadened shallow cavity that will invite inward soft tissue collapse. Obliteration of these large cavities is often best approached with sensible application of filler materials followed by lining with vascularized soft tissue flaps.

In contrast, a sclerotic temporal bone that is also deemed amenable for epitympanic obliteration may be reconstructed with simpler techniques given that these cases may involve comparatively less drilling of canal wall and solid mastoid bone once the cholesteatoma and a limited number of diseased air cells have been eliminated. Mastoid obliteration in a sclerotic temporal bone thus may be completed with a much smaller volume of filler and simple application of a liner and any preserved native canal wall epithelium.

41.3.2 Obliteration Materials

Choosing obliteration materials is often dependent upon a surgeon's bias and background as well as the nature of the underlying tympanomastoid defect. If the defect is small, the choice of obliteration materials tends to be more forgiving.

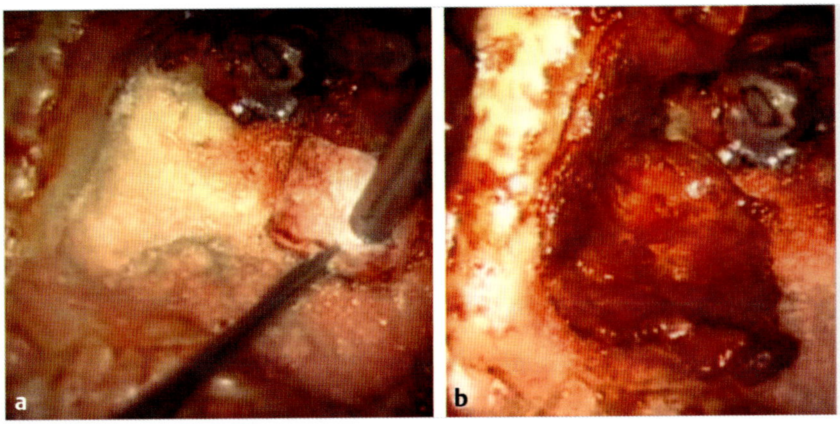

Fig. 41.1 Application of bone paté. (a) Bone paté harvested from the outside of the mastoid cavity is densely packed with a suction cannula and cotton pledget, with multiple applications to fill cavity irregularities (left ear), reduce cavity volume, and generate a smoothly countered platform upon which to apply a soft tissue liner. (b) In this case the middle temporal artery flap was utilized as a liner.

Bone Paté

Bone paté is a commonly used filler material, but it must be covered by a liner to prevent extrusion. Bone paté is abundantly available, in particular from the squamous temporal bone deep to the temporalis muscle. Harvest of bone paté is undertaken by reflecting the temporalis and drilling cortical bone with a cutting bur, followed by collection either using a commercially available reservoir connected to the suction tubing, or, if plentiful, by simply scooping paté from the surgical field into a specimen cup. It is crucial that paté only be harvested from outside of the mastoid so as not to include mucosa or infected material.

After harvest, bone paté is soaked in antibiotic solution while the remaining portions of surgery are completed. For placement, it is essential that the paté is applied into the defect and then densely packed utilizing a suction cannula and cotton pledget (▸ Fig. 41.1). In doing so, it is typical to sequentially apply paté several times in one site to achieve the desired tightly packed density. If bone paté is not densely packed, there is a tendency toward excessive reabsorption that can result in eventual formation of "potholes" within the obliterated cavity.

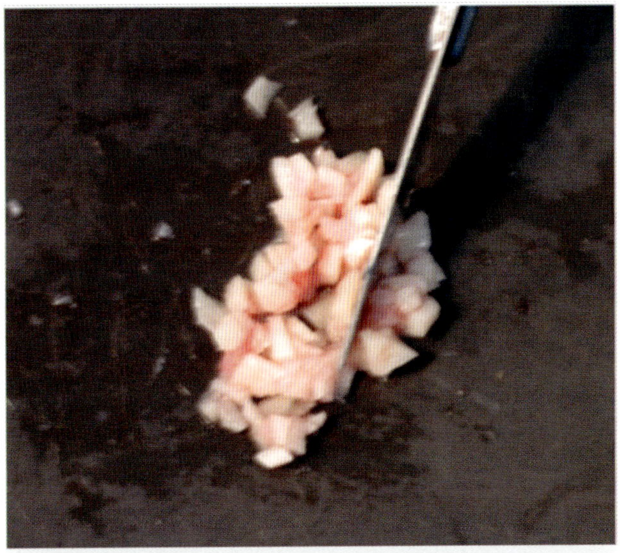

Fig. 41.2 Application of cartilage chips. Cartilage chips are harvested from the tragus and/or concha and morselized with a scalpel blade. Cartilage chips are favored for their high surface area and strong resistance to infection or extrusion.

Cartilage Chips

Auricular cartilage chips are harvested either from the tragus or concha. Once large pieces of cartilage have been acquired from these sites, they are stripped of perichondrium and morselized with a scalpel blade. If there is concern for infection, cartilage chips may be soaked in antibiotic solution, similar to soaking bone paté. After application into the mastoid cavity, a liner is typically applied to prevent extrusion (▸ Fig. 41.2).

Compared with bone paté, cartilage is more resistant to reabsorption and infection and, therefore, it is the authors' filler of choice. The larger size of the cartilage chips results in greater surface area and less need for dense packing. However, in some instances, availability of a sufficient quantity of cartilage may be problematic, especially in a well-pneumatized temporal bone or if cartilage has been used extensively for tympanic membrane reconstruction. In these cases it is possible to combine the cartilage with bone paté or synthetic filler.

Synthetic Materials

Various synthetic materials have been described as fillers in mastoid obliteration, particularly biocompatible ceramics. As noted in Chapter 8, if use of a synthetic material is desired, porous ceramics in a granular form are favored over cements because the latter seem to bear a higher risk of infection. Also, if an extraordinarily large bone defect requires obliteration, osseo-inductive materials, such as bioactive glass (BoneAlive, Boston Medical Products Inc., Westborough, Massachusetts), which are gradually replaced by new bone, may have theoretic advantages. Commercially available xenograft materials, such as demineralized bone matrix (DBX, Osteotech, Inc., Eatontown, New Jersey), are also an option and have been used successfully in small quantities (< 2 ml) by the authors for several years.[14]

Although synthetic materials offer the advantage of being readily available in bulk, they generally share a common tendency to extrude or to become infected. As such, it is favorable to use synthetic materials judiciously and/or in limited combination with autologous materials. Often, it is possible to obliterate the areas deep within the mastoid cavity, such as the sinodural angle and opened retrofacial air cell tract, using synthetic materials, and then to cover these with a layer of cartilage or bone paté that will constitute the outer interface

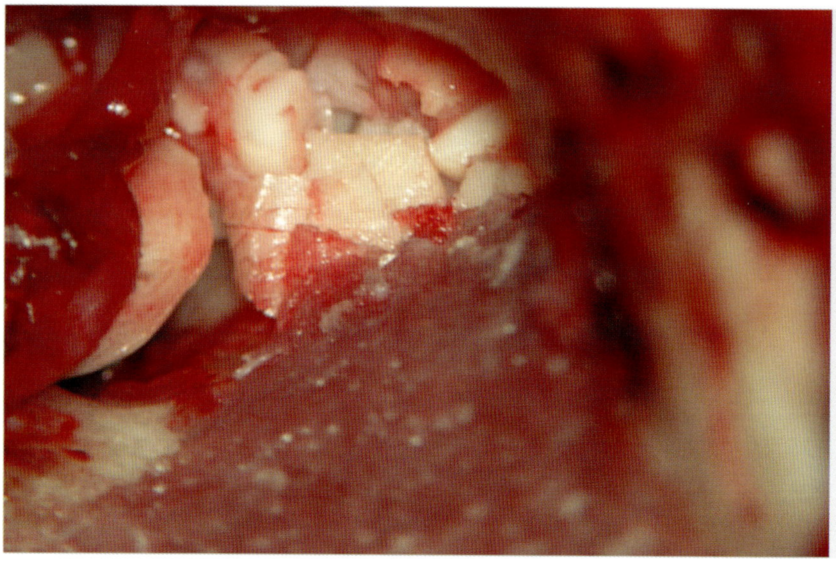

Fig. 41.3 Obliteration with demineralized bone matrix and cartilage chips. Demineralized bone matrix is applied to fill the sinodural angle (left ear), and cartilage chips are then used for obliteration of the more superficial areas near the reconstructed tympanic membrane. Synthetic materials may be useful when additional bulk is required to fill a mastoid cavity.

(▶ Fig. 41.3). If it is deemed necessary to use synthetic fillers in larger quantities, lining with a vascularized soft tissue flap is recommended.

Fascia, Perichondrium, and Pressed Muscle

Thin autologous connective tissues, such as temporalis fascia, pressed skeletal muscle, and auricular perichondrium, can all be used as liners. Such tissue is readily available and easy to process. When very little filler material is required, when there is a large quantity of intact healthy native canal wall epithelium, and/or when the interface with filler materials is small, such as with a sclerotic mastoid defect, these materials generally work well (▶ Fig. 41.4). However, if extensive coverage of filler material is necessary, particularly if the filler is synthetic, non-vascularized grafts may undergo necrosis, infection, and/or delayed epithelialization.

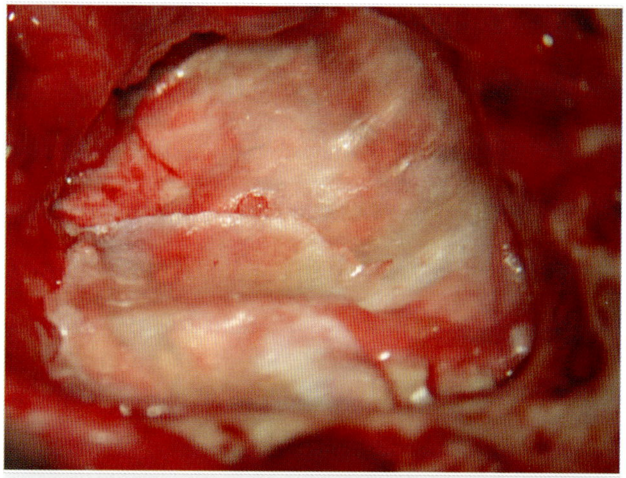

Fig. 41.4 Obliteration with demineralized bone matrix and cartilage chips. Demineralized bone matrix is applied to fill the sinodural angle (left ear), and cartilage chips are then used for obliteration of the more superficial areas near the reconstructed tympanic membrane. Synthetic materials may be useful when additional bulk is required to fill a mastoid cavity.

Soft Tissue Flaps

Rotational soft tissue flaps may variably comprise fascia, periosteum, and/or muscle, having either a distinct or random blood supply. These are pedicled either from a posterior-inferior base or superior-anterior base. In the case of the superior-anterior–based group, thick muscular flaps, such as those composed of temporalis muscle, are best avoided due to the potential for this thick pedicle to obstruct or narrow the external auditory meatus as it enters the tympanomastoid compartment.

Vascular supply to most rotational flaps described for mastoid obliteration is random or variably robust. For example, the commonly used Palva flap does not have a distinct vascular supply and, therefore, it is prone toward shrinkage and less apt to resist infection (▶ Fig. 41.5). Most posterior-inferior-based flaps are randomly fed by branches of the posterior auricular or occipital arteries proximally but tend to be avascular like the Palva flap at the most superior (distal) aspect.

One notable exception to this trend is the authors' favored middle temporal artery flap, a thin pliable anterior-superior–based flap chiefly composed of periosteum, which is based on the axial blood supply of the muscular branch of the superficial temporal artery (▶ Fig. 41.6). The middle temporal artery flap is elevated by releasing the posterior attachment of the temporalis muscle and dissecting in a plane immediately deep to the temporalis muscle. In doing so, the artery is reliably identified by its "train track" appearance (due to the presence of venae comitantes flanking either side). On average, the muscular branch of the middle temporal artery can be identified at a point 9 mm superior and 4 mm posterior to the spine of Henle, where it takes an abrupt turn from its posterior course to then pass toward the vertex of the skull. ▶ Table 41.1 depicts some of the characteristics of various soft tissue flaps that have been described for mastoid obliteration.

The authors' favored usage of soft tissue flaps involves the combination of the middle temporal artery flap and an inferior musculoperiosteal flap.[10] The middle temporal artery is applied as lining for the obliterated sinodural angle as well as coverage

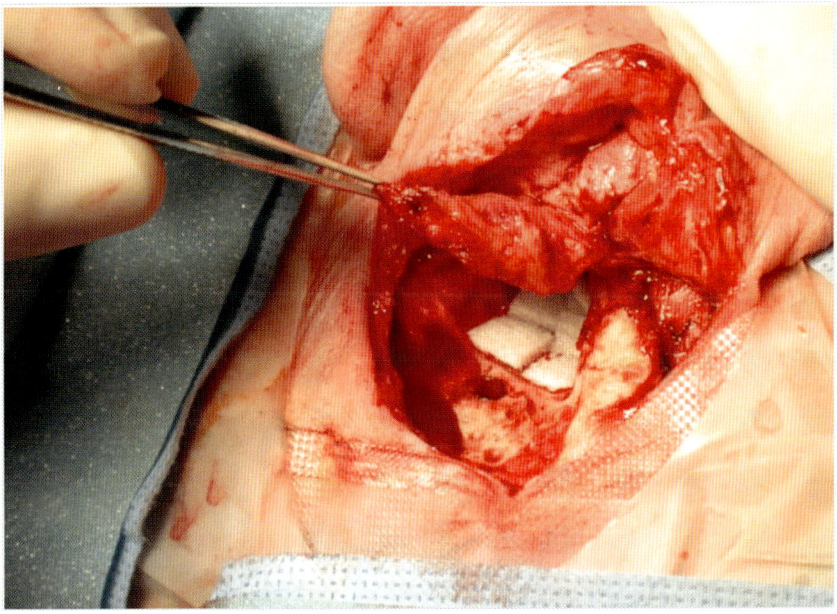

Fig. 41.5 Palva flap. A Palva flap consists of muscle, fascia, and periosteum that is hinged on the posterior aspect of the pinna (left ear). Although useful in some cases as a source of soft tissue obliteration, it lacks a robust vascular supply and therefore may be prone toward delayed shrinkage and fibrosis.

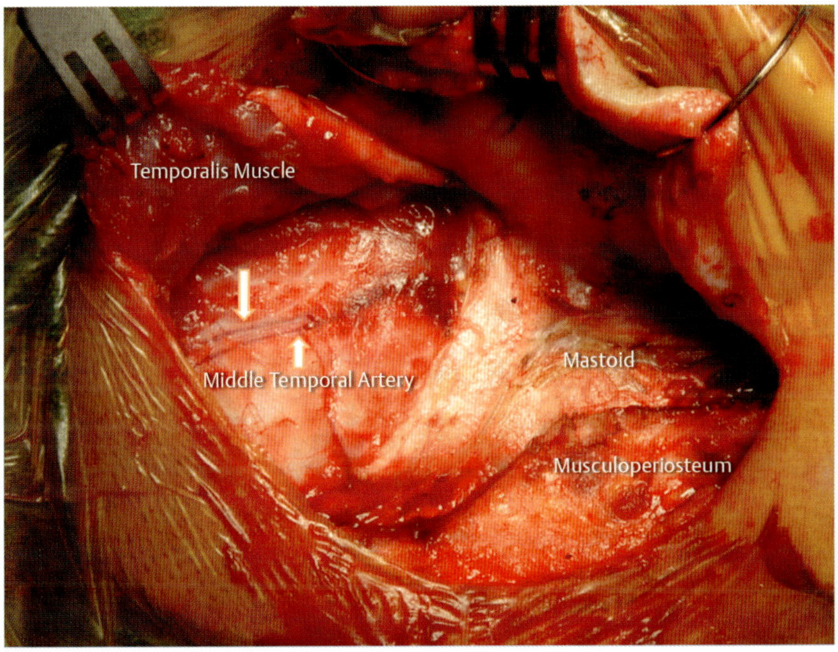

Fig. 41.6 Middle temporal artery flap. The middle temporal artery flap is harvested (right ear) by releasing the posterior attachment of the temporalis muscle and identifying the vessel in a plane immediately deep to the muscle fibers (block arrows). The artery has a typical "railroad track" appearance running within the periosteum. After identification of the artery, it will provide an axial blood supply to a large anteriorly based flap (3 cm x 6 cm) that is thin and pliable. (Image courtesy of Professor Marcus Atlas, Perth, Australia.)

for the tegmen and epitympanum. The inferior musculoperiosteal flap, which tends to have more bulk, is applied to fill the mastoid tip defect and the inferior aspect of the central mastoid defect (▶ Fig. 41.7). This flap is typically held in place with a 3.0 Vicryl stay suture that secures the base of the flap to the soft tissue inferior to the native external auditory canal (parotid fascia).

Skin Grafts

Full or split-thickness skin grafts may be used to line the bone of a mastoid cavity to promote rapid healing and to slightly reduce cavity irregularities; nevertheless, skin grafts in general do not impart significant obliterative effects. If vascularized soft tissue flaps are utilized, it is possible to apply small split-thickness skin grafts over the vascularized soft tissue of a rotational flap (▶ Fig. 41.8). This is particularly advocated when there is very little residual native canal wall or tympanic membrane epithelium present. The use of skin grafts in tympanomastoid surgery is further discussed in Chapter 48.

41.3.3 Surgical Application

Through a postauricular skin incision, the contents of the mastoid cavity are elevated and removed, typically in a single continuous skin flap. Confident removal of all epithelium from the mastoid is necessary if obliteration is to be performed. Drilling and shaping of the mastoid cavity is undertaken according to the desired obliterative scheme. If the epitympanum is deemed safe for obliteration, it may not be necessary to completely

Table 41.1 Soft tissue flaps used in mastoid obliteration

Flap	Composition	Blood Supply	Advantages	Disadvantages
Palva[15]	Musculoperiosteum, hinged on posterior aspect of pinna	Random	Ease of harvest	Avascular, delayed shrinkage and fibrosis, blind rotation into cavity
Hong Kong[11]	Vascularized temporalis fascia	Middle temporal artery (superficial branch)	Thin and pliable, vascularized, anteriorly based	Lacks bulk, difficulty filling mastoid tip in large cavity, blood supply may be cut during prior surgery
Middle temporal artery[8,10,16]	Vascularized periosteum (+/– thin sheet of muscle)	Middle temporal artery (muscular branch)	Thin and pliable, vascularized, anteriorly based	Difficulty filling mastoid tip in large cavity, blood supply may be cut during prior surgery
Temporalis muscle (Musculoperiosteum)[17]	Temporalis muscle	Middle temporal artery and deep temporal artery	Ease of harvest, abundance of tissue	Overly bulky, risk of blocking view of epitympanum and risk of meatal stenosis
Temporoparietal fascia[18,19]	Inferiorly based temporoparietal fascia	Random via superficial temporal and occipital arteries	Thin and pliable, abundance of tissue	Risk of alopecia, scalp numbness, variable blood supply
Inferior musculoperiosteal[9,10,20]	Inferiorly based muscle, fascia, and mastoid periosteum	Random via occipital and posterior auricular arteries	Abundance of tissue, useful for inferior aspect of mastoid cavity, ease of harvest	Avascular at distal tip of flap, risk of mastoid bleeding during harvest, scalp numbness

lower the posterior canal wall bone and facial because as the goal is to "raise" the mastoid and epitympanum up to the level of the natural canal wall and tympanic annulus via obliteration. If the epitympanum is to be exteriorized or if the majority of the canal wall bone has been previously removed, the technique of aggressive canal wall-down drilling, as outlined in Chapter 35, is followed.

Further flap elevation is undertaken until the middle ear space is entered. The authors favor tympanic membrane reconstruction with a large composite perichondrium and cartilage island flap harvested from the tragus. If the epitympanum is to be obliterated, it can be helpful to perform ossiculoplasty at the same stage because the prosthesis will support a cartilage graft at the desired natural annulus height. To estimate this height, a 2-mm partial (PORP) or 4-mm total ossicular replacement prosthesis (TORP) is used, as outlined in Chapter 29. Once the cartilage graft and prosthesis are in position, their placement will serve as a target height for the obliteration materials (▶ Fig. 41.9).

In cases where the epitympanum is to be exteriorized alongside mastoid obliteration, the margin of the tympanic membrane will be rotated medially, as is typical for a modified radical mastoidectomy, such that the tympanic and mastoid segments of the facial nerve serve as rough boundaries of the neotympanic membrane and for the newly reduced volume of the middle ear cleft. In this instance, the surgeon has the option of a Type III stapes columella reconstruction with tympanic membrane graft placement directly onto the superstructure versus placement of a major or minor columella (autograft or synthetic) according to various techniques discussed in Part 5, Roundtable on Ossiculoplasty. If ossicular reconstruction is not planned, Type IV tympanoplasty with exteriorization of the oval window is preferable to tympanoplasty that shields both the oval and round windows, according to the middle ear acoustic principles described in Chapter 9. Alternatively, the surgeon may wish to place Silastic sheeting in the middle ear and stage ossiculoplasty, especially if there is a risk of residual mesotympanic cholesteatoma.

41.4 Postoperative Care

After application of obliteration materials, the residual cavity is packed with ribbon gauze coated in antibiotic ointment, which also fills the external auditory meatus to stent the meatoplasty. If skin grafts are utilized, a thin (0.005-mm) non-reinforced sheeting of Silastic is applied as a barrier between the ribbon gauze and the grafts. Patients are treated with oral antibiotics for 10 days and examined in clinic 2–3 weeks later, at which point the ribbon gauze and Silastic sheeting are removed and excessive secretions and debris are suctioned. If the obliteration involves a large surface area that must heal, it may be repacked with ribbon-gauze on a serial basis every 2 weeks until it reaches near-complete epithelialization. If the cavity is small, repacking may be unnecessary and the patient is simply started on a combination antibiotic/steroid-containing otic drop for several days. Patients are advised to adhere to water precautions until complete epithelialization is confirmed. Premature cessation of postoperative care before healing is complete may result in failure to rehabilitate a cavity. Most obliterated cavities will be completely epithelialized by 2–3 months postoperatively.

41.5 Complications

41.5.1 Residual Cholesteatoma

Perhaps the most feared complication of mastoid obliteration is bulky coverage of residual cholesteatoma, which could

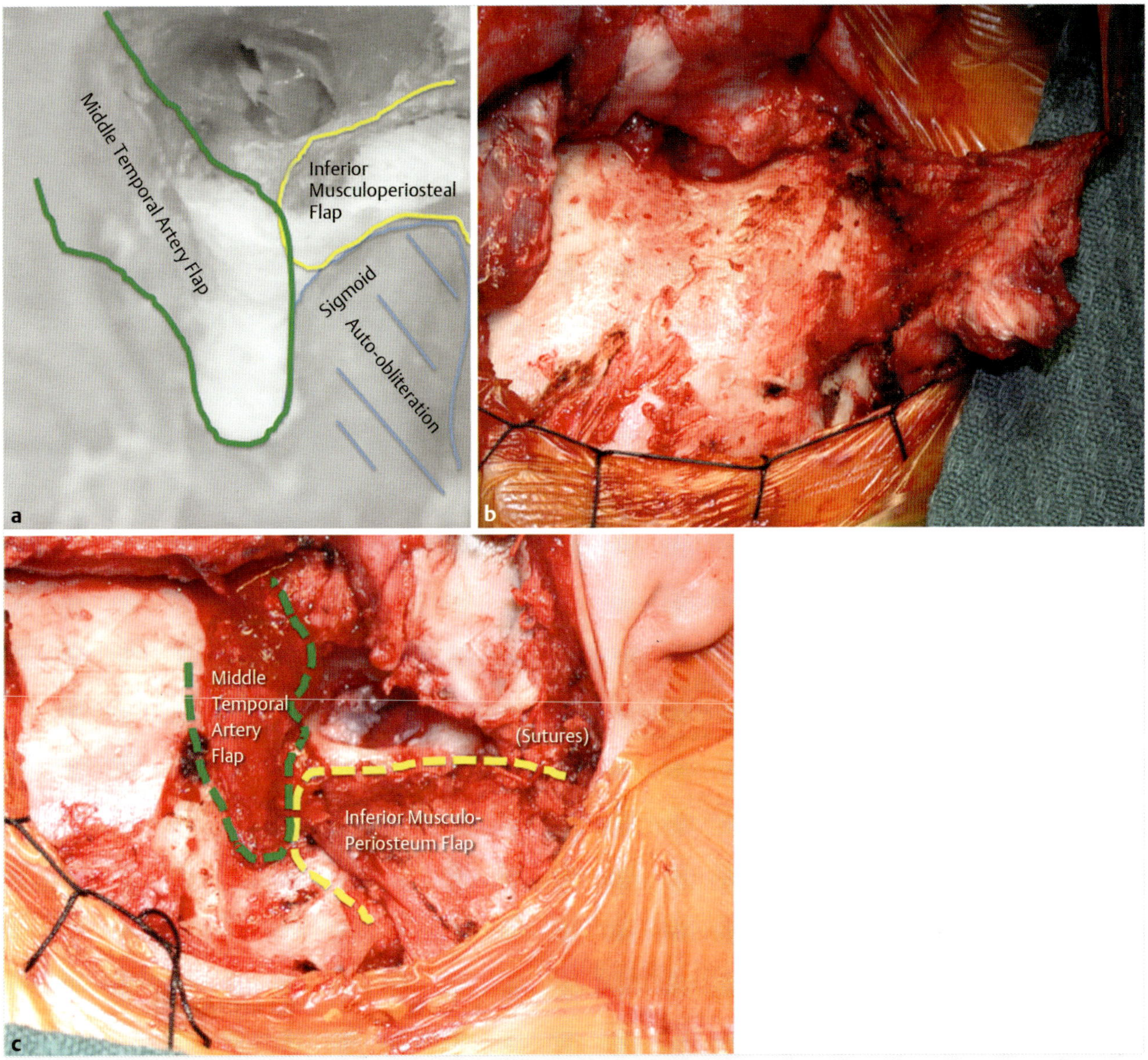

Fig. 41.7 Mastoid obliteration with vascularized soft tissue flaps (large cavity technique). (a) Scheme of obliteration is depicted in a right ear, which involves application of pressed bone paté that is lined with a combination of the middle temporal artery (green) and inferior musculoperiosteal (yellow) flaps. In this approach, the epitympanum is exteriorized, the mastoid tip is amputated from the digastric muscle, and the retrosigmoid aspect of the cavity is allowed to auto-obliterate (blue). This scheme is ideal for a large cavity from a well-pneumatized mastoid. (b) Intraoperative view of inferiorly based musculoperiosteal flap. (c) Intraoperative view of the obliterated cavity following rotation of soft tissue flaps. The inferior flap (yellow) is secured in place at its base with a single suture to the adjacent parotid fascia. Suturing is not required to inset the middle temporal artery flap (green). (Images courtesy of Professor Marcus Atlas, Perth, Australia.)

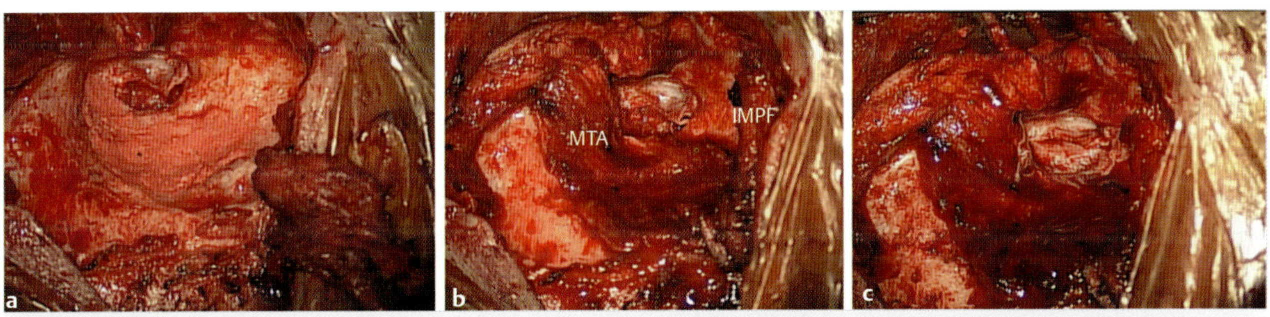

Fig. 41.8 Mastoid and epitympanic obliteration with cartilage tympanoplasty and split-thickness skin grafting (large cavity technique). (a) Bone paté is densely packed into the epitympanum and mastoid of a right ear resulting in a smooth platform upon which to apply soft tissue flaps. (b) The middle temporal artery flap (MTA) is rotated to cover the bone paté, and the inferior musculoperiosteal flap (IMP) is sutured to the parotid fascia to fill the inferior defect after mastoid tip amputation. (c) Final intraoperative view after cartilage tympanoplasty and application of split skin grafts.

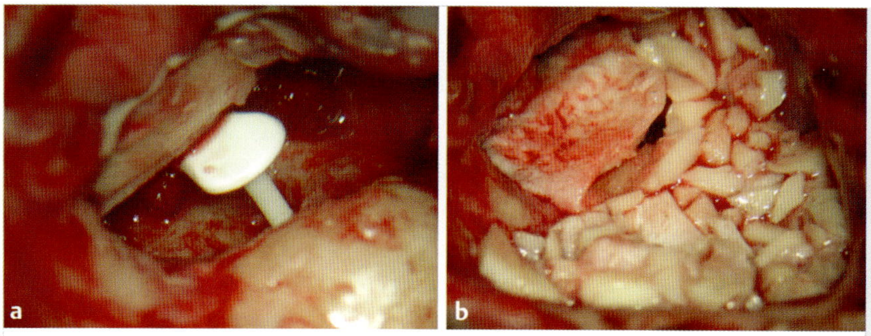

Fig. 41.9 Mastoid obliteration with preservation of middle ear volume using ossicular replacement prosthesis (small cavity technique). (a) The tympano-ossicular mechanism is reconstructed with a 4-mm PORP and a 9-mm composite perichondrium and cartilage island graft with a midline fold to act as a pseudo-malleus. This will set the neo-tympanic membrane height roughly at the place of the natural tympanic ring. (b) The mastoid cavity and epitympanum (left ear) are filled with cartilage chips and then covered with pressed perichondrium or a thin vascularized soft tissue flap.

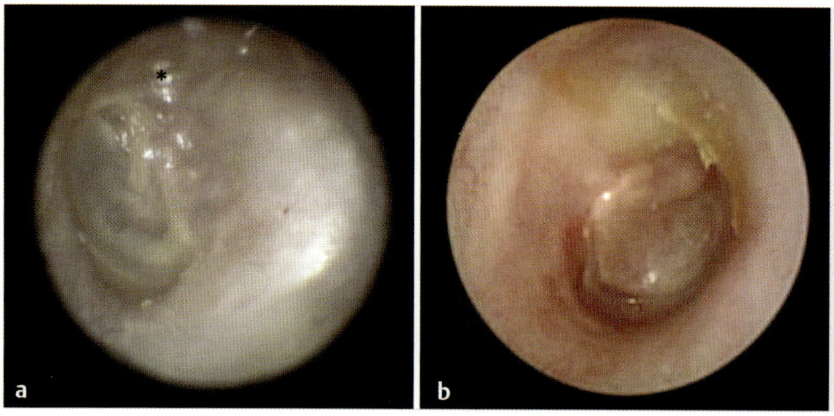

Fig. 41.10 Postoperative view of healed ears following mastoid cavity obliteration. These ears were obliterated using bone paté and vascularized soft tissue flaps. (a) Note the presence of an exteriorized epitympanum (asterisk) in a left ear that underwent mastoid cavity obliteration. (b) This right ear underwent concurrent obliteration of the mastoid cavity and epitympanum utilizing bone paté and the middle temporal artery flap alongside reconstruction of a subtotal tympanic membrane perforation utilizing a large underlay composite cartilage and perichondrium island graft.

potentially go undetected until quite large and even result in an intracranial complication. Although this complication is certainly possible, actual reports of this happening are scarce in the literature and it must be remembered that similar complications can also occur after standard canal wall-up and canal wall-down mastoid surgeries. In the authors' experience, having worked at institutions where mastoid obliteration has been undertaken for over two decades, rare instances of recurrent cholesteatoma within an obliterated mastoid have typically presented in a manner similar to standard cholesteatoma, with granulation tissue, otorrhea, and an expanding cyst. Like all cholesteatoma surgeries, ultimately the safety of mastoid obliteration is dependent upon the wisdom and judgment of the surgeon in determining when and how to proceed. If there is concern for residual cholesteatoma, it may be best to perform staged obliteration, schedule second-look surgery, and/or obtain diffusion-weighted magnetic resonance imaging (MRI) 1–2 years postoperatively.[21]

41.5.2 Infection

Infection following mastoid obliteration is possible, especially if a large amount of filler is required, synthetic materials are used, or there is an abundance of non-vascularized soft tissue. Although *Pseudomonas aeruginosa* infection is commonplace in a chronic ear, *Staphylococcus aureus* appears to be much more frequently encountered in revision canal wall-down mastoidectomy surgery.[22] When the index of suspicion for infection is high, preoperative culture acquisition is wise and culture-directed antibiotic therapy can be preventative. Some centers advocate perioperative treatment with intravenous antibiotics for several doses following mastoid obliteration. Furthermore, when soft tissue flaps have been harvested, it is possible to have wide areas of exposed bone underlying the postauricular incision that lack periosteum or other soft tissue cover; thus, meticulous wound closure and possible placement of a wound drain may prevent postauricular wound dehiscence.

41.5.3 Extrusion and Delayed Reabsorption of Fillers

When bone paté and synthetic materials are used, there is a fair possibility of partial extrusion or delayed reabsorption that can result in defects and irregularities of an obliterated cavity. It has been hypothesized that application of vascularized soft tissue flaps may reduce this occurrence. In the authors' experience, taking care to very densely pack bone paté and/or to combine bone paté or synthetic materials with available cartilage chips will reduce the likelihood and severity of filler loss.

41.6 Outcomes

If properly executed, mastoid cavity obliteration should result in a smoothly epithelialized surface lacking any fissures that could accumulate debris or infection (▶ Fig. 41.10). Favorable outcomes following mastoid obliteration using a variety of techniques have been reported, with success rates for creating a stable ear ranging from 70% to 100%.[6,7,8,9,10,11] Such outcomes should be viewed favorably in light of the fact that many of the cases depicted in these reports had already failed past canal wall-down mastoid surgery and thus represent some of the most difficult chronic ears. By obliterating with soft tissue flaps, O'Sullivan and Atlas reported a reduction in cavity volume to an average of 1.6 ml in 100 patients with postoperative follow-up ranging from 6 months to 4 years.[8] Utilizing a scheme of partial obliteration with bone paté and cartilage plates, Beutner et al. reported an average postoperative cavity volume of 3.1 ml in 26 patients with an average follow-up of 6 years. Additionally, they reported a reduction of caloric-effect vertigo in all of the patients (54%) who had been experiencing this preoperatively based on postoperative caloric testing.[23]

Dornhoffer et al reported changes in quality of life following mastoid obliteration as depicted by the Glascow Benefit Inventory.[24] These findings demonstrated a statistically significant improvement in overall quality-of-life scores and improvements within most subcategories. Furthermore, > 90% of subjects reported that they would recommend the procedure to a family member. Gluth et al. reported an 85% success rate of attempted conventional hearing aid usage after mastoid cavity revision and obliteration among 20 subjects who had been completely unable to wear a hearing aid preoperatively.[25]

41.7 Conclusion

In summary, various mastoid obliteration schemes exist, and these typically involve the application of filler and liner materials with the goals of reducing cavity volume and eliminating irregularities that could lead to retention of debris and chronic instability. In general, surgeons are advised to avoid bulky obliteration over areas deemed to be at high risk of underlying residual cholesteatoma and are discouraged from excessive application of fillers and non-vascularized soft tissue other than cartilage. Whichever method is used, there appears to be a common trend of achieving dry, stable ears and in improving a patient's quality of life.

References

[1] Gluth MB, Metrailer AM, Dornhoffer JL, Moore PC. Patterns of failure in canal wall down mastoidectomy cavity instability. Otol Neurotol. 2012;33(6):998–1001.

[2] Males AG, Gray RF. Mastoid misery: quantifying the distress in a radical cavity. Clin Otolaryngol Allied Sci. 1991;16(1):12–14.

[3] Sadé J, Weinberg J, Berco E, Brown M, Halevy A. The marsupialized (radical) mastoid. J Laryngol Otol. 1982;96(10):869–875.

[4] Wormald PJ, Nilssen EL. The facial ridge and the discharging mastoid cavity. Laryngoscope. 1998;108(1 Pt 1):92–96.

[5] Dornhoffer JL, Friedman AB, Gluth MB. Management of acquired cholesteatoma in the pediatric population. Curr Opin Otolaryngol Head Neck Surg. 2013;21(5):440–445.

[6] Dornhoffer JL. Surgical modification of the difficult mastoid cavity. Otolaryngol Head Neck Surg. 1999;120(3):361–367.

[7] Hung T, Leung N, van Hasselt CA, Liu KC, Tong M. Long-term outcome of the Hong Kong vascularized, pedicled temporalis fascia flap in reconstruction of mastoid cavity. Laryngoscope. 2007;117(8):1403–1407.

[8] O'Sullivan PG, Atlas MD. Use of soft tissue vascular flaps for mastoid cavity obliteration. Laryngoscope. 2004;114(5):957–959.

[9] Ramsey MJ, Merchant SN, McKenna MJ. Postauricular periosteal-pericranial flap for mastoid obliteration and canal wall down tympanomastoidectomy. Otol Neurotol. 2004;25(6):873–878.

[10] Singh V, Atlas M. Obliteration of the persistently discharging mastoid cavity using the middle temporal artery flap. Otolaryngol Head Neck Surg. 2007;137(3):433–438.

[11] van Hasselt CA. Toynbee Memorial Lecture 1994: Mastoid surgery and the Hong Kong Flap. J Laryngol Otol. 1994;108(10):825–833.

[12] Black B, Kelly S. Mastoidectomy reconstruction: Revascularizing the canal wall repair. Am J Otol. 1994;15(1):91–95.

[13] Wilson KF, Hoggan RN, Shelton C. Tympanoplasty with intact canal wall mastoidectomy for cholesteatoma: Long-term surgical outcomes. Otolaryngol Head Neck Surg. 2013;149(2):292–295.

[14] Leatherman BD, Dornhoffer JL. The use of demineralized bone matrix for mastoid cavity obliteration. Otol Neurotol. 2004;25(1):22–25, discussion 25–26.

[15] Palva T. Reconstruction of ear canal in surgery for chronic ear. Arch Otolaryngol. 1962;75:329–334.

[16] Fagan PA, Rodrigues SJ. Middle temporal artery flap in mastoid surgery. Otol Neurotol. 2004;25(3):242–244.

[17] Turner J. Soft tissue technique in musculoplasty obliteration of mastoidectomy cavities. Laryngoscope. 1972;82(7):1145–1159.

[18] Cheney ML, Megerian CA, Brown MT, McKenna MJ. Mastoid obliteration and lining using the temporoparietal fascial flap. Laryngoscope. 1995;105(9 Pt 1):1010–1013.

[19] East CA, Brough MD, Grant HR. Mastoid obliteration with the temporoparietal fascia flap. J Laryngol Otol. 1991;105(6):417–420.

[20] Gibb AG, Tan KK, Sim RS. The Singapore swing. J Laryngol Otol. 1997;111(6):527–530.

[21] Li PM, Linos E, Gurgel RK, Fischbein NJ, Blevins NH. Evaluating the utility of non-echo-planar diffusion-weighted imaging in the preoperative evaluation of cholesteatoma: A meta-analysis. Laryngoscope. 2013;123(5):1247–1250.

[22] Gluth MB, Tan BY, Santa Maria PL, Atlas MD. Unique microbiology of chronically unstable canal wall down tympanomastoid cavities: Considerations for surgical revision. J Laryngol Otol. 2013;127(5):458–462.

[23] Beutner D, Helmstaedter V, Stumpf R, et al. Impact of partial mastoid obliteration on caloric vestibular function in canal wall down mastoidectomy. Otol Neurotol. 2010;31(9):1399–1403.

[24] Dornhoffer JL, Smith J, Richter G, Boeckmann J. Impact on quality of life after mastoid obliteration. Laryngoscope. 2008;118(8):1427–1432.

[25] Gluth MB, Friedman AB, Atcherson SR, Dornhoffer JL. Hearing aid tolerance after revision and obliteration of canal wall down mastoidectomy cavities. Otol Neurotol. 2013;34(4):711–714.

42 Skull Base Approaches in Chronic Ear Surgery

J. Walter Kutz Jr. and Brandon Isaacson

Abbreviations used in this chapter:

COM: chronic otitis media
CROS: contralateral routing of offside signaling
CSF: cerebrospinal fluid
CT: computed tomography
DWI: diffusion-weighted imaging
MRI: magnetic resonance imaging

42.1 Introduction

Chronic otitis media (COM) with or without cholesteatoma typically presents with hearing loss and otorrhea that may be tolerated by some patients until more bothersome or concerning symptoms, such as dizziness, otalgia, facial paralysis, or deafness occur. By the time the patient seeks evaluation, the disease may have advanced beyond the boundaries of the mastoid and middle ear and may involve the petrous apex, perilabyrinthine air cell tracts, the internal auditory canal, the posterior fossa, the carotid artery, or the jugular foramen. The surgeon should be familiar with multiple skull base approaches to facilitate management of extensive COM.

This chapter will review the presentation and differential diagnosis of advanced chronic otitis media. The common surgical approaches for access to the petrous apex, internal auditory canal, and jugular foramen will be discussed. Postoperative care and rehabilitation options will be reviewed.

42.2 Patient Selection

The selection of the appropriate skull base approach depends on the type of lesion and location of the disease, as well as the hearing status and medical status of the patient. Preoperative hearing status should be determined with a comprehensive audiogram because some skull base approaches result in profound deafness in the operated ear. Temporal bone abscesses and cholesterol granulomas may only require the creation of a drainage pathway, whereas cholesteatoma and neoplasms often require more extensive access to attempt a complete excision. Complete eradication of the disease process may not always be possible. The surgeon in select circumstances may elect to leave cholesteatoma behind when resection could result in facial paralysis, vascular injury, or profound hearing loss. Periodic staged procedures may be required to evacuate accumulated debris in these cases.

42.3 Presentation and Differential Diagnosis

Chronic ear disease usually presents with hearing loss and otorrhea that can be treated with standard tympanoplasty with or without mastoidectomy. Symptoms such as otalgia, retro-orbital pain, vertigo, diplopia, facial paralysis, lower cranial nerve deficits, or profound hearing loss suggest more extensive disease. Petrous apicitis may present with Gradenigo's triad of retro-orbital pain, abducens nerve palsy, and chronic otorrhea.[1,2] Profound sensorineural hearing loss, with or without vertigo, implies direct involvement of the labyrinth. Hoarseness or dysphagia suggests involvement of the jugular foramen. Appropriate use of computed tomography (CT) and magnetic resonance imaging (MRI) will confirm the extent of the disease and allow for surgical planning.[3]

The differential diagnosis for COM is extensive (▶ Table 42.1). Cholesteatoma is common and often presents with a posterior-superior retraction pocket and debris collecting under the scutum. A chronically draining perforation that is unresponsive to ototopical antibiotics should raise suspicion for a more serious underlying problem, such as a cholesteatoma, petrositis, or neoplasm. If granulation tissue is identified that is not associated with a definite cholesteatoma and not responsive to ototopical antibiotic/steroid treatment, a biopsy is warranted to evaluate for a neoplasm. Deep otalgia should raise suspicion of a more serious problem, such as petrositis or a neoplasm.

42.4 Petrous Apex Drainage Pathways

The petrous apex is the pyramid-shaped medial aspect of the temporal bone that is bounded laterally by the otic capsule, tensor tympani muscle, and petrous carotid artery. Most individuals have a marrow-filled or sclerotic petrous apex, with only a small minority having aeration. A number of pre-existing pathways to the petrous apex can be used to access disease. Selection of a surgical approach for apical disease is facilitated by dividing the petrous apex into anterior and posterior segments using a parallel line through the internal auditory canal (▶ Fig. 42.1).[4]

Table 42.1 Differential diagnosis of chronic suppurative otitis media

Inflammatory disorders	Neoplasms
Chronic suppurative otitis media	Squamous cell carcinoma
Cholesteatoma	Endolymphatic sac tumor
Apical petrositis	Middle ear adenoma
Sigmoid sinus thrombosis	Lymphoma
Epidural abscess	Glomus tumor
Otitis externa	Langerhans's cell histiocytosis
Malignant otitis externa	Chondrosarcoma
Wegener's granulomatosis	Osteosarcoma
Eosinophilic otitis media	Rhabdomyosarcoma
Tuberculous otitis media	Adenocarcinoma
Cholesterol granuloma	Adenoid cystic carcinoma
Syphilis	Metastasis

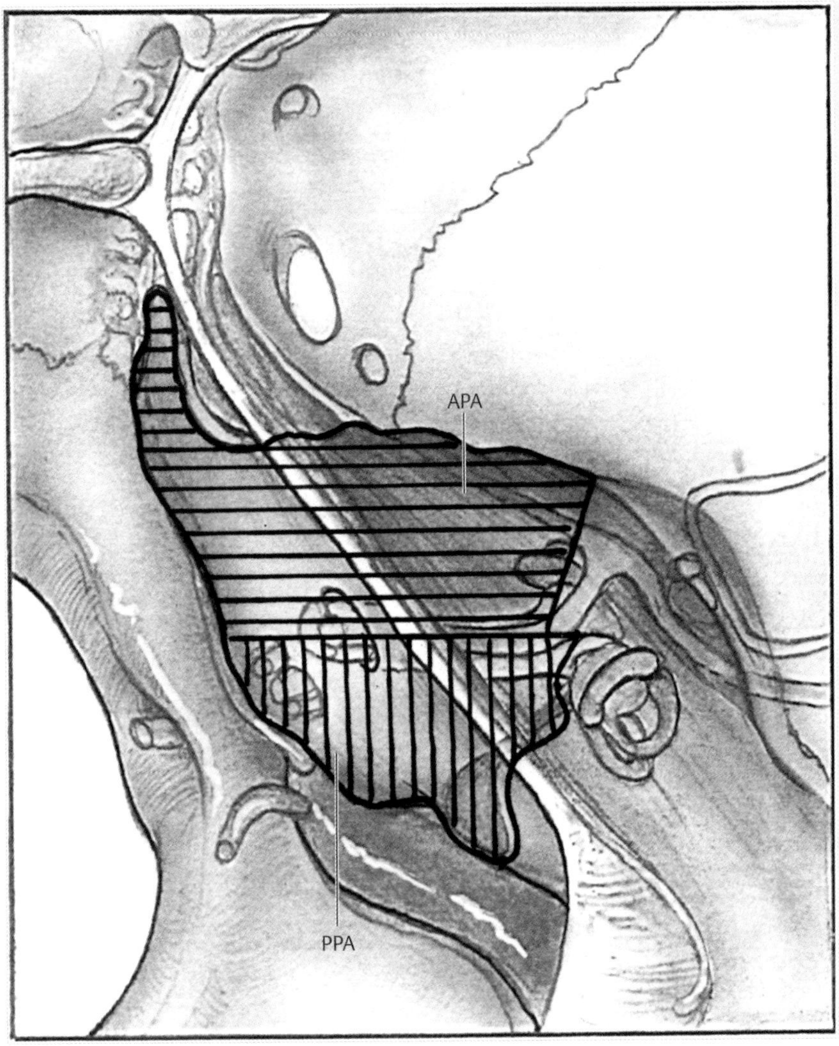

Fig. 42.1 Petrous apex. The petrous apex can be divided into an anterior (APA) and posterior (PPA) compartment by the internal auditory canal.

Three pathways (sinodural angle, subarcuate, infralabyrinthine) to the posterior petrous apex are accessible via a standard postauricular, complete mastoidectomy approach (▶ Fig. 42.2). The sinodural angle and subarcuate tracts provide an avenue for drainage of the superior aspect of the posterior petrous apex. The sinodural angle tract is opened after skeletonizing the posterior and superior semicircular canals, transverse sigmoid sinus junction, and the posterior aspect of the mastoid tegmen. The petrous ridge and superior petrosal sinus are followed into the posterior petrous apex. The subarcuate approach requires skeletonization of the semicircular canals and mastoid tegmen. An opening into the superior aspect of the posterior petrous apex is created by removing the bone through the arch of the superior semicircular canal. Bleeding from the subarcuate artery is typically encountered during this approach. A 2- or 3-mm bur is used to open the subarcuate tract, with care being taken not to enter the vestibule and semicircular canals.[4] Lee used CT scans of 58 temporal bones in patients with aerated petrous apices to estimate the dimensions of the subarcuate tract, which was approximately 4.88 mm by 4.9 mm.[5] Blue-lining the canals may provide additional reference for the surgeon to maximize the opening into the petrous apex via the subarcuate tract.[4]

The transmastoid infralabyrinthine approach provides access to the inferior aspect of the posterior and, occasionally, the anterior petrous apex when the jugular bulb is low. The vertical facial nerve, sigmoid sinus, and the ampullated end of the posterior semicircular canal provide the boundaries for the infralabyrinthine approach. Excessive bleeding from the sigmoid sinus or jugular bulb, audiovestibular dysfunction from otic capsule violation, facial paresis, and cerebrospinal fluid (CSF) leak are all potential complications of this approach.[4]

The transtemporal (infracochlear, pericarotid, and complete apicectomy), transnasal, and extradural middle fossa approaches provide access to the anterior petrous apex (▶ Fig. 42.3). The infracochlear approach allows access to the inferior aspect of the anterior petrous apex. The inferior basal turn of the cochlea, vertical petrous carotid artery, and the anterior aspect of the jugular bulb are the boundaries of the infracochlear approach. The infracochlear approach necessitates removal of the inferior tympanic osseous annulus and a portion of the inferior canal wall. The pericarotid approach and complete apicectomy approach provide access to the superior aspect of the anterior petrous apex. The boundaries of the pericarotid approach are the horizontal petrous carotid artery, the ascending basal turn of the cochlea, and the middle fossa dura. Exposure and removal of the medial wall of the semicanal of

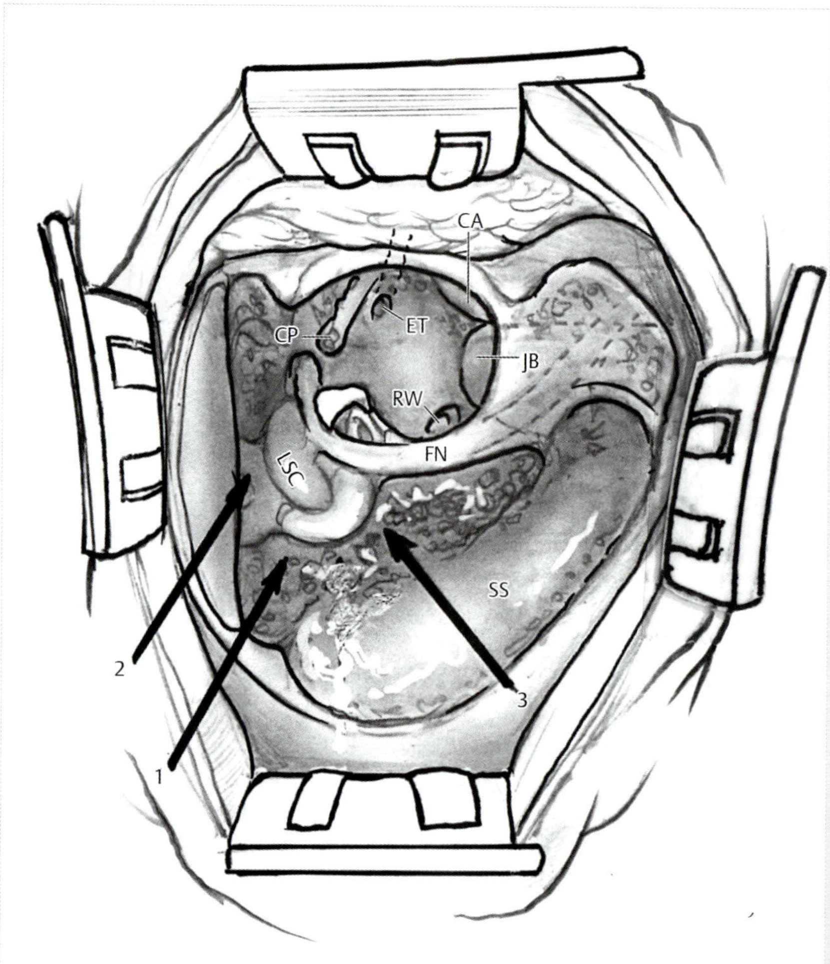

Fig. 42.2 Posterior tracts to petrous apex. Three pathways (1, sinodural angle; 2, subarcuate; 3, infralabyrinthine) to the posterior petrous apex are accessible via a standard postauricular, complete mastoidectomy approach. SS, sigmoid sinus; LSC, lateral semicircular canal; FN, facial nerve; RW, round window; ET, Eustachian tube, CA, carotid artery; CP, cochleariform process; JB, jugular bulb.

the tensor tympani muscle is required to expose the anterior petrous apex via the pericarotid approach. A complete apicectomy is an extension of the pericarotid approach, described by Ramadier and Lempert, and requires removal of the anterior canal wall and mandibular condyle.[4] The medial wall of the glenoid fossa is opened up to the horizontal segment of the petrous carotid artery. A less radical variation of the complete apicectomy that preserves the anterior canal wall and retracts the glenoid contents anteriorly can be utilized to provide wide access of the anterior petrous apex.[4]

The petrous apex typically abuts the posterior lateral wall of the sphenoid sinus. An endoscopic transnasal sphenoidotomy in some cases will permit access to the anterior petrous apex.[6] The extradural middle fossa approach provides wide access to the superior aspect of the anterior and posterior petrous apex. The greater superficial petrosal nerve, arcuate eminence, and the petrous ridge are the boundaries of the petrous apex as viewed from the middle fossa approach.[7]

42.5 Classification of Petrous Apex Cholesteatoma

42.5.1 Congenital

Congenital cholesteatoma is thought to arise from embryonic tissue from the abnormal development of the first brachial groove.[8,9] Cholesteatoma has a linear growth pattern, unlike a true neoplasm. Congenital petrous apex cholesteatoma often presents in a delayed fashion as otoscopy is often normal even in symptomatic patients. Vestibular symptoms and sensorineural hearing loss, as opposed to conductive loss, occur secondary to erosion into the otic capsule or internal auditory canal. Patients typically present with slowly progressing facial paresis or long-standing paralysis secondary to internal auditory canal or Fallopian canal involvement. Diplopia or facial anesthesia may occur with medial cholesteatoma extension into Dorello's canal or Meckel's cave, respectively.[10]

42.5.2 Acquired

Neglected or obscured middle ear and mastoid cholesteatomas, on rare occasion, can spread to the petrous apex via the previously described preformed pathways or by erosion through the otic capsule.[11] Inflammation and infection typically associated with chronic otitis media result in increased epithelial turnover, which leads to progressive cholesteatoma expansion and erosion of adjacent bone. Patients with a known history of prior cholesteatoma are at risk for apical extension regardless of the previous surgical approach (canal wall-up/down, tympanoplasty, etc.); however, canal wall-down mastoidectomy has a lower recurrence rate. Apical extension of cholesteatoma may still occur after canal wall-down mastoidectomy secondary to

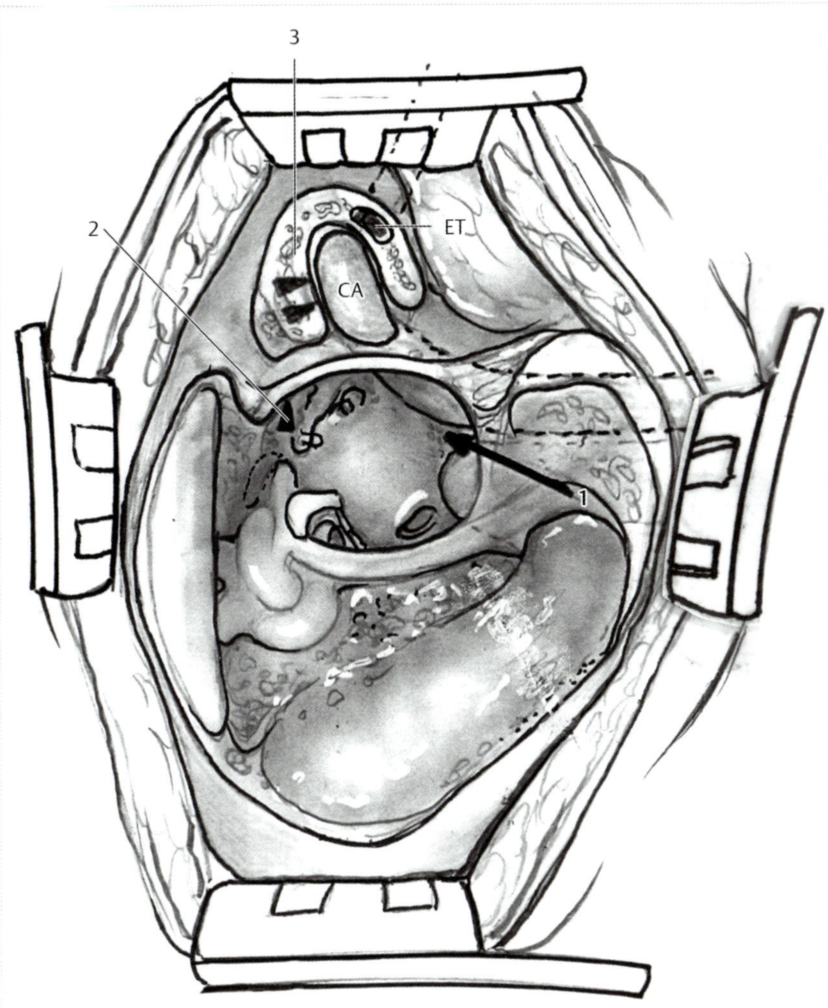

Fig. 42.3 Anterior tracts to petrous apex. The transtemporal (1, infracochlear; 2, supracochlear; 3, transglenoid) approaches provide access to the anterior petrous apex. The transnasal and extradural middle fossa approaches (not pictured) also can be used to approach the anterior petrous apex. CA, carotid artery; ET, Eustachian tube.

spread along preformed pathways from residual disease in the mastoid or the middle ear.[9,11]

Acquired petrous apex cholesteatoma is readily identified with CT but is sometimes not identified until the time of surgery. Imaging rarely alters management but is important when discussing potential outcomes and complications with patients prior to treatment. Preoperative imaging for cholesteatoma or chronic otitis media is indicated in patients with long-standing symptoms, sensorineural/mixed hearing loss, vestibular symptoms, facial nerve symptoms, facial anesthesia, otalgia, or prior temporal bone surgery or trauma.[3]

42.5.3 Extent

Classifying the extent and location of a petrous cholesteatoma is important for surgical planning and for patient counseling regarding prognosis for hearing and facial nerve function. A number of classification systems have been reported for defining the location and extent of petrous apex cholesteatoma. The Moffat-Smith system uses the lesion location relative to the labyrinth.[12] Supralabyrinthine, infralabyrinthine, and massive labyrinthine disease refer to cholesteatoma extending superior, inferior, or through the otic capsule, respectively, without extension into the petrous apex. Extension of the cholesteatoma into the petrous apex in each of the above three categories adds the additional designation of "apical" (i.e., supralabyrinthine-apical). A cholesteatoma confined to the petrous apex without otic capsule invasion is designated as apical disease.[12]

42.6 Surgical Technique

42.6.1 Translabyrinthine Approach

The translabyrinthine approach allows wide access to perilabyrinthine air cell tracts, the petrous apex, the internal auditory canal, and the posterior fossa. The approach itself results in profound sensorineural hearing loss because the labyrinth is removed, so most candidates should have non-serviceable preoperative hearing. Severe postoperative vertigo and imbalance often occur, requiring hospitalization for a few days and vestibular rehabilitation.

The patient is placed in a supine position and facial nerve monitoring is utilized. The incision is performed 1–2 cm from the postauricular sulcus. The mastoid periosteum is divided along the linea temporalis and then toward the mastoid tip. The periosteum is then elevated until the external auditory canal is visualized. A cortical mastoidectomy is performed and the tegmen mastoideum, sigmoid sinus, and posterior fossa dura are identified. Dissection continues medially until the antrum, lateral semicircular canal, and short process of the incus are identified. The extent of the disease will dictate the extent and location of bone removal. If the cholesteatoma involves the perilabyrinthine air cells, the petrous apex, or the internal auditory canal, a labyrinthectomy may be performed.

The semicircular canals should be removed in a systematic fashion by first identifying the membranous labyrinth of the lateral semicircular canal. The lateral semicircular canal should be opened on the superior aspect of the canal to prevent injury to the second genu of the facial nerve. The superior canal is then identified near the ampullated end and followed posterior to the common crus. The posterior semicircular canal is then identified at the common crus and is opened toward the ampullated end. Removal of the inferior ampullated end of the posterior canal requires drilling medial to the second genu of the facial nerve. During a labyrinthectomy the facial nerve is at greatest risk along the medial portion of the distal tympanic segment. Once the labyrinth has been removed, dissection continues medially to the internal auditory canal or petrous apex. The jugular bulb can be at risk, especially if the jugular bulb is more superior than usual. If CSF is encountered, the Eustachian tube can be obliterated and the external auditory canal closed. All open air cell tracts should be closed with bone wax. If CSF is encountered, an abdominal fat graft should be used. If no CSF is encountered, postoperative imaging for recurrent disease may be easier to interpret without fat packing.

42.6.2 Variations of the Translabyrinthine Approach

Transotic Approach

The transotic approach is used to remove disease that involves the cochlea or anterior petrous apex. The facial nerve is not transposed, so dissection occurs on both the mastoid and middle ear side of the facial nerve. The posterior external auditory canal is removed to improve visualization of the middle ear and sinus tympani. The cochlea is removed, so profound sensorineural hearing loss is expected. If CSF is encountered, the Eustachian tube is obliterated and the external auditory canal is closed. This creates a blind cavity that can be followed by serial imaging to ensure cholesteatoma has not reformed.[13]

Trancochlear Approach

The transcochlear approach is similar to the transotic approach, with the differentiating step being the transposition of the facial nerve posteriorly. Transposing the facial nerve usually results in some degree of permanent facial paresis, so the patient should be counseled preoperatively. This approach is useful if disease is medial to the facial nerve and involves the jugular foramen. If possible, it is preferable to work on either side of the Fallopian canal rather than transposing the nerve to prevent chronic facial paresis. This technique has been referred to as the "Fallopian-bridge technique."[14,15,16] Profound sensorineural hearing loss occurs with the transcochlear approach, so appropriate preoperative counseling is essential.

Transcrusal Approach

A transcrusal approach is helpful in patients with serviceable hearing who have extension of disease medial to the semicircular canals. The superior and posterior semicircular canals can be removed by exposing the membranous labyrinth at each end of the canal and then occluding the canals with bone pate and bone wax. It is important to prevent occluding materials from entering the vestibule. The canals can then be removed, resulting in improved access to the petrous apex, perilabyrinthine air cell tracts, and clivus. Sensorineural hearing loss is possible because the labyrinth has been violated.[17,18,19,20]

Pearls and Pitfalls

- Preoperative comprehensive audiometry should be obtained to establish hearing status because the approach will result in profound sensorineural hearing loss.
- CSF fistula management should be considered, including obliteration of the Eustachian tube, closure of the external auditory canal, and use of abdominal fat graft.
- If disease involves the cochlea or jugular foramen, a transotic or transcochlear approach should be considered.
- The transcochlear approach requires transposition of the facial nerve and, likely, chronic facial paresis.
- The transcrusal approach is useful to gain improved access to the petrous apex, with the potential for hearing preservation.

42.6.3 Middle Fossa Approach

The middle fossa approach provides varying degrees of exposure to the petrous apex, clivus, ventral brainstem, and anterior cerebellopontine angle. The standard and extended middle fossa approaches provide excellent exposure of the internal auditory canal from the porus acousticus to the fundus.[21] The extended middle fossa approach entails greater exposure of the anterior and posterior petrous apex. The boundaries of the middle fossa approach are the lateral wall of Meckel's cave and petrous ridge medially, the superior semicircular canal posterior laterally, and the greater superficial petrosal nerve anterior laterally.[22] The Kawase approach, which requires down-fracturing the zygoma, provides access to the ventral pons by removing the anterior petrous apex down to the level of the horizontal petrous carotid artery.[23,24]

The primary disadvantage of the middle fossa approach is an increased risk of facial nerve injury because of its anterior-superior location in the internal auditory canal; however, several studies have demonstrated no long-term difference with other skull base approaches to the internal auditory canal.[25,26] Temporal lobe injury from prolonged retraction or injury to the vein of Labbé is also an important consideration when using this approach.[27] The middle fossa approach does not permit visualization of the inferior cerebellopontine angle. The middle fossa approach may be combined with the pre-sigmoid approaches to address lesions that extend into multiple intracranial compartments.[28]

A variety of skin incisions may be used for the middle fossa approach. Once the skin and subcutaneous tissues are elevated, the temporalis muscle is cut just proximal to its origin from the temporal line to provide a site of attachment during closure. The temporalis muscle is elevated anteriorly and inferiorly and is secured with retractors or hooks. The zygoma and osseous external auditory meatus provide landmarks for the craniotomy bone flap. A 4 by 4 cm craniotomy bone flap that is centered at the zygomatic root is elevated. The inferior edge of the craniotomy is lowered to the middle fossa floor to provide additional visualization. The dura is elevated off the floor of the middle fossa from posterior to anterior to prevent injury to the greater superficial petrosal and facial nerves. The dura is elevated from the petrous ridge posteriorly to the dura of Meckel's cave anteriorly. The greater superficial petrosal nerve, arcuate eminence, petrous ridge, middle meningeal artery, and foramen ovale all serve as landmarks.[7,29]

A lateral-to-medial technique, described by Fisch, begins by blue-lining the superior semicircular canal and then identifying the internal auditory canal at a 60-degree angle.[30] William House identified the fundus of the internal auditory canal by tracing the greater superficial petrosal nerve to the geniculate ganglion.[31] Jackler and Gladstone described a medial-to-lateral technique that begins with drilling at the petrous ridge and identifying the internal auditory canal at the porous acousticus and following it laterally to the fundus.[32] Once tumor removal is complete, air cells are waxed and muscle or fat is used to obliterate the defect.

Pearls and Pitfalls

- The middle fossa approach provides wide access to superior aspects of both the anterior and posterior petrous apex. Inferior petrous apex disease is not as readily accessible with this approach.
- The middle fossa approach is a hearing-preservation approach. Patients with anacusis may be better served with a presigmoid approach.
- The bone flap should be centered at the zygomatic root.
- Cauterization or clipping of the middle meningeal artery provides additional working space.
- Identifying and placing a retractor on the petrous ridge is a mandatory step of the middle fossa approach.
- Identifying the greater superficial petrosal nerve and blue-lining the superior semicircular canal provides consistent landmarks for identifying the internal auditory canal.

42.6.4 Combined Petrosal Approach

The combined approach provides exposure for lesions that extend in the middle and posterior fossa and typically uses a transtemporal approach (retrolabyrinthine, translabyrinthine, and transcochlear) in addition to a middle fossa craniotomy.[33]

A large postauricular C-shaped incision is typically utilized for the combined petrosal approach that allows for a middle fossa craniotomy as well as a transtemporal approach. Leaving the skin flap attached to most of the temporalis muscle and periosteum facilitates prevention of pseudomeningocele formation and incisional CSF leaks. A stair-stepped C-shaped incision parallel to the skin incision is made through the temporalis muscle and mastoid periosteum down to the mastoid tip. The composite skin periosteal flap is then elevated to the osseous external auditory meatus. Retractors are placed and a complete canal wall-up mastoidectomy is performed, with care being taken to minimize the opening of the aditus ad antrum. The tegmen and sigmoid sinus are identified along the labyrinth and vertical facial nerve. The facial recess is not opened to reduce the risk of CSF otorrhea. The sigmoid sinus and middle fossa dura are decompressed down to the semicircular canals, which are then skeletonized. Decompression of the retrosigmoid and lateral middle fossa dura allows for additional room for retraction.

A retrosigmoid combined middle fossa craniotomy is then performed, with care being taken around the transverse sinus. Bur holes on either side of the transverse sinus provide an additional measure of safety when elevating this bone flap. A horizontal middle fossa durotomy is created, and the vein of Labbé is identified. An incision is then made along the inferior temporal lobe dura down to the superior petrosal sinus. A vertical presigmoid dura incision just anterior to the sigmoid sinus is then made up to the level of the superior petrosal sinus. The superior petrosal sinus is then divided after placement of liga-clips or sutures. The tentorium is divided, with care taken not to injure the trochlear nerve, Dandy vein, superior cerebellar artery, and vein of Labbé.[28] Prolonged retraction of the temporal lobe dura poses a risk of injury or thrombosis of the vein of Labbé, but intermittent release of the retractor or division of the sigmoid sinus may prevent this.[27]

The middle fossa retrosigmoid craniotomy bone flap is secured into place with titanium plates at the completion of tumor removal. Titanium mesh, bone cement, or methyl methacrylate can all be utilized to reconstruct the osseous defect created with the combine petrosal approach. The dura is partially re-approximated with sutures. All exposed air cells, including the zygomatic root, retrofacial, facial recess, and mastoid tip, are sealed with bone wax. A piece of bone from the middle fossa decompression is shaped to the approximate size of the opening in the aditus ad antrum. This bone chip is placed over the aditus ad antrum and secured into place with additional bone wax. The retrolabyrinthine cavity is filled with strips of abdominal fat, which are placed partially through the dural openings. The composite periosteal skin flap is then closed in a water-tight fashion in three layers. A pressure dressing is placed for three* days.[28]

Pearls and Pitfalls

- The combined petrosal approach allows exposure of both the middle and posterior fossa from Meckel's cave to the foramen magnum.
- This approach is indicated for cerebellopontine angle epidermoids with intact hearing.
- The vein of Labbé must be identified by opening the middle fossa dura prior to dividing the tentorium.
- The trochlear nerve should be identified prior to cutting the medial edge of the tentorium.
- The primary advantages of the combined approach are decreased brain retraction, which eliminates the need for a staged approach, improved exposure, which allows for a more complete excision, and the possibility of hearing preservation (retrolabyrinthine, transcrusal).
- A disadvantage of the combined petrosal approach is sacrifice of hearing if either the translabyrinthine or the transcochlear approach is required. There is an increased risk of CSF leak if hearing preservation is attempted because it is more difficult to block the antrum with an intact ossicular chain.

42.6.5 Intratemporal Fossa Approach

The intratemporal fossa approach provides access to the jugular foramen, infralabyrinthine temporal bone, anterior petrous apex, glenoid fossa, entire petrous carotid artery, nasopharynx, Eustachian tube, parasellar region, parapharyngeal space, and the mid- and lower clivus. This approach is most commonly used for jugular foramen tumors (paraganglioma, schwannoma, meningioma), but in rare instances, the intratemporal fossa approach can be used for extensive cholesteatoma.

Facial and lower cranial nerve monitoring are utilized. A large postauricular, C-shaped incision is performed. The ear canal is transected and closed in a blind-sac fashion. The carotid artery, jugular vein, and lower cranial nerves are identified in the neck and traced to the jugular foramen. The jugular vein is suture-ligated if the jugular bulb is involved with disease. A wide mastoidectomy is performed, and the tegmen, sigmoid sinus, and pre- and post-sigmoid dura are identified. A facial recess is created, and the incudostapedial joint is disarticulated and the tensor tympani tendon is sectioned. The canal skin, tympanic membrane, malleus, and incus are removed and discarded. The external auditory canal is removed to the level of the mastoid segment of the facial nerve. This allows excellent exposure of the carotid artery, hypotympanum, sinus tympani, and inferior tympanic bone. If the facial nerve does not impede visualization, the facial nerve can remain in the Fallopian canal and dissection can proceed on either side of the nerve. If the cholesteatoma is extensive, the facial nerve can be removed out of the Fallopian canal, from the geniculate ganglion to the stylomastoid foramen, along with the digastric muscle and periosteum. The periosteum is then sutured to the parotid gland, allowing the facial nerve to be anterior to the area of dissection. Transposing the facial nerve will often result in permanent facial paresis, so this should be discussed preoperatively. The mandible can be displaced anteriorly with a self-retaining retractor to improve access to the jugular foramen. The bone medial to the facial nerve is then removed, allowing wide access to the jugular foramen and hypotympanum. If the jugular vein was ligated, the proximal sigmoid sinus can be occluded with extra luminal packing. The resulting defect can be filled with an abdominal fat graft.

Pearls and Pitfalls

- Facial nerve transposition often results in permanent facial paresis and should be discussed preoperatively.
- The facial nerve can often be left in the Fallopian canal, preventing the possibility of paresis from transposition.
- If the jugular bulb is entered, brisk bleeding from the inferior petrosal sinus is encountered. Gentle packing should be utilized for hemostasis to prevent injury to the lower cranial nerves.
- If the external auditory canal is closed, postoperative imaging, including diffusion-weighted MRI, should be used for surveillance of cholesteatoma development.

42.6.6 Subtotal Petrosectomy Approach With Blind Sac Closure

Subtotal petrosectomy is indicated in cases of extensive petrous bone cholesteatoma with destruction of the external auditory canal, CSF leakage, extensive middle ear disease, or encasement of the intratemporal facial nerve. The entire temporal bone air cell system and the external auditory canal are removed. The labyrinth, cochlea, or the entire otic capsule are removed in cases with massive labyrinthine or apical extension.[34]

Ear canal and postauricular injections will reduce bleeding during the ear canal over-closure. A standard postauricular incision is used, followed by a complete mastoidectomy with removal of the superior and posterior external auditory canal. The retrofacial, infracochlear, infralabyrinthine, and sinodural air cells are opened, and the semicircular canals are skeletonized in cases where the otic capsule is going to be preserved. The facial nerve is skeletonized from the geniculate to the stylomastoid foramen. A labyrinthectomy and/or cochlectomy are performed as needed, followed by meticulous removal of all cholesteatoma matrix. Small dural defects can be sutured or closed with muscle plugs. The cavity is then copiously rinsed with antibiotic irrigation. The cavity is often filled with a fat graft, which is easily differentiated from residual disease using diffusion-weighted MRI.[35,36]

Obliteration of the Eustachian tube and over-closure of the ear canal with the modified Rambo or blind sac technique is an essential step of the subtotal petrosectomy approach that reduces the risk of CSF leak.[37] The modified Rambo approach uses a laterally based tragal skin flap, which is elevated to the level of the tragal cartilage after making 6 o'clock and 12 o'clock incisions in the external auditory meatus. The tragal skin is then transected medially at the osseocartilaginous junction, which allows complete mobilization laterally after separating the skin flap from the underlying tragal cartilage. A semicircular incision is made in the concha, with care being taken to preserve the underlying cartilage. The skin anterior and medial to the conchal incision, including the entire canal skin, tympanic membrane, and lateral ossicular chain, are removed. The leading edge of the tragal skin flap is then sutured to the cut edge of the undermined conchal skin.

Pearls and Pitfalls

- The subtotal petrosectomy approach can be used for almost any petrosal cholesteatoma.
- Advantages of this approach are the wide exposure, lack of otorrhea, decreased incidence of CSF leak, and no need to clean a mastoid cavity.
- The modified Rambo ear canal over-closure technique provides a water-tight closure and excellent cosmesis.
- Disadvantages of this approach are that the clinician can no longer use otoscopy to monitor for recurrence and there is risk of obliterating over residual disease. This approach also results in a maximum conductive hearing loss or anacusis if the otic capsule is removed.

The modified Rambo closure provides a two-layer closure and has excellent cosmesis. The blind sac closure requires transection of the meatal skin just lateral to the osseocartilaginous junction. The meatal skin is then dissected from the underlying cartilage and is everted through the external meatus. Interrupted sutures are then used to close the everted skin, which is then displaced medially. The remnant medial canal, tympanic membrane, and lateral ossicular chain are removed. Meticulous removal of all skin in the canal is vitally important as residual skin will develop into cholesteatoma.[37]

42.7 Postoperative Care

Postoperative vestibular dysfunction, hearing loss, facial paralysis, and lower cranial nerve neuropathies are possible. Vestibular dysfunction is usually treated with vestibular rehabilitation and should be started as soon as possible after surgery.[38,39,40] Benzodiazepines for a few days can be helpful, but long-term use should be avoided because delayed compensation is a possibility.

Hearing loss can be sensorineural, conductive, or mixed. For conductive and mixed losses, ossiculoplasty may still be performed in many cases. In cases resulting in single-sided deafness, a contralateral routing of offside signaling (CROS) hearing aid or a bone-anchored hearing aid are good options.[41,42,43] A bone-anchored hearing aid is particularly useful in patients who have intact inner ear function but a closed external auditory canal.[44] However, many patients do not pursue rehabilitation options because they do not perceive a severe disability with single-sided deafness.[45]

In patients with facial paralysis, eye care is paramount. The use of judicious artificial tears and ocular lube at night is essential. In patients with significant lagophthalmos, a gold or platinum weight should be considered. If facial function returns, the weight can be removed. Often a lid-tightening procedure is performed in conjunction with the placement of the weight. If the facial nerve was sacrificed during the procedure, direct anastomosis or a cable-graft should be performed. Recovery of the nerve can take up to a year to be complete. If nerve function has not returned in a year, facial nerve reanimation procedures can be performed. Gracilis muscle free-tissue transfer with neuronal anastomosis to the masseter nerve provides excellent midface movement in patients with long-standing facial paralysis.[46,47] Facial nerve rehabilitation exercises are initiated once facial movement is observed.[48,49]

Lower cranial nerve neuropathies are uncommon, but can result in serious complications, such as aspiration pneumonia. Early identification during the postoperative period allows for avoidance of oral intake and speech pathology evaluation. In severe cases, a gastrostomy tube or tracheotomy may be required. Hoarseness from vocal cord paralysis may be treated with a vocal cord medialization procedure.

42.8 Complications

Complications of skull base surgery can be devastating and life-threatening. Preoperative counseling is essential, so postoperative expectations are appropriate. Unlike certain neoplasms, surgical treatment of most cases of COM should avoid purposeful facial nerve or hearing sacrifice, unless there is preoperative facial paralysis or profound hearing loss.

Facial nerve paralysis is a socially and functionally challenging complication in skull base surgery.[50,51] Avoiding facial nerve injury with knowledge of temporal bone anatomy and intraoperative facial nerve monitoring are the best preventative measures. If the patient wakes with a facial paralysis, the surgeon should wait a few hours to allow the effects of local anesthesia to dissipate. If the paralysis is persistent, and the facial nerve was identified and confidently preserved, oral steroids should be initiated and electrophysiologic testing can be performed in three days.

If the facial nerve was not identified during surgery, surgical exploration should be considered. During exploration, the nerve may be found intact. Stimulating the nerve proximal to the area in question can be helpful to confirm continuity of the nerve. Another possibility during exploration is finding an injured facial nerve. If $< 50\%$ of the nerve circumference is transected, re-approximation with a small nylon suture can be considered. If the nerve is completely or $> 50\%$ transected, the nerve endings should be freshened and re-approximated with suture or fibrin glue.

Facial nerve injuries are stressful for both the patient and the surgeon. Consulting a colleague if a facial nerve injury occurs should be strongly considered. In some cases of advanced cholesteatoma, the facial nerve may be involved with cholesteatoma and is paretic before surgery. In these circumstances, resection of the facial nerve and a cable-graft may be beneficial depending on the preoperative level of dysfunction.[52,53,54]

Sensorineural hearing loss can occur as a result of the approach or as an unexpected complication. Violating the labyrinth or cochlea can result in profound sensorineural hearing loss. If a labyrinthine injury is detected in a timely fashion and closed with fascia, hearing loss may be prevented. In extensive cholesteatoma, a labyrinthine fistula may be present. In most circumstances, the matrix can be removed from the fistula; however, some surgeons would argue to leave matrix behind if a large fistula is present.[55,56,57]

Sensorineural hearing loss may also occur with aggressive manipulation of the ossicular chain and subluxation of the stapes. It is advisable to remove disease involving the stapes last, so an inadvertent footplate injury could be closed with fascia and the case could be completed. Drill contact with the ossicular chain is another cause of sensorineural hearing loss. Brief contact of a high-speed otologic drill can create a severe to profound sensorineural hearing loss.[58] This can be avoided by carefully avoiding the ossicles while drilling or by using a lower-speed drill when working around the ossicles.

Cerebrospinal fluid fistula or dural defects can occur with skull base surgery for the treatment of chronic otitis media.[59] This can be prevented by repairing any defects during the surgery with various techniques and materials. Many defects can be repaired with a transtemporal approach using muscle, fascia, cartilage, fibrin glue, and bone cements. Defects involving the tegmen tympani often require a middle fossa craniotomy for adequate exposure in cases where the ossicular chain is preserved.[7,60,61] Abdominal fat can be utilized to help prevent postoperative CSF fistulas. Routine use of a lumbar drain is controversial.[62,63,64,65,66] If a CSF fistula occurs, lumbar drainage for a few days will often result in closure of the fistula. If the fistula

Table 42.2 Hearing, facial nerve outcomes, and recurrence rates after removal of petrous apex cholesteatoma

Study	n	Preoperative HB Grade I - II (%)	Postoperative HB Grade I - II (%)	Preoperative serviceable hearing (%)	Postoperative serviceable hearing (%)	Hearing preservation rate (%)	Recurrence (%)
Pyle and Wiet 1991[69]	10	5 (50)	7 (70)	5 (50)	3 (30)	60	3 (30)
Atlas, Moffat, and Hardy 1992[52]	14	7 (50)	7 (50)	8 (57.1)	0 (0)	0	1 (7.1)
Axon, Fergie, Saeed, et al 1999[9]	25	11 (44)	11 (44)	9 (36)	3 (12)	33.3	7 (28)
Grayeli, Mosnier, El Garem, et al 2000[70]	19	13 (68.4)	12 (63.2)	9 (47.4)	3 (15.8)	33.3	2 (10.5)
Omran, De Denato, Piccirillo, et al 2006[10]	93	49 (52.6)	45 (48.4)	59 (63.4)	10 (10.8)	16.9	2 (2.2)
Moffat, Jones, and Smith 2009[12]	43	23 (53.4)	24 (55.8)	22 (51.2)	6 (14)	27.2	2 (4.6)
Aubry, Kania, Sauvaget, et al 2010[71]	28	18 (64.2)	24 (85.7)	13 (46.4)	5 (17.8)	38.4	8 (28.6)
Senn Haeusler, Panosetti, and Caversaccio 2011[72]	21	15 (71.4)	19 (90.4)	17 (80.9)	14 (66.6)	82.4	4 (19)
Song, An, and Ahn 2011[53]	13	7 (53.8)	8 (61.5)	8 (61.5)	3 (23)	37.5	0 (0)

is persistent, re-exploration of the surgical site may be required. If the patient has profound sensorineural hearing loss, a subtotal petrosectomy with obliteration of the Eustachian tube and over-closure of the external auditory canal may be performed.[34] In cases of cholesteatoma, postoperative surveillance with diffusion-weighted MRI will be required.[36,67]

Meningitis is an uncommon but potentially life-threatening complication. Use of perioperative antibiotics and strict sterile technique can be helpful to prevent meningitis. Signs and symptoms of meningitis should be discussed with the patient because prompt identification and the initiation of treatment provide the patient the best chance for a favorable outcome. A prolonged course of culture- and sensitivity-specific parenteral antibiotics is used to treat bacterial meningitis.[68]

Vascular injury can lead to severe neurological complications, including cerebrovascular accident, blindness, venous infarct, and death. The sigmoid sinus plate may be eroded by the disease process, making it susceptible to inadvertent injury. Most injuries to the sigmoid sinus can be controlled with absorbable gelatin packing and gentle pressure; however, an extensive injury may require ligation of the sinus. If this is the dominant sinus, venous outflow will be affected, possibly resulting in a hydrocephalus or brain edema. The carotid artery courses through the middle ear and petrous apex and is at risk. Intraoperative injury to the carotid artery requires intraoperative repair or immediate evaluation and possible treatment through angiography.

42.9 Outcomes

The overarching goal in the management of petrous bone cholesteatoma, as with other benign skull base pathology, is to perform as complete an excision as possible while minimizing morbidity. Patients with petrous bone cholesteatomas have a high incidence of facial nerve and audiovestibular dysfunction at presentation in addition to otorrhea, otalgia, and, rarely, recurrent meningitis and other cranial neuropathies. Outcomes with respect to recurrence rate, facial nerve function, and hearing preservation vary significantly across centers, surgical approach, and extent of resection (▶ Table 42.2).

Facial nerve outcomes depend a great deal on the presence, severity, and duration of pretreatment dysfunction. The surgical approach, extent of cholesteatoma, and completeness of resection are other modifying factors that affect facial nerve outcomes.[10] The labyrinthine and geniculate segments are the two most commonly involved portions of the facial nerve in patients with petrous bone cholesteatoma.[53] Patients with long-standing complete facial nerve paralysis (> 1 year) rarely if ever achieve satisfactory function (House-Brackmann Grade I-II) and will typically benefit from static or dynamic re-animation procedures. Patients presenting with lesser degrees of facial paresis can recover function after removing cholesteatoma, along with decompression of the affected segment of the facial nerve. The vast majority of patients presenting with normal facial function show no long-term significant decrement in function. Extensive encasement or mobilization of the facial nerve often results in temporary postoperative paresis that can take up to a year to recover. Post-treatment facial nerve outcomes vary significantly across series (44% to 90.4%), with the results typically being the same or better than the reported preoperative level of functioning.[9,10,52,53,69,70,71]

Hearing preservation in patients with petrous bone cholesteatoma depends on the extent of disease, level of pretreatment dysfunction, surgical approach, and extent of resection. Serviceable hearing varies widely across published series (36% to 80.9%). As expected, patients undergoing exteriorization procedures showed higher rates of hearing preservation.[17,69,72]

Recurrence of disease varies significantly across series and surgical approaches (zero to 30%).[31,32,57,58,59,60,61] Recurrence rates in these reports were likely underestimated, as some patients were lost to follow-up and a number of patients underwent obliteration procedures, where clinical exam is not useful in post-treatment surveillance.

42.10 Diffusion-Weighted MRI

Non-echo planar diffusion-weighted imaging (DWI) is a promising form of MRI that allows detection of cholesteatomas as small as 2 mm.[35,36,67] DWI uses the concept of Brownian motion, which is typically seen in tissues with high water content, to visualize cholesteatoma debris, that has a low water content. Mass-like recidivistic cholesteatoma is filled with squamous debris, which is easily visualized with DWI.[35,36] Sheet-like recidivistic disease, which can cover a small or substantial portion of the resection cavity, is not readily visualized with DWI unless significant squamous debris is present. DWI was not universally employed in many of the larger reported series of petrous cholesteatomas, so its efficacy in evaluating for recurrence has not been validated in this population of patients.

References

[1] Lee YH, Lee NJ, Kim JH, Song JJCT. CT, MRI and gallium SPECT in the diagnosis and treatment of petrous apicitis presenting as multiple cranial neuropathies. Br J Radiol. 2005;78(934):948–951.

[2] Murakami T, Tsubaki J, Tahara Y, Nagashima T. Gradenigo's syndrome: CT and MRI findings. Pediatr Radiol. 1996;26(9):684–685.

[3] Corrales CE, Blevins NH. Imaging for evaluation of cholesteatoma: Current concepts and future directions. Curr Opin Otolaryngol Head Neck Surg. 2013;21(5):461–467.

[4] Chole RA. Petrous apicitis: surgical anatomy. Ann Otol Rhinol Laryngol. 1985;94(3):251–257.

[5] Lee A, Hamidi S, Djalilian H. Anatomy of the transarcuate approach to the petrous apex. Otolaryngol Head Neck Surg. 2009;140(6):880–883.

[6] Aubry K, Kania R, Sauvaget E, Huy PT, Herman P. Endoscopic transsphenoidal approach to petrous apex cholesteatoma. Skull Base. 2010;20(4):305–308.

[7] Kutz JW, Jr, Scoresby T, Isaacson B, et al. Hearing preservation using the middle fossa approach for the treatment of vestibular schwannoma. Neurosurgery. 2012;70(2):334–340, discussion 340–341.

[8] Michaels L. An epidermoid formation in the developing middle ear: *Possible source of cholesteatoma. J Otolaryngol. 1986;15(3):169–174.

[9] Axon PR, Fergie N, Saeed SR, Temple RH, Ramsden RT. Petrosal cholesteatoma: Management considerations for minimizing morbidity. Am J Otol. 1999;20(4):505–510.

[10] Omran A, De Denato G, Piccirillo E, Leone O, Sanna M. Petrous bone cholesteatoma: Management and outcomes. Laryngoscope. 2006;116(4):619–626.

[11] Bartels LJ. Facial nerve and medially invasive petrous bone cholesteatomas. Ann Otol Rhinol Laryngol. 1991;100(4 Pt 1):308–316.

[12] Moffat D, Jones S, Smith W. Petrous temporal bone cholesteatoma: A new classification and long-term surgical outcomes. Skull Base. 2008;18(2):107–115.

[13] Browne JD, Fisch U. Transotic approach to the cerebellopontine angle. 1992. Neurosurg Clin N Am. 2008;19(2):265–278, vivi.

[14] Nonaka Y, Fukushima T, Watanabe K, et al. Less invasive transjugular approach with Fallopian bridge technique for facial nerve protection and hearing preservation in surgery of glomus jugulare tumors. Neurosurg Rev. 2013;36(4):579–586, discussion 586.

[15] Pensak ML, Jackler RK. Removal of jugular foramen tumors: The Fallopian bridge technique. Otolaryngol Head Neck Surg. 1997;117(6):586–591.

[16] Satar B, Yazar F, Ceyhan A, Arslan HH, Aydin S. Analysis of jugular foramen exposure in the Fallopian bridge technique. Skull Base. 2009;19(3):203–207.

[17] Hong SJ, Lee JH, Jung SH, Park CH, Hong SM. Can cochlear function be preserved after a modified translabyrinthine approach to eradicate a huge cholesteatoma extending to the petrous apex? Eur Arch Otorhinolaryngol. 2009;266(8):1191–1197.

[18] Kaylie DM, Horgan MA, Delashaw JB, McMenomey SO. Hearing preservation with the transcrusal approach to the petroclival region. Otol Neurotol. 2004;25(4):594–598, discussion 598.

[19] Horgan MA, Anderson GJ, Kellogg JX, et al. Classification and quantification of the petrosal approach to the petroclival region. J Neurosurg. 2000;93(1):108–112.

[20] Brandt MG, Poirier J, Hughes B, Lownie SP, Parnes LS. The transcrusal approach: A 10-year experience at one Canadian center. Neurosurgery. 2010;66(5):1017–1022.

[21] Brackmann DE, House JR, III, Hitselberger WE. Technical modifications to the middle fossa craniotomy approach in removal of acoustic neuromas. Am J Otol. 1994;15(5):614–619.

[22] Wigand ME, Haid T, Berg M. The enlarged middle cranial fossa approach for surgery of the temporal bone and of the cerebellopontine angle. Arch Otorhinolaryngol. 1989;246(5):299–302.

[23] Kawase T, Shiobara R, Toya S. Anterior transpetrosal-transtentorial approach for sphenopetroclival meningiomas: surgical method and results in 10 patients. Neurosurgery. 1991;28(6):869–875, discussion 875–876.

[24] Kawase T, Toya S, Shiobara R, Mine T. Transpetrosal approach for aneurysms of the lower basilar artery. J Neurosurg. 1985;63(6):857–861.

[25] Isaacson B, Telian SA, El-Kashlan HK. Facial nerve outcomes in middle cranial fossa vs translabyrinthine approaches. Otolaryngol Head Neck Surg. 2005;133(6):906–910.

[26] Satar B, Jackler RK, Oghalai J, Pitts LH, Yates PD. Risk-benefit analysis of using the middle fossa approach for acoustic neuromas with > 10 mm cerebellopontine angle component. Laryngoscope. 2002;112(8 Pt 1):1500–1506.

[27] Lustig LR, Jackler RK. The vulnerability of the vein of labbé during combined craniotomies of the middle and posterior fossae. Skull Base Surg. 1998;8(1):1–9.

[28] Oghalai JS, Jackler RK. Anatomy of the combined retrolabyrinthine-middle fossa craniotomy. Neurosurg Focus. 2003;14(6):e8.

[29] Sennaroglu L, Slattery WH, III. Petrous anatomy for middle fossa approach. Laryngoscope. 2003;113(2):332–342.

[30] Fisch U. Transtemporal surgery of the internal auditory canal. Report of 92 cases, technique, indications and results. Adv Otorhinolaryngol. 1970;17:203–240.

[31] House WF. Surgical exposure of the internal auditory canal and its contents through the middle, cranial fossa. Laryngoscope. 1961;71:1363–1385.

[32] Jackler RK, Gladstone HB. Locating the Internal Auditory Canal during the Middle Fossa Approach: An Alternative Technique. Skull Base Surg. 1995;5(2):63–67.

[33] Bambakidis NC, Kakarla UK, Kim LJ, et al. Evolution of surgical approaches in the treatment of petroclival meningiomas: A retrospective review. Neurosurgery. 2008;62(6) Suppl 3:1182–1191.

[34] Coker NJ, Jenkins HA, Fisch U. Obliteration of the middle ear and mastoid cleft in subtotal petrosectomy: Indications, technique, and results. Ann Otol Rhinol Laryngol. 1986;95(1 Pt 1):5–11.

[35] Jindal M, Riskalla A, Jiang D, Connor S, O'Connor AF. A systematic review of diffusion-weighted magnetic resonance imaging in the assessment of postoperative cholesteatoma. Otol Neurotol. 2011;32(8):1243–1249.

[36] Ketelslagers K, Somers T, De Foer B, Zarowski A, Offeciers E. Results, hearing rehabilitation, and follow-up with magnetic resonance imaging after tympanomastoid exenteration, obliteration, and external canal overclosure for severe chronic otitis media. Ann Otol Rhinol Laryngol. 2007;116(9):705–711.

[37] Meyerhoff WL, Stringer SP, Roland PS. Rambo procedure: Modification and application. Laryngoscope. 1988;98(7):795–796.

[38] Vereeck L, Wuyts FL, Truijen S, De Valck C, Van de Heyning PH. The effect of early customized vestibular rehabilitation on balance after acoustic neuroma resection. Clin Rehabil. 2008;22(8):698–713.

[39] El-Kashlan HK, Shepard NT, Arts HA, Telian SA. Disability from vestibular symptoms after acoustic neuroma resection. Am J Otol. 1998;19(1):104–111.

[40] Herdman SJ, Clendaniel RA, Mattox DE, Holliday MJ, Niparko JK. Vestibular adaptation exercises and recovery: Acute stage after acoustic neuroma resection. Otolaryngol Head Neck Surg. 1995;113(1):77–87.

[41] Hol MK, Bosman AJ, Snik AF, Mylanus EA, Cremers CW. Bone-anchored hearing aids in unilateral inner ear deafness: An evaluation of audiometric and patient outcome measurements. Otol Neurotol. 2005;26(5):999–1006.

[42] House JW, Kutz JW, Jr, Chung J, Fisher LM. Bone-anchored hearing aid subjective benefit for unilateral deafness. Laryngoscope. 2010;120(3):601–607.

[43] Linstrom CJ, Silverman CA, Yu GP. Efficacy of the bone-anchored hearing aid for single-sided deafness. Laryngoscope. 2009;119(4):713–720.

[44] McLarnon CM, Davison T, Johnson IJ. Bone-anchored hearing aid: Comparison of benefit by patient subgroups. Laryngoscope. 2004;114(5):942–944.

[45] Andersen HT, Schrøder SA, Bonding P. Unilateral deafness after acoustic neuroma surgery: Subjective hearing handicap and the effect of the bone-anchored hearing aid. Otol Neurotol. 2006;27(6):809–814.

[46] Terzis JK, Noah ME. Analysis of 100 cases of free-muscle transplantation for facial paralysis. Plast Reconstr Surg. 1997;99(7):1905–1921.

[47] Gousheh J, Arasteh E. Treatment of facial paralysis: dynamic reanimation of spontaneous facial expression-apropos of 655 patients. Plast Reconstr Surg. 2011;128(6):693e–703e.

[48] Teixeira LJ, Soares BG, Vieira VP, Prado GF. Physical therapy for Bell's palsy (idiopathic facial paralysis). Cochrane Database Syst Rev. 2008(3):CD006283.

[49] Pereira LM, Obara K, Dias JM, Menacho MO, Lavado EL, Cardoso JR. Facial exercise therapy for facial palsy: systematic review and meta-analysis. Clin Rehabil. 2011;25(7):649–658.

[50] Ryzenman JM, Pensak ML, Tew JM, Jr. Facial paralysis and surgical rehabilitation: a quality of life analysis in a cohort of 1,595 patients after acoustic neuroma surgery. Otol Neurotol. 2005;26(3):516–521, discussion 521.

[51] Coulson SE, O'dwyer NJ, Adams RD, Croxson GR. Expression of emotion and quality of life after facial nerve paralysis. Otol Neurotol. 2004;25(6):1014–1019.

[52] Atlas MD, Moffat DA, Hardy DG. Petrous apex cholesteatoma: Diagnostic and treatment dilemmas. Laryngoscope. 1992;102(12 Pt 1):1363–1368.

[53] Song JJ, An YH, Ahn SH, et al. Surgical management options and postoperative functional outcomes of petrous apex cholesteatoma. Acta Otolaryngol. 2011;131(11):1142–1149.

[54] Siddiq MA, Hanu-Cernat LM, Irving RM. Facial palsy secondary to cholesteatoma: analysis of outcome following surgery. J Laryngol Otol. 2007;121 (2):114–117.

[55] Gocea A, Martinez-Vidal B, Panuschka C, Epprecht P, Caballero M, Bernal-Sprekelsen M. Preserving bone conduction in patients with labyrinthine fistula. Eur Arch Otorhinolaryngol. 2012;269(4):1085–1090.

[56] Moon IS, Kwon MO, Park CY, et al. Surgical management of labyrinthine fistula in chronic otitis media with cholesteatoma. Auris Nasus Larynx. 2012;39 (3):261–264.

[57] Ikeda R, Kobayashi T, Kawase T, Oshima T, Sato T. Risk factors for deterioration of bone conduction hearing in cases of labyrinthine fistula caused by middle ear cholesteatoma. Ann Otol Rhinol Laryngol. 2012;121(3):162–167.

[58] Jiang D, Bibas A, Santuli C, Donnelly N, Jeronimidis G, O'Connor AF. Equivalent noise level generated by drilling onto the ossicular chain as measured by laser Doppler vibrometry: a temporal bone study. Laryngoscope. 2007;117 (6):1040–1045.

[59] Wootten CT, Kaylie DM, Warren FM, Jackson CG. Management of brain herniation and cerebrospinal fluid leak in revision chronic ear surgery. Laryngoscope. 2005;115(7):1256–1261.

[60] McMurphy AB, Oghalai JS. Repair of iatrogenic temporal lobe encephalocele after canal wall down mastoidectomy in the presence of active cholesteatoma. Otol Neurotol. 2005;26(4):587–594.

[61] Kari E, Mattox DE. Transtemporal management of temporal bone encephaloceles and CSF leaks: review of 56 consecutive patients. Acta Otolaryngol. 2011;131(4):391–394.

[62] Allen KP, Isaacson B, Purcell P, Kutz JW, Jr, Roland PS. Lumbar subarachnoid drainage in cerebrospinal fluid leaks after lateral skull base surgery. Otol Neurotol. 2011;32(9):1522–1524.

[63] al-Mefty O. Prolonged lumbar spinal drainage after the resection of tumors of the skull base: *A cautionary note. Neurosurgery. 1992;30(1):144.

[64] Bien AG, Bowdino B, Moore G, Leibrock L. Utilization of preoperative cerebrospinal fluid drain in skull base surgery. Skull Base. 2007;17(2):133–139.

[65] Moza K, McMenomey SO, Delashaw JB, Jr. Indications for cerebrospinal fluid drainage and avoidance of complications. Otolaryngol Clin North Am. 2005;38(4):577–582.

[66] Roland PS, Marple BF, Meyerhoff WL, Mickey B. Complications of lumbar spinal fluid drainage. Otolaryngol Head Neck Surg. 1992;107(4):564–569.

[67] Dremmen MH, Hofman PA, Hof JR, Stokroos RJ, Postma AA. The diagnostic accuracy of non-echo-planar diffusion-weighted imaging in the detection of residual and/or recurrent cholesteatoma of the temporal bone. AJNR Am J Neuroradiol. 2012;33(3):439–444.

[68] Allen KP, Isaacson B, Kutz JW, Purcell PL, Roland PS, Roland PS. The association of meningitis with postoperative cerebrospinal fluid fistula. J Neurol Surg B Skull Base. 2012;73(6):401–404.

[69] Pyle GM, Wiet RJ. Petrous Apex Cholesteatoma: Exteriorization vs. Subtotal Petrosectomy with Obliteration. Skull Base Surg. 1991;1(2):97–105.

[70] Grayeli AB, Mosnier I, El Garem H, Bouccara D, Sterkers O. Extensive intratemporal cholesteatoma: Surgical strategy. Am J Otol. 2000;21(6):774–781.

[71] Aubry K, Kovac L, Sauvaget E, Tran Ba Huy P, Herman P. Our experience in the management of petrous bone cholesteatoma. Skull Base. 2010;20(3):163–167.

[72] Senn P, Haeusler R, Panosetti E, Caversaccio M. Petrous bone cholesteatoma removal with hearing preservation. Otol Neurotol. 2011;32(2):236–241.

43 Implantable Hearing Devices and Chronic Otitis Media

Robert J.S. Briggs, Robert Mlynski, and Henrik Smeds

Abbreviations used in this chapter:

AMEI: active middle ear implant
AOM: acute otitis media
BAHA: bone-anchored hearing aid
BC-FMT: bone conduction-floating mass transducer
CI: cochlear implant
COM: chronic otitis media
CSF: cerebral spinal fluid
CT: computed tomography
DACS: Direct Acoustic Cochlear Stimulator
EAC: external auditory canal
ECoG: electrocochleography
FMT: floating mass transducer
MRI: magnetic resonance imaging
RS: receiver stimulator
VORP: vibrating ossicular replacement prosthesis

43.1 Introduction

Implantable hearing devices have now become standard of care for the rehabilitation of many hearing loss conditions. Devices include cochlear implants (CIs), bone conduction systems, and also active middle ear implants (AMEIs). These are suitable for a variety of types of hearing loss, ranging from severe to profound sensorineural hearing loss, mixed conductive and sensorineural loss, or purely conductive loss.

Chronic otitis media (COM) may be a predisposing cause for the hearing impairment or it may be coincidental. Either way, the presence of active or inactive COM presents significant challenges in terms of management of the ear to ensure suitability for, and safety of, the implanted hearing device. The most common conditions to manage prior to implantation include tympanic membrane perforations, a radical mastoid cavity, and chronic mucosal disease of the middle ear.

Cochlear implants and AMEIs consist of a postaural receiver stimulator (RS) package and electronic cable with either an electrode in the inner ear (for CIs) or an actuator that drives the ossicular chain, round window, or stapes footplate (for AMEIs). Some AMEIs, like CIs, are partially implantable with a combination of internally implanted and externally worn components, such as the Vibrant Soundbridge (Med-El Corporation, Innsbruck, Austria) and Maxum (Ototronix, Houston, Texas). Totally implantable varieties of AMEIs have also been developed, such as the Esteem (Envoy Medical, Saint Paul, Minnesota), which has an implanted subcutaneous microphone; however, chronic ear disease has been set apart as a contraindication for implantation of the Esteem device by the manufacturer.

Bone conduction hearing aids, such as the Baha system (Cochlear Corporation, Sydney, Australia), use a postauricular osseointegrated screw fixture with a percutaneous connector. Recently, however, transcutaneous implantable bone conduction systems such as the Baha Attract (Cochlear Corporation, Sydney, Australia), BONEBRIDGE (Med-El Corporation, Innsbruck, Austria) and Sophono Alpha 2 MPO (Sophono Corporation, Boulder, Colorado), have become available. These are also positioned posterior to, or within, the mastoid and do not involve the middle ear cleft. Bone conduction implants offer the advantage of potential placement away from the infected tympanomastoid compartment while maintaining the ability to directly stimulate the cochlea and overcome any underlying conductive hearing loss.

The aim of management of an ear with COM in relation to an implantable device is first to eradicate any active disease, such as a chronic infection or cholesteatoma, or inactive disease, such as a dry perforation or retraction, and, second, to create a safe, stable ear with either an aerated tympanomastoid middle ear cleft or an obliterated ear with blind sac closure of the external auditory canal (EAC), with or without Eustachian tube plugging and soft tissue obliteration of the mastoid cavity.

Important principles are to achieve secure soft tissue cover of the postauricular RS package, without any incision crossing the package and no contact between the tympanic membrane or the skin of the EAC and the prosthesis, electrode cable, or actuator. At any point where there is contact, the soft tissue cover should be a thick vascularized layer. This will prevent extrusion of the postauricular RS package, the cable, or the actuator and will also prevent reactivation of infection; hence, eradication of biofilm is essential.

This chapter will provide an overview of the aims and surgical techniques utilized in patients with COM for the eradication of disease and creation of safe, stable ears with the various types of implanted devices described above.

43.2 Patient Selection

Most commonly, patients present with a sequela of long-standing COM, such as severe to profound sensorineural hearing loss, no longer helped by hearing aids, in which case cochlear implantation is indicated. Alternatively, they may present with conductive or mixed hearing loss, which may be suitable for an AMEI or a bone-anchored hearing solution. The type of COM may vary from a central perforation that is dry to one with active discharge. There may be gross atelectasis or frank cholesteatoma, or an open mastoid cavity or old fenestration cavity that may have active granulation and infection, or there may be a radical cavity.

One important factor relating to preimplantation COM surgery is that this may correct a conductive hearing loss and will optimize the use of conventional hearing aids and give a better assessment of the hearing level. The audiologic indications for cochlear implantation continue to evolve as the outcomes achieved with implants progressively improve. Indeed, there is now some overlap with the indications for AMEIs.

Bone-anchored hearing solutions, whether passive percutaneous, transcutaneous, or active (such as the BONEBRIDGE) are usually an option for patients with a conductive or mixed hearing loss with a mild sensorineural component, where the use of conventional hearing aids is not beneficial due to previous ear

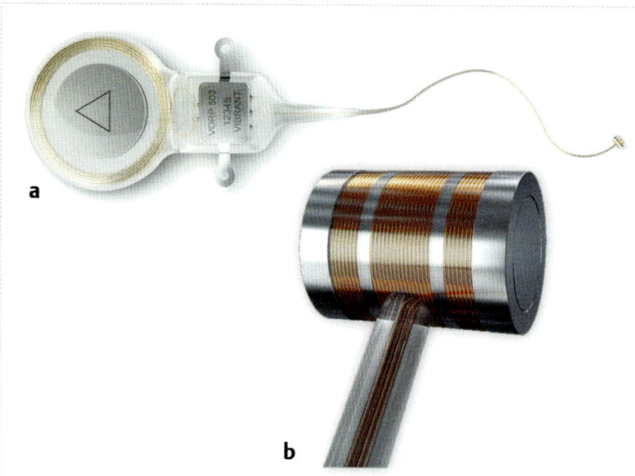

Fig. 43.1 (a) The implantable part of the Vibrant Soundbridge, the VORP, consists of a coil and a magnet to hold the audio processor, a demodulator, and a conductor link to (b) the FMT, a vibrating device converting the electrical signals into mechanical energy. It can be positioned on the ossicular chain or the round window. (Used with permission from Med-El Corporation, Innsbruck, Austria.)

surgery, canal stenosis, chronic discharge, or congenital ear malformations such as atresia of the EAC. They may also be an option in single-sided deafness. For these devices to provide adequate benefit, the bone conduction thresholds need to be reasonably good, with best results achievable if normal.

An AMEI, such as the Vibrant Soundbridge (▶ Fig. 43.1), may be an option for patients with COM, as conventional hearing aids are sometimes insufficient after several surgical procedures and with poorly functioning middle ears.[1] Typically, patients present with a radical cavity and a mixed hearing loss, an acquired stenosis of the EAC/lateralization of the TM, or after failed tympanoplasties and chronic otitis externa from hearing aid use. The Vibrant Soundbridge offers the option of a direct stimulus via the round window in cases where a normal, or at least adequate, middle ear is lacking. Coupling options to the stapes or footplate are also possible. Vibroplasty, a term used to describe tympano-ossicular reconstruction that incorporates the floating mass transducer (FMT) of the Vibrant Soundbridge, is potentially indicated for children older than 3 years or adult patients with an otherwise non-reconstructable conductive hearing loss or mixed hearing loss with a stable bone-conduction threshold above approximately 50 dB at 500–4000 Hz. Especially in patients with a mild to severe sensorineural hearing loss, monosyllabic word scores > 50% are essential for a benefit with this device. The option of using the Vibrant Soundbridge for a round window application, or by prosthesis-coupling options, has widened the initial indications. However, in patients with a history of COM, an AMEI is indicated only after previous failed attempts of tympanoplasty and use of conventional hearing aids.

In terms of preoperative investigation, both a high-resolution computed tomography (CT) scan and magnetic resonance imaging (MRI) are valuable in patients with COM. Both modalities help demonstrate the extent of previous surgery and remaining bony and soft tissue anatomy as well as the presence of active infectious disease. Particularly for cochlear implantation, T2-weighted MRI is important to exclude fibrosis or ossification in the scala tympani basal turn. Preoperative cone-beam CT is an alternative to conventional CT for preoperative imaging. As the field of view is limited, it is particularly suitable for evaluations prior to implanting AMEIs and postoperative evaluation in cases of functional problems.[2]

Although MRI-compatible (in general to 1.5 tesla), all types of implants with an integrated magnet will give a shadow effect on postoperative MRI. This must be considered in patient selection as it might make future evaluation of the internal auditory canal or structures in the posterior fossa difficult. In reality, it is rare that this excludes implant candidates, but it may apply to side selection. The older Vibrant Soundbridge systems are not MRI-compatible as the FMT contains a magnet and, thus, is at risk of movement. The latest Vibrant Soundbridge 503 is MRI compatible at 1.5 tesla.

In the majority of cases with COM, a two-stage surgical approach is utilized to ensure the eradication of infection or cholesteatoma and stable healing. If the aim is an aerated middle ear cleft, an initial tympanomastoidectomy is performed using the surgeon's preferred technique that would be predicted to have the greatest chance of long-term stability. Alternatively if the aim is obliteration of the middle ear cleft, a radical mastoidectomy and blind sac closure are performed, with or without fat or muscle packing of the cavity. The CI or AMEI is then placed at a second-stage procedure. A single-stage procedure can sometimes be safely performed if there is no active infection or cholesteatoma. Most often this would involve the implant being placed in combination with a blind sac closure and obliteration, for example, when there is a dry, clean mastoid cavity. The choice of technique may influence the passive hearing and should, therefore, be discussed with the patient.

43.3 Eradication of COM Prior to Implantation

43.3.1 Tympanic Membrane Perforation

A chronic tympanic membrane perforation needs to be repaired prior to implantation to establish a protected middle ear cleft. Cartilage grafting may help stabilize the tympanic membrane in the case of poor underlying Eustachian tube function. Alternatively, removal of the perforated tympanic membrane remnants together with the canal skin, annulus, and the lateral ossicles may be considered, with closure of the EAC in a blind sac as described below. Even if adding complexity to the procedure, this usually heals without complications and the result is independent of Eustachian tube function and healing properties of the tympanic membrane. Unless the perforation is small and the middle ear mucosa clearly healthy, it is recommended that a cortical mastoidectomy and a posterior tympanotomy are performed at the time as the myringoplasty. This is straightforward when a postaural approach is being used and may improve healing, especially if the middle ear is actively infected (▶ Fig. 43.2).

Although performing a staged procedure should be the general rule in an infected ear, to ensure that the middle ear stays aerated with a healed tympanic membrane and eradication of infection or bacterial colonization, implantation at the same

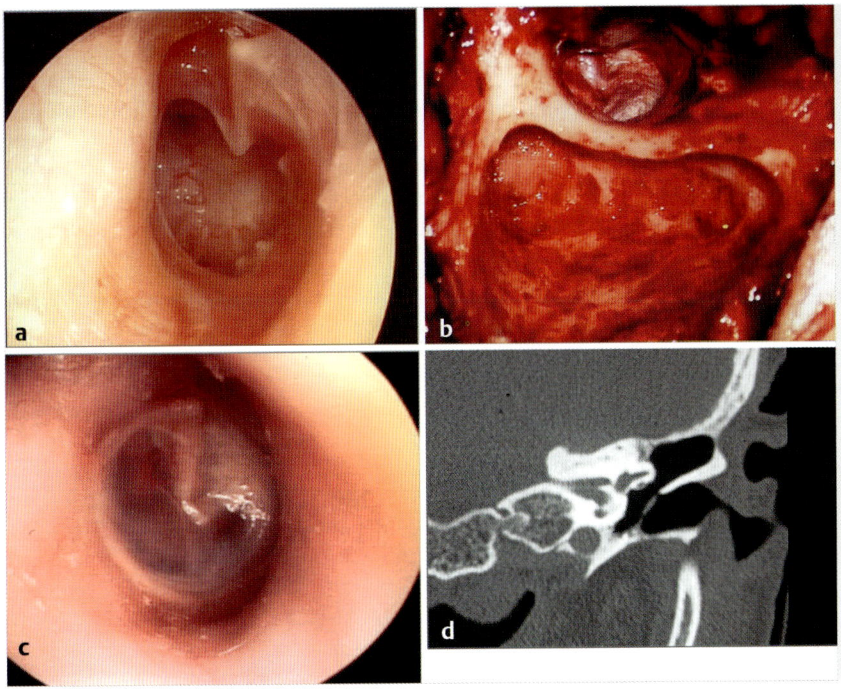

Fig. 43.2 (a) Subtotal tympanic membrane perforation. (b) On-lay myringoplasty and canal wall-up mastoidectomy. (c) Healed tympanic membrane. (d) Coronal view CT scan showing an aerated middle ear cleft.

stage as repairing the perforation may be an option in the case of a long-standing, stable non-infected ear. There may be situations where two surgeries are contraindicated, such as in a patient where additional anesthesia should be avoided or where postponing the implantation of the hearing device creates a considerable handicap. If a single-stage procedure is considered, a blind sac closure rather than a tympanoplasty may be preferable as the more conservative option.

It is a common situation that a child has a ventilation tube in place through the tympanic membrane at the time of cochlear implantation. The tube can be removed at the time of implantation or alternatively left in situ to extrude spontaneously. Either approach seems to work well, with very little risk of developing a chronic perforation or infection of the implant. A well-aerated middle ear has a healthy mucosa, and there seems to be little risk of developing either a new episode of otitis media with effusion when the perforation heals or episodes of acute otitis media (AOM) with discharge through the ventilation tube where it is not removed at the time of implantation. Kennedy and Shelton[3] reviewed the management of ventilation tubes in children receiving CIs and concluded that various approaches were safe.

43.3.2 Tympanic Membrane Retraction and Atelectasis

"Retraction disease" has a pathophysiology in which recurrent problems are common. Localized retractions in the attic or pars tensa regions may be managed by a limited tympanoplasty prior to implantation, aiming to stabilize the tympanic membrane. This is preferably done as a staged procedure but may be performed with implantation if very limited. For cases with larger retractions, removal of all epithelium and amputating the EAC with a blind sac closure may provide a safer alternative. An atelectatic tympanic membrane may be a substantial challenge. Avoidance of retraction onto the electrode cable or any part of the implant is essential. Cartilage grafting, particularly to the posterior-superior quadrant, may help provide long-term stability.

43.3.3 Cholesteatoma

The presence of cholesteatoma in an ear is clearly incompatible with long-term stability of a CI or an AMEI. It is essential that there is complete eradication of squamous epithelium from the middle ear cleft and reconstruction or obliteration such that recurrence will not occur. In some circumstances (e.g., small attic cholesteatoma) the surgeon may elect to use a canal wall-up technique, aiming to preserve a normal ear canal and aerated middle ear. Given the unpredictable nature of cholesteatoma and its tendency to recur, conversion to a radical cavity with blind sac closure of the meatus is very reasonable. Regardless of which procedure is used, the standard is to use a two-stage approach, with the implant being placed at the second stage after confirmation that there is no residual cholesteatoma. In cases with labyrinthine or cochlear fistulas with imminent cochlear fibrosis, the placement of a dummy electrode should be considered. The replacement of the dummy electrode by an active electrode is performed during the second-stage procedure.

43.3.4 Open Mastoid Cavity

In cases of a pre-existing radical cavity after surgical treatment for cholesteatoma or a fenestration procedure, eradication of all epithelial lining of the tympanomastoid cavity is essential (▶ Fig. 43.3). Any attempt to implant a CI or position a Vibrant Soundbridge in close proximity to skin is very likely to lead to complications of infections or extrusion of the array. Techniques that cover the array or actuator with cartilage or muscle have been described, resulting in a "cavity reduction"; however, complete epithelial removal is likely to be a safer long-term solution.

43.4 Surgical Technique

When the extent or recurrent nature of tubotympanic disease indicates that achievement of an aerated middle ear cleft is predicted to fail or has failed, or where there is an existing canal wall-down cavity or cholesteatoma with significant bony canal erosion, then the appropriate procedure is a radical mastoidectomy combined with removal of all tympanic membrane remnants and bony canal skin, with eversion and blind sac closure of the external auditory meatus. It should be noted that this is not a true subtotal petrosectomy, as it is often described. Care is taken not to remove all bone over the mastoid segment of the facial nerve (facial ridge) as a perineurium without a bony cover will adhere to the soft tissues used for obliteration and make a second-stage procedure potentially more complicated.

The blind sac closure is usually combined with obliteration of the cavity, either with a vascularized rotational flap or with an autologous fat graft. The Eustachian tube is plugged. To facilitate secure closure of the Eustachian tube, the tensor tympani muscle can be elevated from its semicanal and rotated into the Eustachian tube after mucosal elevation and the plugging further reinforced with bone pate and muscle or fascia. Bone wax or other foreign material is ideally avoided. For the mastoid cavity obliteration, if the middle ear cleft is actively infected, then it is preferable to use a vascularized soft tissue flap without non-vitalized filler materials; however, if the cavity has been dry and free of infection, then autologous (abdominal) fat may be used.

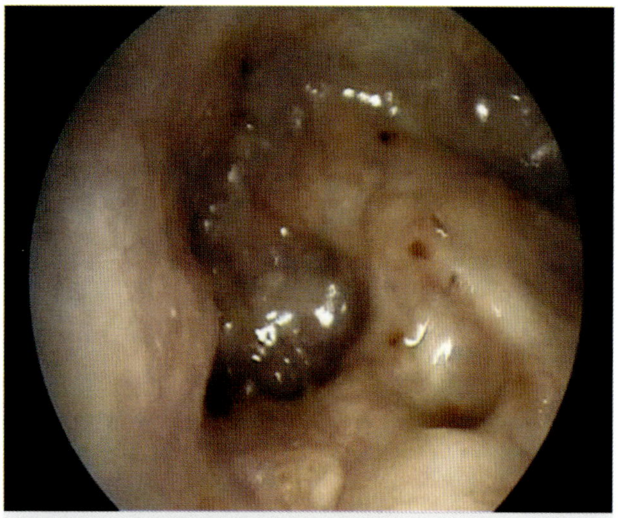

Fig. 43.3 A left ear radical cavity Type IV.

43.4.1 Blind Sac Closure

Using a postauricular approach, the technique is to divide the skin of the EAC circumferentially at the level of the cartilaginous-bone junction. A subperichondrial plane is developed over the tragal cartilage, and the skin is dissected in a lateral direction creating a "skin tube" that can be everted from the meatus. During the procedure, it is important to avoid tears in the skin as these may heal with epithelium trapped under the skin. The everted skin edges are transfixed with a vertical mattress suture. This maintains eversion of the amputated, closed canal and ensures secure healing, avoiding skin entrapment. Initially, the everted meatus will project slightly; however, with healing it will become cosmetically acceptable and be positioned slightly medial to the conchal bowl (▶ Fig. 43.4).

To secure and stabilize the medial aspect of the everted meatus, a purse string–type resorbable suture can be placed. The medial aspect should be further reinforced with a periosteal and muscle flap, superiorly-anteriorly based or inferiorly-posteriorly based (or a combination of the two), which is rotated into the area under the amputated canal. Care should be taken to position and secure the flap anteriorly toward the temporomandibular joint; the flap may be sutured to the medial aspect of the tragus.

The final result is an absent or short, clean EAC, sometimes healed with a "skin bud" at the bottom. The mastoid cavity and middle ear cleft should be free of squamous epithelium and any pathology associated with it. The everted meatus may be dressed with antibiotic cream during healing.

43.4.2 Mastoid Obliteration

It should be noted that obliteration of a closed mastoid cavity is a different scenario than obliteration of an open mastoid cavity

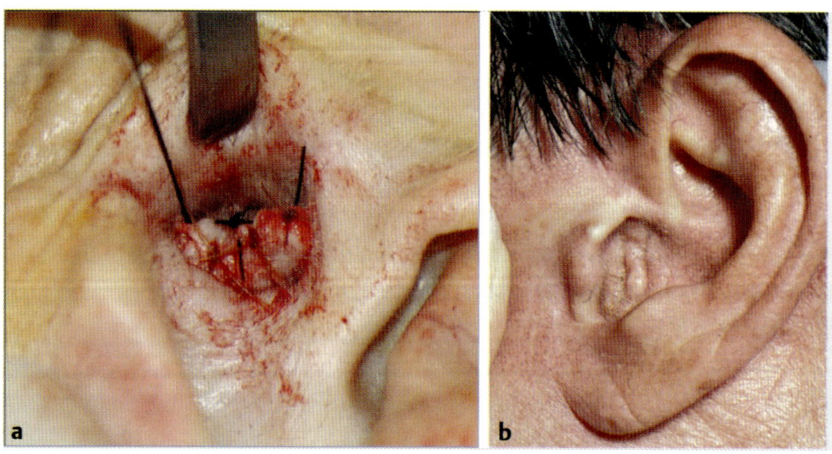

Fig. 43.4 Blind sac closure. (a) The external auditory canal skin is everted out of the meatus and sutured. (b) Once healed, the meatus is closed with a short, or, as in this case, an absent auditory canal.

(as is described in Chapter 41); however, techniques involving rotational soft tissue flaps may apply to both situations. The aim of "closed mastoid obliteration" is to create a clean, non-aerated environment, thus reducing the risks of infection associated with introduction of a foreign material. This also achieves secure cover of the electrode cable or actuator, avoiding the risk of exposure and extrusion (▶ Fig. 43.5). Obliteration of the created surgical cavity in the mastoid and the tympanum with abdominal fat or muscle flaps is a traditional way of closing the defect in cases where a large aerated volume would be disadvantageous, such as when a large area of the dura is exposed or when there is risk of cerebrospinal fluid (CSF) leak. In this situation the aim of the obliteration is complete eradication of any aerated space, and this, of course, requires a simultaneous closure of the Eustachian tube.

In the case of chronic otitis surgery prior to implantation of an active hearing device, the cavity often consists of a radical mastoidectomy. The bone is usually intact over the middle and posterior fossa dura. However, and with secure closure of the amputated ear canal, the anatomical condition of the created cavity is stable. In this situation, if Eustachian tube function is normal, without tubotympanic infection, one can consider leaving the cavity aerated (i.e., not obliterating the Eustachian tube). One advantage with this approach is that in a staged procedure there is nothing obstructing the mesotympanum, giving easier access to the stapes or round window region when implanting. Another advantage is that, in a cavity with a blind sac closure where it is not possible to clinically control/inspect the middle ear, leaving the cavity aerated makes CT interpretation easier. Some centers have advocated cavity reduction and reinforcement procedures, with cover of the electrode cable with fascia flaps or cartilage grafts.

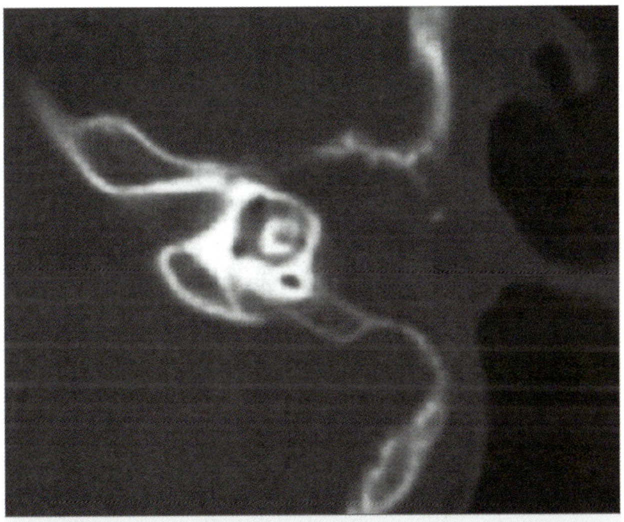

Fig. 43.5 CT scan of an obliterated left mastoid cavity prior to second-stage implantation.

43.4.3 CI Insertion

Following an obliteration procedure, the CI insertion is usually performed 3 to 6 months later, once healing is complete and there is minimal chance of residual active infection. The RS package positioning under the scalp should be planned so that the postauricular incision is not directly over the hardware, although the incision is made through the previous scar. It may be possible to develop a skin flap to allow an offset periosteal incision and create a pocket for the RS package. The mastoid cavity is explored by elevation of the soft tissue obliteration, commencing in the region of the sinodural angle. Often there is considerable venous ooze, which can be controlled with a diamond bur. As the usual landmarks are absent, and it is safest to approach the mesotympanum superiorly. The mastoid tegmen is followed anteriorly, and then the dissection is carried medially until the lateral semicircular canal is identified. This allows safe identification of the horizontal (tympanic) segment of the facial nerve and, hence, the stapes and round window niche.

For correct cochleostomy placement or round window electrode insertion, it is important that the access is equivalent to the usual facial recess approach and that the true round window membrane is identified. This may require further lowering of the facial ridge if this was not adequately performed during the primary procedure. Sometimes a small amount of the soft tissue in the mastoid cavity needs to be removed for adequate access. Electrode insertion can then proceed in the routine manner. A tissue seal is placed as usual and the electrode cable is coiled in the mastoid cavity. The previous soft tissue obliteration then refills the cavity and holds the electrode cable in position (▶ Fig. 43.6).

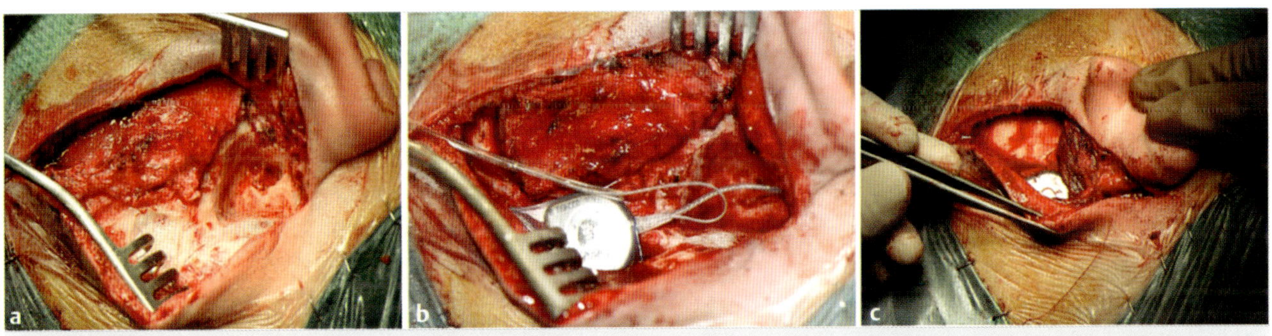

Fig. 43.6 A right ear single-stage cochlear implantation and mastoid obliteration. (a) A radical mastoidectomy combined with removal of all tympanic membrane remnants. (b) Prior to cochlear implantation, an anteriorly based temporal muscle flap is prepared. (c) The muscle flap rotated into the mastoid cavity.

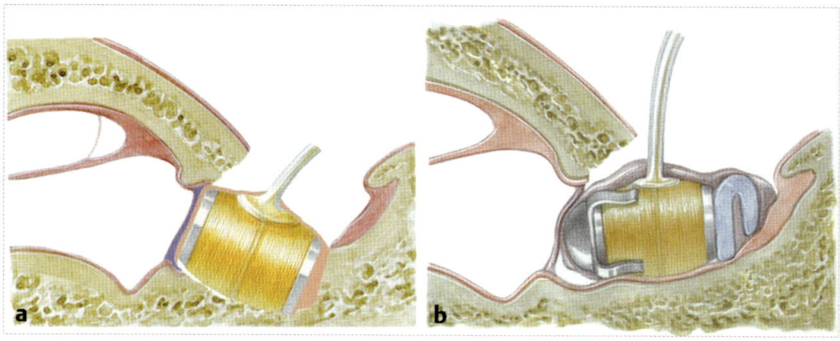

Fig. 43.7 (a) Positioning of the FMT in a round window vibroplasty. The lip of the round window niche is removed, exposing the membrane. (b) In cases of a narrow round window niche or an unfavorable angle not allowing a perpendicular placement, a round window coupler may be attached to the FMT. The FMT is stabilized with cartilage. (Used with permission from Med-El Corporation, Innsbruck, Austria.)

43.4.4 AMEI Surgery

The surgical approach in AMEI surgery depends on the preexisting anatomical condition and pathology causing the hearing loss. There is now significant experience with Vibrant Soundbridge surgery in patients with COM,[4,5,6,7,8,9,10,11] and a round window application of the FMT (a round window vibroplasty) is possible in patients with COM and previous unsuccessful attempts at reconstructive surgery, extensive ossicular chain defects, or radical cavities. Depending on the existing findings, a vibroplasty may be performed as a one-stage procedure (for instance, in a case with an acquired stenosis of the EAC). However, a staged procedure is often recommended, either to create a stable middle ear cleft or an obliteration prior to implantation as described above.

At the second stage the skin incision is made through the previous scar, ideally with an offset and traverse periosteal incision, creating periosteal flaps. The thickness of the skin flap above the implant should not exceed 7 mm to ensure later attachment of the audio processor and prevent reduced high-frequency signal transmission due to distance. Care is taken to place the coil of the vibrating ossicular replacement prosthesis (VORP) cranially from the temporal line. An implant bed should be drilled to prevent the VORP from later movement and displacement, causing a breakage of the conductor lead. The implant bed consists of two flat, deepening regions: one circular for the center magnet of the coil and one rectangular for the demodulator unit, with a passage for the conductor lead. Repeated placement of the template helps to create a flat and stable implant bed. The implant bed should be placed in a dorsal position in relation to the ear, with the thickened part of the conductor link entering the mastoid in the sinodural angle. The placement of the implant into its bed is performed after a decision is made where and how to position the FMT and after preparation of the placement site is completed.

In case of a preserved posterior canal wall, an extended posterior tympanotomy is performed, sometimes with a rerouting of the chorda tympani to create sufficient space for placement and maneuvering of the FMT. The use of a sizer kit is helpful. If previously obliterated, the soft tissues are elevated out of the mastoid and retracted anteriorly; sometimes a small amount of soft tissue needs to be resected to optimize visualization of the middle ear. Depending on the type of previous surgery or existing COM, the FMT may be positioned differently, and applying the FMT to the round window, instead of to the incus, has proven to be a good option (▶ Fig. 43.7a). The bony overhang of the round window niche is gradually reduced with a diamond bur, and, commonly, a mucosal fold is removed, exposing the true round window membrane. A FMT sizer is used to check the position, and the clip on the FMT is removed with scissors. The FMT is best positioned perpendicularly, in direct contact to the round window membrane, with or without a round window coupler (▶ Fig. 43.7b). The use of graft material, such as fascia or perichondrium, should be avoided given that it reduces coupling efficiency and promotes FMT migration.[12]

Having ensured membrane contact, the FMT is stabilized with cartilage. A correct position can be evaluated by touching the stapes/footplate, validating movement of the FMT. Electrocochleography (ECoG) has been used to further ensure the position.[13,14] The round window technique is recommended if FMT coupling to oval window pathways is not favorable. Alternatives are FMT attachment to the stapes itself or attachment with a coupling prosthesis (▶ Fig. 43.8). If the stapes superstructure is missing, an oval window coupler can be positioned on the footplate (▶ Fig. 43.9).[15,16] Stapes or oval window couplers may also be used in second-stage procedures or after a previous obliteration.[10]

In cases of otosclerosis and sensorineural hearing loss, effective rehabilitation can be achieved by connecting the FMT to the long process of the incus in conjunction with a stapes prosthesis (▶ Fig. 43.10). As in the classical Vibrant Soundbridge application, the FMT must be firmly secured to the long incus process. The axis of the FMT should be parallel to the axis of the stapes prosthesis.[6,17]

The surgical procedure of the DACS (direct acoustic cochlear stimulator) system (Cochlear Corporation, Sydney, Australia), currently in clinical trial use only, is more challenging and requires an ear without previous tympanomastoid surgery. The surgery involves several steps, including fixation of the mounting system within the mastoid, removing the stapes superstructure through a posterior tympanotomy, positioning the actuator in the middle ear, perforating the stapes footplate, and fixing a stapes piston to the artificial incus.[18]

43.4.5 Bone-Anchored Hearing Systems

The concept of bone-anchored hearing is well established and is a good option in patients with a conductive or mixed hearing loss when reconstruction is not an option, in patients with problems related to the use of conventional hearing aids, or in patients with single-sided deafness.[19]

Passive Bone-Anchored Hearing Systems

For percutaneous bone-anchored devices in patients with COM, the titanium screw fixture is inserted approximately 5–6 cm posterior and superior to the EAC meatus. A straight incision is

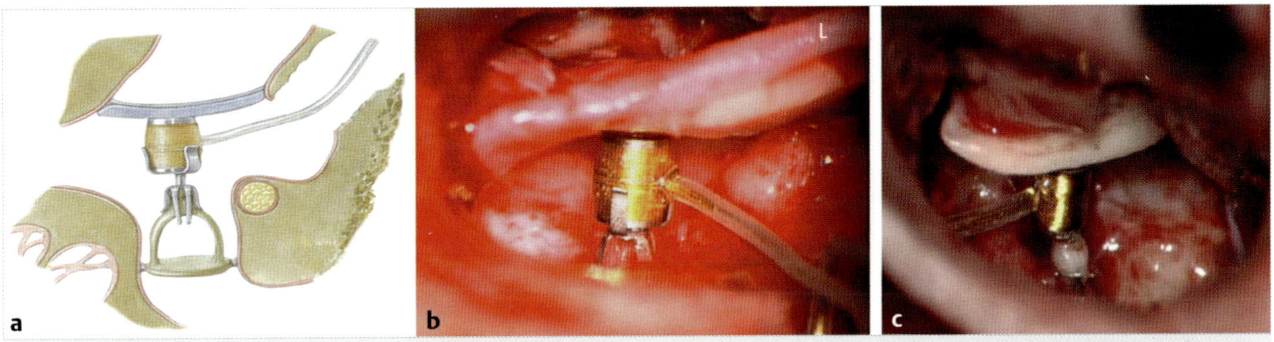

Fig. 43.8 (a) FMT positioning in cases with an intact stapes, here with a coupling prosthesis. (b) FMT interpositioned with a coupling prosthesis between the stapes head and cartilage perichondrium island graft in a left ear, with partial cavity obliteration. (c) FMT connected to the stapes head using the regular clip attached to the device. Right ear view through the EAC with elevated meatal flap. (8a used with permission from Med-El Corporation, Innsbruck, Austria)

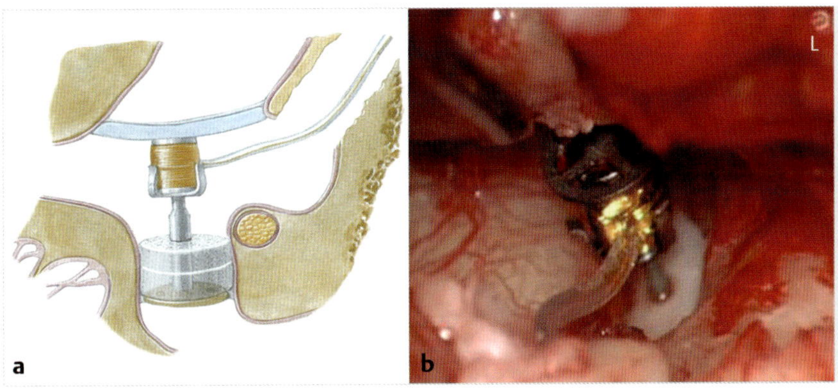

Fig. 43.9 (a) The FMT attached to an oval window coupler with a cartilage shoe on the stapes footplate. Care is taken to have good cartilage interpositioning toward the tympanic membrane. (b) Left ear view with elevated meatal flap in a partially obliterated cavity. (9a used with permission from Med-El Corporation, Innsbruck, Austria.)

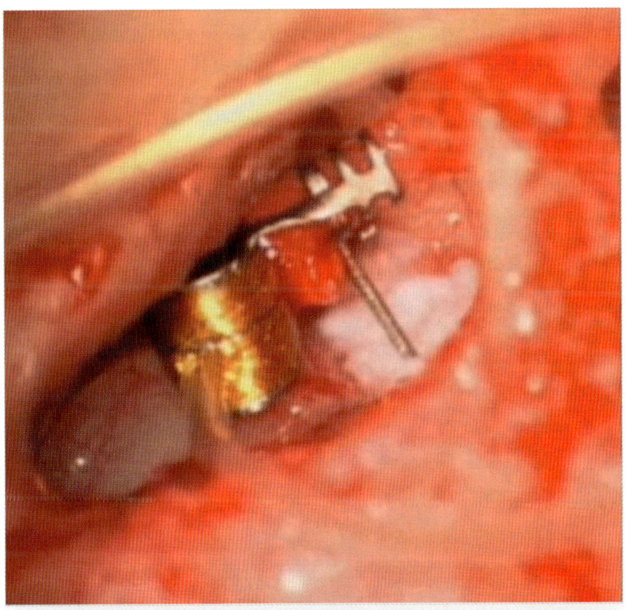

Fig. 43.10 The FMT attached to the long incus process in a single stage with partial stapedectomy and a titanium stapes piston in a left ear using a mastoidectomy and posterior tympanotomy approach.

made down to bone. After having checked bone thickness with a guide drill, usually to 4 mm, the hole is widened with a countersink drill and the implant screwed in. In the past, the overlying soft tissues were thinned extensively and the percutaneous abutment fixed to periosteum at a second stage with a split-thickness skin graft. However, the procedure is now usually performed in one stage (in adults) using longer abutments and little or no soft tissue removal, with good results.[20]

Recently, transcutaneous bone-anchored solutions, such as the Sophono Alpha[21] or the Baha Attract (▶ Fig. 43.11), have become available and may prove to be a good option for patients in whom skin problems related to a percutaneous abutment can be anticipated or for improved cosmesis. In these devices, an implantable magnet is fixed to the bone, and the vibrations from the audio processor, kept in place by an external magnet, are transmitted through intact skin. Bone conduction hearing thresholds are reported to be equal to or better than 30 dB as some vibratory energy is lost due to the dampening effect of the skin.

Active Bone-Anchored Hearing Systems

The Bonebridge is an active bone conduction implant consisting of an internal implantable component with a coil, a magnet, and a demodulator connected to a relatively large actuator, the bone conduction-floating mass transducer (BC-FMT). The audio processor is worn externally, attached with a magnet (▶ Fig. 43.12a). As with other bone conduction hearing devices, suitable patients have a conductive or mixed hearing loss with a mild-to-moderate sensorineural component. Also, patients with single-sided sensorineural deafness with normal hearing in the other ear may be candidates.

A preoperative CT scan is mandatory to plan the positioning of the BC-FMT in the sinodural angle and also to position the two retention screws, making sure to avoid the dura and the sigmoid sinus. After a postaural incision and an off-set pericranial fascia incision, a subperiosteal pocket is created for the receiver coil. The skin flap needs thinning if exceeding 7 mm. A recess with a diameter of 15.8 mm and a necessary depth of 8.7 mm is drilled in the bone for the BC-FMT, with the temporal line and ear canal as reference points. Two holes are drilled with a guide and the BC-FMT fixed with screws; the use of a torque wrench to 10 N cm is recommended (▶ Fig. 43.12b; ▶ Fig. 43.12c).[22] In cases with severe temporal bone malformations or radical cavities, the BC-FMT may be placed in the retrosigmoid region. Identification of the placement site using navigational systems might be used in complex cases.

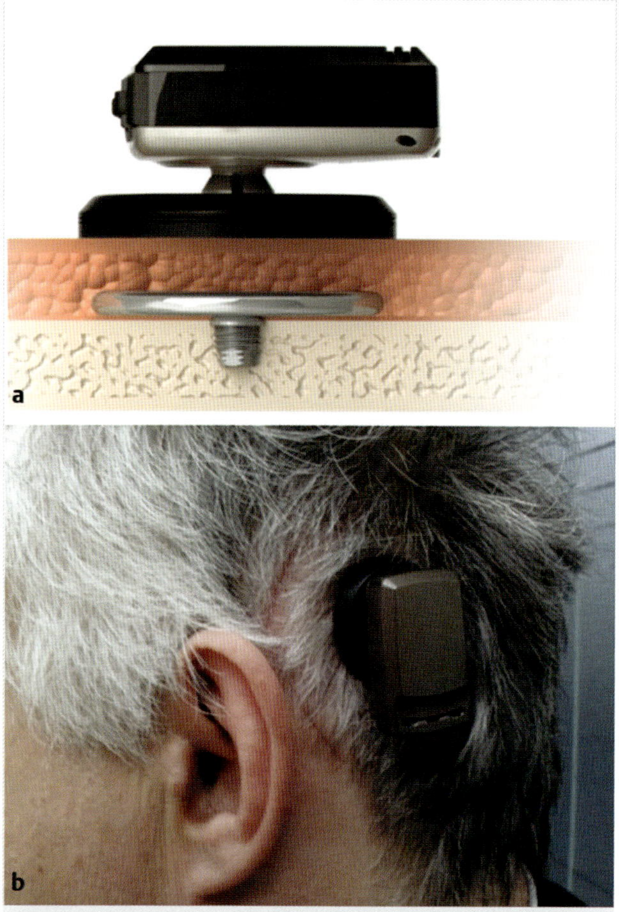

Fig. 43.11 (a) The transcutaneous bone-anchored hearing aid consists of an internal part with an implant magnet attached to a conventional osseointegrated titanium screw. The sound processor is attached with an external magnet. (b) Loading at 4 weeks after surgery. (11a used with permission from Cochlear Corporation, Sydney, Australia.)

43.5 Postoperative Care

43.5.1 Imaging

For CIs a standard "cochlear view" X-ray is usually performed the same day or the day after the implantation to verify a correct position of the electrode prior to turning it on. The same applies to AMEIs, despite the fact that normal X-ray is limited to defining a baseline for future imaging in case of reduced implant function. Using cone-beam CT is a good alternative for postoperative CI and AMEI imaging as this technique, with small radiation exposure, allows creation of high-resolution multi-plane projections and seems to produce less metal artifacts. This is especially valuable in AMEIs because it allows evaluation of the positioning of the actuator in the middle ear.[2] In the case of the Vibrant Soundbridge, as the FMT is positioned in the round window niche in patients with COM, this technique permits a very precise estimation of the location in relation to the round window membrane.

A specific imaging challenge is the follow-up after obliteration and implantation to exclude residual cholesteatoma. CT can be used but is not particularly sensitive for differentiating soft tissue, fat, or muscle from cholesteatoma. In complicated cases, such as in an ear with an atelectatic tympanic membrane or frank cholesteatoma, it may be an advantage not to obliterate a closed ear, instead leaving a large aerated volume behind the closed EAC. In this case, a residual cholesteatoma will appear as

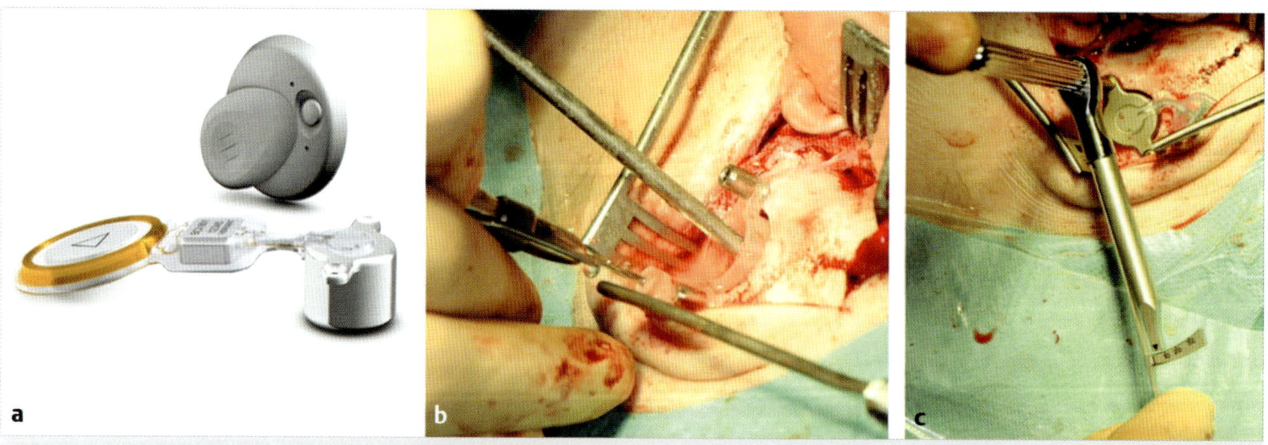

Fig. 43.12 (a) The BONEBRIDGE is an active bone conduction implant. It consists of an implanted part, with a receiver coil, a demodulator, and a transducer (the BC-FMT). The audio processor is the external part worn on the head. (b) The sizer is used to verify the depth for the BC-FMT and as a guide for drilling two fixation holes. (c) The BC-FMT is secured with screws using a torque wrench. (12a used with permission from Med-El Corporation, Innsbruck, Austria.)

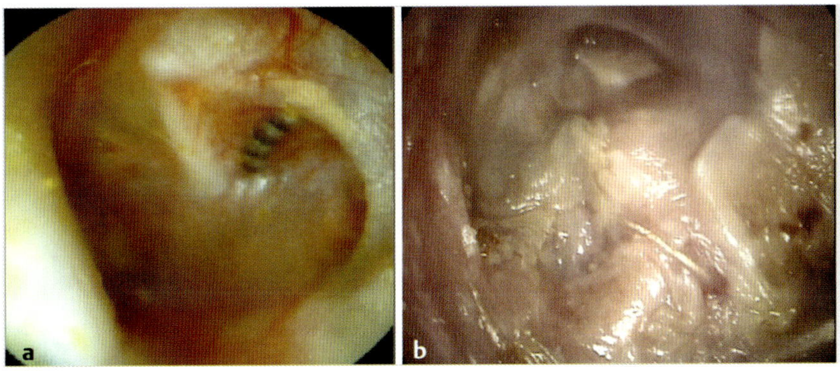

Fig. 43.13 Retracted tympanic membrane draping (a) the array of a CI and (b) the FMT of a Vibrant Soundbridge.

a rounded mass on CT instead of being imbedded in other soft tissue, making diagnostics easier.

With appropriate diffusion sequences, MRI is more sensitive; however, the presence of the implant creates significant problems. As previously mentioned, despite the fact that CIs are MRI-compatible, in general to 1.5 tesla, everything with an integrated magnet will show a significant artifact on postoperative MRI. Some of the models have a magnet that may be temporarily explanted during the MRI procedure. MRI is contraindicated in patients with a Vibrant Soundbridge. For standard bone-anchored devices, postoperative imaging is not a problem; for those with an active or transcutaneous solution, and thus an internal magnet, a considerable artifact will appear on MRI. It is important to consider a possible future need of single or repeated MRI scans when considering bone-anchored hearing solutions, especially in the pediatric population.[23]

In all cases of a closed ear, imaging, in general a CT scan, should at least be performed at 1 and 3years after surgery, and the threshold for additional examinations should be low.

43.5.2 Antibiotic Therapy

For implant surgery in a well-healed, previously obliterated ear, intravenous antibiotics are usually used only as a one-dose prophylaxis immediately prior to surgery. In the case of active infection, intravenous administration is continued during the hospital stay and a course of oral antibiotics may be considered after discharge in the first postoperative week. This also applies to one-stage obliteration-implantation surgery.

43.6 Complications

The presence of COM and performing an obliteration of an ear adds a significant degree of complexity to any implant surgery, cochlear implantation as well as vibroplasty, and does require sufficient experience in lateral skull base surgery. Complications do occur, both in relation to primary surgery and in the long-term postoperative period, and it is important that patients are counseled accordingly preoperatively.

43.6.1 AOM or COM Occurring in the Presence of an Implant

Acute otitis media may occur in an implanted ear. Despite the fact that AOM is common in childhood, it is generally believed that it is less common in children with implanted ears, a situation possibly related to a mastoidectomy having been performed. Fortunately, it is rare that chronic infection of the prosthesis results, and possibly this is because the RS package is protected by fibrous encapsulation. An AOM in a child (or, rarely, an adult) with an implantable hearing device may present with otalgia and typical findings of the tympanic membrane, but also a postauricular red swelling. This finding looks similar to an acute mastoiditis, but is clinically to be regarded as a local abscess. Although conservative treatment may be considered in mild cases, surgical drainage, either by incision or needle aspiration, should be considered, together with ventilation tube placement. Intravenous antibiotics are administered, and a prolonged oral course considered depending on microbiology and clinical response.

It is unusual to develop COM in the presence of an implant. A well-performed CI or AMEI usually preserves the EAC and leaves the tympanic membrane untouched, resulting in a well-aerated middle ear and mastoid with intact Eustachian tube function. In the unusual case of a retraction developing in an ear with previous hearing device implantation, presenting with the tympanic membrane draping the tympanic segment of the electrode (▶ Fig. 43.13a) or FMT (▶ Fig. 43.13b), it is the authors' experience that a limited tympanoplasty can be performed. The retraction is elevated and the electrode covered with cartilage. In the case of more extensive retraction or a breakdown of the posterior bony canal wall, with the electrode extruding into the EAC (▶ Fig. 43.14), a more aggressive approach may be necessary, with explantation and obliteration. Explantation is necessary when the electrode cable is irreversibly involved with the disease (often in the case of a CI with partial extrusion from the cochlea). Sometimes reimplantation may be performed at the same procedure. If done at a later stage, depending on the extent of disease and individual patient needs, a dummy electrode should be inserted to prevent cochlea obliteration.

43.6.2 Cholesteatoma

The most obvious danger when obliterating an ear is entrapment of skin and subsequent cholesteatoma formation. Having closed the EAC, this is a potentially dangerous situation because cholesteatoma growth can go on for a long time without symptoms or a possibility of diagnosing it. In the literature post-obliteration cholesteatomas are sometimes found accidentally doing a CT scan for other reasons. Any late loss in hearing performance or need for change in the mapping of the implantable

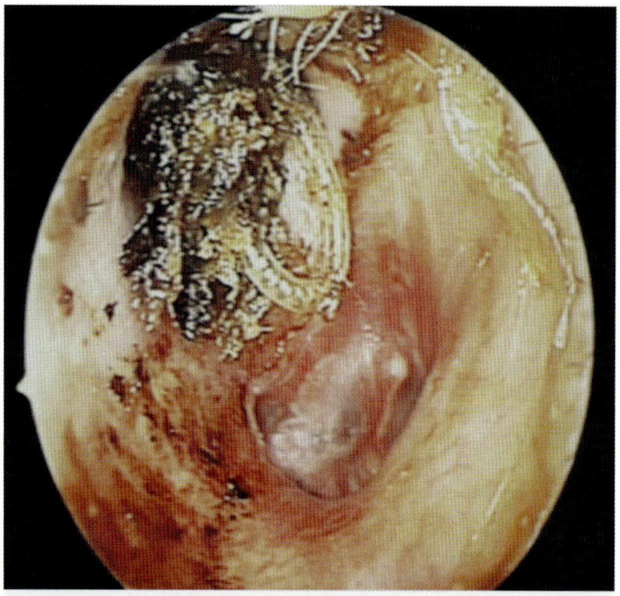

Fig. 43.14 Any part of an implant may extrude through skin unless the soft tissues are thick and well vascularized. In this case, the electrode of a cochlear implant has broken through the skin due to a defect in the bony part of the external auditory canal.

hearing device needs to be assessed with the suspicion of recurrent/residual disease.

Other risks related to closing the EAC and obliterating the cavity include skin breakdown of the EAC, requiring a revision meatoplasty, and autologous fat infection.

43.6.3 Incidence of Complications in the Literature

Leung and Briggs[24] reported on a series of 17 patients, where two needed revision of the obliteration prior to implantation (due to incomplete Eustachian tube plugging and breakdown of the blind sac closure) and two of the patients required revision of the CI (due to migration of the RS package and thinning of the postaural skin with threatening exposure). Vincenti and colleagues[25] presented radiological follow-up in 12 patients, indicating no long-term sign of cholesteatoma, but did report one residual cholesteatoma found at second-stage cochlear implantation and one case of EAC breakdown. Free et al.[26] described complications in two patients in a series of 32 one-stage cochlear implantations and simultaneous obliterations (one electrode extrusion and one CSF collection); however, this was with a shorter follow-up period. Barañano and colleagues[27] reported on 39 surgeries in adults and children with a complication rate of 15.4%, including 3 adult abscesses requiring explantation and reimplantation, development of subcutaneous emphysema in one case, one patient with EAC closure granulations requiring revision prior to implantation, and one case of electrode extrusion.

Reported complications in relation to round window application of the Vibrant Soundbridge in combination with obliteration (Linder et al.,[4] Beltrame et al.,[5] Baumgartner et al.,[7] Böheim et al.,[8] Marino et al.,[9] Verhaert et al.,[10] Colletti et al.[11]; 121 patients total) included recurrent cholesteatoma (n=1), prolonged healing of the postauricular area or meatus (n=5), skin breakdown over the RS package or meatus (n=3), late sensorineural hearing loss requiring CI (n=1), FMT migration requiring revision surgery (n=6), and device failure requiring replacement (n=2).

Early clinical trials of the BONEBRIDGE have shown few and minor adverse events, all of which resolved at the end of a 3-month study period. No change in residual hearing thresholds was seen after surgery.[22]

43.7 Outcomes

The very good hearing outcome for cochlear implantation COM recipients is similar to those without previous chronic ear disease. During preoperative counseling, the normal aspects of CI hearing rehabilitation should be discussed with the patient.

The reported hearing results for round window application of the Vibrant Soundbridge are very good and are often reported to give a 15–40 dB functional gain, with the peak values at 1.5–2 kHz. Baumgartner et al.[7] and Böheim et al.[8] reported significant monosyllable word recognition improvement, from 6% to 67%. In the largest study, Colletti and colleagues[11] reported on stable and good to very good long-term results in 91% of the patients. No significant change in residual hearing in relation to implantation was reported.

Bone-anchored devices very often give a good improvement of hearing perception scores. In comparison between transcutaneous bone-anchored systems, such as the Sophono or Baha Attract, and traditional percutaneous solutions, the audiologic results seem better with percutaneous bone-anchored hearing.[28] However, for each individual the benefits of fewer skin-related problems have to be balanced against the reduced gain due to attenuation through intact skin. It is reasonable to limit the use of transcutaneous solutions to patients with a sensorineural component of 30 dB or less on average. Active bone conduction implants, such as the BONEBRIDGE, combine the advantages of intact skin and powerful stimulation and have in early clinical trials been shown to be effective, with significant improvement in speech perception scores[22]; it is, however, a more expensive implant.

43.8 Conclusion

Isolating the tympanomastoid cleft is important in cases of preexisting COM or other unfavorable conditions to ensure a safe implantation and long-term survival of an implantable hearing device. After removal of disease, the techniques used often include a blind sac closure of the EAC and a soft tissue obliteration of the surgical cavity. A staged procedure is recommended to ensure healing and eradication of disease prior to implantation; however, a single-stage procedure may be performed if conditions are favorable.

The medical complications resulting in revision surgery include residual cholesteatoma, recurrent retraction or perforation of the tympanic membrane, and extrusion of the electrode cable as well as postauricular skin flap necrosis. Follow-up of patients with an obliterated ear often include a second look in cases of a staged procedure, but postoperative CT is important.

Published results of hearing outcomes include limited series of patients with good CI hearing, similar to normal CI recipients. Vibroplasty often gives very good hearing outcome in recipients with mixed hearing loss, in general with overclosure in the mid-frequencies; however, the surgery is challenging and the outcome is very dependent on optimal positioning of the FMT. Revision surgery and repositioning may become necessary. Bone-anchored hearing devices can be placed in a less complicated surgery and have very predictable outcomes. The application of bone-anchored hearing devices and AMEIs regularly provide good rehabilitative hearing results on aided sound field and speech reception thresholds, as well as good speech reception scores if candidates are carefully selected.

References

[1] Colletti V, Soli SD, Carner M, Colletti L. Treatment of mixed hearing losses via implantation of a vibratory transducer on the round window. Int J Audiol. 2006;45(10):600–608.

[2] Mlynski R, Nguyen TD, Plontke SK, Kösling S. Presentation of floating mass transducer and Vibroplasty Couplers on CT and Cone Beam CT. Eur Arch Otorhinolaryngol. 2013

[3] Kennedy RJ, Shelton C. Ventilation tubes and cochlear implants: What do we do? Otol Neurotol. 2005;26(3):438–441.

[4] Linder T, Schlegel C, DeMin N, van der Westhuizen S. Active middle ear implants in patients undergoing subtotal petrosectomy: New application for the Vibrant Soundbridge device and its implication for lateral cranium base surgery. Otol Neurotol. 2009;30(1):41–47.

[5] Beltrame AM, Martini A, Prosser S, Giarbini N, Streitberger C. Coupling the Vibrant Soundbridge to cochlea round window: Auditory results in patients with mixed hearing loss. Otol Neurotol. 2009;30(2):194–201.

[6] Mlynski R, Mueller J, Hagen R. Surgical approaches to position the Vibrant Soundbridge in conductive and mixed hearing loss. Oper Tech Otolaryngol–Head Neck Surg. 2010;21:272–277.

[7] Baumgartner WD, Böheim K, Hagen R, et al. The vibrant soundbridge for conductive and mixed hearing losses: European multicenter study results. Adv Otorhinolaryngol. 2010;69:38–50.

[8] Böheim K, Mlynski R, Lenarz T, Schlögel M, Hagen R. Round window vibroplasty: long-term results. Acta Otolaryngol. 2012;132(10):1042–1048.

[9] Marino R, Linton N, Eikelboom RH, Statham E, Rajan GP. A comparative study of hearing aids and round window application of the vibrant sound bridge (VSB) for patients with mixed or conductive hearing loss. Int J Audiol. 2013;52(4):209–218.

[10] Verhaert N, Mojallal H, Schwab B. Indications and outcome of subtotal petrosectomy for active middle ear implants. Eur Arch Otorhinolaryngol. 2013;270(4):1243–1248.

[11] Colletti L, Mandalà M, Colletti V. Long-term outcome of round window Vibrant SoundBridge implantation in extensive ossicular chain defects. Otolaryngol Head Neck Surg. 2013;149(1):134–141.

[12] Rajan GP, Lampacher P, Ambett R, et al. Impact of floating mass transducer coupling and positioning in round window vibroplasty. Otol Neurotol. 2011;32(2):271–277.

[13] Radeloff A, Shehata-Dieler W, Rak K, et al. Intraoperative monitoring of active middle ear implant function in patients with normal and pathologic middle ears. Otol Neurotol. 2011;32(1):104–107.

[14] Colletti V, Mandalà M, Colletti L. Electrocochleography in round window Vibrant Soundbridge implantation. Otolaryngol Head Neck Surg. 2012;146(4):633–640.

[15] Beleites T, Neudert M, Beutner D, Hüttenbrink KB, Zahnert T. Experience with vibroplasty couplers at the stapes head and footplate. Otol Neurotol. 2011;32(9):1468–1472.

[16] Huber AM, Mlynski R, Müller J, et al. A new vibroplasty coupling technique as a treatment for conductive and mixed hearing losses: A report of 4 cases. Otol Neurotol. 2012;33(4):613–617.

[17] Kontorinis G, Lenarz T, Mojallal H, Hinze AL, Schwab B. Power stapes: An alternative method for treating hearing loss in osteogenesis imperfecta? Otol Neurotol. 2011;32(4):589–595.

[18] Busch S, Kruck S, Spickers D, et al. First clinical experiences with a direct acoustic cochlear stimulator in comparison to preoperative fitted conventional hearing aids. Otol Neurotol. 2013;34(9):1711–1718.

[19] Kompis M, Caversaccio MD, eds. Implantable Bone Conduction Hearing Aids. Adv Otorhinolaryngo. Basel, Karger, 2011;vol 71.

[20] Hultcrantz M. Outcome of the bone-anchored hearing aid procedure without skin thinning: a prospective clinical trial. Otol Neurotol. 2011;32(7):1134–1139.

[21] Siegert R, Kanderske J. A new semi-implantable transcutaneous bone conduction device: Clinical, surgical, and audiologic outcomes in patients with congenital ear canal atresia. Otol Neurotol. 2013;34(5):927–934.

[22] Sprinzl G, Lenarz T, Ernst A, et al. First European multicenter results with a new transcutaneous bone conduction hearing implant system: Short-term safety and efficacy. Otol Neurotol. 2013;34(6):1076–1083.

[23] Doshi J, Schneiders S, Foster K, Reid A, McDermott AL. Magnetic resonance imaging and bone anchored hearing implants: Pediatric considerations. Int J Pediatr Otorhinolaryngol. 2014 Feb;78(2):277–9.

[24] Leung R, Briggs RJ. Indications for and outcomes of mastoid obliteration in cochlear implantation. Otol Neurotol. 2007;28(3):330–334.

[25] Vincenti V, Pasanisi E, Bacciu A, Bacciu S. Long-term results of external auditory canal closure and mastoid obliteration in cochlear implantation after radical mastoidectomy: a clinical and radiological study. Eur Arch Otorhinolaryngol. 2014 Aug;271(8):2127–30.

[26] Free RH, Falcioni M, Di Trapani G, Giannuzzi AL, Russo A, Sanna M. The role of subtotal petrosectomy in cochlear implant surgery—a report of 32 cases and review on indications. Otol Neurotol. 2013;34(6):1033–1040.

[27] Barañano CF, Kopelovich JC, Dunn CC, Gantz BJ, Hansen MR. Subtotal petrosectomy and mastoid obliteration in adult and pediatric cochlear implant recipients. Otol Neurotol. 2013;34(9):1656–1659.

[28] Hol MK, Nelissen RC, Agterberg MJ, Cremers CW, Snik AF. Comparison between a new implantable transcutaneous bone conductor and percutaneous bone-conduction hearing implant. Otol Neurotol. 2013;34(6):1071–1075.

44 Endoscopic Ear Surgery

David D. Pothier and Alejandro Rivas

Abbreviations used in this chapter:

EES: endoscopic ear surgery
TEES: transcanal endoscopic ear surgery

44.1 Introduction

The development of the rigid rod endoscope by Hopkins in the 1950s opened a new path for surgery in almost every branch of the discipline. Although endoscopes have been used for centuries, early devices comprised a light source that directed light through the lumen of a tube through which body cavities could be viewed directly. These devices allowed the inspection of the bowel, esophagus, bladder, and airways in a way that had not been possible before. Given the limitation of the necessarily narrow diameter of the lumen of these rudimentary endoscopes, however, there was little potential for surgical procedures to be carried out endoscopically.

The "Hopkins rod" revolutionized endoscopy by applying optics to the problem, along with the relatively new technology of light-carrying fibers. These new endoscopes allowed for a wide field of view with good illumination; this combination propelled endoscopy to new levels of utility. Endoscopes have had a long history in surgery, including otolaryngology, but, until recently, have had less widespread acceptance in the field of otology.

Early uses for endoscopes in otology were as an aid to microscopic surgery[1] and for the second-look inspection of mastoid cavities through a "stab-incision," in which a canal wall-up procedure had been performed.[2] Other early uses included photography[3] and exploration of the middle ear.[4,5] Despite the advantages of the endoscope in obtaining a wide field of view and a superior access to obscure areas of the middle ear, the use of narrower-diameter endoscopes[1] made endoscopic surgery, as such, technically challenging. In the early 1990s, Tarabichi published the first series of cases that had been managed exclusively using an endoscopic approach,[6,7] followed by a publication on the long-term results of this work.[8]

Since these early days of endoscopic ear surgery (EES), also often referred to as totally transcanal EES (TEES), other institutions have taken on the technique and published the results of their work.[9,10,11]

44.2 Principles of EES

Even though the origin of cholesteatoma is within the middle ear and it merely extends into the mastoid system, it is often thought of as a mastoid disease rather than a middle ear disease. This is likely because of the need to perform a cortical or even an extended mastoidectomy to gain access to the anterior epitympanum and to the facial recess so as to address disease in the sinus tympani through a posterior tympanotomy. While this is now accepted practice, it has become the necessary result of the natural access route to the middle ear, the ear canal being too narrow to allow for adequate access with the microscope.

The mastoid performs a vital physiological function in terms of gas exchange and as a buffer for fluctuations in middle ear pressure. The seemingly unwarranted destruction of this often uninvolved and often healthy system to allow access to the middle ear is particularly apparent when removing disease limited to the middle ear or epitympanum. Given that the rates of residual disease in the mastoid are relatively low[12] when compared with regions of the middle ear, such as the retrotympanum, it seems disproportionate to damage large volumes of healthy bone and mucosa merely to facilitate access to the middle ear. Endoscopic ear surgery takes advantage of the endoscope to gain access to all areas of the middle ear without resorting to the need to damage healthy tissue to achieve adequate exposure.

44.3 Patient Selection

In addition to the reduction in damage to healthy tissue, TEES eliminates the need for a postauricular incision or endaural incision to allow access to the surgical field. Although the skin incisions associated with traditional open ear surgery are seldom considered important, patients hold a great deal of value in being able to avoid a painful incision as well as a scar; indeed, when discussing EES with many patients, the issue of the scar and the need for the removal of sutures become key points of discussion, perhaps surprisingly given the gravity of the issues surrounding cholesteatoma surgery. This is an indication of the importance of the skin incision to many patients.

Access to the anterior epitympanum and sinus tympani are notoriously difficult using the microscope, which, although providing a very clear magnified view of the surgical field, is limited by the line-of-sight view inherent in its design. Thus, it is disease in these areas that is more appropriately addressed by EES. Although the advantages are greatest in these anatomical regions, the benefits of the endoscope are apparent in all parts of the middle ear. As a result of the superior view offered by the endoscope, it can be argued that the question of patient or case selection should not be decided in terms of the type, nature, or extent of disease, but, rather, which tool should be used where and at what point during the surgery. Performing a mastoidectomy to remove extensive cholesteatoma from the mastoid is not best undertaken with an endoscope, and the middle ear is not best suited to the microscope. Therefore, it is useful to address disease within the middle ear endoscopically and then switch to a microscope to remove disease that is beyond the reach of an entirely endoscopic approach. Preoperative imaging will help the surgeon plan the expected flow of the operation (▶ Fig. 44.1).

44.4 Anatomy

The use of the endoscope in the management of middle ear disease has allowed the more careful examination of the hidden structures of the mesotympanum and epitympanum. In many cases, these insights amount to rediscoveries of anatomical

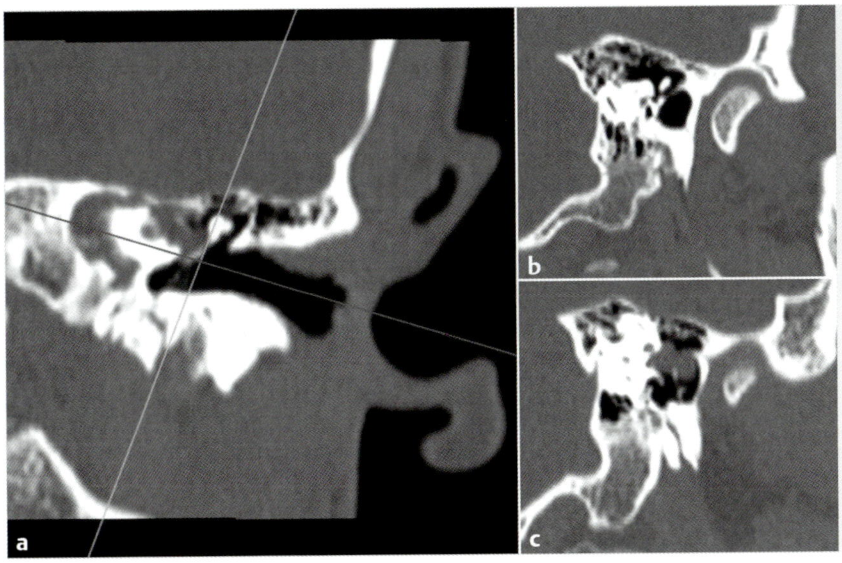

Fig. 44.1 Multiplanar reconstruction of a high-resolution CT scan along the plane of the external auditory canal. (a) The plane is set along the plane of the external auditory canal, parallel to the direction of approach of the endoscope. This allows slices to be constructed that match what is expected at each stage of the endoscopic surgery. (b) At the level of the tympanic ring and scutum. (c) Mesotympanum showing the relationship of cholesteatoma to important structures.

features that have been previously described, but were not able to be fully understood in the context of middle ear surgery given that they were not easily identified during surgery with the operating microscope (▶ Fig. 44.2).

The sinus tympani is a notoriously difficult area to access with a microscopic view. The posterior tympanotomy was developed to improve access to this area, but this dissection provides access through the facial recess rather than the sinus tympani itself. Although this improves access to disease in the sinus tympani, the facial nerve that lies between the two structures prevents direct access even through a wide posterior tympanotomy. Although it has been possible to undertake a retrofacial approach to the sinus tympani, the close proximity of the posterior semicircular canal and the variable course of the vertical segment of the facial nerve make this surgical approach very challenging. In cases of a shallow sinus tympani, even a retrofacial approach may not be sufficient to access disease in this area.

The wide angle of view and the use of angulated endoscopes have allowed a more detailed examination of the sinus tympani that informs surgical planning. In their work on describing the morphology of the sinus tympani, Marchioni et al[13] describe a classification system of the sinus tympani in relation to its depth relative to the facial nerve (▶ Fig. 44.3) and its morphology relative to surrounding structures, subdividing it into normal shape, confluent shape, and partitioned shape. Knowledge of these configurations allows disease to be removed from the sinus tympani with greater confidence owing to the benefits of a comprehension of the complex interrelationships between structures such as the styloid eminence, ponticulus, and subiculum (see Chapter 7).

Although originally described by Aimi et al[14] in 1978, the anatomy of the anterior and posterior tympanic isthmus came to the attention of endoscopic surgeons who were now able to clearly assess these areas without any disruption of the surrounding anatomy (▶ Fig. 44.4). Marchioni et al describe the endoscopic anatomy of the ventilation pathways of the middle ear, with particular attention being paid to the endoscopic anatomy of the anterior and posterior tympanic isthmus, showing the role that blockage of these routes for ventilation of the epitympanum and mastoid air cell system has on the development of retraction of the tympanic membrane and cholesteatoma (see Chapter 7).[15] This is described in greater detail in another paper by the same group with emphasis on the improved access afforded by the endoscope when assessing these areas.[16] Prussak's space plays a major role in the development of cholesteatoma, with its genesis in the pars flaccida; although the pathways for ventilation of this space have been described previously, the endoscopic anatomy of this region of the middle ear has expanded knowledge of the physiology of the ventilation of the middle ear[17,18] and has provided advantages in ear surgery designed to improve ventilation along with the extirpation of middle ear disease.

Another structure that has been, until recently, considered of limited importance beyond obscure anatomical knowledge is the tensor fold, a mucosal structure that originates at the cog of the epitympanum and extends to the tendon of the tensor tympani. Depending on the morphology of the anterior epitympanum and the supratubal recess, this structure can range from near horizontal to near vertical and can play an important role in the dysventilation of the epitympanum, given its proximity to the Eustachian tube.[15,19]

44.5 Required Equipment Recommendations

44.5.1 Endoscopes

Diameter

The choice of endoscope involves a necessary trade-off between the field of view it provides and its diameter. Smaller-diameter endoscopes can be used more easily than wider endoscopes alongside other instruments in the ear canal, but they produce a far smaller image and are able to supply less light owing to their limited ability to carry sufficient fiberoptic light bundles alongside their lenses. Current technology limits the surgeon to a choice of diameters ranging from 2.7 mm to 4 mm. Most endoscopic ear surgeons favor the 3-mm diameter rigid endoscope as a good compromise between view and bulk.

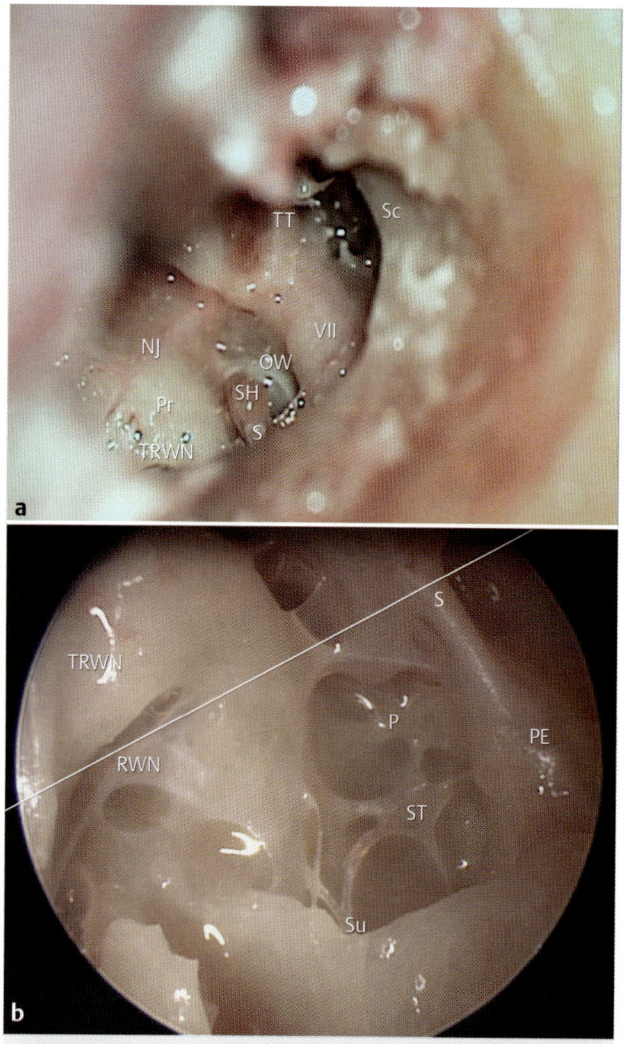

Fig. 44.2 Microscopy versus endoscopy. (a) A transcanal view using a postauricular approach to the left ear with optimal positioning to view the retrotympanum. (b) Endoscopic view of the same ear using a 45-degree endoscope. The white line shows the posterior limit of the microscopic view. The following structures are visible: VII, facial nerve; OW, oval window niche; NJ, Jacobson's nerve; Pr, promontory; TRWN, tegmen of the round window niche; RWN, round window niche; SH, stapes head; S, stapedius tendon; Sc, scutum; TT, tensor tympani tendon; PE, pyramidal eminence; P, ponticulus (rudimentary in this specimen); ST, sinus tympani; Su, subiculum.

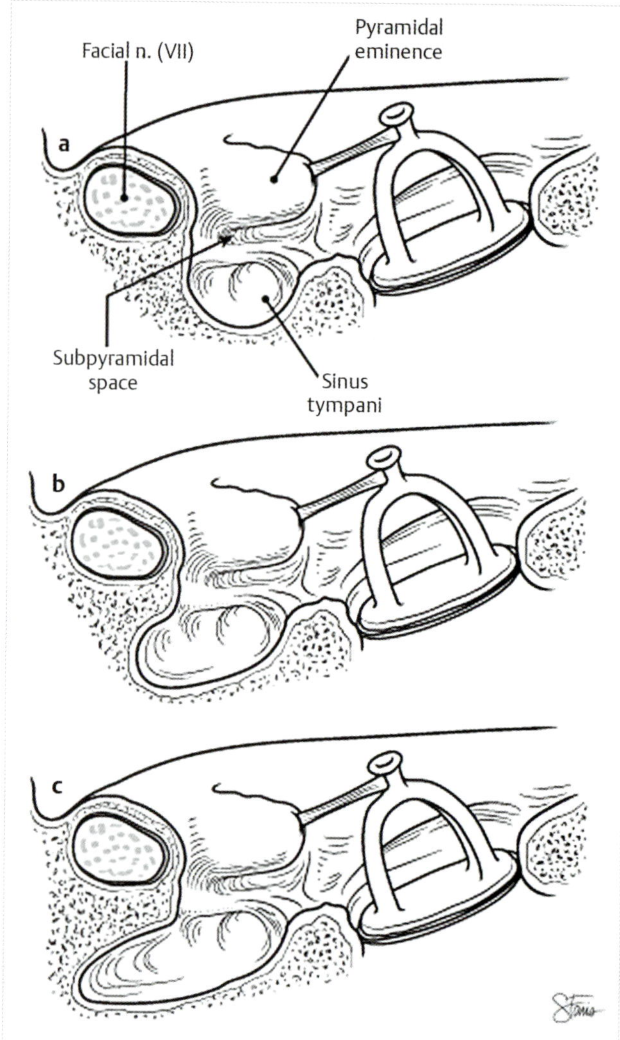

Fig. 44.3 Classification of the morphology of the sinus tympani based on depth. (a) Limited sinus tympani. (b) Deep sinus tympani with medial extension with respect to the facial nerve. (c) Deep sinus tympani with posterior extension with respect to the facial nerve.

Length

Traditional oto-endoscopes have been manufactured to a length of 6 cm. These endoscopes are very useful for the examination and photodocumentation of ears in the outpatient department but are of little use in EES. Using the endoscope as a surgical tool requires that the endoscope and camera head attached to the endoscope are as unobtrusive as possible. Short endoscopes cause the surgeon's hands to occupy the same area of the operative field, interfering with the endoscope and making it very difficult to direct the surgical instruments to the intended place when the endoscope is obstructing the trajectory of the instrument. For this reason, it is preferable to use an endoscope that is between 14 cm and 18 cm in length (▶ Fig. 44.5). This allows the endoscope to be further from the operative area than the hand that holds the instrument and, consequently, causes no difficulties with maneuverability.

Angles

Most EES is performed with a 0-degree endoscope. The wide field of view allows access to all but the most hidden areas on of the epitympanum and retrotympanum; indeed, the entire middle ear space of some ears can be completely inspected without the need to convert to an angled endoscope. If the anatomy of the patient dictates the need for an angled endoscope to achieve a suitable view of disease, the choice will be between a 30-degree, 45-degree, or, in rare circumstances, a 70-degree endoscope. The choice of angle is dependent on personal preference, but a good rule of thumb is that the smallest angle that produces a satisfactory view should be used. The 70-degree endoscope is particularly difficult to control in the middle ear and should be reserved for cases where extensive removal of disease has already taken place (▶ Fig. 44.6).

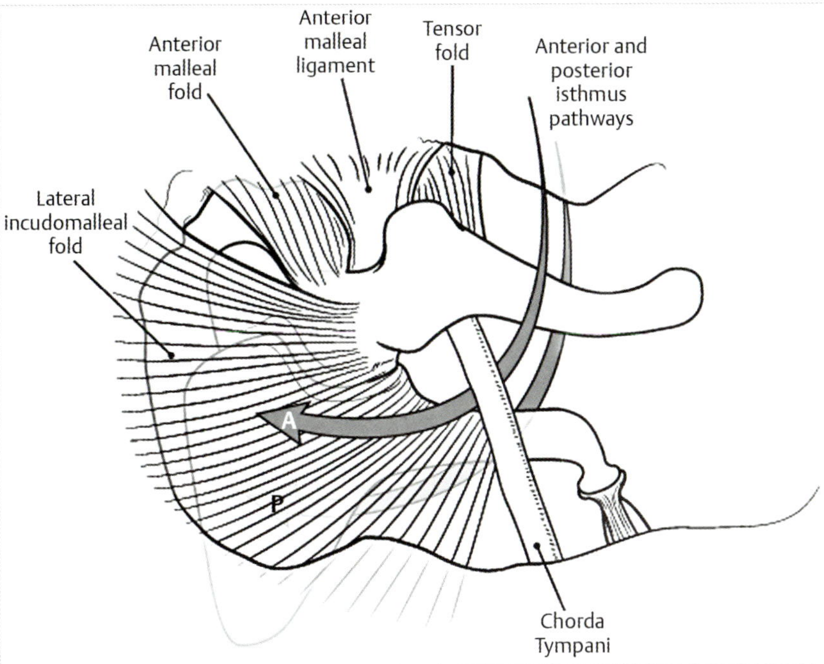

Fig. 44.4 Anterior and posterior tympanic isthmus. The anterior isthmus and posterior isthmus afford communication between the mesotympanum and the epitympanum.

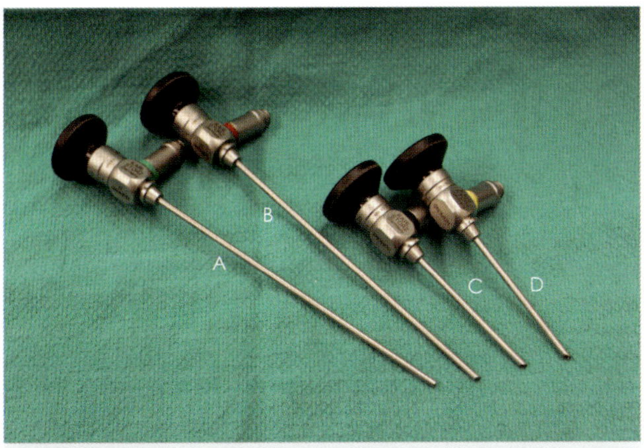

Fig. 44.5 Endoscope lengths. Traditionally, endoscopes designed for use in the ear have been short (~6 cm in length). Although these are valuable for examining the ear and for photodocumentation, the newer 14-cm endoscopes (a) and (b) are easier to use for surgical applications. The shorter endoscopes (c) and (d) are more difficult to use in combination with a surgical instrument.

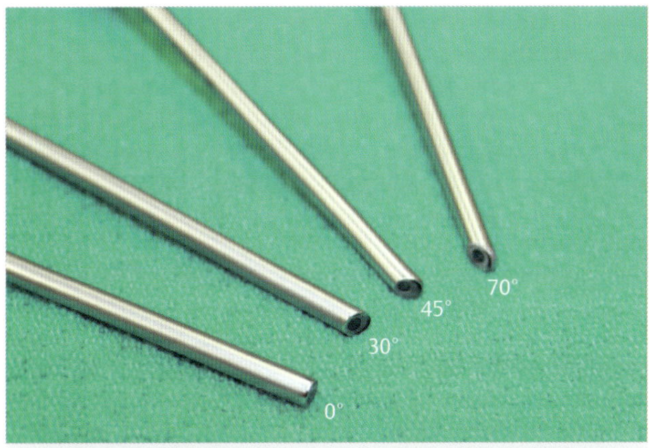

Fig. 44.6 Endoscope angles. Rigid endoscopes are commonly produced with angles of view of 0, 30, 45, and 70 degrees. The majority of EES is performed with a combination of 0- and 45-degree endoscopes. The range of angles is shown from smallest (0 degrees) on the left of the image to the largest (70 degrees) on the right.

44.5.2 Other Surgical Instruments

To take full advantage of the around-the-corner view of the endoscope, it is useful to have access to instruments with angled distal tips. The endoscope produces a field of view of approximately 70 degrees, even in the case of a 0-degree endoscope[20]; this field is of a similar breadth for endoscopes with angled lenses, but the direction of the center of this field is angled away from the midline. It is this property that allows for the narrow isthmus of the external auditory canal to be bypassed while maintaining the broad field of view of the mesotympanum.

When performing endoscopic surgery, it can be frustrating to use instruments designed to be used with a microscope and which are correspondingly designed to work in a line-of-sight fashion. Medical equipment manufacturers have been quick to meet the need of surgeons operating with an endoscope by developing suction cannulas and elevators designed to be used with the enhanced view provided by the endoscope (► Fig. 44.7a; ► Fig. 44.7b). The advantages of instruments that incorporate a suction component within a dissection instrument are of considerable use when dealing with areas that are bleeding (► Fig. 44.7c).

The use of the traditional high-speed otologic drill during EES presents some difficulties, including the accumulation of bone dust and the need for constant irrigation. It is often best for the surgical assistant to apply irrigation and suction while the primary surgeon performs the drilling. Although the use of drills in EES is common, it is usually easy to remove sufficient

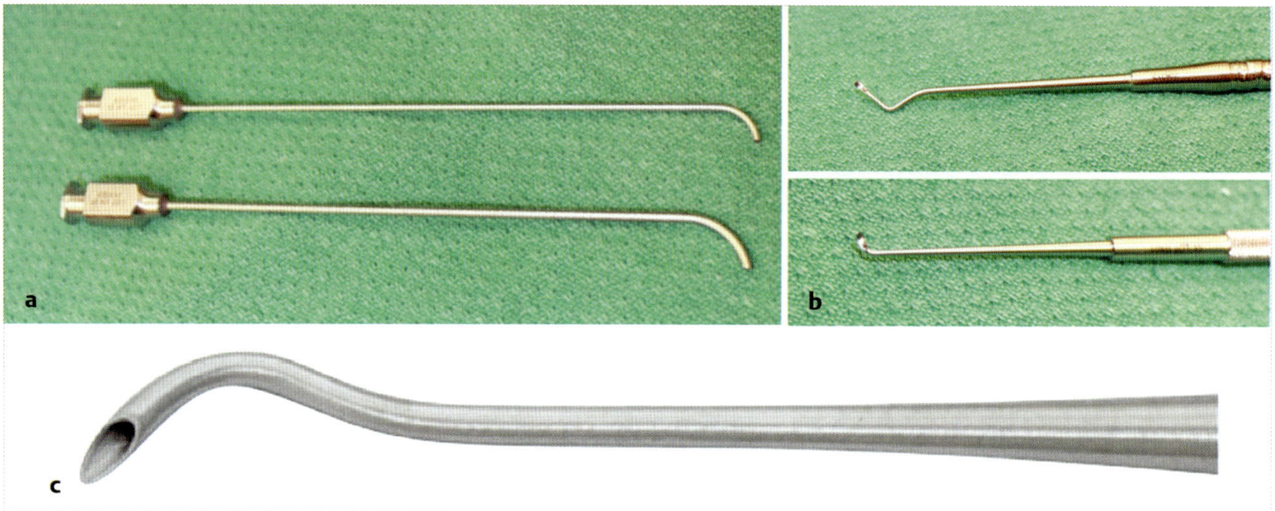

Fig. 44.7 Specialized instruments. (a) Suction cannulas have been modified with curved ends to facilitate access. (b) Curved dissectors are useful for improving access to anatomical areas that are not in direct view. Those with a double curve (above) are valuable in removing disease in the epitympanum, whereas those with a single curve (below) are particularly useful to access the sinus tympani and other structures of the retrotympanum. (c) Suction dissector.

bone in cases of limited disease with a standard middle ear bone curette. In cases of microscopic atticotomy, this would not be possible because the amount of bone that would need to be removed to gain sufficient line-of-sight access would be too large to make its removal with a curette a practical proposition. In the case of EES, however, the relatively small amount of bone removal required to fully address the mesotympanum and epitympanum is quite limited and can be removed with little difficulty using simple instruments.

If more bone needs to be removed in the case of more extensive disease, it may be necessary to preserve much of the scutum and use the microscope to perform a limited cortical mastoidectomy to remove what is left of the disease, following its endoscopic removal from the mesotympanum and epitympanum. If the surgeon chooses to continue an endoscopic dissection to the limit of the disease, this usually requires powered dissection of some kind.

The use of drills in EES has been mentioned, but many surgeons find that using bone dissection instruments that have no rotating parts to be easier to use alongside an endoscope. The technology of ultrasonic bone curettes has allowed the technique of EES to be of value without the need for mastoidectomy, even in cases of advanced disease. Kakehata et al[21] describe the indications for this type of bony dissection in a case series of 43 patients, some with extensive disease.

44.6 Surgical Technique

44.6.1 Tympanoplasty

Tympanoplasty can be performed endoscopically using any of the established techniques. Most commonly an underlay technique is favored owing to the relatively straightforward steps and the rapid healing in the postoperative period. EES has its major advantages in the pursuit of cholesteatoma, but it also has important advantages in tympanoplasty owing to the ability to be able to see the entire annulus in a single view and, as a result, being able to address perforations that are situated primarily in the anterior-inferior segment of the tympanic membrane (▶ Fig. 44.8). A common problem encountered during tympanoplasty is the inability to gain access to the anterior recess owing to a large anterior prominence of the ear canal; this is easily bypassed with an endoscope, even one without an angled lens. Employing a 30-degree endoscope will be sufficient to provide a clear view of any perforation.

In cases of large or subtotal perforations, a lateral graft tympanoplasty can be used to allow the anterior prominence to be lowered with a bone curette or bone drill. Although this is seldom required, the security of a firm base on which to lay the graft, in the form of the fibrous remnant of the tympanic membrane, can be of value.

One technique that lends itself to an endoscopic approach is the cartilage butterfly tympanoplasty,[22] in which a disc of cartilage is fashioned to a size slightly larger than the perforation, with a shallow groove running along its edge; this is inserted into the perforation with one of the resulting flanges of cartilage medial to the tympanic membrane and one lateral to it. The tympanic membrane heals around the graft, with the cartilage taking a fusiform shape after 4 to 6 weeks (▶ Fig. 44.9).

The interlay tympanoplasty is a combination of the underlay and the lateral graft technique and is also uniquely suited to TEES. A standard tympanomeatal flap is raised, but the middle ear is not entered at the level of the fibrous annulus; instead, the squamous layer is separated off the fibrous layer of the tympanic membrane. This plane is then extended around the perforation. The squamous layer is not elevated past the anterior annulus to reduce the risk of anterior blunting of the canal. A graft, usually perichondrium from the tragus, is placed over the perforation on top of the fibrous layer. The squamous layer is then replaced along with the ear canal skin (▶ Fig. 44.10).

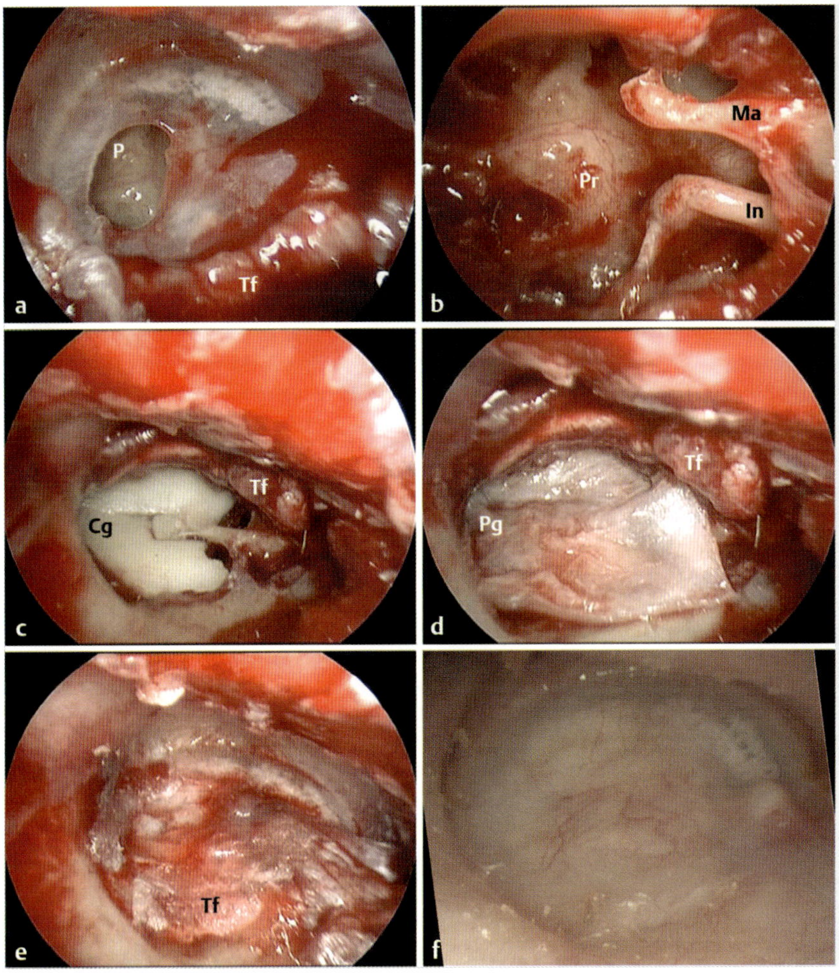

Fig. 44.8 Lateral to malleus underlay endoscopic tympanoplasty. (a) Left ear with anterior-inferior central tympanic membrane perforation (p). The tympanomeatal flap (Tf) is raised off the bone of the posterior canal wall to the level of the annulus, that is elevated to gain access to the middle ear. (b) The tympanic membrane is completely elevated off the malleus (Ma) to gain access to the anterior portion of the tympanic cavity. (c) After the ventilation pathways are opened, a cartilage graft (Cg) is placed to reconstruct the drum, followed by (d) a perichondrium graft (Pg). (e) The tympanomeatal flap is then returned to its original position. (f) Three-month postoperative result. P, perforation; Tf, tympanomeatal flap; Pr, promontory; Ma, malleus; In, incus; Cg, cartilage graft; Pg, perichondrium graft.

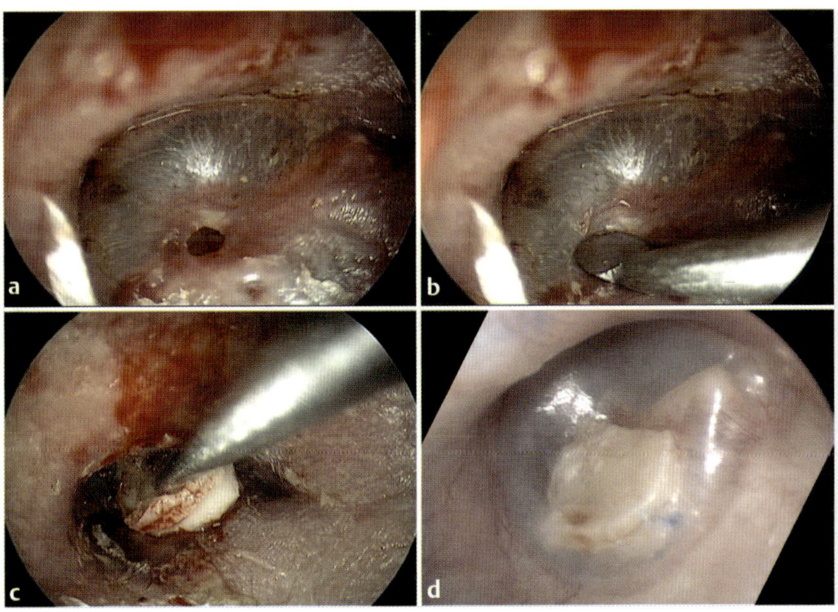

Fig. 44.9 Butterfly endoscopic tympanoplasty. (a) Left ear with small central perforation. (b) The squamous layer of the tympanic membrane is elevated from the fibrous layer, 3 mm away from the center of the perforation toward the periphery. (c) A composite cartilage graft with perichondrium on each side, measuring 2 mm larger in diameter than the perforation, is snapped in the perforation. Notice the shallow groove along the center of the graft that allows the edges of the graft to spread, similar to a pressure equalizing tube. (d). Three-month postoperative result.

44.6.2 Cholesteatoma Dissection

The greatest value of EES lies in the management of cholesteatoma. The ability to examine all areas of the mesotympanum, particularly the areas where cholesteatoma develops initially, allows the surgeon to undertake a disease-pursuant approach and be sure of direct removal of disease. The transcanal approach involves a front-to-back dissection of the cholesteatoma sac, concentrating on exposing the limits of the disease with the stepwise removal of bone, usually in the area of the scutum.

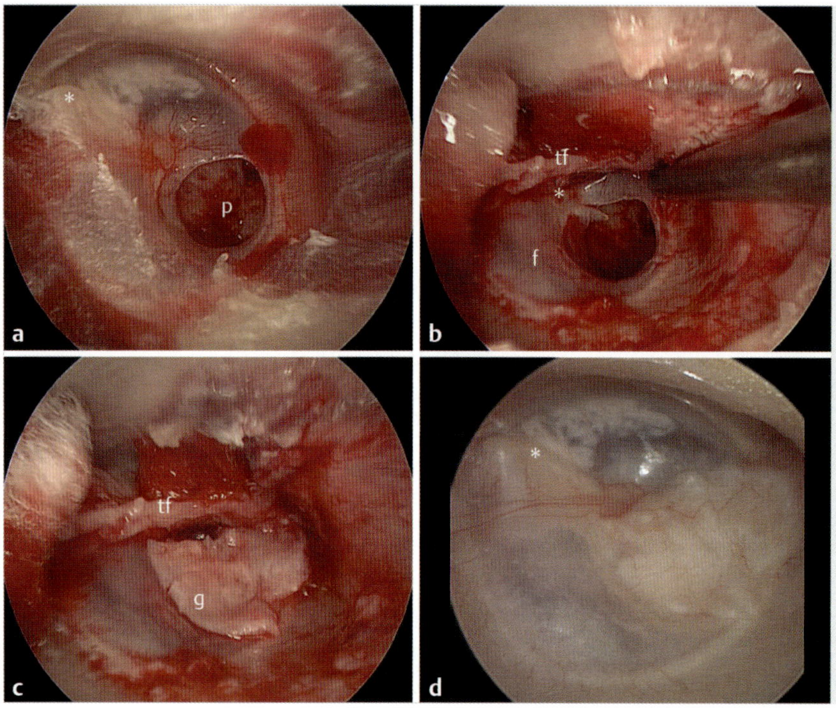

Fig. 44.10 Interlay endoscopic tympanoplasty. (a) Right ear with posterior-inferior tympanic membrane perforation (p). (b) The tympanomeatal flap (tf) is raised off the bone of the posterior canal wall to the level of the fibrous annulus. The squamous layer of the tympanic membrane is elevated from the fibrous layer (f). The squamous layer is elevated around the entire margin of the perforation and the malleus (*) as needed. (c) Graft material is used. In this case a composite cartilage/perichondrium graft (g) was inserted between the layers. The squamous layer will subsequently be returned to its original position along with the tympanomeatal flap. (d) Six-month postoperative result. Notice the composite graft healed in the posterior-inferior quadrant. p, perforation; (*), malleus; tf, tympanomeatal flap; f, fibrous layer of the tympanic membrane; g, cartilage/perichondrium composite graft.

Owing to the one-handed nature of EES, the need to control bleeding is of major importance. Most surgeons take great care in the preparation of the patient prior to commencing surgery. A good working relationship with the anesthesiologist is essential for controlling blood pressure and heart rate. Hypotensive anesthesia accompanied by a reverse Trendelenburg position will reduce the need for suctioning the ear to clear accumulated blood. Of equal importance is the careful preparation of the ear itself, with a mixture of local anesthetic and epinephrine, usually at a concentration of 1:100 000. It may be useful to prepare the area of the postauricular or endaural incision in case the need to open the ear arises. It is also useful to infiltrate the tragus at this early stage to allow a bloodless dissection when harvesting graft material. When taking the tragal graft it is important to leave a rim of cartilage (usually ~3 mm) on the lateral edge to prevent cosmetic and functional deformities of the tragus.[23]

Once the canal has been cleaned and inspected, the canal itself is infiltrated, with care being taken to ensure that the entire canal is blanched all the way to the annulus.

The tympanomeatal flap can be positioned in any configuration required to provide adequate access to the middle ear; the endoscope affords a view of the entire canal, so it is only necessary to raise the flap from the posterior canal wall. The elevation of the tympanomeatal flap often offers the most difficulty for surgeons just learning the technique of TEES; the judicious use of epinephrine-soaked cottonoids to assist with the elevation of the flap and the use of saline irrigation of the operative field will reduce bleeding considerably. Packing the flap against the tympanic membrane once it has been reflected anteriorly will tamponade the bleeding and the surgery thereafter will be essentially bloodless in most cases.

The cholesteatoma is then pursued until its furthest extent is reached. If this is beyond the limit of easy endoscopic dissection, it may be sensible to convert to a combined technique, using the microscope to remove the residual cholesteatoma sac from the mastoid antrum after the middle ear has been cleared of disease using the endoscope. Debate continues regarding the point at which this decision to use a combined open approach should be made, but the general principle is that the scutum should be taken down only to the point where it can be repaired. This is usually performed with a composite tragal cartilage/perichondium graft. Where there is involvement of the ossicles in disease but the ossicular chain remains intact, there is some evidence that the use of a transcanal endoscopic approach may reduce the need to remove the ossicles to ensure confident clearance of disease (▶ Fig. 44.11).[24]

Following disease extirpation and reconstruction of the bony defect, the ear canal can be packed with absorbable dressings or removable dressings inserted under direct vision using the endoscope. No head bandage is necessary unless an open approach has also been used, in which case the use of a head bandage is a personal preference.

44.7 Postoperative Care

The postoperative care of a patient who has undergone EES differs from traditional ear surgery from the time that the ear canal is packed. In all cases of open ear surgery, the skin of the ear canal lateral to the tympanomeatal flap is raised off the underlying bone along with the cartilaginous portion of the ear canal. During the postauricular approach this takes place when the pinna is reflected anteriorly and held in position by a self-retaining retractor, with or without a length of ribbon gauze placed through the canal. During an endaural approach, this skin is retracted posteriorly as the cartilaginous ring is widened to provide access to the bony canal. In the case of EES, this skin never leaves the canal, reducing morbidity and the chance of epithelial inclusion cysts.

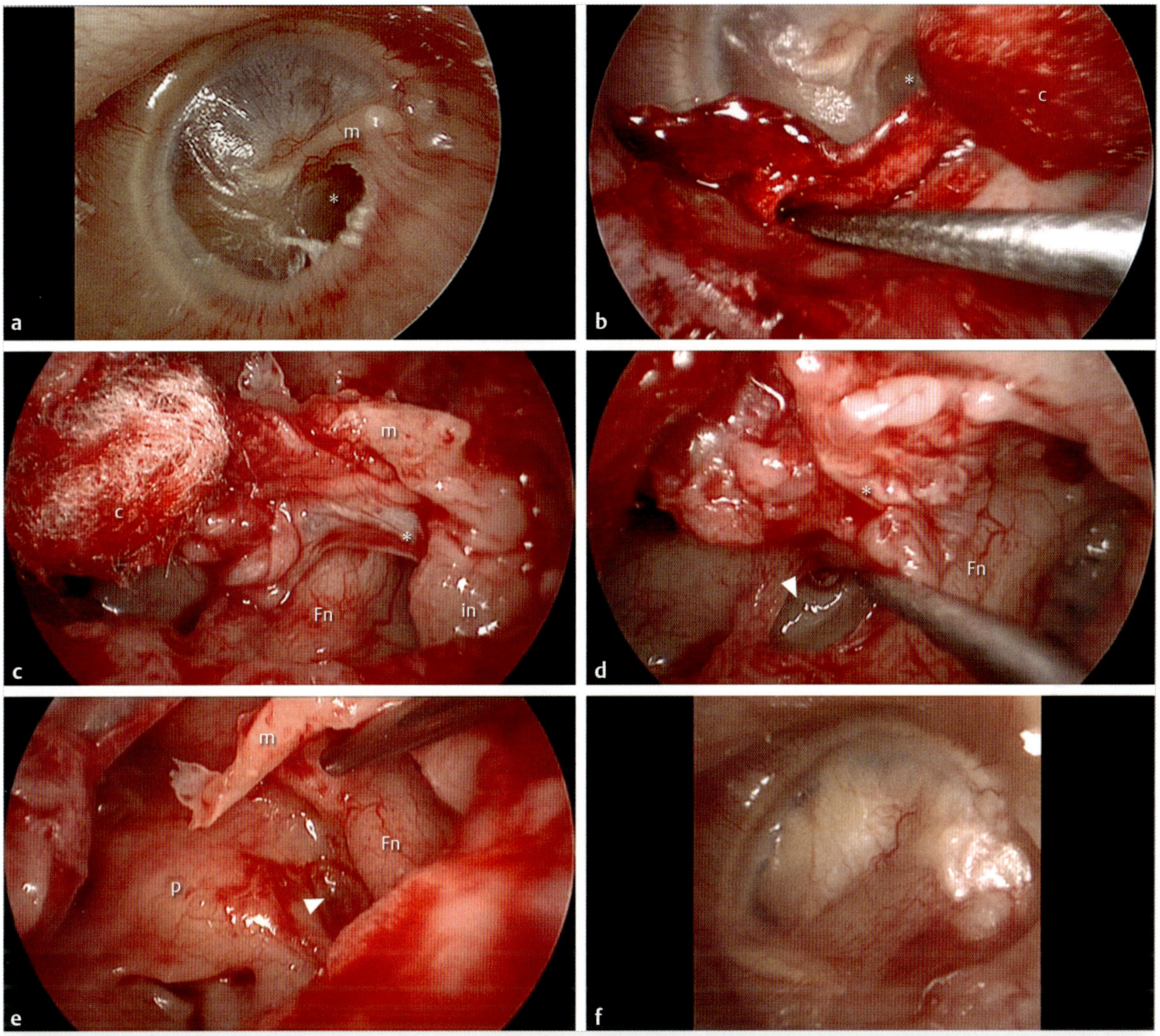

Fig. 44.11 Transcanal endoscopic cholesteatoma removal. (a) Left ear with posterior epitympanic cholesteatoma. Notice the cholesteatoma (*) eroding the scutum. (b) The tympanomeatal flap is raised off the bone of the posterior canal wall to the level of the annulus, that is elevated to gain access to the middle ear. Dissection is carried out using cotton balls (c) with epinephrine to control bleeding. (c) The tympanic membrane is completely elevated off the malleus (m), and the cholesteatoma (*) is isolated and dissected away from a dehiscent facial nerve (Fn) and the ossicles. Note how the cholesteatoma is elevated in one piece, even from the undersurface of the malleus (m) and eroded incus (in). (d) The cholesteatoma is elevated away from the stapes footplate (arrow) using a small round dissector. (e) Tympanic cavity after complete resection of the cholesteatoma. Note the partial erosion of the stapes footplate (arrow), evidenced by its bluelined surface. (f) Nine-month postoperative result. (*), cholesteatoma; m, malleus; c, cotton ball; in, incus with erosion of the long process; Fn, dehiscent facial nerve; arrow, stapes footplate; p, promontory.

Simple analgesia is usually sufficient for most patients during the postoperative period as very little soft tissue trauma has taken place and healing is usually rapid. Practice varies regarding follow-up, but most surgeons will remove the ear canal dressing 1–2 weeks postoperatively.

44.8 Complications and Pitfalls

44.8.1 Barriers to the Technique

EES is technically demanding and requires experience in the use of an endoscope prior to commencing any surgery. It has been noted that there seems to be a strong correlation between levels of experience with nasal endoscopic surgery and the ability to comfortably introduce EES into practice. For otologists who have been subspecialized for some time and who have not been trained in any endoscopic technique, the adoption of EES, perhaps one of the most technically challenging forms of endoscopic surgery, will be very difficult indeed. This is not to say that this is not possible for certain surgeons; the learning curve will vary considerably from surgeon to surgeon. The ability to interpret three-dimensional anatomy from a two-dimensional image comes naturally to some, yet others find this more difficult. Again, experience with endoscopy in other areas is helpful.

Learning to operate with one hand may not come naturally to many surgeons even though current otologic practice often demands a one-handed approach; for example, stapes surgery and transcanal microscopic myringoplasty are often performed in this way. It is interesting to note that neither of these techniques involves injury to soft tissue or extensive drilling of bone and, thus, like EES, are not associated with much bleeding.

44.8.2 Morbidity

EES is not without morbidity, but the profile of potential complications is inherently no different than what would be expected for traditional microsurgery; the tympanomeatal flap, removal of bone, and surgery within the middle ear space all contribute to postoperative pain, but the judicious use of tragal cartilage/perichondrium as a graft material all reduce the soft tissue injury usually inherent in ear surgery. Care should be taken, however, to maintain an anterior rim of tragal cartilage to avoid any cosmetic or functional complications.[13]

44.9 Outcomes

The exclusive use of the endoscope as a tool for the removal of cholesteatoma has only been studied intensively in the last few years. The wealth of data on the rates of residual and recurrent disease that are plentiful for microscopic approaches are not yet widely available for EES. Despite this, there are a number of publications that strongly suggest that rates of residual disease are likely to be substantially lower than cases where a microscope is used alone.

Both Badr-El-Dine[25] and Ayache[26] published studies where standard microscopic procedures were undertaken to remove cholesteatoma; at the point of completion, endoscopes were introduced and the surgical field reexamined. Both studies showed a high rate of residual disease that had been missed during extensive microscopic clearance. These findings suggest that rates of residual disease can be expected to be lower in cases where the endoscope has been employed. Tarabichi,[8] Marchioni,[11] and Migirov[9] have all reported series of patients undergoing EES, with rates of residual disease comparable to or below those published for series where the microscope was used in isolation.

44.10 Conclusion

The idea of using the endoscope in the ear has been around for some time; the work by Thomassin using early oto-endoscopes to assist with microscopic procedures opened the way for surgeons such as Tarabichi to take the advantages of endoscopes to their natural conclusion and develop the field of TEES. This field will still be very much under development for some time when compared with how long the microscope has been the mainstay of otologic surgery. The technology must now catch up with the technique. The popularity of EES has risen exponentially in recent years, reflecting the interest that modern otologists have in improving surgical exposure, respecting the anatomy and physiology of the ear, and tackling disease without causing unnecessary harm to the patient.

References

[1] Thomassin JM, Korchia D, Doris JM. Endoscopic-guided otosurgery in the prevention of residual cholesteatomas. Laryngoscope. 1993;103(8):939–943.

[2] McKennan KX. Endoscopic "second look" mastoidoscopy to rule out residual epitympanic/mastoid cholesteatoma. Laryngoscope. 1993;103(7):810–814.

[3] Nomura Y. Effective photography in otolaryngology-head and neck surgery: endoscopic photography of the middle ear. Otolaryngol Head Neck Surg. 1982;90(4):395–398.

[4] Poe DS, Rebeiz EE, Pankratov MM. Evaluation of perilymphatic fistulas by middle ear endoscopy. Am J Otol. 1992;13(6):529–533.

[5] Takahashi H, Honjo I, Fujita A, Kurata K. Transtympanic endoscopic findings in patients with otitis media with effusion. Arch Otolaryngol Head Neck Surg. 1990;116(10):1186–1189.

[6] Tarabichi M. Endoscopic management of acquired cholesteatoma. Am J Otol. 1997;18(5):544–549.

[7] Tarabichi M. Endoscopic middle ear surgery. Ann Otol Rhinol Laryngol. 1999;108(1):39–46.

[8] Tarabichi M. Endoscopic management of cholesteatoma: Long-term results. Otolaryngol Head Neck Surg. 2000;122(6):874–881.

[9] Migirov L, Shapira Y, Horowitz Z, Wolf M. Exclusive EES for acquired cholesteatoma: Preliminary results. Otol Neurotol. 2011;32(3):433–436.

[10] Presutti L, Marchioni D, Mattioli F, Villari D, Alicandri-Ciufelli M. Endoscopic management of acquired cholesteatoma: Our experience. J Otolaryngol Head Neck Surg. 2008;37(4):481–487.

[11] Marchioni D, Villari D, Mattioli F, Alicandri-Ciufelli M, Piccinini A, Presutti L. Endoscopic management of attic cholesteatoma: A single-institution experience. Otolaryngol Clin North Am. 2013;46(2):201–209.

[12] Yung MW. The use of middle ear endoscopy: *has residual cholesteatoma been eliminated? J Laryngol Otol. 2001;115(12):958–961.

[13] Marchioni D, Mattioli F, Alicandri-Ciufelli M, Presutti L. Transcanal endoscopic approach to the sinus tympani: Aclinical report. Otol Neurotol. 2009;30 (6):758–765.

[14] Aimi K. The tympanic isthmus: Its anatomy and clinical significance. Laryngoscope. 1978;88(7 Pt 1):1067–1081.

[15] Marchioni D, Alicandri-Ciufelli M, Molteni G, Artioli FL, Genovese E, Presutti L. Selective epitympanic dysventilation syndrome. Laryngoscope. 2010;120 (5):1028–1033.

[16] Marchioni D, Mattioli F, Alicandri-Ciufelli M, Molteni G, Masoni F, Presutti L. Endoscopic evaluation of middle ear ventilation route blockage. Am J Otolaryngol. 2010;31(6):453–466.

[17] Marchioni D, Piccinini A, Alicandri-Ciufelli M, Presutti L. Endoscopic anatomy and ventilation of the epitympanum. Otolaryngol Clin North Am. 2013;46 (2):165–178.

[18] Marchioni D, Grammatica A, Alicandri-Ciufelli M, Aggazzotti-Cavazza E, Genovese E, Presutti L. The contribution of selective dysventilation to attical middle ear pathology. Med Hypotheses. 2011;77(1):116–120.

[19] Marchioni D, Mattioli F, Alicandri-Ciufelli M, Presutti L. Endoscopic approach to tensor fold in patients with attic cholesteatoma. Acta Otolaryngol. 2009;129(9):946–954.

[20] Van Gompel JJ, Tabor MH, Youssef AS, et al. Field of view comparison between two-dimensional and three-dimensional endoscopy. Laryngoscope. 2014 Feb;124(2):387–90.

[21] Kinney SE. Five years experience using the intact canal wall tympanoplasty with mastoidectomy for cholesteatoma: Preliminary report. Laryngoscope. 1982;92(12):1395–1400.

[22] Eavey RD. Inlay tympanoplasty: Cartilage butterfly technique. Laryngoscope. 1998;108(5):657–661.

[23] Pothier DD, Charaklias N. Tragal cartilage harvesting and "in the ear" earphones: A pilot study. J Laryngol Otol. 2006;120(9):1–3.

[24] Marchioni D, Alicandri-Ciufelli M, Molteni G, Villari D, Monzani D, Presutti L. Ossicular chain preservation after exclusive endoscopic transcanal tympanoplasty: Preliminary experience. Otol Neurotol. 2011;32(4):626–631.

[25] Badr-el-Dine M. Value of ear endoscopy in cholesteatoma surgery. Otol Neurotol. 2002;23(5):631–635.

[26] Ayache S, Tramier B, Strunski V. Otoendoscopy in cholesteatoma surgery of the middle ear: What benefits can be expected? Otol Neurotol. 2008;29 (8):1085–1090.

45 Eustachian Tuboplasty

Ilkka Kivekäs, Juha Silvola, and Dennis S. Poe

Abbreviations used in this chapter:

CT: computed tomography
ICA: internal carotid artery
LVP: levator veli palatini
TVP: tensor veli palatini

45.1 Introduction

The Eustachian tube in humans is a complex and dynamic organ with a small, but proportionately long, lumen and relatively weak muscles of dilation, all of which make it commonly prone to dysfunction.[1] It is believed that the principal function of the Eustachian tube is to provide for adequate ventilation of the middle ear, but it is also recognized for its role in clearing secretions from the middle ear with its mucociliary flow and, when closed, for protecting against reflux of material and sound from the nasopharynx.[1]

Eustachian tube dysfunction is believed to be chiefly due to inadequate opening of the lumen. Failure of adequate tubal dilation is known to be associated with chronic negative middle ear pressure, difficulties with equalization of middle ear pressure, and otitis media with effusion. Over time, complications of tympanic membrane retraction may occur, including adhesive otitis media, cholesteatoma, and tympanic membrane perforation. These diseases affect roughly 1% to 3% of the population.[2]

The rates of developing pressure changes within the middle ear in the absence of a patent Eustachian tube have been recently measured in humans. Three healthy volunteers who avoided swallowing or yawning for up to 2 hours demonstrated steadily decreasing pressures down to 150 daPa on successive tympanometry measurements.[3] Eleven patients undergoing parotidectomy who volunteered to have a catheter placed into the mastoid for 24 hours demonstrated similar rates of progressively negative middle ear pressure over time although three subjects showed increasing pressure from an initially negative baseline. The reasons for rising pressure within the middle ear space remain uncertain and under investigation.[4]

Assumptions have been made in the past that Eustachian tube function may be limited by its narrowest static lumen, which, although occurring in the cartilaginous portion just adjacent to the bony-cartilaginous junction, has been previously thought to be within the osseus portion.[5] Surgical procedures intended to improve its dilatory function have been attempted since the 18th century,[6] focusing on widening the osseous portion of the Eustachian tube using approaches from the middle ear, preauricular region, and even by middle fossa craniotomy. Poor long-term results (even with stenting) and life-threatening complications led to abandonment of these approaches. In the past three decades, submillimeter and slow-motion endoscopic evaluations of the Eustachian tube have demonstrated an association between Eustachian tube dysfunction and pathology affecting the dynamic dilatory process within its cartilaginous portion. Disorders involving the nasopharyngeal orifice of the Eustachian tube and the area in which the mucosal surfaces are in approximation at rest, termed the functional valve, are now believed to be the principal source of Eustachian tube dilatory dysfunction.[7]

Mucosal disease, with edema and other inflammatory changes within the cartilaginous Eustachian tube, is thought to be the most common cause for dilatory dysfunction. The source of the inflammation remains uncertain, but associations have been made with adenoid hypertrophy, reflux, allergic rhinitis, and chronic rhinosinusitis.[6,8] A mechanism for adenoid hypertrophy causing functional obstruction has been observed in which the swollen inflamed torus tubarius becomes compressed between the enlarged adenoid and the lateral pharyngeal wall during swallowing, thrusting it anteriorly to cover the tubal orifice at the time that it should be dilating.[9] Disorders of the muscles, such as limited movements of the tensor veli palatini (TVP), early relaxation of the levator veli palatini (LVP), or lack of coordination between the two, have been observed. The LVP is the first to contract during swallows or yawns and it medially rotates the torus tubarius, holding it in position as a scaffold against which the relatively weak final dilator of the Eustachian tube, the TVP, then contracts. Lastly, benign or malignant tumors of the nasopharynx should be considered in cases of Eustachian tube dysfunction, especially in adults with unilateral middle ear effusion.

Chronic Eustachian tube dysfunction, despite maximal efforts to control possible underlying etiologies, may imply that the mucosa has become irreversibly injured. The reasons for the persistent disease remain uncertain. Bacterial biofilms have been identified in the middle ear and adenoid of patients with middle ear effusions, and these may play some role in mucosal disease within the Eustachian tube.[10,11]

Patients in whom medical therapy failed are commonly offered tympanostomy tubes or adenoidectomy, but a substantial number fail to improve after extrusion of one or more tubes. Although tympanostomy tubes are known to be effective in relieving negative middle ear pressure, non-adherent tympanic membrane retraction, effusion, atelectasis, or other symptomatic Eustachian tube dysfunction, tube insertion does not treat the underlying problem. In addition, tympanostomy tube insertion carries some risk of complications, including otorrhea and recurrent infections (10 to 26%), tympanic membrane perforation (2%), and cholesteatoma (1%).[12] Adenoidectomy may provide significant relief for children with otitis media with effusion associated with adenoid hypertrophy, especially if the adenoid is in contact with the torus tubarius.[13] Endoscopic-assisted adenoidectomy permits careful but more complete removal of the tissue in contact with the torus tubarius and allows for light cauterization of the "cobblestoned" hyperplastic mucosa that may also involve the torus.

Eustachian tuboplasty has received increasing attention as a safe and potentially effective surgical option for patients with Eustachian tube dilatory dysfunction. This chapter discusses the three surgical options to restore Eustachian tube dilatory function: laser-assisted tuboplasty, microdebrider (powered-shaver) tuboplasty, and balloon dilation tuboplasty.

45.2 Patient Selection

Patients who have failed maximal medical therapy and conventional surgical treatment, if appropriate, may be candidates for Eustachian tuboplasty. Patients may typically have persistent otitis media with effusion despite having had one or more tympanostomy tubes; recalcitrant non-adherent tympanic membrane retraction; troublesome or symptomatic negative pressure within the middle ear (documented on a tympanogram); or difficulties with pressure equalization during flights, scuba diving, or with other rapid changes in altitude. These patients usually have associated subjective symptoms, such as a sensation of ear pressure, otalgia, or conductive hearing loss.

Caution is needed for patients whose only complaint is a sensation of ear pressure or fullness, despite having normal tympanometry; the absence of objective ear pathology; or failure to improve with a tube. In such cases, the underlying problem is something other than Eustachian tube dilatory dysfunction and further evaluation is indicated. The most common differential diagnosis is temporomandibular joint disorder with associated musculoskeletal effects. It is noteworthy that the medial pterygoid muscle, which is immediately adjacent to the TVP muscle, may cause discomfort that radiates to the ear and Eustachian tube. Furthermore, a patulous Eustachian tube, Minor's third labyrinthine window syndrome, semicircular canal dehiscence syndrome, and endolymphatic hydrops need to be considered in the differential diagnosis.

The authors have not selected younger children for Eustachian tuboplasty because it remains unknown whether reflux of pathogens is an important cause of acute otitis media and at what age they may outgrow the tendency to reflux. Eustachian tuboplasty may be indicated in adults with recurrent acute otitis media if there is significant evidence for mucosal inflammation or other compromise around the tubal orifice and valve area.

When performing tympanoplasty in patients highly suspected for Eustachian tube dilatory dysfunction, a tympanostomy tube is sometimes placed during the primary procedure. Alternatively, a Eustachian tuboplasty may be performed 4 to 6 weeks in advance or might be combined with the tympanoplasty procedure. There is some evidence that Eustachian tuboplasty with balloon dilation may take 4 to 8 weeks postoperatively to reach an optimal benefit.[14]

45.3 Preoperative Examination

A comprehensive history and physical examination are important in the evaluation of Eustachian tube dysfunction. Patients should be questioned about inflammatory disorders, such as allergies, chronic rhinosinusitits, laryngopharyngeal reflux, or vasomotor rhinitis. Tobacco use or smoke exposure also negatively affects mucociliary clearance.

Typically, the tympanic membrane appears abnormal and there may also be middle ear effusion. Tympanometry findings include type B or C curves, unless the patient's complaints are limited to air travel, scuba diving, or driving through mountains. A thorough endoscopic-assisted examination, assessing the nasal mucosa, nasopharynx, pharynx, larynx, hypopharynx, and subglottic space for signs of inflammation or underlying allergy, as well as granulomatous, laryngopharyngeal reflux, or other diseases, should be performed in addition to evaluating the Eustachian tube in detail.

The Eustachian tube orifice can be readily identified just posterior to the inferior turbinate by the prominence of the torus tubarius, also known as the posterior cushion. It is important to differentiate between the tubal orifice and the fossa of Rosenmüller just posterior to the torus tubarius. An important surgical landmark is where the internal carotid artery (ICA) courses just deep to the apex of the fossa; in some cases it may be located immediately under the mucosa.[15] The condition of the Eustachian tube mucosa and the function of the peritubal muscles should be evaluated. To best inspect the tubal valve during swallowing and yawning, the endoscope should be directed down the longitudinal axis of the lumen, which courses approximately 45 degrees laterally and superiorly from the floor of the nasal cavity (▶ Fig. 45.1). Optimal views can be obtained by angling a fiberoptic endoscope, sometimes even by passing it through the contralateral nares and behind the vomer, or by passing a 30- or 45-degree angled rigid endoscope through the ipsilateral nasal cavity.

Preoperative high-resolution, non-contrasted computed tomography (CT) imaging, including temporal bone and nasopharynx CT imaging, is currently recommended before proceeding with balloon dilation. This test helps to exclude other possible pathologies that may compromise Eustachian tube function, including nasal and sinus diseases, middle ear disease,

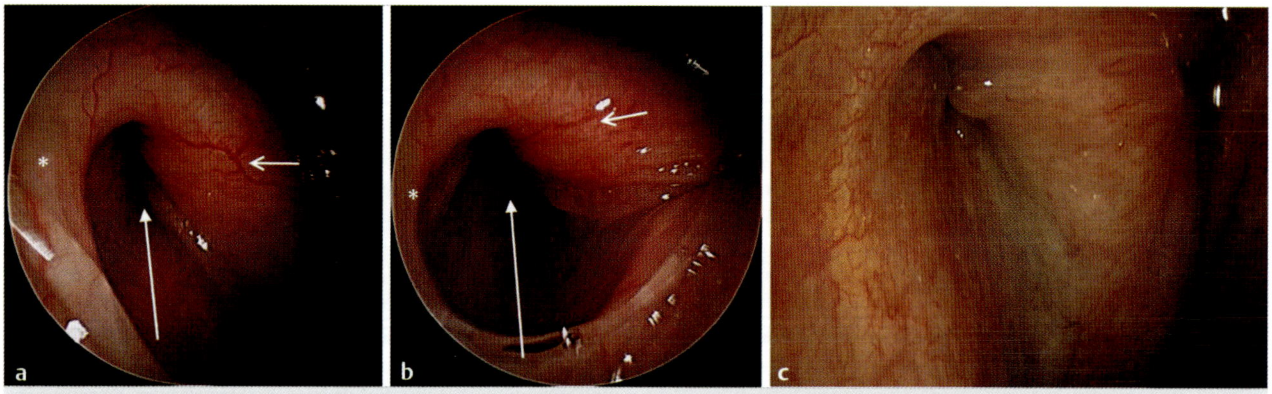

Fig. 45.1 (a) Normal Eustachian tube in resting position. An asterisk is on the lateral cushion, a short arrow is on the medial cushion, and a longer arrow points to the lumen. (b) Normal Eustachian tube in its maximal opening. An asterisk is on the lateral cushion, a short arrow is on the medial cushion, and a longer arrow points to the lumen. (c) Swollen Eustachian tube mucosa with small polyps in the lumen.

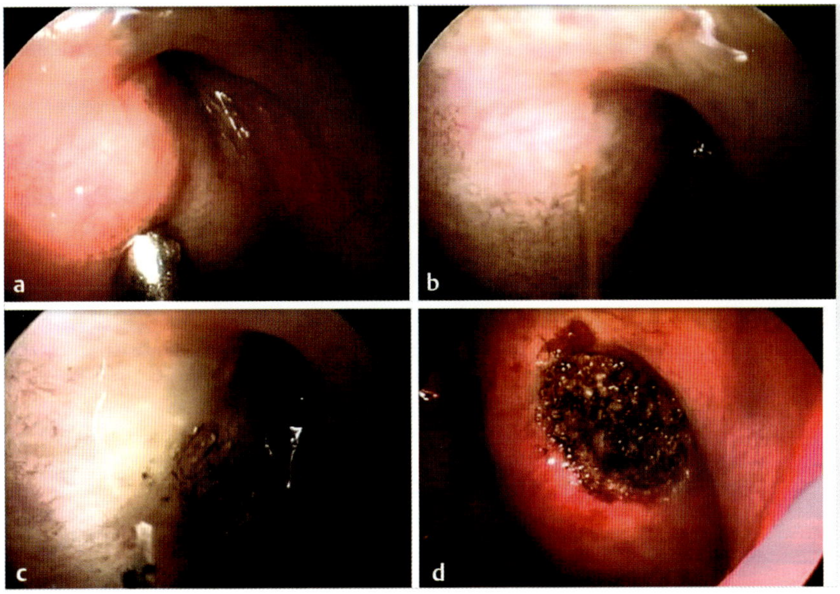

Fig. 45.2 Laser-assisted tuboplasty. (a) The suction is pushing the medial cushion and allows a better view to the valve area of the Eustachian tube. (b) Mucosa of the medial cushion is cauterized with a laser tip. (c) In most cases, only the top layer of mucosa is cauterized, but in more severe Eustachian tube dysfunction, the deeper layer of the mucosa is also cauterized. (d) The Eustachian tube after a laser-assisted approach.

and nasopharyngeal tumors. Additionally, the position of the internal carotid canal should be assessed for any possibilities of an aberrant course that may bring it into proximity with the cartilaginous Eustachian tube. The distance between the Eustachian tube and the ICA is lowest at the osseous portion of the Eustachian tube, where the artery can even be dehiscent into the lumen. The distance between the nasopharyngeal orifice of the Eustachian tube and ICA is an average of 23 mm, but, in certain cases, it may be as little as 10 mm with an aberrant ICA.[15] Presently, balloon dilation is not being performed in patients with significant dehiscence of the ICA into the bony Eustachian tube, even though the balloon catheter should theoretically be introduced only into the cartilaginous portion.

45.4 Surgical Technique

Currently, there are three commonly used surgical approaches to restore Eustachian tube dilatory function: laser-assisted tuboplasty, microdebrider (powered-shaver) tuboplasty, and balloon dilation tuboplasty. Any of these procedures can be combined with sinonasal surgery (e.g., septoplasty, inferior turbinectomy, adenoidectomy) for treatment of disease or for access.

45.4.1 Laser-Assisted Eustachian Tuboplasty

This procedure is based on the hypotheses that dilation of the lumen by surgical debulking may facilitate the dilatory function of the TVP muscle and that removal of irreversibly thickened mucosa may allow it to regrow in a healthier and thinner state.

The surgery may be performed with local or general anesthesia. Nasal vasoconstriction is carried out with a topical decongestant spray, and submucosal injection of lidocaine with epinephrine is performed along the luminal surface of the torus tubarius. The Eustachian tube orifice can be viewed with a 30- or 45-degree 4-mm diameter endoscope, and the operation performed while watching a surgical video monitor.

Different kinds of lasers have been used with similar success rates, including diode, waveguide-delivered CO_2, KTP, and argon lasers. The surgeon should choose the laser with which he or she is familiar. A few examples of laser setups are as follows: a 980-nm contact tip diode laser with power settings of 7 W, continuous pulse mode with 0.2 seconds on and 0.08 seconds off; an argon ion laser with power settings of 3 W, continuous mode; or a CO_2 laser with power settings of 12 W with a 0.05-second pulse.

Kujawski introduced the laser cauterization of inflamed mucosa and submucosa along the luminal side of the posterior-medial wall, where the inflammatory disease is typically most prominent.[8] Cauterization begins from the leading edge of the torus tubarius and continues up to the valve region, and, in cases with disease extending well into the valve, submucosal ablation of the valve region may be done. If a patient is under general anesthesia, distending forceps may be used to achieve a better view and gain better access to the valve region. Cartilage is exposed; if a prominent cartilaginous bulge compromises the lumen, it can be removed by sharp dissection via laser vaporization. Complete circumferential cauterization is avoided, and only the lumen of the posterior-medial wall of the Eustachian tube should be cauterized to avoid synechiae formation (▶ Fig. 45.2). The ICA lies in increasingly close proximity to the Eustachian tube as it courses superiorly, and care should always be made to protect and avoid the artery.

Another technique for laser-assisted tuboplasty was introduced by Yanez et al, which employs a KTP laser to create horizontal full-thickness cross-hatches through the luminal mucosa into the cartilage.[16] This technique is based on the hypothesis that weakening of the spring of the medial cartilaginous lamina will facilitate the dilatory effort of the TVP muscle.

Depending on the extent of the cauterized area, the posterior cushion may demonstrate significant swelling postoperatively, so intraoperative tympanostomy is often recommended.

45.4.2 Microdebrider Eustachian Tuboplasty

This operation is done with general anesthesia because sufficient local anesthesia may be difficult to administer. Sinus surgery may be done during the same operation if needed, but it may be preferable to perform the tuboplasty first given that bleeding from the nasal cavity may inconveniently obscure the Eustachian tube lumen.[17] Thorough nasal vasoconstriction should be performed before the operation. A submucosal injection of lidocaine with epinephrine is placed along the posterior Eustachian tube cushion and anterior cushion. To determine the best blade angle, 0-, 15-, and 30-degree microdebrider blades are passed through the nasal cavity. A 2.9-mm or 4.0-mm blade may be used depending on the size of the nasal cavity. In the narrowest cases, the endoscope may be passed through the contralateral nostril. Hypertrophic mucosa and submucosa are removed from the midpoint of the torus tubarius, continuing superiorly into the Eustachian tube as high as necessary toward the valve or until becoming limited by the size of the lumen.

In most cases, removal of diseased mucosa measuring roughly 1 cm over the luminal surface of the torus is enough. Tissue removal is carried out until reaching the cartilage. If resection of any cartilage is needed, it is done sharply. The cartilage serves additionally as an important landmark as it runs between the lumen and the ICA, in effect providing some protection. Care should be taken to avoid injury of the mucosa of the anterior cushion to avoid circumferential scarring that may lead to obstruction and synechiae.

45.4.3 Eustachian Tube Balloon Dilation

Eustachian tube balloon dilation has been mostly carried out under general anesthesia, but it is possible to perform the procedure under local anesthesia using smaller balloons with lesser dilation pressures and shorter dilation times. However, adequate local anesthesia to the deeper part of the Eustachian tube is difficult, and it may cause unnecessary pain for the patient or lead to inadequate intervention. Meticulous nasal topical vasoconstriction is carried out to avoid causing any mucosal damage to the nose and to prevent bleeding that could deteriorate the view to the Eustachian tube lumen. We prefer 4-mm, 30- or 45-degree endoscopes. Different sizes of balloons have been used ranging from 3 mm to 7 mm, with the smaller ones being designed specifically for tuboplasty and larger ones for sinuplasty. The most commonly used balloon in our experience is 6 mm, and the size may be determined based on the size of the Eustachian tube orifice and the severity of the disease.

The surgical anatomy of the Eustachian tube should be familiar to the surgeon. The Eustachian tube initially curves slightly posterior-medially around the bulge of the torus tubarius before coursing more posterior-laterally toward the ear. The authors employ a sinuplasty balloon system (Acclarent, Inc., Palo Alto, California) that has a 70-degree frontal sinus guide catheter through which the balloon catheter will be inserted. The tubal orifice may be opened gently by pushing medially on the torus with the guide catheter, allowing for a view deep into the lumen before beginning the insertion. Failure to medially rotate the posterior cushion could result in laceration of the anterior-medial wall mucosa, with bleeding or creation of a false passage into the submucosal tissue as the catheter advances. The balloon catheter is passed through the lumen gently and slowly, until meeting the expected slight resistance as the catheter engages the isthmus at a depth of approximately 24 mm from the orifice. There is a yellow marker 31 mm from the tip of the catheter that should not pass into the tubal lumen. The catheter should never be inserted forcefully. The guide catheter is allowed to rest on the floor of the nasal cavity, where it helps to stabilize the balloon catheter, preventing it from extruding from the lumen during inflation. The balloon catheter should not have any kinks in it as these can interfere with the inflation and deflation. There is usually no need for using a guidewire, but if one were to be employed, it would have to be removed prior to inflation to open the lumen of the balloon catheter, allowing for decompression of any air that might become trapped within the tubal lumen and the middle ear space.

The catheter is inflated to12 atm and maintained in place for 2 minutes, during which time the pressure often falls to 10 atm. After the 2 minutes, the balloon is deflated and removed. Alternatively, if a deeper dilation is desired but not achieved with the initial dilation, the balloon may be deflated after 1 minute, inserted to the desired depth, and re-inflated for another minute. Small mucosal tears are commonly visible after the dilation and are considered self-limited and not significant (▶ Fig. 45.3).

45.5 Postoperative Care

Patients are asked to refrain from nose-blowing for seven to ten days after balloon dilation to avoid the possibility of air emphysema in the malar area. Postoperative saline irrigations may be used to decrease mucosal drying after Eustachian tube surgery. Preoperative medical therapy, such as corticosteroid nasal spray or other ongoing management of possible underlying disease (e.g., allergies, chronic rhinosinusitis, reflux) should be continued to prevent recurrence of Eustachian tube dysfunction.

45.6 Complications

Laser and microdebrider tuboplasties have been used for over a decade. No major complications have been reported; minor complications have been rare but include postoperative epistaxis, synechiae, and local granuloma. Postoperative pain is mild and is generally limited to 2 days of a sore throat.

As balloon dilation is a relatively new technique compared with the other surgical options, there are a limited number of published studies reporting adverse event rates. However, it appears that its complication rate is lower than for laser or microdebrider tuboplasty. Complications have included excessive intraoperative bleeding and malar emphysema, probably from a false passage. Postoperatively, pain appears to be less than with laser or microdebrider techniques, but there have not been any reports assessing or describing postoperative pain.

45.7 Outcomes

There is currently no "gold standard" test for Eustachian tube function, which remains a problem for objectively evaluating

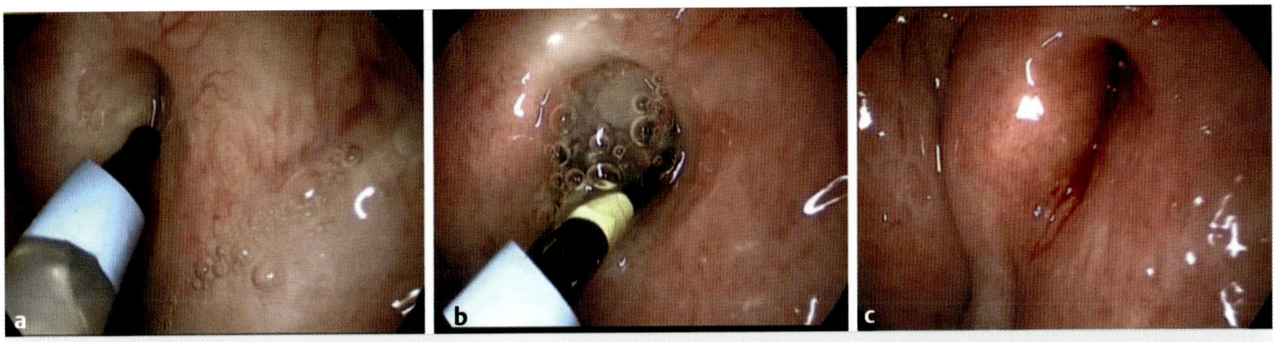

Fig. 45.3 Balloon dilation of the Eustachian tube. (a) The tubal orifice may be opened gently by pushing medially on the torus with the guide catheter, allowing for a deeper view into the lumen before beginning the insertion of the balloon catheter. (b) The balloon catheter is passed through the lumen gently until the yellow marker is at the tubal orifice. Insertion should be easy, and there should be no resistance. The balloon is then inflated to 10–12 atm for 2 minutes. (c) Eustachian tube after balloon dilation demonstrating some trace of blood that could be from a minor mucosal laceration from the dilation.

Eustachian tube dysfunction or the outcome of surgical interventions. Multiple tests and methods of assessment have been used to examine certain aspects of Eustachian tube function pre- and postoperatively, including video endoscopic assessment; sonotubometry; tubomanometry; tympanometry; the Valsalva maneuver; the pressure chamber test; the passive tube opening test; the Bluestone nine-step inflation-deflation test; and otomicroscopic tympanic membrane evaluation. A combination of these tests, rather than any individual test, may better reflect the true function of the Eustachian tube.

Because a large number of different tests are in use, the heterogeneity in Eustachian tube function tests across studies creates difficulty in comparing their findings. Also, the indication for surgical treatment has been inconsistent between studies. In some studies, patients without objective findings have been treated surgically, even if preoperative evaluation by Valsalva maneuver, tympanometry, and pressure chamber tests have been normal.[18,19]

Laser tuboplasty has been in use since 1997, making it the modern surgical procedure on the Eustachian tube with the greatest longevity.[8] Depending on the severity of the indications and the length of follow-up, the success rate has ranged from 38% to92%.[8,16,18,19,20,21] In the most severe cases, such as with persistent nasosinus pathology, Samter's triad, granulomatous disease, or other refractory mucosal disorders, temporary improvement may be obtained but recurrence of tubal dysfunction is more common. The best success rates have been achieved with patients whose suspected underlying inflammatory pathology has been adequately controlled. The least favorable long-term success appears to be with middle ear effusions, followed by negative middle ear pressure, and the best results are with those in whom the symptoms are limited to pressure equalization problems. These manifestations of symptoms may represent a spectrum of severity of Eustachian tube dysfunction. The results appear to be correspondingly better in patients with mild to moderate disease burden seen preoperatively.

The microdebrider approach is less commonly used. There is only one small study assessing the outcome and feasibility of microdebrider tuboplasty[17] that looked at Eustachian tube outcomes although the tuboplasty was done concurrently with sinonasal surgery in all cases. Results were comparable to those of the laser tuboplasty studies, with over 3 months of follow-up (mean, 13 months). Subjective symptoms improved in 70% of cases, and tympanometry values improved in 65% of cases; however, the effect of microdebrider tuboplasty was not clear because of the concomitant sinus surgery. In earlier studies, Stoikes and Dutton have shown that sinus surgery itself has a positive impact on patients with Eustachian tube symptoms.[22] Studies where only microdebrider tuboplasty has been done are still lacking, as is a comparison between approaches, where sinus surgery is done with or without tuboplasty.

The newest approach for treatment of Eustachian tube dysfunction is balloon dilation. Preliminary results from balloon dilation Eustachian tuboplasty have been assessed for feasibility, safety, and clinical application. In a pilot study on eleven patients with chronic otitis media with effusion lasting 5 or more years, postoperatively 11/11 (100%) were able to perform a Valsalva maneuver whereas they had previously been unable to do so. However, the rate declined to 63.6% by the end of the follow-up period of 6–14 months.[23] Similar results have been reported by Ockermann et al, where 12/12 were able to perform the Valsalva maneuver 8 weeks postoperatively, and by Schöder et al, where 13/15 (87%) were able to perform the Valsalva maneuver 12 months postoperatively.[24,25] Resolution of otitis media with effusion occurred in all of the 5/11 (45.4%) who had intact tympanic membranes (no perforations or tubes) in the study by Poe et al.[23] Ockermann et al demonstrated improvement in Eustachian tube scores, from a preoperative value of 1.1 to a postoperative value of 7.5.[24] The Eustachian tube score included subjective measurements of Eustachian tube function in swallowing, the Valsalva maneuver, and tubomanometry results at 30, 40, and 50 mbar levels and varied from 0 to 10 (where 0 describes the worst results and 10 describes the best results). In the study by McCoul et al, there was improvement in tympanometry results in 34/35 (97%) cases in a 6-week follow-up period.[26]

The longest follow-up results (mean > 2.5 years, range, 1.5–4.2 years) have been presented by Silvola et al, in which 41 patients suffering from middle ear effusion or tympanic membrane atelectasis for at least 5 years and with an inability to perform a Valsalva maneuver were treated with balloon dilation. Postoperatively, patients could do a Valsalva maneuver in 80% of cases; the tympanometry results improved to normal (type A) in 79% of cases; effusion, retraction, or atelectasis improved to normal in 90% of cases; and Eustachian tube mucosal inflammation scores decreased significantly in 70% of cases.[27]

It has been proposed that the reduction afforded by laser-assisted tuboplasty of inflamed tissue volume from the posteromedial wall of the lumen and posterior cushion, where the inflammation is usually maximal, would facilitate Eustachian tube dilation. Removal of the hypertrophic mucosa and submucosal tissue permitted regrowth with healthier, thinner epithelium and thinner submucosal scar.[20] Kujawski et al described a comparative analysis between preoperative and postoperative biopsy specimens in 18 patients, and there was a reduction in inflammatory cells and new fibrosis in the submucosa, with a normal pseudostratified epithelium 6 months after surgery.[8]

It is still unclear how balloon dilation enhances the Eustachian tube function. It has been observed with histology that in some cadaver specimens balloon dilation caused some microfractures within the cartilage of the Eustachian tube. It was additionally proposed that the compressive forces might induce deterioration of the surrounding connective tissue architecture.[24] Another hypothesis is that the compression of irreversibly injured hypertrophic mucosa and submucosa may permit healing with thinner and healthier layers.[23] In a previous study, mucosal inflammation was rated using a 4-point scale, where 1 consisted of normal mucosa and 4 consisted of severe erythema and edema and inability to dilate the lumen open. Mucosal inflammation within the Eustachian tube decreased from 2.9 to 1.7 after balloon dilation, which was statistically significant.[23,27]

In our preliminary histological samples, we have found the presence of significant lymphocytic infiltration and even follicles within the submucosa within the tubal lumen. There is commonly loss of the cilia in areas, indicating chronic inflammation preoperatively. Histological samples taken after balloon dilation have shown that the lymphocyte infiltration is markedly reduced and has been replaced, in part, by thinner fibrotic tissue. The injured epithelium has regenerated with healthy pseudocolumnar ciliated epithelium. Endoscopically observed thinning of the Eustachian tube mucosa supports this histological finding. Therefore, dilation of the cartilaginous Eustachian tube could induce permanent widening of the lumen, thereby reducing the work required for the muscles of dilation, especially the TVP muscle. In some cases, fibrotic synechiae within the lumen have been observed preoperatively and they have been loosened or removed by balloon dilation.

45.8 Conclusion

Balloon dilation of the Eustachian tube is a new, safe, and promising approach for surgical treatment of Eustachian tube dilatory dysfunction. It appears that the results of balloon dilation may be even better than conventional laser tuboplasty, and it is better-tolerated with a lower complication risk. The cost of balloon dilation is higher than the cost of laser tuboplasty, and comparative studies between the two different approaches are lacking. Microdebrider tuboplasty may be a consideration in a case with sinonasal disease and concomitant sinus surgery, but more data will be needed to assess the value of tuboplasty from studies in which concomitant surgery was not performed.

References

[1] Bluestone CD. Impact of evolution on the Eustachian tube. Laryngoscope. 2008;118(3):522–527.

[2] Browning GG, Gatehouse S. The prevalence of middle ear disease in the adult British population. Clin Otolaryngol Allied Sci. 1992;17(4):317–321.

[3] Pau HW, Sievert U, Just T, Sadé J. Pressure changes in the human middle ear without opening the Eustachian tube. Acta Otolaryngol. 2009;129(11):1182–1186.

[4] Gaihede M, Dirckx JJ, Jacobsen H, Aernouts J, Søvsø M, Tveterås K. Middle ear pressure regulation—complementary active actions of the mastoid and the Eustachian tube. Otol Neurotol. 2010;31(4):603–611.

[5] Miura M, Sando I, Balaban CD, Takasaki K, Haginomori S. Estimated locations of the narrowest portion of the Eustachian tube lumen during closed and open states. Ann Otol Rhinol Laryngol. 2002;111(3 Pt 1):255–260.

[6] McCoul ED, Lucente FE, Anand VK. Evolution of Eustachian tube surgery. Laryngoscope. 2011;121(3):661–666.

[7] Poe DS, Metson RB, Kujawski O. Laser Eustachian tuboplasty: A preliminary report. Laryngoscope. 2003;113(4):583–591.

[8] Kujawski OB, Poe DS. Laser Eustachian tuboplasty. Otol Neurotol. 2004;25(1):1–8.

[9] Poe DS, Abou-Halawa A, Abdel-Razek O. Analysis of the dysfunctional Eustachian tube by video endoscopy. Otol Neurotol. 2001;22(5):590–595.

[10] Kania RE, Lamers GE, Vonk MJ, et al. Characterization of mucosal biofilms on human adenoid tissues. Laryngoscope. 2008;118(1):128–134.

[11] Hall-Stoodley L, Hu FZ, Gieseke A, et al. Direct detection of bacterial biofilms on the middle-ear mucosa of children with chronic otitis media. JAMA. 2006;296(2):202–211.

[12] Kay DJ, Nelson M, Rosenfeld RM. Meta-analysis of tympanostomy tube sequelae. Otolaryngol Head Neck Surg. 2001;124(4):374–380.

[13] Nguyen LH, Manoukian JJ, Yoskovitch A, Al-Sebeih KH. Adenoidectomy: Selection criteria for surgical cases of otitis media. Laryngoscope. 2004;114(5):863–866.

[14] Ockermann T, Reineke U, Upile T, Ebmeyer J, Sudhoff HH. Balloon dilatation Eustachian tuboplasty: A clinical study. Laryngoscope. 2010;120(7):1411–1416.

[15] Bergin M, Bird P, Cowan I, Pearson JF. Exploring the critical distance and position relationships between the Eustachian tube and the internal carotid artery. Otol Neurotol. 2010;31(9):1511–1515.

[16] Yañez C. Cross-hatching: a novel technique for Eustachian tuboplasty. Preliminary report. Otolaryngol Head Neck Surg. 2010;142(5):688–693.

[17] Metson R, Pletcher SD, Poe DS. Microdebrider eustachian tuboplasty: A preliminary report. Otolaryngol Head Neck Surg. 2007;136(3):422–427.

[18] Jumah MD, Jumah M, Pazen D, Sedlmaier B. Laser Eustachian tuboplasty: Efficiency evaluation in the pressure chamber. Otol Neurotol. 2012;33(3):406–412.

[19] Caffier PP, Sedlmaier B, Haupt H, Göktas O, Scherer H, Mazurek B. Impact of laser Eustachian tuboplasty on middle ear ventilation, hearing, and tinnitus in chronic tube dysfunction. Ear Hear. 2011;32(1):132–139.

[20] Poe DS, Grimmer JF, Metson R. Laser Eustachian tuboplasty: Two-year results. Laryngoscope. 2007;117(2):231–237.

[21] Sedlmaier B, Pomorzev A, Haisch A, Halleck P, Scherer H, Göktas O. The improvement of middle ear ventilation by laser ablation of the epipharyngeal eustachian tube: a prospective study. Lasers Med Sci. 2009;24(5):793–800.

[22] Stoikes NF, Dutton JM. The effect of endoscopic sinus surgery on symptoms of Eustachian tube dysfunction. Am J Rhinol. 2005;19(2):199–202.

[23] Poe DS, Silvola J, Pyykkö I. Balloon dilation of the cartilaginous Eustachian tube. Otolaryngol Head Neck Surg. 2011;144(4):563–569.

[24] Ockermann T, Reineke U, Upile T, Ebmeyer J, Sudhoff HH. Balloon dilation Eustachian tuboplasty: A feasibility study. Otol Neurotol. 2010;31(7):1100–1103.

[25] Schröder S, Reineke U, Lehmann M, Ebmeyer J, Sudhoff H. [Chronic obstructive eustachian tube dysfunction in adults: long-term results of balloon *eustachian tuboplasty] HNO. 2013;61(2):142–151. German.

[26] McCoul ED, Anand VK. Eustachian tube balloon dilation surgery. Int Forum Allergy Rhinol. 2012;2(3):191–198.

[27] Silvola J, Kivekäs I, Poe DS. Balloon Dilation of the Cartilaginous Portion of the Eustachian Tube. Otolaryngol Head Neck Surg. 2014;125-130.

46 Tympanic Membrane Tissue Engineering

Shin-ichi Kanemaru

Abbreviations used in this chapter:

bFGF: basic fibroblast growth factor
HL: hearing level
TM: tympanic membrane

46.1 Introduction

Although various treatments for tympanic membrane (TM) perforation have been used, almost all of them, especially in cases of larger TM perforations, are surgical treatments, such as myringoplasty or tympanoplasty. Previous studies have demonstrated the ability to repair small, chronic TM perforations using collagen sheets or other types of patches.[1,2] For larger perforations spanning greater than one-third of the TM, however, conventional surgical treatment is usually still required. These surgeries require a skin incision and harvesting of autologous tissue, which is then used as repair material for the TM. Traditional otosurgical treatments may demand that patients endure some combination of anesthesia, hospitalization and/or bed rest, the high price of a surgical operation, and restrictions on daily life. In addition, these surgical techniques often pose other risks, including the development of iatrogenic cholesteatoma, otitis media, sensorineural hearing loss, and dysgeusia.

Given the disadvantages associated with conventional surgical treatments, research has been performed to investigate the causes of healing arrest in chronic TM perforations and the mechanisms involved in this process.[3,4,5] Acute small perforations of the TM usually heal spontaneously while chronic perforations and large perforations are less likely to do so. However, if given an adequate arrangement of scaffolding and growth factors to support the healing process, large chronic TM perforations may regenerate. Recent progress in regenerative medicine has provided us with various kinds of scaffolds and growth factors that make it possible to accelerate this type of tissue repair.[6,7]

Because the TM generally demonstrates good regenerative capabilities, we hypothesized that a better selection of scaffolds and other extrinsic factors, applied under the appropriate conditions, could bring out its maximum regenerative potential. According to the principles of in situ tissue engineering, regeneration of tissues/organs requires the introduction of three elements: cells, scaffolds, and regulatory factors, under suitable conditions.[6,7] In the TM regenerative scheme described here, scaffolding (in the form of a gelatin sponge) and a regulatory factor (basic fibroblast growth factor [bFGF]) are provided, while cells are endogenously supplied from the mechanically disrupted edge of the perforation. Mechanical disruption of the perforation edge may be the trigger to stimulate progenitor/tissue stem cells in this region of the TM.[8] This is another significant advantage of this novel therapy, as cell transplantation would make it difficult to widely and easily apply this therapy as an outpatient treatment.

By applying the principles of modern tissue engineering, we developed a novel, minimally invasive therapy for regenerative repair of large or total TM perforations (▶ Fig. 46.1) that may represent a new stage in the advancement of otologic surgery. In what follows, a description of TM regeneration is provided in the framework of our recently published prospective clinical trial.[9]

46.2 Patient Selection

The criteria used to screen patients for TM regeneration are:

- Dry TM and tympanic cavity without active inflammation during the previous 6 months.
- Proper aeration and no regions of soft tissue density in the mastoid and tympanic cavities based on temporal bone CTs.
- Intact ossicular chain.
- No cholesteatoma and no invasion of epithelia to tympanic cavity.

During our study we selected 140 patients with 158 chronic TM perforations from outpatients with a dry TM and tympanic cavity without active inflammation during the previous 6 months. The diseases affecting these patients included chronic otitis media (n=95), postoperative re-perforated TM (n=16), traumatic perforation (n=21), and iatrogenic TM perforation following insertion of a ventilation tube (n=26). Eighteen patients had bilateral TM perforations.

Patients ranged in age from 10 to 91 years, with an average age of 59 years. The patients consisted of 59 males and 81 females. The TM perforations were classified into three groups based on the size of the perforation, as follows: < 1/3 as Grade I (n=39), 1/3 to 2/3 as Grade II (n=69), and > 2/3 as Grade III (n=50).

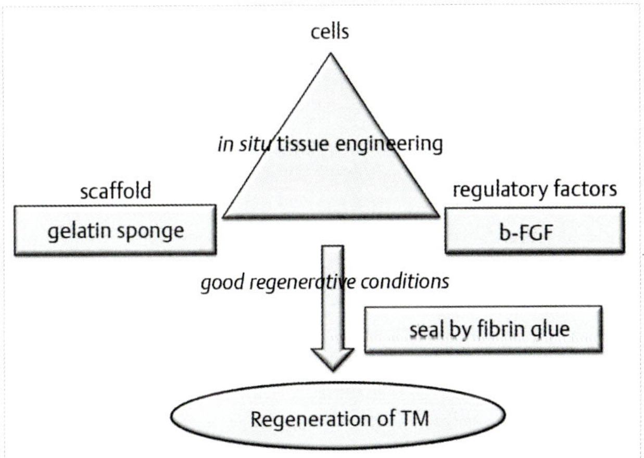

Fig. 46.1 Strategy for regeneration of the TM. Based on the concept of in situ tissue engineering, we introduce just two of these elements, gelatin sponge for scaffolding and bFGF for a regulatory factor, as cells are expected to be endogenously supplied from the mechanically disrupted edge of the perforation. For creating optimal regenerative conditions, we seal the gelatin sponge with fibrin glue.

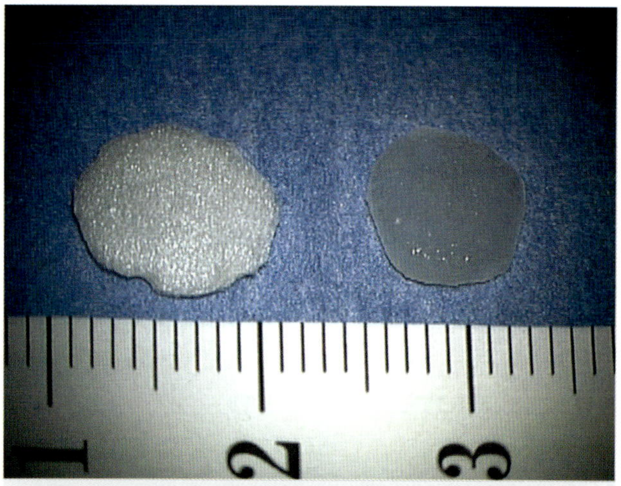

Fig. 46.2 Gelatin sponge. Left side: Trimmed gelatin sponge; right side: Trimmed gelatin sponge with bFGF.

46.3 Materials

Materials used for TM regeneration include gelatin sponge (Spongel, Astellas Pharma Inc., Tokyo, Japan) (▶ Fig. 46.2), basic fibroblast growth factor (bFGF, Fibrast, Kaken Pharma Co., Ltd, Tokyo, Japan), and fibrin glue (Bolheal, Kaketsuken, Kumamoto, Japan; Beriplast, CSL Behring K.K., Tokyo, Japan).

Basic-FGF is one of the few commercially produced growth factors available for clinical applications. It is usually used for the treatment of skin ulcers or decubitus ulcers because it has strong inductive effects on both fibroblasts (from which the name comes) and blood capillaries.[10,11] This former property is particularly suitable for TM regeneration because the pars tensa, which represents the largest part of the TM, consists of an intermediate layer of fibrous tissue produced by fibroblasts.[11] The capillary-inducing ability of bFGF may also foster improvements in local regenerative conditions. Although several reports have tested the use of growth factors and repair materials for improving TM regeneration in animal models,[2,12] an ideal combination of factors and materials has yet to be determined. The results of these controlled studies, however, suggest that bFGF may be suitable to act as the regulatory factor for optimal TM regeneration.

Given the limitations of sheet-form scaffolds, we use gelatin sponge as our scaffold material of choice. Gelatin sponge is made of a protein extracted from the collagen found inside connective tissues of animals and is often used for its hemostatic properties in medical procedures. Gelatin sponge has a high affinity for living tissues and is absorbed in vivo within a few months.[13,14] Another benefit of gelatin sponge is that it can fit into any size/shape of TM perforation and is easy to handle because of its gel form. Observations of the regenerative processes occurring in the TM reveal that cells will grow into a gelatin sponge and can occupy a large space. Therefore, with this technique a portion of the gelatin sponge extends into the TM, whereas another portion remains outside of the regenerating TM, providing a large surface area for cell growth. Gelatin sponge that remains in the tympanic cavity following TM regeneration is gradually absorbed and disappears within 3 months. A gelatin sponge works not only as a scaffold for the regeneration of the TM, but also as a sustained release substrate for bFGF.[14,15] These characteristics make it particularly advantageous for use in regeneration of the TM.

In the final step of our procedure, we seal the gelatin sponge with fibrin glue to insulate it from the outside and create optimal regenerative conditions. Not only does the fibrin glue help to keep the sponge in place, it also prevents cells from drying out and provides a barrier to infection, thus providing ideal culture conditions in vivo.

46.4 Surgical Technique

The tympanic region is fully anesthetized by applying a cotton ball soaked in 4% lidocaine to the perforation, in contact with the residual TM, for 15 minutes. Mechanical disruption of the perforation edge is then created under the microscope with a myringotomy knife. A gelatin sponge that is larger than the perforation is immersed in bFGF (5–30 µg of trafermin, a genetic recombinant, used at 100 µg/mL) and inserted into the perforation in contact with the edge of the TM. In our study, this was applied to 148 ears and saline, inserted in a similar fashion, was used as a control in 10 ears. Fibrin glue is then dripped over the sponge. ▶ Fig. 46.3 illustrates this process.

46.5 Postoperative Care

After this procedure, patients are advised not to blow their nose and/or sniff strongly. During the first follow-up visit at 3 weeks, crust over the TM is removed. For cases in which complete closure of the TM perforation is not achieved, the above treatment is repeated up to 4 times at three-week intervals. There is no additional special care required after this treatment.

46.6 Complications

In 25 cases, post-treatment otorrhea was observed after a few days. Sixteen of the 140 patients in our study were administered antibiotic drops. Slight retraction of the TM was observed in 12 cases 3 months after treatment. Two patients with aural fullness had to be treated by surgical puncture of the TM. In 4 cases, small cholesteatomas (epithelial pearl) were observed in the regenerated TM and were subsequently removed.

46.7 Outcomes

The effectiveness of this treatment for TM repair has been evaluated 3 weeks and 3 months after treatment using indicators such as closure rate, hearing level, improvement of tinnitus, and aural fullness. ▶ Fig. 46.4 illustrates some of the key outcomes in the treatment group versus the control group. ▶ Fig. 46.5 depicts a case that illustrates the typical process of healing with TM regeneration.

46.7.1 Rate of Closure of TM Perforations

The overall rate of complete closure of the TM perforations with 4 or less treatments was 87.2% (129/148) in the bFGF group and

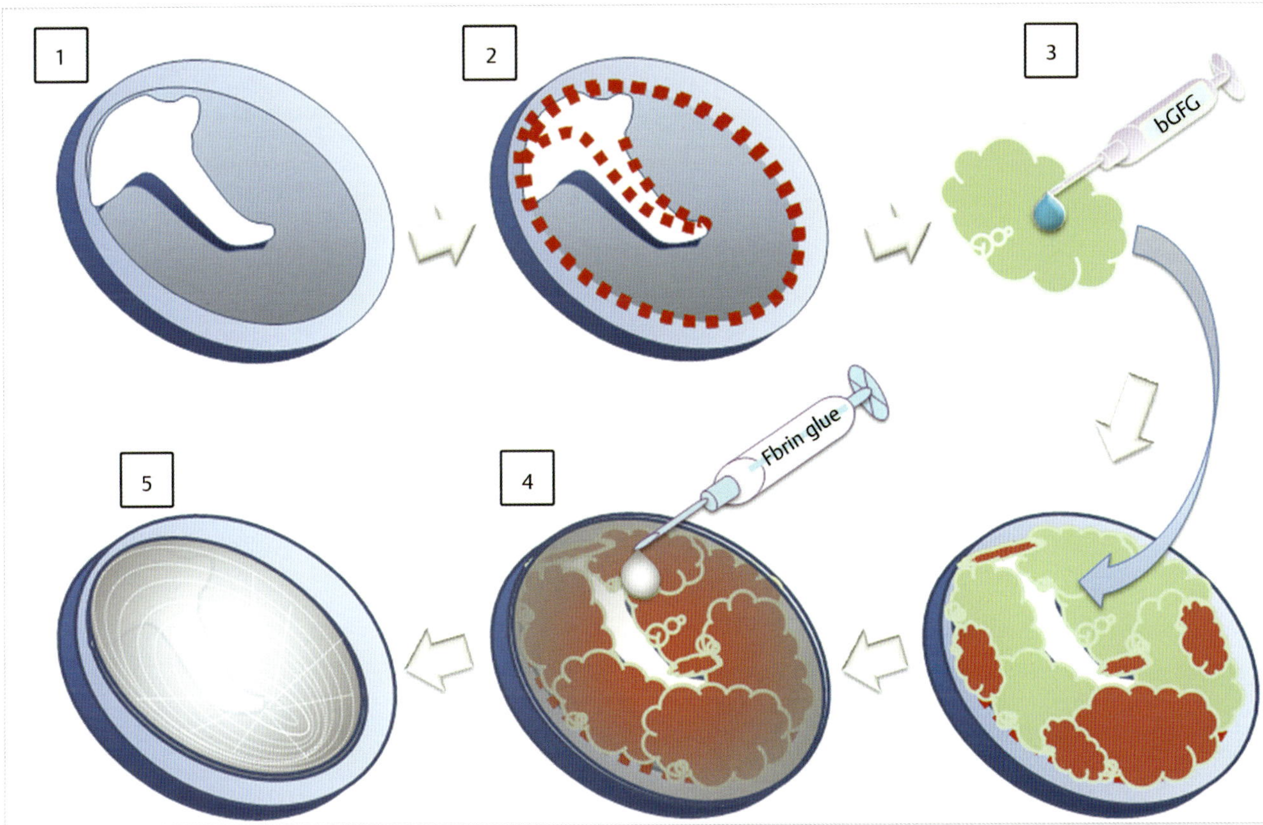

Fig. 46.3 Schematic diagram showing the method of TM regeneration. (1) TM perforation. (2) A mechanical disruption of the TM perforation edge is created under the microscope following local anesthesia with 4% lidocaine. (3) A gelatin sponge immersed in bFGF is placed over the perforation, in contact with the residual TM. (4) A gelatin sponge that has absorbed blood and changed color. Fibrin glue is dripped over the sponge. (5) At 3 weeks after treatment, residual crust is removed. In cases of incomplete closure of the TM perforation, the treatment is performed repeatedly.

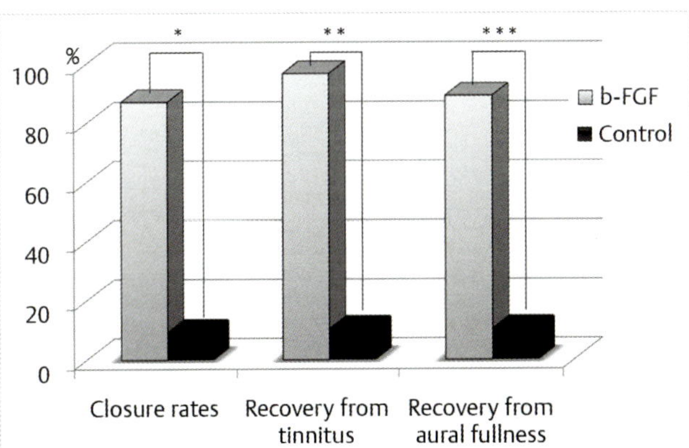

Fig. 46.4 Bar graphs comparing the TM perforation closure rates and recovery from tinnitus and aural fullness between the control and bFGF treatment groups. The bFGF group showed superior recovery compared with the control group for all conditions. (Mann-Whitney U test: $^{*}p<0.001$, $^{**}p<0.001$, $^{***}p<0.001$).

10% (1/10) in the control group (▶ Table 46.1). The number/rate of cases in which the TM perforation was able to close completely after 1 treatment, 2 treatments, 3 treatments, or 4 treatments was 86 (66.7%), 21 (16.3%), 13 (10.0%), and 9 (7.0%), respectively, in the bFGF group. In the control group, complete closure of the TM perforation was achieved in only 1 case (Grade I) after 4 treatments. In 19 cases (12.8%) in the bFGF group and 9 cases (90%) in the control group, the TM perforation had not perfectly closed by the end of the fourth treatment.

Otorrhea was observed after treatment in 13 of the 19 cases in the bFGF group with incomplete TM closure. Eight of these 19 cases resulted from postoperative re-perforation of the TM. The TM perforations in 4 cases were the result of thermal injury. It is worthy to note that successful closure was not achieved in any of the cases in which the TM perforation was caused by thermal injury. It is also very difficult for postoperative cases, especially after canal wall-down tympanoplasty, to regenerate the TM. We conjectured that very few tissue stem cells remain in regions that suffered thermal injuries or surgery. Knutsson et al tried to detect the progenitor/stem cell markers α_6-integrin, β_1-integrin, and cytokeratin19 in human TMs.[8] They concluded that possible progenitor cells were found in the umbo, the annular region, and along the malleus. It follows that the handle of the malleus, the umbo, and the annular ligament should be kept as much as possible for preservation of tissue stem/progenitor cells in tympanoplasty.

46.7.2 Hearing Improvement

One of the primary goals of TM repair is to restore a patient's hearing to optimal levels. With traditional surgical treatment

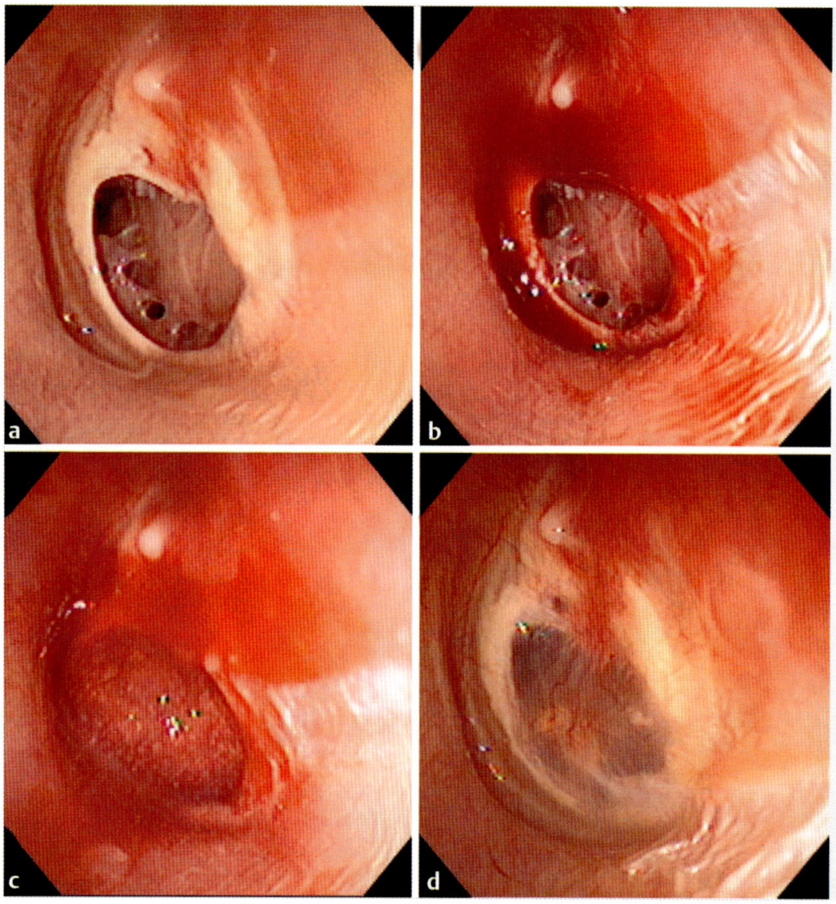

Fig. 46.5 The process of TM regeneration. (a) An 81-year-old female with chronic otitis media persisting for more than 75 years presented with a large, dry, Grade III perforation. (b) Disruption of the perforation edge. (c) Gelatin sponge with bFGF was placed over the perforation and sealed with fibrin glue. (d) At 3 months after the treatment, the TM was perfectly regenerated. The regenerated TM becomes a near-normal TM with hyper-vascularity.

Table 46.1 Results of TM regeneration

Grade		Total n=148	Grade I n=37	Grade II n=64	Grade III n=47
Closure rates		87.2% (129/148)	94.6% (35/37)	85.9% (55/64)	83.0% (39/47)
Number of treatments		1–4 (Average:1.57)	1–4 (Average:1.31)	1–4 Average:1.31)	1–4 (Average:1.95)
Average HL improvement	NA	19.7 dB	14.1 dB	20.6 dB	24.5 dB
	LA	31.7 dB	28.7 dB	31.1 dB	35.3 dB
Adverse events	TO	n=25	n=3(1*)	n=10(6*)	n=12(9*)
	RTM	n=10	n=2	n=5	n=5
	Chole	n=4	n=0	n=2	n=2

Grade I: PS (tympanic membrane perforation size) < 1/3. Grade II: 1/3 < PS < 2/3. Grade III: 2/3 < PS. NA, average hearing level at 0.5, 1 and 2 kHz; LA, average hearing level at 0.125, 0.25 and 0.5 kHz; TO, temporary otorrhea; *, administration of antibiotic ear drops; RTM, slight retraction of tympanic membrane; Chole, cholesteatoma.

strategies, it is quite difficult to improve hearing levels to the point that there is no air-bone gap, even in cases involving simple perforations. This failure may be attributed to factors such as a bulky reconstructed TM, detachment of the TM from the malleus, or re-perforation. Reconstruction of the TM using autologous tissue, such as the temporalis fascia, may not sufficiently improve hearing levels because the reconstructed TM is different from the original.

The majority of the TM comprises three layers: the epithelial layer, the fibrous (intermediate) layer, and the mucosal layer. For restoration of optimal hearing levels, it is desirable to maintain this structure. The intermediate layer is especially

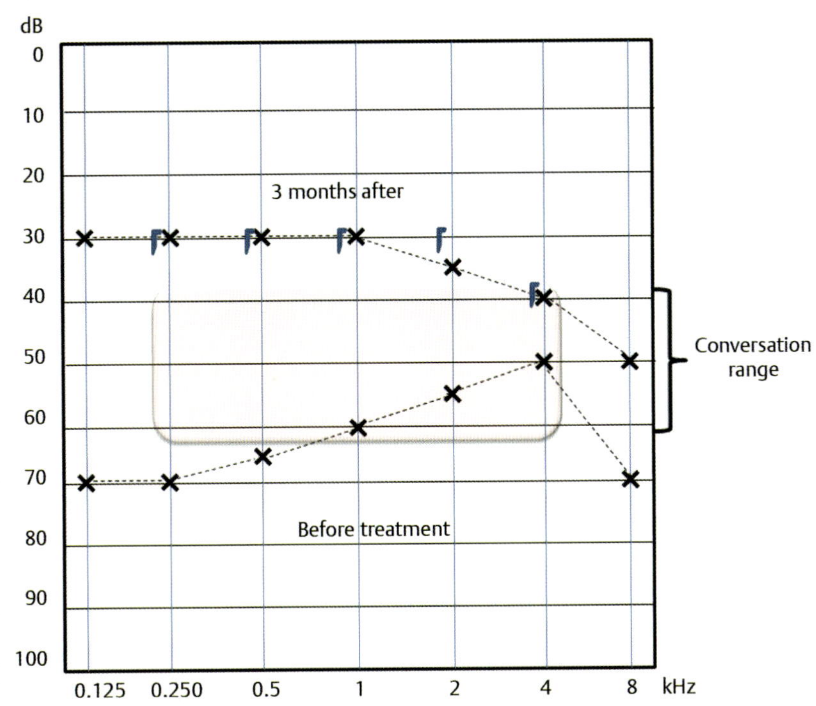

Fig. 46.6 Hearing after TM regeneration. After the treatment, hearing levels improve to the point that there is almost no air-bone gap. The patient did not need to wear a hearing aid and her maximum speech discrimination score improved from 85% (90 dB) to 100% (70 dB).

important for improving the strength of the TM and for sustaining blood capillaries (further details of TM healing are discussed in Chapter 3). Our study suggests that TM regeneration is associated with the formation of many new blood capillaries and hypertrophic tissue by 3 weeks post-treatment. Subsequently, the regenerated regions of the TM become thinner and are morphologically reshaped to appear more like a normal TM over time (▶ Fig. 46.5).

Pure-tone audiometry was measured in all patients prior to and 3 months after treatment. Average hearing levels showed improvement in all patients of the bFGF group with successful TM regeneration (▶ Table 46.1; ▶ Fig. 46.6). Of note, hearing levels showed remarkable gains in the lower frequency ranges: 125 Hz, 250 Hz, and 500 Hz.

46.7.3 Tinnitus and Aural Fullness

Prior to treatment, many patients reported subjective symptoms: 71.5% (113/158) had tinnitus and 58.9% (93/158) had aural fullness. Of patients from both the bFGF and control groups that had complete closure of their TM perforations, 96.7% (88/91) and 89.2% (66/74), respectively, noticed improvements in tinnitus and aural fullness. Although 13 patients had temporal deterioration in tinnitus a few days immediately following treatment, the tinnitus improved in 10 of these patients within 3 months. Aural fullness was still reported by 8 patients after treatment.

46.7.4 Duration of Procedure

The time required to perform each procedure, excluding local anesthesia, ranged from 7 to 25 minutes. There were 17 cases in which difficulties arose during the treatment: 10 cases of Grade II and 7 cases of Grade III. In these 17 cases, it was very difficult to observe the anterior-inferior edge of the perforation due to a protrusion of the anterior-inferior wall of the external auditory meatus.

46.8 Conclusion

We have developed a new regenerative treatment for perforation of the TM using a combination of bFGF, gelatin sponge, and fibrin glue, without the need for conventional surgical procedures. This is an innovative therapy with the benefits of being an easy, simple, safe, cost-effective, and minimally invasive outpatient procedure.

Tympanic membrane perforations are not always regenerated with this treatment strategy after one round; however, in roughly 90% of cases we achieved perfect regeneration within 4 rounds of treatment. As a general rule, the more times a surgical treatment is repeated, the worse the condition becomes, and it grows increasingly difficult to achieve success. But there is very little disadvantage to performing our treatment repeatedly because, in each consecutive round of the procedure, the mechanical disruption is created at a new perforation edge that has been regenerated by the previous round of treatment. Therefore, even when repeated treatments are necessary, scar formation, that would normally prevent tissue regeneration, is minimized.

References

[1] Hakuba N, Taniguchi M, Shimizu Y, Sugimoto A, Shinomori Y, Gyo K. A new method for closing tympanic membrane perforations using basic fibroblast growth factor. Laryngoscope. 2003;113(8):1352–1355.

[2] Weber DE, Semaan MT, Wasman JK, Beane R, Bonassar LJ, Megerian CA. Tissue-engineered calcium alginate patches in the repair of chronic chinchilla tympanic membrane perforations. Laryngoscope. 2006;116(5):700–704.

[3] Johnson AP, Smallman LA, Kent SE. The mechanism of healing of tympanic membrane perforations. A two-dimensional histological study in guinea pigs. Acta Otolaryngol. 1990;109(5–6):406–415.

[4] Laurent C, Hellström S. Extracellular matrix components reflect the dynamics of a healing tympanic membrane perforation—a histochemical study. Int J Biochem Cell Biol. 1997;29(1):221–229.

[5] Somers T, Goovaerts G, Schelfhout L, Peeters S, Govaerts PJ, Offeciers E. Growth factors in tympanic membrane perforations. Am J Otol. 1998;19(4):428–434.

[6] Lokmic Z, Mitchell GM. Engineering the microcirculation. Tissue Eng Part B Rev. 2008;14(1):87–103.

[7] Macri L, Silverstein D, Clark RA. Growth factor binding to the pericellular matrix and its importance in tissue engineering. Adv Drug Deliv Rev. 2007;59(13):1366–1381.

[8] Knutsson J, von Unge M, Rask-Andersen H. Localization of progenitor/stem cells in the human tympanic membrane. Audiol Neurootol. 2011;16(4):263–269.

[9] Kanemaru S, Umeda H, Kitani Y, Nakamura T, Hirano S, Ito J. Regenerative treatment for tympanic membrane perforation. Otol Neurotol. 2011;32(8):1218–1223.

[10] Virag JA, Rolle ML, Reece J, Hardouin S, Feigl EO, Murry CE. Fibroblast growth factor-2 regulates myocardial infarct repair: Effects on cell proliferation, scar contraction, and ventricular function. Am J Pathol. 2007;171(5):1431–1440.

[11] Vrabec JT, Schwaber MK, Davidson JM, Clymer MA. Evaluation of basic fibroblast growth factor in tympanic membrane repair. Laryngoscope. 1994;104(9):1059–1064.

[12] Kato M, Jackler RK. Repair of chronic tympanic membrane perforations with fibroblast growth factor. Otolaryngol Head Neck Surg. 1996;115(6):538–547.

[13] Rohanizadeh R, Swain MV, Mason RS. Gelatin sponges (Gelfoam) as a scaffold for osteoblasts. J Mater Sci Mater Med. 2008;19(3):1173–1182.

[14] Komura M, Komura H, Kanamori Y, et al. An animal model study for tissue-engineered trachea fabricated from a biodegradable scaffold using chondrocytes to augment repair of tracheal stenosis. J Pediatr Surg. 2008;43(12):2141–2146.

[15] Takemoto S, Morimoto N, Kimura Y, et al. Preparation of collagen/gelatin sponge scaffold for sustained release of bFGF. Tissue Eng Part A. 2008;14(10):1629–1638.

47 Chronic Otitis Media in the Setting of Congenital Ear Disease

Bradley W. Kesser

Abbreviations used in this chapter:

CAA: congenital aural atresia
CSF: chloramphenicol/sulfanilamide/fungizone
CT: computed tomography
MRI: magnetic resonance imaging

47.1 Introduction

Chronic otitis media, defined by the presence of a tympanic membrane perforation or cholesteatoma, is rare in the setting of congenital middle ear abnormalities. Chronic otitis media may take several forms: middle ear cholesteatoma in congenital aural atresia (CAA), ear canal cholesteatoma secondary to congenital stenosis of the external auditory canal, tympanic membrane perforation or cholesteatoma as a postoperative complication of CAA surgery, or congenital cholesteatoma. This chapter reviews the clinical characteristics and management of these entities with emphasis on diagnosis and imaging of these rare lesions. Acquired ear canal cholesteatoma will not be discussed, but many of the principles of management of ear canal cholesteatoma in congenital ear canal stenosis apply to the management of acquired ear canal cholesteatoma. Meatoplasty and canalplasty techniques are addressed in Chapter 20.

47.2 Middle Ear Cholesteatoma in CAA

With only a single reported patient in the literature, middle ear cholesteatoma in CAA is extremely rare.[1] Logically, it does not seem possible for skin to become trapped in the middle ear space when the ear canal did not open, an eardrum did not develop, and ectoderm/skin never invaginated into the temporal bone from the branchial apparatus. If Michaels's [Epidermoid Formation Theory of congenital cholesteatoma] (see below) is true however, then it is theoretically possible for epithelial cells to become trapped in the tympanic cavity.[2]

The diagnosis in this single pediatric patient was made only at the time of surgery for CAA when an unusual soft tissue mass was noted in the middle ear space (▶ Fig. 47.1). This soft tissue was not expansile and did not appear to be skin, but on pathological examination, keratin was identified (▶ Fig. 47.2).

Preoperatively, the high-resolution temporal bone computed tomography (CT) scan showed a discrete rounded density in the middle ear space (▶ Fig. 47.3) that was not expansile or erosive. In almost all patients with CAA, opacification in the epitympanum or mastoid represents either fluid or mesenchymal tissue, not cholesteatoma. Nevertheless, any opacification in an ear with CAA needs close scrutiny with a follow-up CT scan in one year, especially in the ear with stenosis of the canal and opacification lateral to the middle ear space (see below). Opacification in an ear with CAA disqualifies the patient from surgical repair (the opacity in the above patient was small and limited, with no bone erosion and otherwise favorable anatomy); if the opacification is fluid, the Eustachian tube may be immature, and hearing results will be poor. Interestingly, acute otitis media in patients with CAA is rare, and patients generally do not develop "classic" acute otitis media symptoms. Although it is certainly possible to have fluid in the middle ear space, the patient will, in general, not have pain because there is no tympanic membrane.

If the opacification is mesenchymal tissue, this tissue will impede the vibratory capacity of the ossicles and prevent a good hearing outcome. This tissue will remain unchanged on serial radiographic examinations. Although Eustachian tube dysfunction in CAA is rare, any opacification of the middle ear

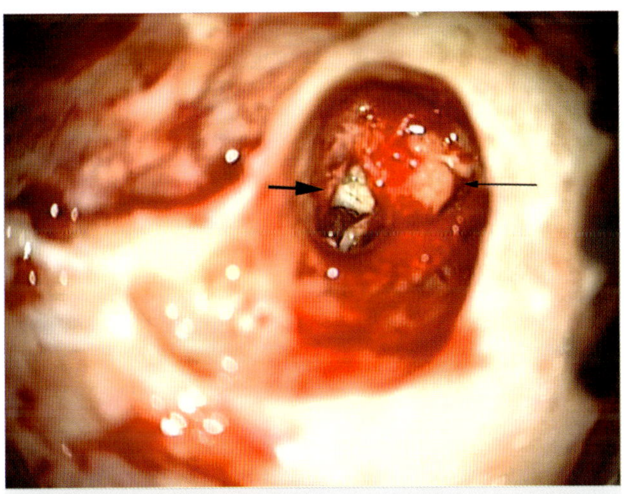

Fig. 47.1 Intraoperative otomicroscopic image showing cholesteatoma (large arrow) medial to the ossicular mass (small arrow).

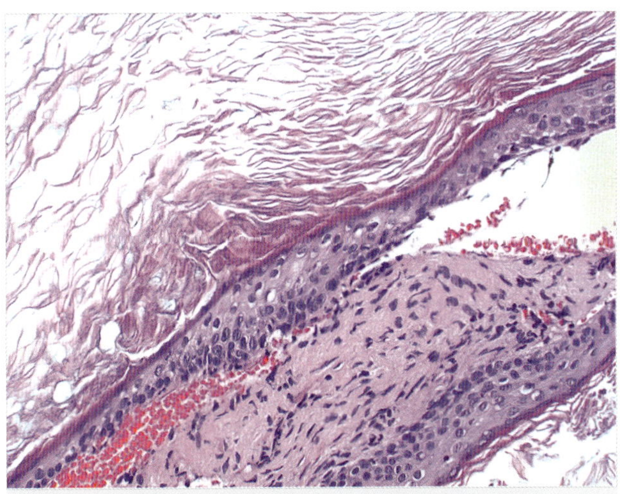

Fig. 47.2 Microscopic hematoxylin and eosin stain of soft tissue mass showing keratinaceous debris consistent with cholesteatoma.

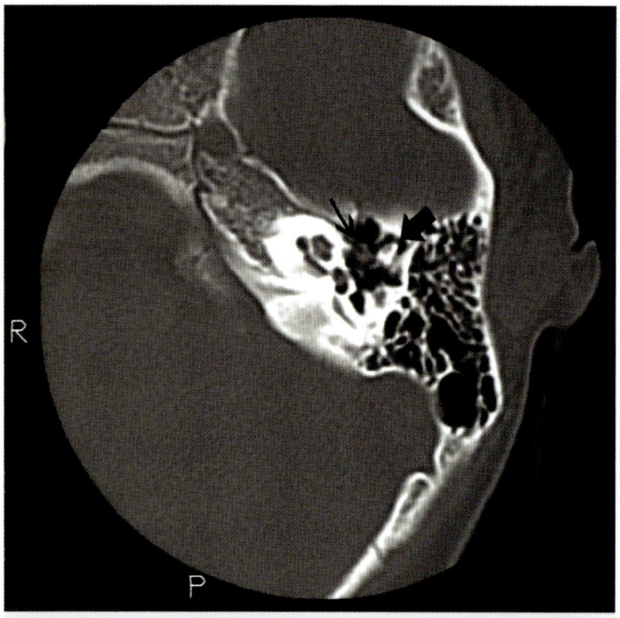

Fig. 47.3 Axial high-resolution CT scan of the temporal bone showing subtle soft tissue mass (small arrow) medial to the ossicular chain (large arrow).

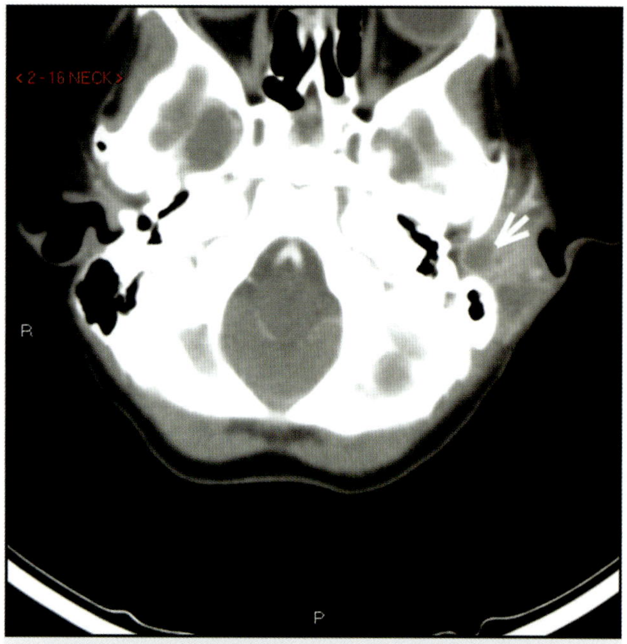

Fig. 47.4 Axial high-resolution CT scan of the left temporal bone showing subcutaneous abscess (arrow) created by infected ear canal cholesteatoma in the lateral ear canal.

or mastoid is a relative contraindication to surgery, but must be followed with a second CT scan (generally in 1 year) to ensure it is not expansile and does not erode or remodel bone. Alternatively, magnetic resonance imaging (MRI) with diffusion-weighted sequences can often differentiate between cholesteatoma and fluid or soft (mesenchymal) tissue.[3,4]

In summary, opacification in the middle ear space of the patient with CAA should raise minimal concern for cholesteatoma (as mentioned, this is extremely rare in the middle ear and much more common laterally, in a stenotic ear canal, as described below). Features of cholesteatoma include a rounded density exhibiting bony remodeling or bony expansion. Opacification extending from a stenotic ear canal into the middle ear is more concerning. Options for evaluation include MRI or repeating the high-resolution CT imaging in 9–12 months.

In an ear with CAA, opacification of the middle ear or mastoid in the absence of bony erosion can be followed with repeat high-resolution CT imaging in 1 year. If the scan is stable, the opacification most likely represents fluid or primitive mesenchymal tissue, a relative contraindication to surgical repair of CAA, but a safe ear nonetheless.

47.3 Ear Canal Stenosis and Cholesteatoma

The stenotic ear canal should at least raise the suspicion of the possibility of external auditory canal cholesteatoma. If the ear canal is skin-lined, but the canal is too narrow for the normal migratory pattern of ear canal skin, then skin can become trapped in the narrow canal. Trapped skin builds over time and begins to remodel the surrounding bone. The skin can become infected and develop into a subcutaneous abscess, which needs both drainage and, at a later date, definitive management of the canal cholesteatoma (▶ Fig. 47.4). An ear canal cholesteatoma in congenital stenosis of the external auditory canal can also be asymptomatic. CT scanning for surveillance around the age of 5–6 years is indicated because cholesteatoma in the setting of external auditory canal stenosis, especially in a canal with a diameter measuring 2 mm or narrower, can develop in as many as 91% of ears in patients 12 years or older; no patient with canal openings larger than 4 mm developed cholesteatoma in one study.[5]

Findings on physical examination may include keratin debris noted at the meatus, drainage from the meatus, or pain in the ear. Any ear canal measuring 2 mm or narrower should raise the suspicion of canal cholesteatoma and prompt high-resolution CT scanning of the temporal bone (▶ Fig. 47.5).[5] The recommended age for high-resolution CT imaging for the evaluation of a child's candidacy for CAA repair is generally around the age when surgery is being considered (5–7 years). Some practitioners recommend earlier scanning, but radiation doses cover a greater surface area in smaller children. CT scanning certainly does not need to be performed before the age of 3 years, even in the patient with canal stenosis. On the other hand, drainage from a stenotic ear canal should prompt earlier CT scanning, but canal cholesteatoma is often not seen or identified until the age of 4 years.[5]

High-resolution CT shows a rounded density in the lateral temporal bone, medial to the meatus. The rounded density remodels bone but is not invasive (▶ Fig. 47.6; ▶ Fig. 47.7). The patient may also have a rudimentary tympanic membrane that can bulge into the middle ear space (▶ Fig. 47.8).

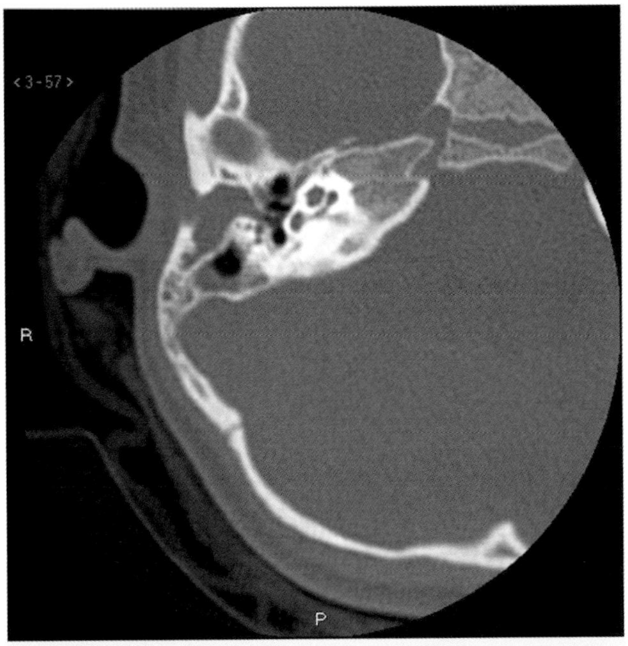

Fig. 47.5 Axial high-resolution CT scan of the right temporal bone showing opacification within a stenotic ear canal, with bony expansion of the lateral temporal bone, sparing the middle ear space.

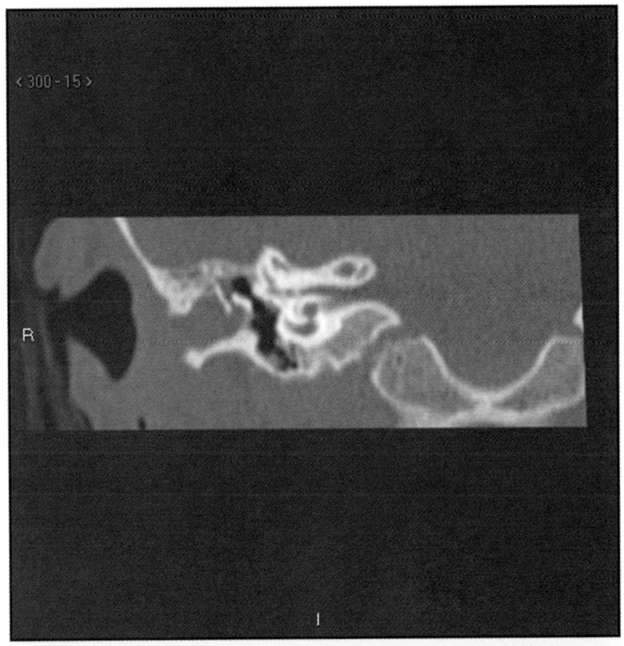

Fig. 47.6 Coronal high-resolution CT scan of the right temporal bone (same patient) showing opacification with bony expansion of the external auditory canal.

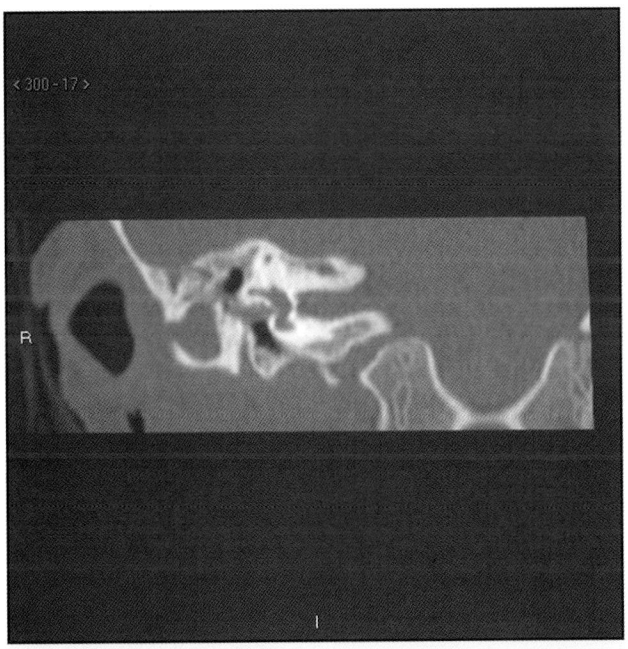

Fig. 47.7 Coronal high-resolution CT scan of the right temporal bone anterior to the section in ▶ Fig. 47.6, showing the rounded density of a canal cholesteatoma.

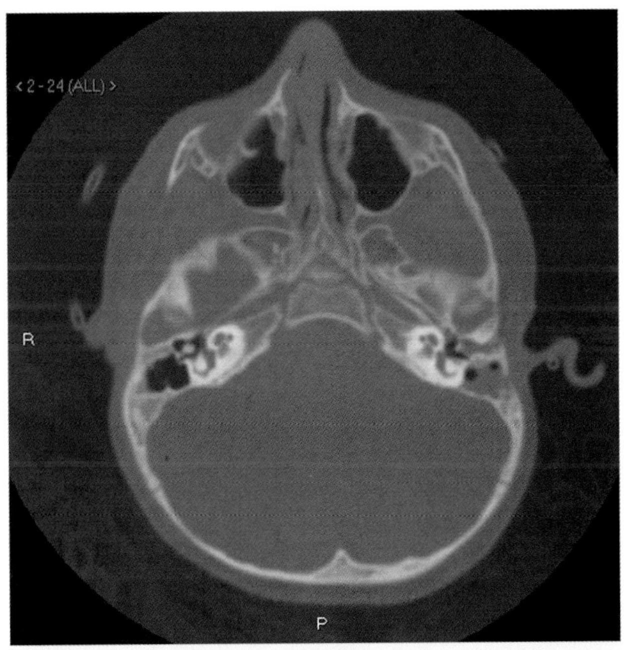

Fig. 47.8 Axial high-resolution CT scan of the temporal bone showing left ear canal cholesteatoma bulging into the middle ear space.

A linear opacification running in the bony canal without bony erosion is sometimes seen extending from the meatus to the middle ear or rudimentary tympanic membrane (▶ Fig. 47.9). Surgical exploration has shown this to be a fibrous band down to the mesotympanum and not cholesteatoma. This fibrous band can be a helpful landmark to the middle ear when drilling the canalplasty, but care must be taken as the drilling proceeds medially, as this band may be connected to the manubrium of the malleus.

Surgical management of ear canal cholesteatoma requires a postauricular incision, with standard mastoid periosteal incisions along the linea temporalis and perpendicular down to the mastoid tip. The periosteum is elevated to the posterior canal skin, and the skin is incised transversely at the bony-

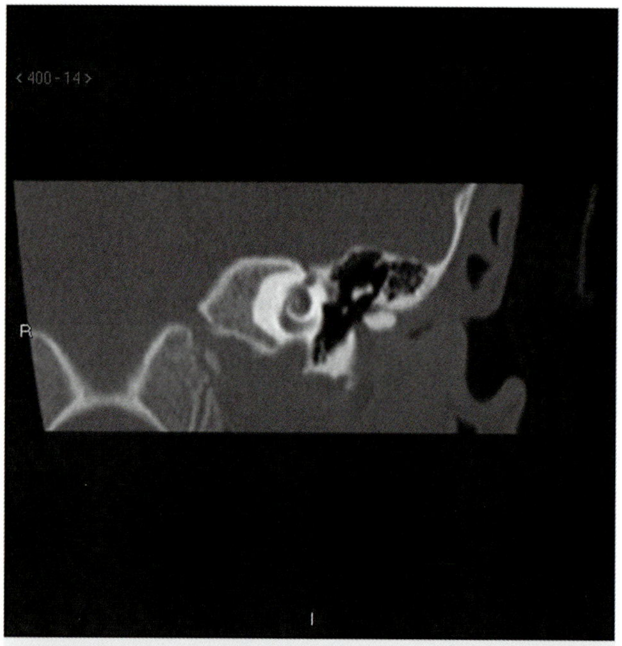

Fig. 47.9 Coronal high-resolution CT scan of the left temporal bone showing a thin linear opacity extending from the lateral canal to the mesotympanum in a patient with ear canal stenosis. This linear density was not cholesteatoma. Note the lack of bony expansion or remodeling.

cartilaginous junction. When the canal is entered, squamous debris is identified and removed (▶ Fig. 47.10). The debris is suctioned to the medial bony canal or to a rudimentary tympanic membrane. Once the squamous debris is removed, the eardrum can be assessed and elevated with a standard tympanomeatal flap, and the middle ear and ossicles evaluated.

The canal must still be addressed so that the cholesteatoma does not recur. Canal skin can be elevated medially and a canalplasty performed, widening the canal superiorly, inferiorly, and anteriorly. Mastoid air cells should not be opened. Alternatively, the stenotic canal can be addressed as an atretic ear, with removal of the canal skin (or saving a strip of canal skin anteriorly) and drilling the canal superiorly to identify the tegmen. Once identified, the tegmen is followed medially into the epitympanum (as in a standard atresia operation), where the malleus and incus (often fused) are identified. The final area to drill is a bony bridge between the head of malleus/body of incus in the epitympanum and the rudimentary eardrum opening into the mesotympanum. The ossicles are freed from the surrounding bone. Temporalis fascia can be placed medial to the native eardrum remnant, draped over the malleus/incus and up onto the canal wall in a lateral surface fashion. Placement of the skin graft, ear canal packing, and wide meatoplasty proceed similarly to a standard atresia operation.[6]

Prevalence of cholesteatoma in external auditory canal stenosis is high, with estimates ranging from 19% to 50%.[5,7,8] Risk factors and exam findings include a canal 2 mm or narrower (especially in patients 12 years or older), female gender, otorrhea, otalgia, and mastoid swelling or abscess.[5,7,8] Age does seem to be a factor, as older patients with external auditory canal stenosis are more likely to develop cholesteatoma, probably because they come to diagnosis after years of growth and

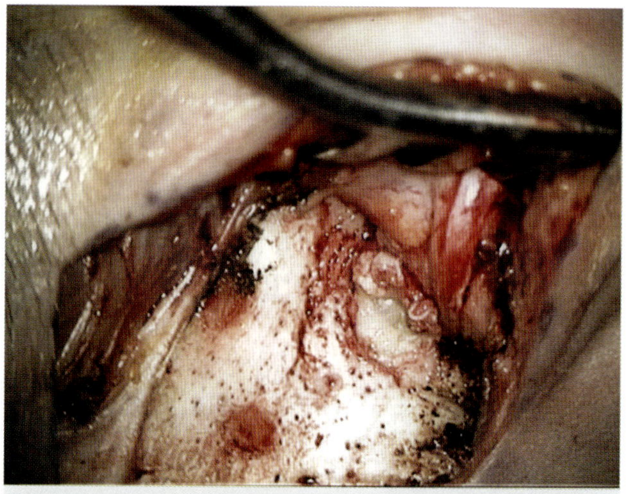

Fig. 47.10 Intraoperative otomicroscopic image of squamous debris filling the stenotic right ear canal of a child with ear canal stenosis and associated cholesteatoma.

manifest more urgent symptoms.[7] No cholesteatoma has been found in children 3 years of age or younger.[5]

47.4 Chronic Otitis Media as a Postoperative Complication of CAA Surgery

47.4.1 Canal Stenosis

Surgery to repair CAA for the purpose of hearing rehabilitation involves drilling the tympanic bone to identify the middle ear space, freeing the ossicular chain from the surrounding bone and atretic plate, placing an overlay temporalis fascia graft for eardrum reconstruction, and using a thin split-thickness skin graft to cover the temporalis fascia graft and bony canal wall. Meatoplasty is performed, and the skin graft is delivered through the newly created meatus and sutured to the native skin of the concha circumferentially.[6,9] Despite meticulous technique, the most common complication of surgery is canal stenosis, which occurs in 15% to 30% of patients.[10,11,12]

Canal stenosis takes two forms: lateral soft tissue stenosis is usually seen within the first 6–12 months after surgery, and bony stenosis secondary to new bone growth is seen during and after puberty. Even though the skin graft in the canal does not migrate, the skin is alive and produces dead skin, which is why the canal requires cleaning 1 to 2 times a year. If the dead skin cannot be cleaned, either because the meatus has stenosed or new bone has formed trapping skin behind the new bone, it accumulates over time, can cause infection and drainage, and can begin to erode the bony canal or push into the middle ear space.

In these two instances where the skin cannot be adequately cleaned (meatal stenosis and new bone growth), a high-resolution CT scan is advised. CT imaging may show lateral soft tissue stenosis with a widely patent medial bony canal (▶ Fig. 47.11). Imaging may also show exuberant new bone growth with opacification (trapped skin) behind the new bone growth just lateral to the middle ear space (▶ Fig. 47.12). For these two

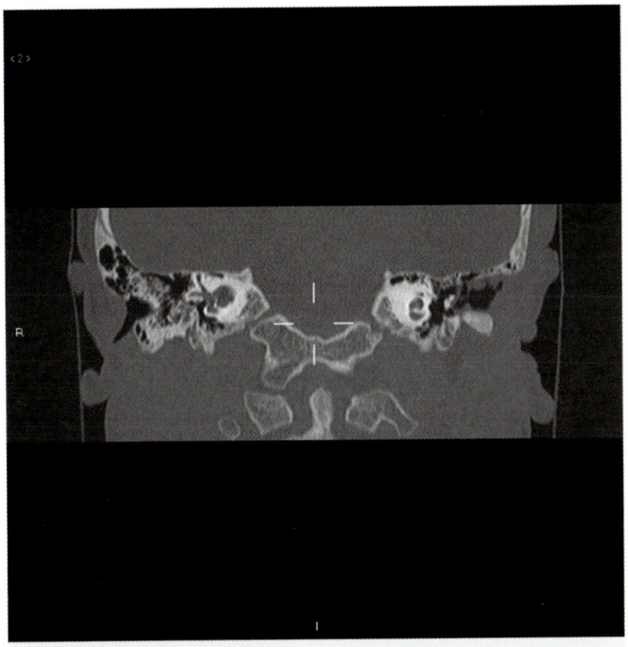

Fig. 47.11 Coronal high-resolution CT of the left temporal bone showing stenosis of the soft tissue of the lateral canal with a widely patent bony medial canal after prior CAA repair. Note debris in the medial, bony canal.

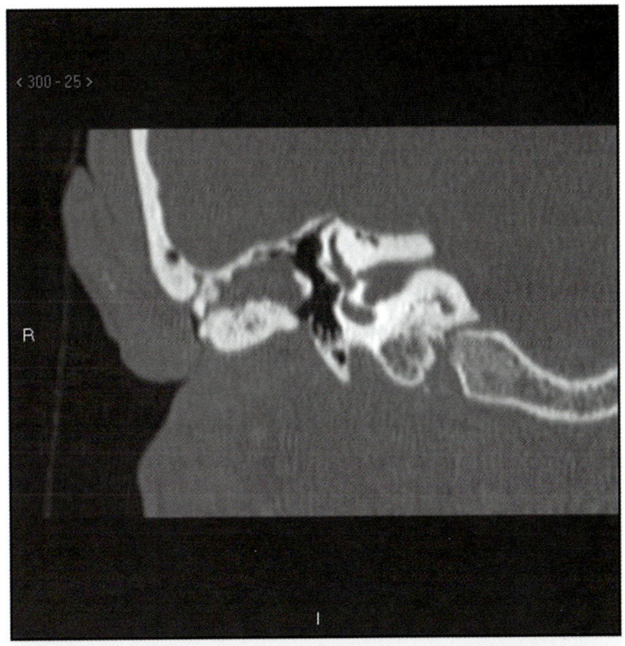

Fig. 47.12 Coronal high-resolution CT of the right temporal bone demonstrating trapped skin medial to new bone growth in a 23-year-old patient who underwent CAA repair 15 years prior to the CT scan.

conditions, revision surgery is recommended. Goals of revision surgery include removal of all accumulated keratin debris, and either closing off the canal (with compulsive technique to remove all epithelium) or reopening the canal by resecting the fibrous tissue, causing the lateral stenosis (and usually skin regrafting) or drilling away the new bone growth (and most often replacing the skin graft).[10]

Lateral Soft Tissue Stenosis

For meatal stenosis, a postauricular approach is used. The posterior canal skin is transected at the bony-soft tissue junction, and the canal lumen is entered. The keratin debris medial to the stenosis is debrided and the tympanic membrane identified. If the tympanic membrane and skin graft in the medial bony canal are healthy, the dead skin is cleaned away, and the medial canal is undisturbed. If the medial skin graft has sloughed and there is mucosalization or inflammation, the area of mucosalization is resected and replaced with a fresh skin graft, or if the area is wide, the medial skin and tympanic membrane are replaced with fresh tissue (a fresh temporalis graft for the tympanic membrane and fresh skin graft for the medial skin).

The meatus is addressed by passing a gimmick through the lateral meatus medially to identify the tract. The fibrous tissue is then resected widely and a new meatus is created. If the meatus is inferior to the bony canal, the auricle can be elevated so that the meatus aligns with the bony canal by excising a strip of postauricular skin and advancing the entire auricle superiorly. Once the fibrous tissue has been excised, a new skin graft can be placed. The new skin graft is anchored in the bony canal with some overlap with the healthy medial skin using Pope Oto-Wicks (Medtronic, Jacksonville, Florida) hydrated with an ototopical antibiotic solution. Once anchored medially, the auricle is elevated and sutured into position. The skin graft is brought out through the newly created meatus and sutured to the native skin of the concha with interrupted 5–0 fast-absorbing gut sutures. Additional Pope Oto-Wicks are placed in the lateral canal and hydrated.

Local injection of a depot steroid (e.g., triamcinolone) and, starting 1 month after surgery, use of a foam earplug coated in a water-soluble lubricant at night (with removal in the morning) or long-term stenting (at least 6 months) can often prevent meatal stenosis.[13] Younger patients and patients with more severe microtia carry a higher risk of postoperative stenosis.[14]

Bony Stenosis

For skin trapped behind new bone growth, a postauricular approach is again used. The posterior canal skin is transected lateral to the new bone growth, and a circumferential incision is made in the canal skin at the bony-soft tissue junction. The medial canal skin is elevated over the new bone medially down to the tympanic membrane if possible. The new bone is drilled away with care to identify the tegmen and follow it medially. If the tympanic membrane is healthy and intact, it may be left in place and a new skin graft placed. If the tympanic membrane shows inflammation or mucosalization, it is carefully elevated off the fused malleus/incus complex and removed. The ossicular chain may or may not be mobile under the tympanic membrane, so care must be taken elevating the eardrum off the ossicles. If the ossicles have refixed, they can be liberated again at this point.

Once the new bone has been drilled away, the middle ear space explored, and the ossicles evaluated for mobility, reconstruction proceeds in a standard fashion with a temporalis fascia graft to drape over the fused malleus/incus and middle ear

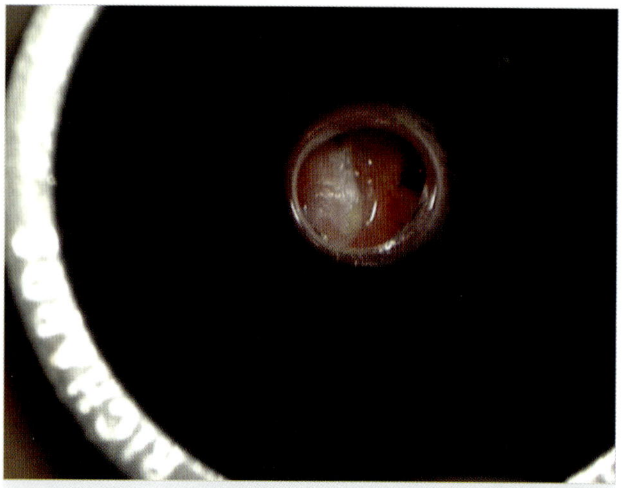

Fig. 47.13 Transcanal otomicroscopic view of a previously operated atretic ear showing the clear line of demarcation between the squamous epithelium of the canal skin graft (left) and the red, moist, shiny mucosa of the medial canal where the skin graft has sloughed and been replaced by mucous membrane (right).

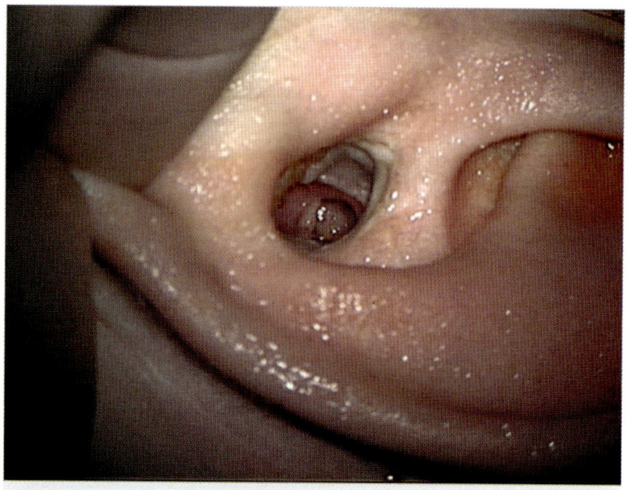

Fig. 47.14 Transcanal otomicroscopic view of a previously operated atretic ear showing a tympanic membrane perforation. Note the mucosalization of the remaining eardrum.

space. The fascia is draped onto the polished canal wall 1–2 mm in all directions. Air cells are packed with autologous temporalis muscle. The skin graft is next placed and anchored with a 0.4-inch Silastic disk. The Pope Oto-Wicks are delivered into the canal and hydrated with a topical antibiotic solution. If the meatus is adequate, the lateral skin graft is delivered through the meatus after the auricle is sutured down and simply packed in place with additional Pope Oto-Wicks.[6,9]

Of note, new bone growth is rarely seen in postpubertal patients. One theory behind the formation of new bone in the postoperative ear is the surge of growth hormone during the pubertal years. If the patient with new bone growth can be temporized until after puberty, recurrence of new bone after revision surgery is very low. Some atresia surgeons advocate waiting until the patient is 12 years of age or older to perform the primary surgery.[14]

47.4.2 Otorrhea and Tympanic Membrane Perforation

In a recent report of 107 revision surgeries for CAA, 20 (19%) were performed for chronic otorrhea and/or infection, with 10 operations secondary to sloughing of the skin graft and mucosalization of the canal (▶ Fig. 47.13), 4 secondary to eardrum perforation (▶ Fig. 47.14), 3 for canal cholesteatoma, and 3 for a combination.[10]

Factors thought to contribute to sloughing of the skin graft and replacement of the skin with mucous membrane include loss of blood supply to the skin graft, exposure to large mastoid air cells, trapping of skin (secondary to new bone growth or meatal stenosis) with resultant infection, and eardrum perforation. A small area of mucosalization/granulation can be treated in the office with silver nitrate cautery and a topical antibiotic powder such as chloramphenicol/sulfanilamide/fungizone (CSF). Small areas can also be resected with a small curette to allow the surrounding skin to re-epithelialize. These small areas of mucosalization (< 1 cm) may cause some moisture in the canal but rarely cause significant otorrhea.

Larger areas will also respond to cauterization and application of CSF powder, but if the area of mucosalization is > 50% of the surface area of the canal, the ear will retain moisture and may drain from time to time. The patient is counseled that the drainage does not necessarily represent infection, it simply is the wrong tissue (mucous membrane) in the wrong place (ear canal). The drainage can be managed and controlled medically, but if bothersome to the patient, revision surgery to remove the mucosalized tissue (which often includes the tympanic membrane) and replace it with a fresh eardrum graft and skin graft as described above can give the patient a dry, skin-lined canal.

Because the canal skin in a surgically repaired atretic ear is simply a skin graft and does not migrate, tympanic membrane perforations in surgically repaired ears will not heal. When exposed to the mucosa of the middle ear, the remainder of the eardrum often mucosalizes and the ear retains moisture. Topical antibiotic drops or powder can keep the drainage controlled, along with dry ear precautions. A paper patch can be tried as well; because the skin does not migrate, the paper patch will stay in place but may not prevent mucosalization and drainage.

Tympanoplasty surgery can also be offered, but because the skin does not migrate in the atretic ear, a simple underlay graft will fail. For the best chance at healing, surgery requires removal of the remaining eardrum and medial canal skin, with a new temporalis fascia graft placed in a lateral graft technique and skin graft. If healthy, the lateral, meatal skin can be saved, and the new medial skin graft can overlap the healthy lateral skin edge by 1–2 mm.

Steps to prevent mucosalization during the primary surgery include drilling and polishing the bone superiorly (along the tegmen) and anteriorly to remove all air cells, opening as few mastoid air cells as possible, plugging any large mastoid air cells with autologous temporalis muscle, ensuring the fascia graft covers the aditus area and does not "fall into" the posterior epitympanum or mastoid antrum, and harvesting a skin graft measuring 0.006 inches (thicker skin grafts are more difficult to work with because they curl and roll; thinner grafts will break down and slough).

Of the 20 ears revised for reasons of drainage/mucosalization, 12 ears had a minimum clinical follow-up of 3 months, with 9 ears dry and epithelialized and 3 ears persisting with otorrhea despite revision surgery; 1 ear underwent 3 revisions, and a persistent mucosalized canal remains. Ultimately, if all else fails, the canal can be closed.[10]

47.5 Congenital Cholesteatoma

A white mass behind an intact tympanic membrane is the classic description of congenital cholesteatoma, which accounts for approximately 2% to 4% of all cholesteatomas; however, congenital cholesteatoma has been reported in the mastoid,[15] the infratemporal fossa,[16] the Eustachian tube,[17] the tympanic membrane,[18] and the facial nerve canal.[19] The criteria for the diagnosis include the following: a white mass medial to a normal tympanic membrane; a normal pars flaccida and pars tensa; no prior history of otorrhea or perforations; and no prior otologic procedures. Prior bouts of otitis media are not grounds for exclusion.[20,21]

Theories behind the formation of congenital cholesteatoma include the Invagination Theory, where inflammation in the middle ear or retraction of the tympanic membrane causes the tympanic membrane or part of the tympanic membrane to invaginate to form a congenital cholesteatoma.[22] The Ectoderm Migration Theory proposes that ectoderm from the primitive external canal passes through or around the tympanic ring to enter the middle ear.[23] Sade introduced the Metaplasia Theory, in which otitis media or another inflammatory middle ear process results in squamous metaplasia, leading to keratin formation.[24] Finally, the most accepted theory behind the formation of congenital cholesteatoma was proposed by Michaels in 1986, the Epidermoid Formation Theory.[2] Michaels identified epithelial cells ("epidermoid formation") in the lateral wall of the embryonic tympanic cavity that normally disappear by 33 weeks of gestation. If the rest of the cells do not involute, congenital cholesteatoma forms.[2,25]

The diagnosis of congenital cholesteatoma is often made by an astute pediatrician who notes the white retrotympanic mass. Children are also referred after failing a school hearing test or hearing test in the pediatrician's office. The hearing loss is conductive in nature as the cholesteatoma exerts a mass effect on the tympanic membrane and ossicles. A typical location is the anterior-superior quadrant of the mesotympanum, although they can also develop posteriorly, even in the mastoid cavity.[1,5,26,27] These posterior mastoid cholesteatomas often reach a large size before they become clinically apparent, growing from the mastoid through the aditus into the epitympanum, where they will again cause conductive hearing loss by mass effect on the incus bone. It has been proposed that these posterior congenital cholesteatomas are more common in the Asian population.[28] In general, disease severity depends on location, patient age, ossicular integrity, and number of anatomic sites involved.[29]

Evaluation and management of congenital cholesteatoma depends on the size and extent of disease. Binocular microscopy shows a white retrotympanic mass (▶ Fig. 47.15) that does not move with pneumatic otoscopy (as opposed to myringosclerosis, which moves with the eardrum on pneumatic otoscopy). Tuning fork testing establishes the nature of the hearing loss, if any. Preoperative audiometry to document hearing levels, degree of hearing loss, and bone conduction thresholds is mandatory. Computed tomography can be helpful and is recommended, but is not necessary, for surgical planning to evaluate size and extent of disease (▶ Fig. 47.16). High-resolution CT can inform decisions about surgical approach (transcanal versus postauricular), the need for mastoidectomy, the possible need to stage the procedure, and the potential hearing outcome. Sound energy may be conducted through a large, erosive congenital cholesteatoma, giving the patient relatively good hearing despite bulky disease. The hearing will be worse after surgery when the cholesteatoma is removed. The stapes superstructure may be eroded with no connection between the footplate and the tympanic membrane.

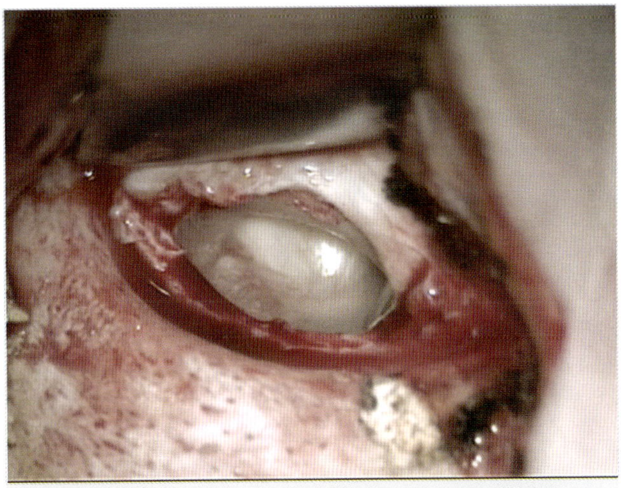

Fig. 47.15 Intraoperative image of a right ear showing a white mass behind an intact tympanic membrane in the anterior-superior quadrant of the middle ear typical of congenital cholesteatoma.

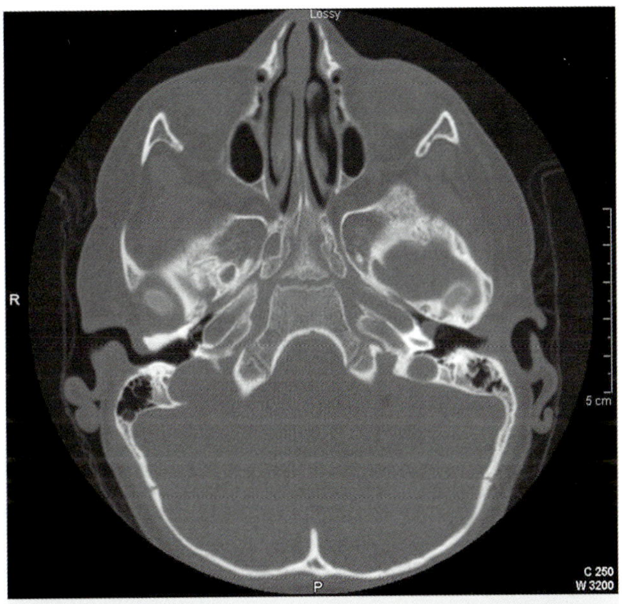

Fig. 47.16 Axial high-resolution CT showing a rounded mass in the anterior mesotympanum consistent with congenital cholesteatoma.

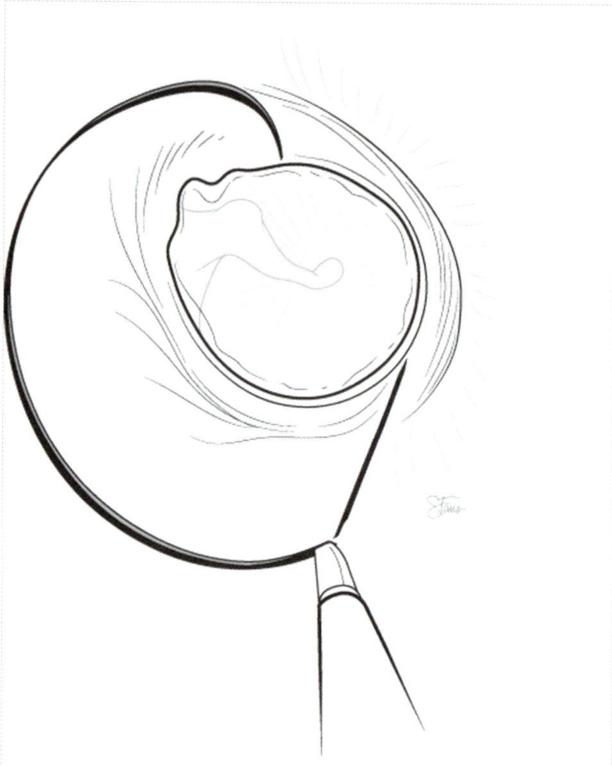

Fig. 47.17 Ear canal incisions (right ear) for an extended tympanomeatal flap to dissect the eardrum off the malleus and reflect it inferiorly attached to the umbo.

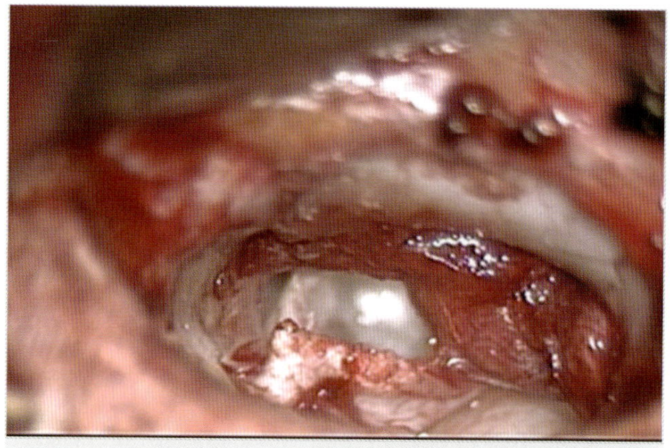

Fig. 47.18 Intraoperative otomicroscopic image of the exposure achieved with an extended tympanomeatal flap dissecting the eardrum off the manubrium and reflecting it inferiorly. The cholesteatoma was incised, and the interior keratin debris was removed, leaving the matrix to be dissected and excised.

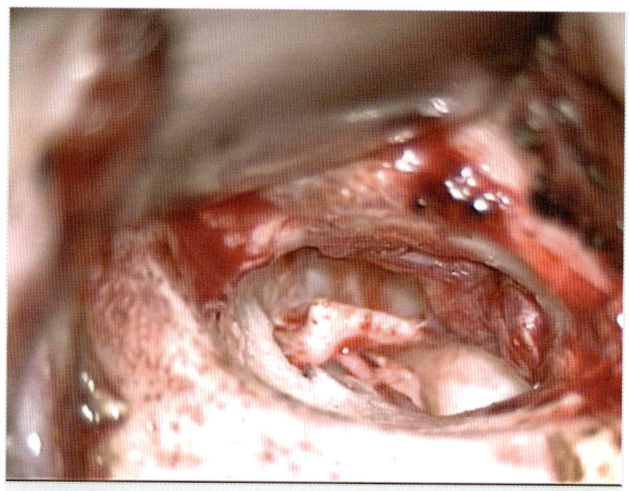

Fig. 47.19 Intraoperative otomicroscopic image of the reflected eardrum and mesotympanum after the cholesteatoma was excised.

Extent of surgery depends on extent of disease. Congenital cholesteatomas have classically been described as closed (cystic; isolated mass) or open (more invasive). Isolated cholesteatoma in the mesotympanum can be approached transcanal with total removal of disease through a tympanomeatal flap. Larger disease in the anterior-superior quadrant can be accessed through a postauricular approach and an extended tympanomeatal flap, where the eardrum is carefully and sharply dissected off the malleus and reflected inferiorly to the umbo (▶ Fig. 47.17; ▶ Fig. 47.18; ▶ Fig. 47.19). Once exposed, the cholesteatoma matrix is incised, the interior contents removed, and the matrix dissected and excised. Larger disease may require more extensive surgery, including mastoidectomy or a staged approach with ossiculoplasty, the details of which are found in this book.

More extensive initial disease, ossicular erosion, and the need for ossicular removal are associated with residual disease. The best chance for completely removing congenital cholesteatoma at initial surgery requires removing involved ossicles if they are eroded; for example, if the congenital cholesteatoma is abutting or enveloping the incus or stapes, or if the congenital cholesteatoma is medial to the malleus or incus.[30] Other risk factors for recidivistic disease include older age at diagnosis,[31] prior atticotomy, and stapes destruction. Extension into the Eustachian tube is a risk factor for a retraction pocket.[32] Hearing outcomes are excellent with limited disease and early diagnosis. More extensive congenital cholesteatomas will require ossicular reconstruction; nevertheless, these patients do not typically have Eustachian tube dysfunction, and hearing results can be maintained long-term with 60% to 70% of patients enjoying closure of the air-bone gap to within 10 dB.[33,34]

47.6 Conclusion

Although chronic ear disease in patients with congenital middle ear abnormalities is rare, it may take several forms, including congenital middle ear cholesteatoma, congenital ear canal cholesteatoma in the setting of congenital external auditory canal stenosis, as a postoperative complication of CAA surgery, or as congenital middle ear cholesteatoma. Evaluation of these lesions requires careful microscopic otoscopy, an index of suspicion, and high-resolution CT imaging to evaluate the presence and extent of disease. Based on imaging findings and the pathophysiology of disease, a rational surgical approach can be undertaken, and the patient and family appropriately counseled on expected outcomes, both short- and long-term, after surgery.

References

[1] Caughey RJ, Jahrsdoerfer RA, Kesser BW. Congenital cholesteatoma in a case of congenital aural atresia. Otol Neurotol. 2006;27(7):934–936.

[2] Michaels L. Origin of congenital cholesteatoma from a normally occurring epidermoid rest in the developing middle ear. Int J Pediatr Otorhinolaryngol. 1988;15(1):51–65.

[3] Li PM, Linos E, Gurgel RK, Fischbein NJ, Blevins NH. Evaluating the utility of non-echo-planar diffusion-weighted imaging in the preoperative evaluation of cholesteatoma: A meta-analysis. Laryngoscope. 2013;123(5):1247–1250.

[4] Vercruysse JP, De Foer B, Somers Th, Casselman J, Offeciers E. Magnetic resonance imaging of cholesteatoma: an update. B-ENT. 2009;5(4):233–240.

[5] Cole RR, Jahrsdoerfer RA. The risk of cholesteatoma in congenital aural stenosis. Laryngoscope. 1990;100(6):576–578.

[6] Kesser B, Jahrsdoerfer R. Surgery for congenital aural atresia. In: A. Julianna Gulya M, Lloyd B. Minor M, Dennis S. Poe M, eds. Surgery of the ear. 6th edition ed. Shelton, CT: People's Medical Publishing House-USA; 2010:413–422.

[7] Mazita A, Zabri M, Aneeza WH, Asma A, Saim L. Cholesteatoma in patients with congenital external auditory canal anomalies: retrospective review. J Laryngol Otol. 2011;125(11):1116–1120.

[8] Casale G, Nicholas BD, Kesser BW. Acquired ear canal cholesteatoma in congenital aural atresia/stenosis. Otol Neurotol. 2014;35(8):1474–1479.

[9] Kesser BW. Repair of congenital aural atresia. In: McKinnon BJ, ed. Operative techniques in otolaryngology-head and neck surgery. Vol. 21, Issue 4 ed. New York: Elsevier, Inc.; 2010:278–86.

[10] Oliver ER, Hughley BB, Shonka DC, Kesser BW. Revision aural atresia surgery: indications and outcomes. Otol Neurotol. 2011;32(2):252–258.

[11] Lambert PR. Congenital aural atresia: Stability of surgical results. Laryngoscope. 1998;108(12):1801–1805.

[12] De la Cruz A, Teufert KB. Congenital aural atresia surgery: Long-term results. Otolaryngol Head Neck Surg. 2003;129(1):121–127.

[13] Moon IJ, Cho YS, Park J, Chung WH, Hong SH, Chang SO. Long-term stent use can prevent postoperative canal stenosis in patients with congenital aural atresia. Otolaryngol Head Neck Surg. 2012;146(4):614–620.

[14] Chang SO, Lee JH, Choi BY, Song JJ. Long term results of postoperative canal stenosis in congenital aural atresia surgery. Acta Otolaryngol Suppl. 2007;558 (558):15–21.

[15] Giannuzzi AL, Merkus P, Taibah A, Falcioni M. Congenital mastoid cholesteatoma: case series, definition, surgical key points, and literature review. Ann Otol Rhinol Laryngol. 2011;120(11):700–706.

[16] Abdel-Aziz M. Congenital cholesteatoma of the infratemporal fossa with congenital aural atresia and mastoiditis: a case report. BMC Ear Nose Throat Disord. 2012;12:6.

[17] Sim MW, Stewart TA, Snissarenko EP, Xu HX. Congenital cholesteatoma involving the Eustachian tube. Int J Pediatr Otorhinolaryngol. 2011;75 (4):600–602.

[18] Shu MT, Lin HC, Yang CC, Chen YC. Congenital cholesteatoma in the tympanic membrane. Ear Nose Throat J. 2010;89(8):E27.

[19] Sina-Khadiv M, Alemi AS, Ziai K, Djalilian HR. Congenital cholesteatoma originating within the facial nerve canal. Otolaryngol Head Neck Surg. 2010;143 (5):708–709.

[20] Levenson MJ, Michaels L, Parisier SC, Juarbe C. Congenital cholesteatomas in children: An embryologic correlation. Laryngoscope. 1988;98(9):949–955.

[21] Levenson MJ, Michaels L, Parisier SC. Congenital cholesteatomas of the middle ear in children: origin and management. Otolaryngol Clin North Am. 1989;22 (5):941–954.

[22] Tos M. A new pathogenesis of mesotympanic (congenital) cholesteatoma. Laryngoscope. 2000;110(11):1890–1897.

[23] Aimi K. Role of the tympanic ring in the pathogenesis of congenital cholesteatoma. Laryngoscope. 1983;93(9):1140–1146.

[24] Sadé J, Babiacki A, Pinkus G. The metaplastic and congenital origin of cholesteatoma. Acta Otolaryngol. 1983;96(1-2):119–129.

[25] Michaels L. An epidermoid formation in the developing middle ear: possible source of cholesteatoma. J Otolaryngol. 1986;15(3):169–174.

[26] Inokuchi G, Okuno T, Hata Y, Baba M, Sugiyama D. Congenital cholesteatoma: posterior lesions and the staging system. Ann Otol Rhinol Laryngol. 2010;119 (7):490–494.

[27] Warren FM, Bennett ML, Wiggins RH, III, et al. Congenital cholesteatoma of the mastoid temporal bone. Laryngoscope. 2007;117(8):1389–1394.

[28] Hidaka H, Yamaguchi T, Miyazaki H, Nomura K, Kobayashi T. Congenital cholesteatoma is predominantly found in the posterior-superior quadrant in the Asian population: Systematic review and meta-analysis, including our clinical experience. Otol Neurotol. 2013;34(4):630–638.

[29] Richter GT, Lee KH. Contemporary assessment and management of congenital cholesteatoma. Curr Opin Otolaryngol Head Neck Surg. 2009;17(5):339–345.

[30] Stapleton AL, Egloff AM, Yellon RF. Congenital cholesteatoma: Predictors for residual disease and hearing outcomes. Arch Otolaryngol Head Neck Surg. 2012;138(3):280–285.

[31] Lim HW, Yoon TH, Kang WS. Congenital cholesteatoma: clinical features and growth patterns. Am J Otolaryngol. 2012;33(5):538–542.

[32] Lazard DS, Roger G, Denoyelle F, Chauvin P, Garabédian EN. Congenital cholesteatoma: Risk factors for residual disease and retraction pockets—a report on 117 cases. Laryngoscope. 2007;117(4):634–637.

[33] Doyle KJ, Luxford WM. Congenital aural cholesteatoma: Results of surgery in 60 cases. Laryngoscope. 1995;105(3 Pt 1):263–267.

[34] Rizer FM, Luxford WM. The management of congenital cholesteatoma: Surgical results of 42 cases. Laryngoscope. 1988;98(3):254–256.

48 Skin Grafting in the Management of Chronic Ear Disease

David H. Jung and Michael J. McKenna

48.1 Introduction

Split-thickness skin grafting has been an important tool in the kit of otologic surgeons for over 100 years. These grafts can be placed primarily at the time of tympanoplasty or tympanomastoidectomy. Split-thickness skin grafts may also be placed secondarily to address post-surgical mastoid cavities or tympanic grafts presenting with myringitis. Although split-thickness skin grafting is not required for epithelialization to occur, it does appear to decrease the time required for complete healing.

48.2 Patient Selection

We use primary split-thickness skin grafts routinely, not only in tympanomastoidectomy surgery, but also in canalplasty and aural atresia repair. In cavities or grafts that remain poorly healing, we also perform secondary split-thickness skin grafting as needed to obtain a dry, safe ear.

48.3 Surgical Technique

48.3.1 Primary Grafts

Our current technique for primary split-thickness skin grafting at the Massachusetts Eye and Ear Infirmary has been passed down from Schuknecht to generations of trainees. The basic setup is shown in ▶ Fig. 48.1. After general anesthesia has been induced, the arm is prepped and mineral oil is applied to the donor site and the battery-powered dermatome. The graft is harvested from the medial aspect of the ipsilateral upper arm (▶ Fig. 48.2). Following harvest, the skin graft is laid flat, epithelial side down, onto OTOSILK graft dressing (Boston Medical Products, Inc., Westborough, Massachusetts) that has been lightly covered with bacitracin. The OTOSILK allows for easy manipulation of the grafts without sacrificing pliability.

The grafts are then cut into smaller pieces, covered with moist gauze, and set aside for later use during surgery. We favor thin grafts given that they better conform to surfaces and appear to survive better over time. As shown in ▶ Fig. 48.3, a 5 cm x 4 cm graft is sufficient for a canal wall-down procedure. The donor site is then covered with a sterile adhesive dressing wrapped with sterile gauze.

Once the tympanomastoid procedure is completed and the fascia and cartilage grafts have been placed (▶ Fig. 48.4), the trimmed skin grafts are brought into the field and placed over the exposed bone and fascia with the epithelial and OTOSILK sides facing up. It is our practice to rotate an inferiorly based periosteal flap over bone paté into a canal wall-down cavity for partial obliteration,[1] and we also place skin grafts over areas of the flap that lie exposed within the cavity. We partially overlap the grafts at the edges (▶ Fig. 48.5). To hold the grafts in place, we apply multiple OTOSILK otologic strips soaked in cortisporin solution in a starburst pattern that covers all the grafts. Pieces of cotton soaked in cortisporin are then gently laid on top of the strips.[2] The otologic strips are then folded back over the cotton to complete the "rosebud" dressing (▶ Fig. 48.6), and lateral strip gauze packing is placed.

48.3.2 Secondary Grafts

Our treatment of secondary skin grafts is similar to that of primary grafts. This procedure can be performed in the office under local anesthesia,[2] but patients often prefer general anesthesia. General anesthesia also allows for more aggressive debridement of granulations as well as the option to exenterate

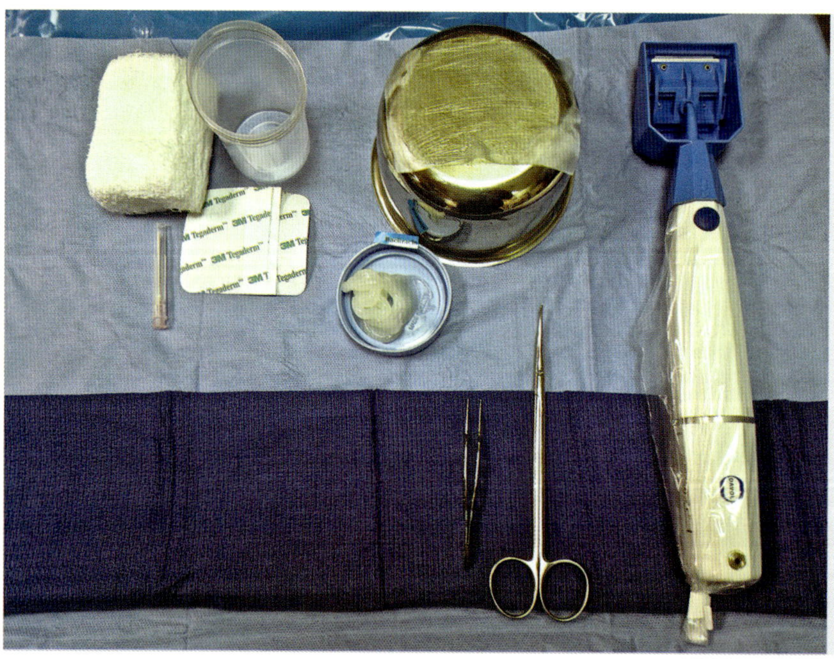

Fig. 48.1 Basic materials for collecting a split-thickness skin graft. OTOSILK graft dressing is lightly coated with bacitracin. A battery-powered dermatome is used to collect the graft after applying mineral oil to the skin and the dermatome blade. Following graft harvest, the site is covered with a plastic adhesive dressing and a needle is used to fenestrate the adhesive to allow egress of blood. The arm is then wrapped with sterile gauze.

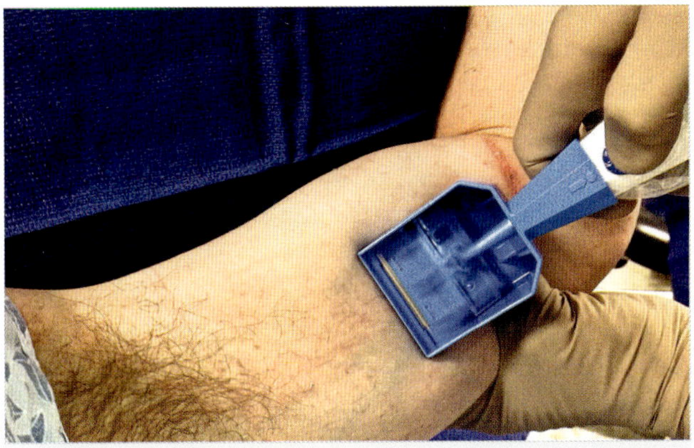

Fig. 48.2 The split-thickness skin graft is harvested from the inner aspect of the ipsilateral upper arm.

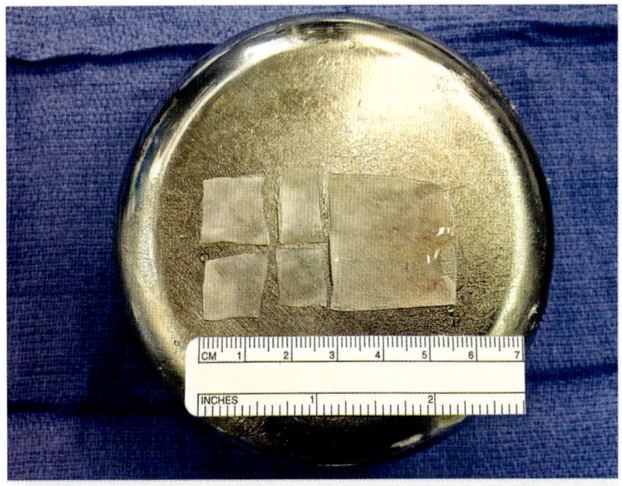

Fig. 48.3 The harvested split-thickness skin graft is laid epithelial side down onto the OTOSILK graft dressing, spread flat, and cut into smaller pieces. A graft of this size will comfortably line a canal wall-down cavity.

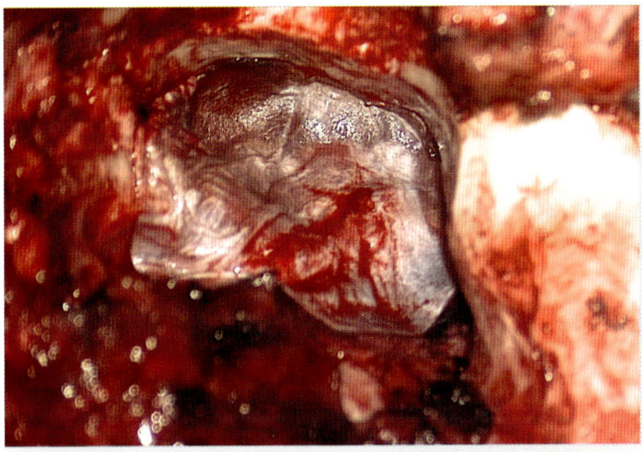

Fig. 48.4 The tympanomastoid cavity immediately prior to grafting. This is a canal wall-down procedure performed on a left ear, and the cartilage and fascia grafts have been placed. Note the inferiorly based periosteal flap that has been rotated forward to partially obliterate the cavity.

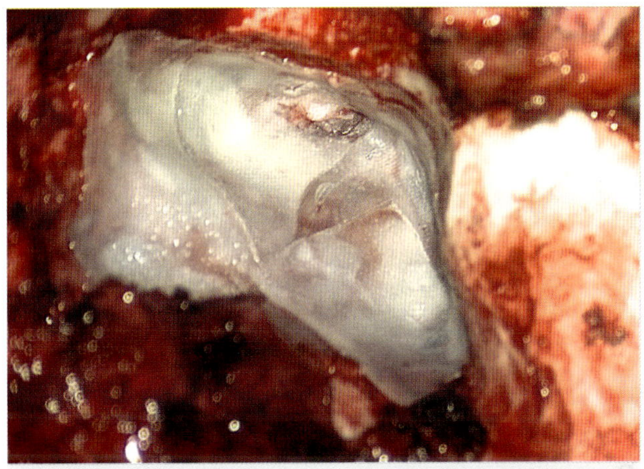

Fig. 48.5 Split-thickness skin grafts placed over the fascia graft, exposed bone within the cavity, and the exposed portion of the inferiorly based periosteal flap.

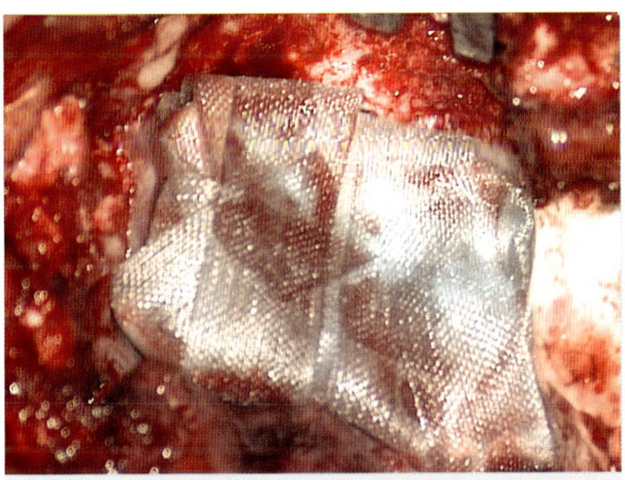

Fig. 48.6 The rosebud dressing. OTOSILK strips have been laid radially to cover the grafts, followed by cotton to hold the grafts in place. The strips have been folded back over themselves to complete the dressing.

remaining mastoid air cells and revise the meatoplasty as necessary. A split-thickness skin graft is harvested as outlined above. All disease is removed using sharp instruments, and the grafts are laid down, followed by a rosebud dressing.

48.4 Postoperative Care

Postoperative care is the same for either primary or secondary grafts. At the 1-week follow-up appointment, the lateral packing is removed and the patient is started on neomycin and polymyxin B sulfates and hydrocortisone otic suspension drops. The patient removes the adhesive arm dressing at home at approximately 7–10 days. Two weeks after the procedure, the rosebud dressing is removed, along with the graft backing strips, taking care not to disturb the grafts. The patient is instructed to switch to neomycin and polymyxin B sulfates and hydrocortisone solution drops until follow-up in 4–6 weeks. Maintenance of the resultant ear canal or mastoid cavity then proceeds as required.

48.5 Complications

Problems with the arm donor site are rare. Typically the donor site has dried by the 1-week post-operative appointment. Hypertrophic scarring of the donor site can, however, be a problem, especially in children. The most common complication involving split-thickness skin grafting within the ear is failure of the grafts to take, the most typical cause of which is infection in the immediate postoperative period.

48.6 Outcomes

Descriptions of split-thickness skin grafting in otologic surgery extend back to the late 1800s. Following the first description of skin grafting by Thiersch, Siebenmann espoused split-thickness skin grafting to speed epithelialization following mastoid surgery.[3] Older reports can be difficult to interpret, as radical mastoid cavities were often considered together with fenestration cavities that were previously free of infection and/or cholesteatoma. In this regard, a report from 1954 described an average healing time for non-grafted fenestration cavities of 4.4 months, whereas cavities generated from both fenestration and tympanomastoidectomy procedures required an average of 1.7 months to heal after secondary split-thickness skin grafting.[4] A more recent report found that secondary split-thickness skin grafting resulted in complete epithelialization of 45 out of 52 cavities presenting with postoperative otorrhea or significant granulation tissue.[3] Although no randomized, controlled studies have been performed for secondary split-thickness skin grafting, the evidence supports the idea that split-thickness skin grafting is a useful technique to address poorly healing cavities and grafts following tympanomastoid surgery.

There is a similarly long history of primary split-thickness skin grafting in chronic ear surgery. In 1925, Mosher reported his method of skin grafting using a paraffin mold to hold the grafts in place.[5] A later retrospective series measuring time to epithelialization claimed an average of 9.3 weeks with split-thickness skin grafting compared with 25.6 weeks in cavities without split-thickness skin grafting.[6] The largest recent retrospective series, in which primary split-thickness skin grafts were used in all 248 cases, reported a 91% infection control rate following tympanomastoid surgery. Notably, all the cases in this series presented with active chronic otitis media, and more than half of these procedures were revisions.[7] Finally, an important recent report described a randomized, controlled study of primary split-thickness skin grafting in primary canal wall-down tympanomastoidectomy performed in patients with active chronic otitis media and cholesteatoma. In this study, the authors reported an average time of 3.2 weeks to epithelialization in grafted cavities, and non-grafted cavities required an average of 6.6 weeks to epithelialize, a difference that was statistically significant. There was no significant difference in complications between the two groups.[8] Overall, the data suggest that primary split-thickness skin grafting promotes healing after tympanomastoid surgery, and that primary split-thickness skin grafting can play a role in an effective surgical strategy when routinely performed.

48.7 Conclusion

Split-thickness skin grafting can speed healing following chronic ear surgery; however, the most important factors in the success of chronic ear surgery are meticulous eradication of all disease and optimization of post-surgical anatomy to minimize the likelihood of recurrent disease. Split-thickness skin grafting may therefore be viewed as a useful adjunct, never a substitute, for a well-performed tympanomastoidectomy. Although cost and logistical concerns currently render such an approach impractical, primary or secondary grafting of cultured epithelium generated from a small (1-cm) skin biopsy may hold future promise in reducing the morbidity of split-thickness skin grafting.[9]

References

[1] Ramsey MJ, Merchant SN, McKenna MJ. Postauricular periosteal-pericranial flap for mastoid obliteration and canal wall down tympanomastoidectomy. Otol Neurotol. 2004;25(6):873–878.

[2] Nadol JB Jr, McKenna MJ. Surgery of the ear and temporal bone. 2nd ed. Philadelphia: Lippincott; 2005.

[3] Morris MS, Mitchell CC, Snell SW, Sperling N. Contemporary skin grafting in otologic surgery. Ear Nose Throat J. 1992;71(12):652–654.

[4] Guilford FR, Wright WK. Secondary skin grafting in fenestration and mastoid cavities. Laryngoscope. 1954;64(7):626–631.

[5] Mosher HP. Method of skin grafting for radical mastoid cavity. Ann Otol Rhinol Laryngol. 1925;34:1297–1299.

[6] Withers BT, Dickson JC, Wattleworth KL. Primary split thickness skin grafting of radical mastoid cavities. Ann Otol Rhinol Laryngol. 1953;62:656–662.

[7] Merchant SN, Wang P, Jang CH, et al. Efficacy of tympanomastoid surgery for control of infection in active chronic otitis media. Laryngoscope. 1997;107(7):872–877.

[8] Wetmore SJ, Bueller HA, Cost JL. Split thickness skin grafting in canal wall down tympanomastoidectomy. Otol Neurotol. 2014;35(1):97–100.

[9] Premachandra DJ, Woodward B, Milton CM, Sergeant RJ, Fabre JW. Long-term results of mastoid cavities grafted with cultured epithelium prepared from autologus epidermal cells to prevent chronic otorrhea. Laryngoscope. 1993;103(10):1121–1125.

Index

Note: Page numbers set **bold** or *italic* indicate headings or figures, respectively.

A

B

C

D

E

N

O

W

Y

Z